PATHOLOGY OF THE COLON, SMALL INTESTINE, AND ANUS

SECOND EDITION

CONTEMPORARY ISSUES IN SURGICAL PATHOLOGY VOLUME 17

SERIES EDITOR

Lawrence M. Roth, M.D.

Professor of Pathology
Director, Division of Surgical Pathology
Indiana University School of Medicine
Indianapolis, Indiana

Previously published

Vol. 1   Pathology of Glomerular Disease
Seymour Rosen, M.D.

Vol. 3   Muscle Pathology
Reid R. Heffner, Jr., M.D.

Vol. 6   Tumors and Tumorlike Conditions of the Ovary
Lawrence M. Roth, M.D., and Bernard Czernobilsky, M.D.

Vol. 7   Pathology of the Testis and Its Adnexa
Aleksander Talerman, M.D., and Lawrence M. Roth, M.D.

Vol. 9   Pathology of the Vulva and Vagina
Edward J. Wilkinson, M.D.

Vol. 10   Pathology of the Head and Neck
Douglas R. Gnepp, M.D.

Vol. 11   Bone Tumors
K. Krishnan Unni, M.B.,B.S.,

Vol. 12   Pathology of the Heart and Great Vessels
Bruce F. Waller, M.D.

Vol. 13   Pathology of the Urinary Bladder
Robert H. Young, M.D.

Vol. 14   Pathology of the Adrenal Glands
Ernest E. Lack, M.D.

Vol. 15   Pathology of the Prostate
David G. Bostwick, M.D.

Vol. 16   Tumors and Tumor-like Conditions of the Kidneys and Ureters
John N. Eble, M.D.

Forthcoming volumes in the series

Vol. 18   Tumors and Tumorlike Lesions of Soft Tissues
Vito Ninfo, M.D., and E.B. Chung, M.D., M.Sc., Ph.D.

PATHOLOGY OF THE COLON, SMALL INTESTINE, AND ANUS

SECOND EDITION

Edited by

H. Thomas Norris, M.D.

Professor and Chairman
Department of Pathology and Laboratory Medicine
East Carolina University School of Medicine
Chief of Pathology
Pitt County Memorial Hospital
Greenville, North Carolina

Churchill Livingstone
New York, Edinburgh, London, Melbourne, Tokyo

Library of Congress Cataloging-in-Publication Data
Pathology of the colon, small intestine, and anus / edited by H.
   Thomas Norris. — 2nd ed.
         p. cm. — (Contemporary issues in surgical pathology ; v. 17)
      Includes bibliographical references and index.
      ISBN 0-443-08729-6
      1. Colon (Anatomy)—Diseases. 2. Intestine, Small—Diseases.
   3. Anus—Diseases. I.Norris, H. Thomas. II. Series.
      [DNLM: 1. Diagnosis, Differential. 2. Intestinal Diseases-
   -pathology.   W1 CO769MS v. 17 / WI 400 P297]
   RC802.9.P37 1991
   616.3'407—dc20
   DNLM/DLC
   for Library of Congress   90-15161
                                                        CIP

Second edition © Churchill Livingstone Inc. 1991
First edition © Churchill Livingstone Inc. 1983

Distributed in the United Kingdom by Churchill Livingstone, Robert Stevenson House, 1–3 Baxter's
Place, Leith Walk, Edinburgh EH1 3AF, and by associated companies, branches, and representatives
throughout the world.

Accurate indications, adverse reactions, and dosage schedules for drugs are provided in this book, but
it is possible that they may change. The reader is urged to review the package information data of the
manufacturers of the medications mentioned.

The Publishers have made every effort to trace the copyright holders for borrowed material. If they
have inadvertently overlooked any, they will be pleased to make the necessary arrangements at the
first opportunity.

Acquisitions Editor: *Beth Kaufman Barry*
Copy Editor: *Ann Ruzycka*
Production Designer: *Patricia McFadden*
Production Supervisor: *Jeanine Furino*

Printed in the United States of America

First published in 1991   7 6 5 4 3 2 1

Contributors

Henry D. Appelman, M.D.
Professor, Department of Pathology, University of Michigan Medical Center, Ann Arbor, Michigan

Harry S. Cooper, M.D.
Professor and Director, Division of Anatomical Pathology, Department of Pathology and Laboratory Medicine, Hahnemann University School of Medicine; Hahnemann University Hospital, Philadelphia, Pennsylvania

Yogeshwar Dayal, M.B., B.S., M.D.
Clinical Professor, Department of Pathology, Tufts University School of Medicine; Senior Pathologist, Department of Pathology, New England Medical Center Hospitals, Boston, Massachusetts

William O. Dobbins III, M.D.
Professor, Department of Internal Medicine, University of Michigan Medical Center; Staff Physician, Department of Gastroenterology, Veterans Administration Medical Center, Ann Arbor, Michigan

Rodger C. Haggitt, M.D.
Professor, Department of Pathology, Adjunct Professor, Department of Medicine, and Director, Division of Hospital Pathology, University of Washington Medical Center, Seattle, Washington

Stanley R. Hamilton, M.D.
Associate Professor, Departments of Pathology and Oncology, The Johns Hopkins University School of Medicine; The Johns Hopkins University Hospital, Baltimore, Maryland

Elson B. Helwig, M.D.
Chairman, Department of Gastrointestinal Pathology, Armed Forces Institute of Pathology, Washington, D.C.

Thomas H. Kent, M.D.
Professor, Department of Pathology, University of Iowa College of Medicine, Iowa City, Iowa

David F. Keren, M.D.
Adjunct Professor of Pathology, Eastern Michigan University, Ypsilanti, Michigan; Medical Director, Warde Medical Laboratory, Ann Arbor, Michigan

Frank A. Mitros, M.D.
Professor, Department of Pathology, University of Iowa College of Medicine, Iowa City, Iowa

H. Thomas Norris, M.D.

Professor and Chairman, Department of Pathology and Laboratory Medicine, East Carolina University School of Medicine; Chief of Pathology, Pitt County Memorial Hospital, Greenville, North Carolina

Robert H. Riddell, M.D., F.R.C.Path., F.R.C.P.(C)

Professor, Department of Pathology, McMaster University School of Medicine; Chief of Service, Anatomical Pathology, Chedoke-McMaster Hospitals, Hamilton, Ontario, Canada

J. Ross Slemmer, M.D.

Chief Resident and Clinical Instructor, Department of Pathology and Laboratory Medicine, Hahnemann University School of Medicine; Hahnemann University Hospital, Philadelphia, Pennsylvania

Foreword

Since the first volume in the *Contemporary Issues in Surgical Pathology* was published in 1983, eighteen volumes have appeared, and the series has been established as an authoritative source for current information that fully covers the latest developments in the field. The volumes published have been organized by specific anatomic site or organ system. The quality of the volumes is a direct result of the efforts of the editors of the individual volumes and their contributors. The response by its readership has been heartening. I would like to thank the many colleagues who have contributed time from their busy schedules in support of this project.

One of the most successful volumes has been *Pathology of the Colon, Small Intestine, and Anus*, edited by Dr. H. Thomas Norris, Professor and Chairman of the Department of Pathology and Laboratory Medicine at East Carolina University School of Medicine. With the publication of this volume, the series has reached a milestone. The first edition of this volume was completely sold out within a relatively short time. The second edition, the first revised edition in the series, brings this popular volume up to date. In this volume, Dr. Norris has again assembled a group of authorities in their subject, who provide a volume that should be of great practical value for the practicing pathologist. I would like to personally thank Dr. Norris for a job well done.

In the future we will continue publishing volumes on subjects not yet covered in the series, as well as adding timely second editions of selected books in the series. Comments and suggestions from the readership of the series will be greatly appreciated.

Lawrence M. Roth, M.D.
Series Editor

Preface

Since this book's initial publication in 1983, there has been an extraordinary increase in knowledge about the subjects covered in this text. The criteria for diagnosis of these lesions has also been refined. Greater insight into the progression of a lesion to a malignancy has been the result of discoveries using contemporary techniques of molecular biology. In addition, a much greater understanding of the pathogenesis of these lesions has developed.

Once again, we review in eleven chapters the latest knowledge on subjects of current interest. All of the authors have extensively reviewed and rewritten their chapters to incorporate this new information. Each author is widely recognized for his expertise in gastrointestinal pathology. Each chapter is designed to give concise but comprehensive coverage of each of its topics, with emphasis on recent advances in knowledge, areas of rapid change, and new techniques.

The general organization of the book is identical to the first edition. The initial chapters deal with various aspects of inflammatory bowel disease. The first chapter deals with the diagnosis of and comparison between ulcerative colitis and Crohn's disease. The second chapter deals with the differential diagnosis of inflammatory bowel disease. This is followed by a chapter on the experimental pathology of inflammatory bowel disease, including immune-mediated aspects of the disease process. A chapter on dysplasia associated with inflammatory bowel disease concludes the chapters on inflammatory bowel disease. The book then changes direction with a re-examination of the spectrum of ischemic bowel disease. The next chapter deals with small bowel biopsy processing and interpretation, with emphasis on malabsorption syndromes. The final five chapters deal with neoplasia of the lower gastrointestinal tract. The relationship between polyps and cancer is extensively reviewed, with emphasis on recent discoveries involved in the development of cancer. The next chapter presents an extensive review of cancer of the colon, focusing on the early stages of development. Neoplasms of the appendix are then reviewed extensively. Neoplastic lesions of the endocrine cells of the gut are discussed in depth. The book ends with a chapter on neoplasms of the anus.

This second edition, the first second edition in Churchill Livingstone's series, *Contemporary Issues in Surgical Pathology,* is a direct response to you, the reader. The first edition was dedicated to informing the reader of specific areas of gastrointestinal pathology in which advances had been particularly dramatic or pivotal in understanding the disease process. This dedication continues in the second edition. It is the expectation of the contributors that the second edition will continue to help refine current practices in gastrointestinal pathology.

A note of special thanks is appropriate to all of the authors who have found time in their hectic schedules to complete their contributions. Once again, their cooperation and contributions have been outstanding.

H. Thomas Norris, M.D.

Contents

1. Diagnosis and Comparison of Ulcerative Colitis and Crohn's Disease
    Involving the Colon   1
    Stanley R. Hamilton

2. The Differential Diagnosis of Idiopathic Inflammatory Bowel Disease 23
    Rodger C. Haggitt

3. Immunopathogenesis of Inflammatory Bowel Disease 61
    David F. Keren

4. Dysplasia in Inflammatory Bowel Disease 85
    Robert H. Riddell

5. Re-examination of the Spectrum of Ischemic Bowel Disease 121
    H. Thomas Norris

6. Small Bowel Biopsy in Malabsorptive States 137
    William O. Dobbins III

7. Polyps of the Colon and Small Intestine, Polyposis Syndromes, and the
    Polyp-Carcinoma Sequence 189
    Thomas H. Kent and Frank A. Mitros

8. Carcinoma of the Colon and Rectum 225
    J. Ross Slemmer and Harry S. Cooper

9. Epithelial Neoplasia of the Appendix 263
    Henry D. Appelman

10. Neuroendocrine Cells and Their Proliferative Lesions 305
    Yogeshwar Dayal

11. Neoplasms of the Anus 367
    Elson B. Helwig

    Index 395

1

Diagnosis and Comparison of Ulcerative Colitis and Crohn's Disease Involving the Colon

Stanley R. Hamilton

Ulcerative colitis (UC) and Crohn's disease (CD) are the two recognized forms of idiopathic inflammatory bowel disease (IBD). Clinically significant involvement of the colon occurs in about one-third of patients with CD. As a result, the distinction between UC and colonic Crohn's disease (CCD) poses a frequent problem for gastroenterologists and surgeons. Because of the widespread use of endoscopy, pathologists are often asked to interpret biopsy specimens taken in an attempt to make this distinction. In some patients, the diagnosis is not clear prior to the time of a resection, and UC and CCD must be distinguished in the surgical specimen.

In the past, distinguishing UC from CCD was largely an intellectual exercise because the medical and surgical therapy for the two diseases were similar. With recent advances, however, this situation has changed. Medical therapy for UC and CD sometimes utilizes different drugs. Of even greater immediate importance to the patient, surgical techniques for continent ileostomy or ileoanal anastomosis with pouch reservoir offer the potential to avoid an ileostomy appliance following colectomy. These newer surgical procedures are, however, usually contraindicated in patients with CD.[1] In addition, the risk of colorectal cancer as a complication of idiopathic IBD is higher in patients with UC than in those with CCD. Colonoscopic surveillance for dysplasia, the precursor lesion to carcinoma, is currently recommended for patients with UC, but the approach to patients with CCD is less standardized.[2] As a consequence of these various considerations, pathologists are under greater pressure than was the case of a few years ago to distinguish UC and CCD in biopsy and resection specimens. This chapter presents pathologic findings that can be helpful in this differential diagnosis.

DEFINITION OF IDIOPATHIC INFLAMMATORY BOWEL DISEASE

Inflammatory diseases of the bowel, with the term used in a generic sense, include a large group of diseases of the small and large intestine in which inflammation has a pathogenetic role. The etiologies of inflammatory diseases of the bowel thus include infectious agents, ischemia, irradiation, toxic materials, and a variety of other causes,[3] as discussed in Chapter 2. *Idiopathic IBD* refers to UC and CD. The first principle in the diagnosis of UC and CCD is that inflammatory diseases of the bowel that are not idiopathic IBD must be excluded. Clinical history, physical findings, laboratory results, and radiographic features, as well as pathologic findings, are considered in patient diagnosis. Recognition that UC and CD are largely diagnoses of exclusion is essential so that patients with inflammatory diseases of the bowel for which specific therapy is available are treated appropriately. Treatment of some forms of inflammatory diseases of the bowel, such as infectious colitis, with the nonspecific anti-inflammatory drugs used for idiopathic IBD can have disastrous consequences for the patient. Therefore, consideration of inflammatory diseases of the bowel other than idiopathic IBD is the important first step in evaluating biopsy and resection specimens.

ULCERATIVE COLITIS AND COLONIC CROHN'S DISEASE IN RESECTION SPECIMENS

LABORATORY PROCEDURES FOR RESECTION SPECIMENS

Accurate diagnosis of UC and CD in resection specimens often depends on accurate documentation of the anatomic distribution of the pathologic findings. As a result, a standardized procedure for examining resection specimens is strongly recommended for surgical pathology laboratories. A number of such procedures have been described.[4, 5] In our laboratory, the resection specimen is brought for processing as soon as possible after removal from the patient. The specimen is then oriented in anatomic position for opening. If the surgeon does not mark the splenic and hepatic flexures, these landmarks can sometimes be identified at either end of the omental attachment to the transverse colon or by the curvature of the colon produced by the mesocolon. The colon is opened along the anterior free taenia, and any small bowel is opened along the anterior aspect of the mesenteric border. The specimen is then stretched slightly and pinned out flat in anatomic position on a 24 × 20 × 2-inch sheet of Styrofoam. The Styrofoam is inverted and floated in a 25 × 21 × 15-inch flat pan (Belart, Pequanock, NJ) containing neutral buffered formalin for overnight fixation of the specimen. Although this fixation procedure is complicated by regulatory requirements to reduce exposure of laboratory personnel to formalin fumes, it remains an important first step for evaluation of resection specimens.

After overnight fixation, the specimen is rinsed thoroughly in running water and photographed. A low-power view of the entire specimen as well as close-up photographs of areas of particular interest are included. Such photographs are often essential for documentation of findings. Photographs of fresh specimens are generally avoided because of light reflection and drying under flood lights as well as rolling of and leakage of blood from unfixed cut edges.

Gross description complements the gross specimen photographs. The anatomic structures in the specimen are noted and measured. Abnormal mucosa, bowel wall, and serosa or pericolonic and perirectal soft tissue are described, and their anatomic locations are noted. Tissue for histopathologic sections is then removed from the resection margins, anatomic landmarks, areas of abnormality, random sites at 10- to 20-cm intervals throughout the length of the specimen, and representative lymph nodes. Each tissue block is labelled with a designation and described as to its source in the gross description. In addition, the site of each block is drawn on extra copies of the specimen photographs, which are retained in the laboratory records. The salient histopathologic findings in the various areas are briefly noted in a paragraph of description included in the surgical pathology report.

The goal of systematic specimen processing is to allow accurate reconstruction of the findings for diagnosis. Documentation of the anatomic distribution of histopathologic findings is often critical for correct diagnosis of difficult cases, as is discussed below.

The surgical pathology report includes the organs and structures in the resection specimen, the type of operation, the classification of the idiopathic IBD, the site of predominant involvement, and any complicating features. A representative report would be: "Terminal ileum, cecum, appendix, colon, rectum, and anus (total proctocolectomy with ileostomy): Active ulcerative colitis predominantly involving the left and transverse colon. Negative for tumor and dysplasia."

Table 1-1. Comparison of Ulcerative Colitis and Crohn's Disease Involving the Colon: Gross Pathology in Resection Specimens

Features	Ulcerative Colitis	Colonic Crohn's Disease
Distribution of gross abnormalities		
Continuous involvement	+++	−/+
Distal predominance	+++	−/+
Rectal involvement	+++	+
Total colonic involvement	+	−/+
Discontinuous, segmental involvement ("skip lesions")	−/+	+++
Right colonic predominance	−/+	+
Relative rectal sparing	−/+	+
Terminal ileal involvement	−/+	+
Anal involvement	−/+	+
Character of colonic mucosal abnormalities		
Loss of mucosal folds	+++	+
Diffuse granularity	+++	+
Prominent vascularity	+++	−/+
Numerous inflammatory polyps	+	−/+
Discrete ulcers	−/+	+++
Serpiginous ulcers	−/+	+
Linear, longitudinal ulcers	−/+	+
Fissuring ulcers	−/+	+
"Cobblestone" appearance	−/+	+
Aphthoid ulcers	−/+	+
Prominent edema	−/+	+
Character of bowel wall abnormalities		
Shortening of colonic length	+++	+
Thickening	−/+	+++
Stricture	−/+	+
Serositis and adhesions	−/+	+
Fistula	−/+	+

+++ = usually present; + = sometimes present; −/+ = usually absent

GROSS PATHOLOGY OF ULCERATIVE COLITIS AND CROHN'S DISEASE INVOLVING THE COLON

The pathologic findings in patients with UC and CCD are dynamic. The findings are influenced by a variety of factors, including severity of activity, duration of disease, and therapy prior to resection. As a result, the pathologic findings of UC or CCD show striking variability among individual patients. In addition, the type of resection determines the type of specimen available for examination: obviously, pathologic findings in the rectum and anus cannot be assessed in an abdominal colectomy specimen, whereas a total proctocolectomy specimen allows pathologic evaluation of the entire large bowel.

The gross pathology[4, 6–8] of *typical* UC and CCD is summarized and compared in Table 1-1. Problem areas are addressed in the later section entitled "Colitis of Indeterminate Type."

UC is characterized by the continuous nature of the gross abnormalities (Fig. 1-1), although sometimes with variability in the severity. Distal predominance of the abnormalities with involvement of the rectum (proctitis) is a usual feature, although there may be exceptional cases with relative sparing of the rectum.[9] In some specimens, involvement of the entire colorectum is

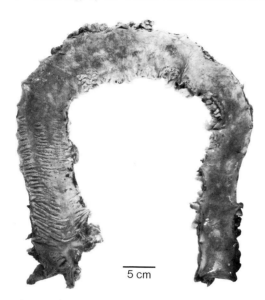

Fig. 1-1. Long-standing ulcerative colitis in a specimen from a total abdominal colectomy with rectal mucosal stripping and ileoanal pull-through procedure. The entire left and transverse colon show smooth featureless mucosa without folds. The right colon is less involved, as some mucosal folds remain. A nodular area of high-grade dysplasia is present in the proximal transverse colon (see Ch. 4).

evident, whereas in other cases the proximal colon is uninvolved. The terminal ileum is normal in the majority of UC resection specimens. Abnormality of the terminal ileum, when present, is usually associated with a rigidly dilated and incompetent ileocecal valve. The incompetence appears to allow colonic contents to backflow a short distance into the terminal ileum, leading to "backwash ileitis." Appendiceal involvement occurs commonly in UC, often in the absence of proximal colonic involvement.[10] Anal abnormalities occur in a minority of specimens and, when present, usually consist of excoriation and acute fissures.

In contrast to UC, the distribution of gross abnormalities in CCD is typically discontinuous or segmental, with "skip lesions" separated by uninvolved colon. The right colon is sometimes the site of predominant involvement, and the rectum is spared in a sizeable proportion of specimens (Fig. 1-2). The terminal ileum is involved in some specimens, often with long lengths affected. The appendix is often abnormal. The anal region is sometimes the site of multiple fistulas, ulcers, chronic fissures, and edematous skin tags. Anal involvement, however, seems less common in the United States than in Great Britain.

In addition to the differences in distribution

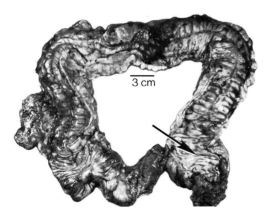

Fig. 1-2. Crohn's disease involving the colon in a specimen from a total proctocolectomy. The distal ascending, transverse, and proximal left colon show linear longitudinally oriented ulcers. The cecum and rectum (arrow) are relatively spared.

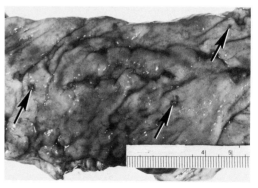

Fig. 1-3. Discrete ulcers in Crohn's disease involving the colon. The central portion of the figure shows an area of irregular ulceration. Aphthoid ulcers surrounded by relatively uninvolved mucosa are also present (arrows).

of gross abnormalities, the character of the lesions also differs in UC and CCD. The colonic mucosa grossly involved by UC usually shows loss of folds associated with generalized granularity, producing "featureless mucosa" (Fig. 1-1). With activity, vascularity is prominent and the mucosa is friable. Ulceration, when present, is within otherwise abnormal mucosa. Numerous inflammatory polyps are present in some specimens.

The characteristic mucosal features of CCD are discrete ulcers surrounded by otherwise grossly uninvolved mucosa (Fig. 1-3). The configuration of the ulcers varies greatly. Ulcers in CCD may be serpiginous, or may be linear and longitudinally oriented, described as "rake" or "railroad track" ulcers (Fig. 1-2). The ulcers may produce sharp crevices into the bowel wall, termed *fissuring*. Interconnecting ulcers surrounding edematous areas of mucosa result in a "cobblestone" mucosa. Tiny, punched-out ulcers in otherwise grossly normal mucosa (Fig. 1-3) are referred to as "aphthoid" ulcers, because of their similarity to oral aphthous ulcers. Striking mucosal and submucosal edema is sometimes seen in CCD.

In typical UC, the colonic length is reduced, but the bowel wall itself is usually of normal thickness. In contrast, thickening of the bowel wall is the rule in CCD, and the colonic length is not usually reduced. Strictures, serosal inflammation sometimes associated with adhesions, and fistulas to other areas of bowel or to other structures such as skin or urinary bladder are seen in typical CCD.

HISTOPATHOLOGY OF ULCERATIVE COLITIS AND CROHN'S DISEASE INVOLVING THE COLON

As described in the preceding discussion of laboratory procedures, the anatomic distribution of pathologic findings is often extremely helpful for accurate diagnosis. The distribution of histopathologic abnormalities generally corresponds to that of the gross abnormalities summarized in Table 1-1. The character of the histopatho-

logic abnormalities in UC and CCD is summarized and compared in Table 1-2.

The granular mucosa devoid of folds in UC typically shows atrophy. Destruction of crypt architecture with shortening and distortion of those crypts that remain is characteristic of UC (Fig. 1-4A). Villous transformation of the mucosal architecture is sometimes present. The lamina propria usually shows increased numbers of chronic inflammatory cells, including plasma cells, eosinophils,[11] and lymphocytes. Active UC is characterized by crypt epithelial infiltration by neutrophils. Destruction of crypt epithelium with accumulation of fibrinoinflammatory exudate in the crypt lumen produces the crypt abscess. Dilated congested blood vessels are prominent with active inflammation, and the epithelium typically shows reduced numbers of goblet cells and reduced quantity of mucin in the remaining goblet cells. Chronic inflammation of the lamina propria is greater with active than inactive disease. Paneth cell metaplasia of the epithelium and thickening of the muscularis mucosae are sometimes seen. Erosions and ulcers, when present, arise within abnormal mucosa. Multinucleated giant cells, usually representing foreign body reaction in areas of ulceration or erosion, may be seen occasionally.

A striking increase in the number and size of lymphoid nodules with prominent germinal centers occurs in the rectum of some specimens. This lymphoid proliferation is referred to as *follicular proctitis* and leads to distortion of remaining crypts (Fig. 1-5). Inflammatory polyps are common in UC and are characterized by proliferation of distorted glands and inflamed granulation tissue, frequently on a stalk of mucosa and submucosa. The proportion of epithelial and stromal structures is highly variable, as some inflammatory polyps are composed only of granulation tissue while others have numerous glands. Finger-like "filiform" inflammatory polyps occur in some cases; the normality of the mucosal architecture in this form of inflammatory polyp is striking. The grossly normal mucosa of the proximal colon in resection specimens of UC without apparent total colonic involvement is commonly abnormal on histopa-

Table 1-2. Comparison of Ulcerative Colitis and Crohn's Disease Involving the Colon: Histopathology in Resection Specimens

Features	Ulcerative Colitis	Colonic Crohn's Disease
Distribution of histopathologic abnormalities See Table 1-1		
Character of mucosal abnormalities		
Atrophy with prominent crypt loss and distortion	+++	+
Diffuse chronic inflammation	+++	+
Prominent vascularity	+++	−/+
Crypt abscesses	+++	+
Depleted epithelial mucin	+	−/+
Paneth cell metaplasia	+	−/+
Thickened muscularis mucosae	+	−/+
"Follicular proctitis"	+	−/+
Numerous inflammatory polyps	+	−/+
Noncaseating epithelioid cell granulomas	−/+	+
Granulomatous inflammation	−/+	+
Fissuring ulcers	−/+	+
Aphthoid erosions or ulcers	−/+	+
Focal active inflammation	−/+	+
Clusters of lymphocytes	−/+	+
Character of bowel wall abnormalities		
Widened, edematous submucosa	−/+	+++
Lymphangiectasia	−/+	+++
Submucosal inflammation and lymphoid aggregates	+	+++
Submucosal fibrosis	−/+	+
Muscularis propria and pericolonic inflammation with lymphoid aggregates ("transmural")	−/+	+++
Noncaseating epithelioid cell granulomas in bowel wall and lymph nodes	−/+	+
Fibrous stricture	−/+	+
Fistula with granulation tissue	−/+	+
Neural hyperplasia	−/+	+
Vasculitis	−/+	+

+++ = usually present; + = sometimes present; −/+ = usually absent

thologic examination: chronic inflammation of the lamina propria and increased epithelial mitotic figures are usually present.

In CCD, the noncaseating epithelioid cell granuloma is the characteristic finding (Fig. 1-4B). Granulomas are found in a majority of cases when a diligent search is carried out. Well-formed granulomas have a demarcated aggregate of epithelioid cells with abundant pink cytoplasm. Multinucleated giant cells formed by fusion of the epithelioid cells are often present in the aggregate. A cuff of chronic inflammatory cells frequently surrounds the accumulation of epithelioid cells. Necrotizing or confluent granu-

lomas are very uncommon and should raise the question of tuberculosis and yersiniosis. Granulomatous inflammation or "microgranulomas" composed of ill-defined collections of chronic inflammatory cells with a heavy admixture of epithelioid cells can also be seen commonly with CCD.

The histopathologic features of the ulcers in CCD are sometimes distinctive. Fissuring ulcers show cleft- or crack-like penetration of the mucosa. The aphthoid erosion or ulcer typically occurs over a pre-existing lymphoid nodule and is surrounded by uninflamed mucosa. Crypt abscesses are common in CCD, but crypt architec-

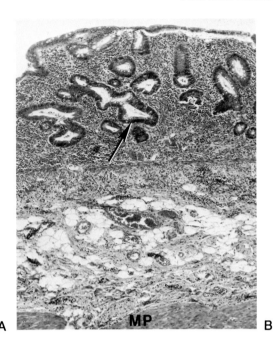
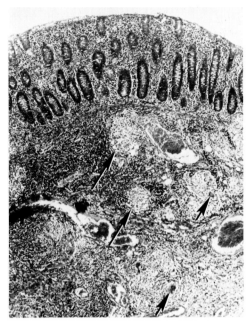

Fig. 1-4. Comparison of histopathology of ulcerative colitis and Crohn's disease involving the colon. **(A)** The mucosa in this specimen of low-grade active ulcerative colitis shows loss of crypts with bizarre configuration (arrow) of those remaining. Epithelial mucin is markedly reduced. The lamina propria shows diffuse chronic inflammation that extends into the superficial submucosa. The deep submucosa and muscularis propria (*MP*) are uninvolved. **(B)** The mucosa in this specimen of active Crohn's disease shows preservation of crypt architecture and epithelial mucin. The lamina propria shows diffuse chronic inflammation that extends into the deep submucosa. Multiple noncaseating epithelioid cell granulomas (long arrows), some with multinucleated giant cells (short arrows), are present. (H&E, × 50.)

ture and epithelial mucin content are frequently maintained (Fig. 1-4B). In addition, crypt abscesses may show contiguous granulomatous inflammation (Fig. 1-6) or granulomas. Diffuse or patchy chronic inflammation may occur in the lamina propria. Focal active inflammation of rectal mucosa with crypt epithelial infiltration by neutrophils, surrounded by a cuff of inflammatory cells amid otherwise uninflamed mucosa, is characteristic of CCD. Clusters of lymphocytes, particularly near the bases of crypts, are sometimes seen but should not be confused with lymphoid nodules.

Histopathologic findings in the bowel wall are particularly helpful in the differential diagnosis of UC and CCD. The submucosa in UC may show inflammation and lymphoid aggre-

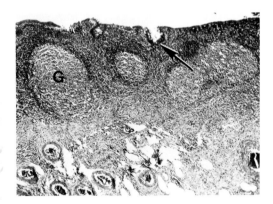

Fig. 1-5. "Follicular proctitis" in ulcerative colitis. The lamina propria of the rectum contains confluent hyperplastic lymphoid nodules with enlarged germinal centers (*G*). Crypts (arrow) are compressed and distorted. (H&E, × 40.)

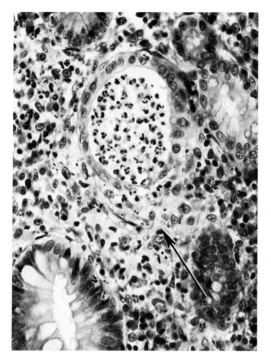

Fig. 1-6. Granulomatous inflammation in Crohn's disease. An ill-defined aggregate of epithelioid cells (arrow) is contiguous with a crypt abscess. (H&E, × 450.)

gates, especially with severe active disease. In contrast, the muscularis propria, serosa, and pericolonic or perirectal soft tissue typically lack inflammation (Fig. 1-7A). Shortening of the colonic length is associated with thickened muscularis propria. Benign strictures in UC, when they occur, show thickening of the muscularis mucosae and muscularis propria rather than fibrosis, as in CCD. By contrast with UC, CCD is characterized by prominent bowel wall abnormalities (Fig. 1-7B). The submucosa is often thickened and edematous with dilated lymphatics, which are usually surrounded by chronic inflammatory cells. Submucosal fibrosis is frequently present. Transmural inflammation with lymphoid aggregates and granulomas in the deeper layers of the colonic wall is a characteristic finding. Granulomas may also be found in regional lymph nodes and in the anus (Fig. 1-8). Narrowing of the colonic lumen owing to stricture is a common finding. Strictures in CD are characterized by fibrous tissue in the bowel

wall and prominent proliferation of smooth muscle fibers in the muscularis mucosae and submucosa. Fistula tracts lined by granulation tissue represent the sequelae of fissuring ulcers that extend into other structures. Mucosal regeneration occurs in some fistula tracts, producing an epithelial lining that may impede closure. Striking neural hyperplasia in the submucosal and myenteric plexi is present in some specimens and has been shown to involve peptidergic nerves.[12] Axonal necrosis has been reported in ultrastructural studies.[13] Inflammation of mural and extramural blood vessels is also found in some cases of CCD.

Involvement of the vermiform appendix is common in both CD and UC. The character of the inflammatory process is similar to that in the colonic mucosa and bowel wall of the two diseases. Appendiceal involvement in UC, however, sometimes occurs in the absence of proximal colonic involvement rather than in continuity with the more distal inflamed regions.[10]

As is apparent from Tables 1-1 and 1-2, there is considerable overlap between many of the pathologic features of UC and CCD. *No one feature, even the occurrence of granulomas, is pathognomonic of either disease.* Some features, when present, are particularly helpful in distinguishing these two forms of idiopathic IBD. These distinguishing characteristics are listed in Table 1-3.

ULCERATIVE COLITIS AND CROHN'S DISEASE IN ENDOSCOPIC BIOPSY SPECIMENS

The widespread use of endoscopy has led to a dramatic increase in the numbers of gastrointestinal biopsy specimens submitted to most surgical pathology laboratories. Colorectal and ileal biopsies are now widely used in the assessment of inflammatory diseases of the bowel.[14] Such biopsies are useful in primary diagnosis to demonstrate and document the presence of inflammatory disease as well as to classify inflammatory disease or to assess its etiology (see Ch. 2). Follow-up biopsies are helpful in evaluating the response of active inflammatory disease to

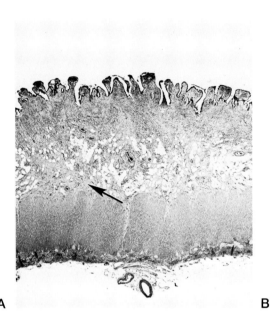 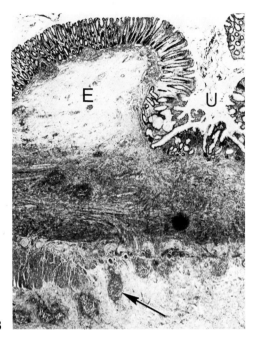

A   **B**

Fig. 1-7. Comparison of histopathology of ulcerative colitis and Crohn's disease involving the colon. **(A)** The mucosa in this specimen of low-grade active ulcerative colitis shows the villiform configuration of the mucosa with chronic inflammation and scarring extending throughout the submucosa (arrow) as a result of previous severe disease. The muscularis propria and serosa, however, are uninvolved. **(B)** The mucosa in this specimen of Crohn's disease shows a healed ulcer (*U*) with destruction of the submucosa and mucosal regeneration on the subjacent scarred muscularis propria. Mucosal architecture in nearby areas is preserved. The bowel wall is thickened owing to submucosal edema (*E*), thickening of the muscularis propria, and transmural lymphoid aggregates (arrow) in the pericolonic connective tissue. (H&E, × 16.)

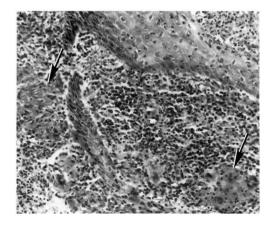

Fig. 1-8. Histopathology of the anus from a patient with Crohn's disease involving the colon. Noncaseating epithelioid cell granulomas (arrows) are present beneath actively inflamed anal squamous epithelium. (H&E, × 160.)

Table 1-3. Pathologic Features in Resection Specimens That Most Reliably Distinguish Crohn's Disease Involving the Colon from Ulcerative Colitis

1. Right-sided predominance
2. Discontinuous, segmental involvement
3. Rectal sparing
4. Discrete ulcers
5. Fissuring ulcers
6. Aphthoid erosions or ulcers
7. Linear ulcers
8. Ileal involvement
9. Fibrous stricture
10. Fistula lined by granulation tissue
*11. Transmural inflammation with lymphoid aggregates
*12. Noncaseating epithelioid cell granulomas
*13. Focal active inflammation in mucosa

* Histopathologic features only

therapy and in assessing the development of dysplasia or malignancy in long-standing idiopathic IBD (see Ch. 4).

LABORATORY PROCEDURES FOR ENDOSCOPIC BIOPSY SPECIMENS

Optimal laboratory procedures for endoscopic biopsy specimens require cooperation between endoscopists and pathologists. The endoscopists' responsibilities start with the sampling procedures, including number of specimens to be taken, number of sites to be sampled, and avoidance of artifactual damage to the tissue. Damage may result from overzealous enema preparation of the patient, endoscopic trauma, dull forceps, rough handling of the tissue, and delayed fixation. Endoscopists are also responsible for providing pathologists with satisfactory clinical history and documentation of the endoscopic findings and biopsy sites, preferably on a diagram.

Pathologists are responsible for selecting an appropriate fixative for biopsy specimens, deciding on a procedure for specimen orientation to be used either at the time of endoscopy or in the laboratory, determining the number of histopathologic sections to be prepared and the stains to be used, and finally, assessing the clinical information as well as the histopathologic findings to provide an accurate diagnosis.

A number of laboratory procedures for endoscopic biopsy specimens have been published.[15–19] In the past, we preferred Hollande fixative owing to the outstanding histopathologic results obtained with its use. Although this fixative is satisfactory for most immunohistochemical procedures on paraffin-embedded tissue, in situ hybridization and procedures requiring DNA extraction cannot be done owing to acid-induced degradation. On the other hand, neutral buffered formalin permits these latter procedures, although sometimes at the expense of optimal histopathology. Plastic embedding of biopsy specimens also has its proponents, but expense seems to be a limitation.

We currently supply neutral buffered formalin containing a small amount of eosin to the endoscopy areas in our institution and physicians'

offices. We ask that biopsy specimens be carefully removed from the forceps with a toothpick and placed directly in the fixative. We prefer that no attempt be made in the endoscopy area to orient the biopsy specimens on a substrate, thereby avoiding additional mechanical trauma to and suboptimal uneven fixation of the tissue fragments. We ask that tissue from endoscopically distinct areas or various anatomic sites be placed in different specimen containers, although we encourage multiple pieces of tissue in each container. A diagram for recording the endoscopic findings and biopsy sites is included on the laboratory requisition sheet along with the request for clinical history.

In the laboratory, the tissue specimens are prepared for paraffin embedding using a tissue processor with optimized times and solutions. At the time of embedding the specimens are oriented to obtain sections perpendicular to the luminal surface. The inclusion of eosin in the buffered formalin fixative seems to assist histotechnologists in orienting the tissue for embedding and in microtome sectioning the embedded tissue. Eight slides of semiserial sections are prepared to include about two-thirds to three-fourths of the tissue thickness in each block. With this procedure, well-oriented sections are usually obtained in at least some slides, and the chances of identifying focal abnormalities are increased. Two slides (Nos. 6 and 8) are stained with hematoxylin and eosin. The unstained slides and blocks are filed for possible later use. [For upper gastrointestinal tract biopsies, we routinely include a periodic acid-Schiff/Alcian blue pH 2.5 stain on slide No. 4 and a Diff-Quik Solution II stain on slide No. 5. The former stain is useful for distinguishing gastric-type and intestinal-type mucin and identifying fungi, and the latter is an easy rapid stain for *Helicobacter* (formerly *Campylobacter*) *pylori*.[20]]

Selection of laboratory procedures to be used for gastrointestinal biopsy specimens obviously depends on resources available in and goals of the particular laboratory. However, multiple tissue sections from each biopsy specimen are essential, and a diagram of the endoscopic findings and biopsy sites is very helpful for optimal interpretation.

As is apparent in the earlier sections on resection specimens, pathologic features helpful in distinguishing UC and CCD include the anatomic distribution of the abnormalities, gross and histopathologic findings in the mucosa, and gross and histopathologic findings in the bowel wall (see Tables 1-1 to 1-3). Endoscopic biopsy specimens have the limitation of providing only a small sample of the histopathologic findings in the mucosa and sometimes the superficial submucosa. The bowel wall findings are essentially unavailable as features in the differential diagnosis. Furthermore, pathologists are dependent on endoscopists' assessments of the distribution of gross abnormalities and the selection of biopsy sites. On the other hand, repeated biopsies over time have the advantage of providing sequential information on the course of inflammatory diseases of the bowel; this information is not available from a resection specimen that represents a single point in the clinical course of the disease.

As was described previously, the pathologic findings in patients with UC and CCD are dynamic, not static. With the recognition that features vary in individual patients, three categories of biopsy findings are useful in the differential diagnosis of UC and CCD: (1) anatomic distribution of biopsy findings; (2) histopathologic characteristics of the inflammation; and (3) histopathologic distribution of nonspecific active inflammation. These features are summarized in Table 1-4.

Table 1-4. Comparison of Ulcerative Colitis and Crohn's Disease Involving the Colon: Histopathology in Endoscopic Biopsies

Features	Ulcerative Colitis	Colonic Crohn's Disease
Anatomic distribution of biopsy findings		
Continuous abnormalities	+++	−/+
Distal predominance	+++	−/+
Rectal biopsy abnormalities	+++	+
Total colonic abnormalities	+	−/+
Abnormalities of endoscopically normal areas	+++	+
Discontinuous, segmental abnormalities	−/+	+++
Right colon predominance	−/+	+
Rectal biopsy without abnormality	−/+	+
Ileal biopsy with active inflammation	−/+	+
Histopathologic characteristics of inflammation		
Active crypt epithelial inflammation and crypt abscesses	+++	+
Prominent vascularity	+++	−/+
Crypt loss & distortion	+++	+
Epithelial mucin depletion	+	−/+
Paneth cell metaplasia	+	−/+
Thickened muscularis mucosae	+	−/+
"Follicular proctitis"	+	−/+
Noncaseating epithelioid cell granuloma	−/+	+
Granulomatous inflammation	−/+	+
Fissuring ulcer	−/+	+
Aphthoid erosion or ulcer	−/+	+
Clusters of lymphocytes	−/+	+
Histopathologic distribution of active inflammation		
Diffuse	+++	+
Patchy	+	+
Focal in rectal biopsy	−/+	+
Disproportionate submucosal involvement	−/+	+

+++ = usually present; + = sometimes present; −/+ = usually absent

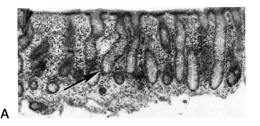

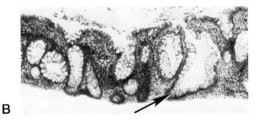

Fig. 1-9. Colonoscopic biopsies from a patient with inactive ulcerative colitis illustrating distal predominance of abnormalities. **(A)** Biopsy from endoscopically normal ascending colon shows mild crypt distortion (arrow) accompanied by chronic inflammation of the lamina propria and increased epithelial mitoses. **(B)** Biopsies from the endoscopically atrophic rectum show thinning of the mucosa with crypt loss and marked distortion (arrow) of those crypts remaining. (H&E, × 65.)

ANATOMIC DISTRIBUTION OF BIOPSY FINDINGS

Knowledge of the anatomic distribution of findings can be very helpful in the differential diagnosis of biopsy specimens. Colonoscopic biopsy specimens in UC typically show continuous abnormalities with distal predominance, including abnormalities on rectal biopsy (Fig. 1-9), although there are exceptions.[9] These distribution characteristics are best recognized when multiple tissue fragments from various anatomic sites are submitted as separate specimens (e.g., separately submitted specimens from the right, transverse, descending, and sigmoid colon as well as the rectum). Histopathologic abnormalities in biopsy specimens taken throughout the colon, including areas that have appeared endoscopically normal, are common in UC. Terminal ileal biopsies obtained through the colonoscope are usually normal or show only nonspecific abnormalities of villous architecture with increased epithelial mitotic figures and mild chronic inflammation; active ileal inflammation is unusual in UC but can be seen with "backwash" ileitis.

By contrast, the biopsy abnormalities in CCD are typically discontinuous or segmental, with abnormal tissue fragments interspersed with histopathologically normal or minimally abnormal fragments from the same anatomic area. Subtle abnormalities in endoscopically normal areas can be identified by morphometry.[21] Right-sided predominance of histopathologic abnormalities and sparing of the rectum are features of CCD. Terminal ileal biopsies can be particularly helpful by demonstrating active inflammation (Fig. 1-10).

HISTOPATHOLOGIC CHARACTERISTICS OF INFLAMMATION IN BIOPSY SPECIMENS

Abnormalities in biopsy specimens are mainly the mucosal histopathologic abnormalities described previously for resection specimens (see Table 1-2). The abnormalities can be characterized as findings representing active inflammation and changes associated with chronicity.

Active inflammation in both UC and CCD is characterized by infiltration of crypt epithelium by neutrophils, often with crypt abscesses. This acute inflammation is accompanied by chronic inflammation of the lamina propria that includes eosinophils, by vascularity, and by reactive epithelial changes. The reactive changes include reduced or depleted mucin, cytologic abnormalities, and increased mitotic figures.

Changes associated with chronicity include mucosal atrophy with shortening, loss and distortion of crypts; fibrosis of the lamina propria; Paneth cell metaplasia of crypt epithelium; and thickening of the mucularis mucosae.

The character of the inflammation in UC is entirely nonspecific. However, in active chronic UC, active inflammation is frequently associated with destruction of crypt architecture and other findings of chronicity, epithelial mucin deple-

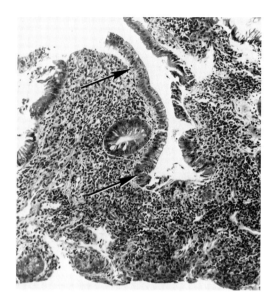

Fig. 1-10. Ileal biopsy from a patient with Crohn's disease. Active inflammation is present, characterized by neutrophils in villous and crypt epithelium (arrows), erosion, and accompanying chronic inflammation of the lamina propria. (H&E, × 145.)

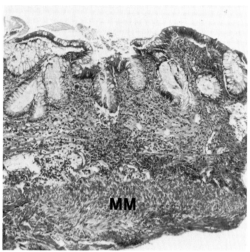

Fig. 1-11. Rectal biopsy from a patient with inactive ulcerative colitis. The specimen shows crypt loss, crypt distortion with branching, "shortfall" with enlarged space between the bottoms of the crypts and the thickened muscularis mucosae (*MM*), and chronic inflammation and fibrosis of the lamina propria. This constellation of findings is characteristic of inactive ulcerative colitis. (H&E, × 70.)

tion, and prominent vascularity. The chronic inflammatory cell population in UC is commonly composed of a large proportion of plasma cells with admixed lymphocytes and eosinophils. Foreign body giant cells and granulomatous inflammation characterized by increased numbers of epithelioid histiocytes occur in some cases of UC. Well-formed granulomas are extremely rare, however. Findings associated with chronicity are common in biopsy specimens from the rectum in UC (Fig. 1-11), even in the absence of active inflammation. This feature is in keeping with the typical distal distribution of the disease. In inactive UC, goblet cell mucin and the chronic inflammatory cell population of the lamina propria may be nearly normal in the presence of marked abnormalities of crypt architecture. Striking lymphoid hyperplasia producing "follicular proctitis" is characteristic of UC (Fig. 1-5).

In contrast to UC, the inflammation that accompanies CCD can be characteristic. The noncaseating epithelioid cell granuloma is the most distinctive finding.[21-24] Granulomatous inflammation (Fig. 1-6), discrete ulcers, fissuring ulcers, and aphthoid erosions or ulcers are also features useful in the recognition of CCD in biopsy specimens. These histopathologic features are described in more detail in the earlier section on histopathology in resection specimens. Finally, clustering of lymphocytes in the lamina propria, especially around the bases of crypts, is also seen in biopsy specimens from patients with CCD.

HISTOPATHOLOGIC DISTRIBUTION OF
NONSPECIFIC ACTIVE INFLAMMATION

Nonspecific active inflammation is acute and chronic inflammation devoid of any distinctive features such as granulomas. In active UC, the chronic inflammation typically has a diffuse pattern of involvement of the lamina propria. That is, the entire lamina propria in the biopsy specimen is relatively uniformly involved by chronic

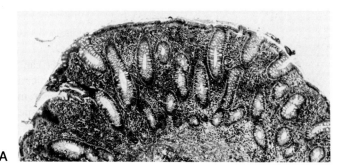

A

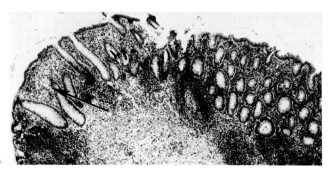

B

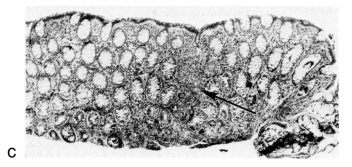

C

Fig. 1-12. Distribution of nonspecific inflammation in biopsies of Crohn's disease involving the colon. **(A)** Diffuse. **(B)** Patchy with relatively spared area (arrow). **(C)** Focal with actively inflamed crypts (arrow) and surrounding chronic inflammation. (H&E, × 55.)

inflammatory cells, although there may be variable intensity from one area to another. Patchy involvement also occurs, represented by chronic inflammation in some areas of the biopsy but its absence in others. This distribution is common in low-grade active UC. Submucosal extension of chronic inflammation below the muscularis mucosae of biopsy specimens can also be seen, particularly with severe inflammation. The submucosal inflammation, however, is usually similar in intensity to that in the overlying mucosa. As is the case for the characteristics of inflammation, the histopathologic distribution in UC is also entirely nonspecific.

CCD may show diffuse, patchy, or focal distribution of nonspecific inflammation (Fig. 1-12). The focal distribution of active inflammation in rectal biopsies is characteristic of CCD.[15, 25] The focal lesion shows infiltration of crypt epithelium by neutrophils, sometimes with crypt abscesses, surrounded by an area of chronic inflammatory cells in the lamina propria. The chronic inflammation is often predominantly lymphocytic, but with some plasma cells and eosinophils. This typical lesion is situated in the midst of otherwise uninflamed rectal mucosa, hence the term *focal*. This focal lesion can be considered as a histopathologic manifes-

Table 1-5. Pathologic Features in Endoscopic Biopsies That Most Reliably Distinguish Crohn's Disease Involving the Colon from Ulcerative Colitis

1. Noncaseating epithelioid cell granulomas
2. Discontinuous, segmental abnormalities
3. Discrete ulcers
4. Fissuring ulcers
5. Aphthoid erosions or ulcers
6. Focal nonspecific active inflammation in rectal biopsy
7. Rectal sparing
8. Disproportionate submucosal inflammation
9. Active inflammation in ileal biopsy

tation of the discontinuity of CCD. Of note, however, focal lesions are commonly seen in the endoscopically normal mucosa proximal to obvious active UC. Submucosal extension of chronic inflammation as a result of the transmural nature of the inflammatory process is identifiable in occasional biopsy specimens of CCD. Disproportionate submucosal inflammation, with more intense inflammation in the submucosa than in the overlying mucosa, suggests CCD.

The features that, when present in biopsy specimens, are particularly helpful in distinguishing CCD from UC are listed in Table 1-5.

COLITIS OF INDETERMINATE TYPE

The term *colitis of indeterminate type* is used to indicate colonic involvement by an inflammatory process for which the etiology or classification has not been determined. The term may be applied in two main clinical settings: a patient presenting with colitis in whom the entire range of diagnostic possibilities must be considered (see Ch. 2) or a patient with idiopathic IBD in whom no firm choice between UC and CCD can be made. The latter setting will be considered in this chapter. The diagnosis of colitis of indeterminate type usually results from atypical combinations of the findings in Tables 1-1 to 1-5. Thus, colitis of indeterminate type is not an entity but an expression of uncertainty regarding diagnosis.

Colitis of indeterminate type applies to a relatively small percentage of patients with idiopathic IBD.[26] In the vast majority of patients, differentiation between UC and CCD can be made on the basis of clinical, radiographic, and pathologic findings. Pathologists, however, may use the term often in reporting on biopsy specimens, because of the limitations inherent in biopsy diagnosis, as described previously. Colitis of indeterminate type is often a temporary pathologic classification. Examination of a colectomy specimen or of sequential biopsy specimens usually results eventually in categorization of idiopathic IBD as UC or CCD. It should be kept in mind, however, that patients with both UC and CD have been reported in the literature.[27, 28]

Three main factors contribute to the difficulty in the differential diagnosis of UC and CCD: effects of therapy, inactivity of disease, and fulminant colitis ("toxic megacolon").

EFFECTS OF THERAPY

The beneficial effects of a variety of therapeutic measures on active UC and CCD can be easily recognized clinically. The effects of therapy on pathologic findings have received less attention. In a study of rectal biopsies in UC, anti-inflammatory drugs appeared to result in a decrease in crypt abscesses but an increase in mucosal edema.[29] This reduction in active inflammation was associated with increased numbers of goblet cells, decreased epithelial injury, and decreased mucosal leukocytes, including eosinophils. However, the population of inflammatory cells affected by various drugs varies.[30] Salicylazosulfapyridine (sulfasalazine-azulfidine) led to reduced numbers of plasma cells, while oral prednisone appeared to reduce neutrophils. Both plasma cells and neutrophils decreased in number with 6-mercaptopurine, but this decrease was associated with increased numbers of mast cells and macrophages. Numbers of lymphocytes in the chronic inflammatory infiltrate were not affected by any of the drugs studied. In another publication, azathioprine was found to reduce mucosal plasma cells in UC.[31] These various studies indicate that changes in histopathologic characteristics of inflammation in UC can occur with anti-inflammatory therapy. Thus, features generally useful in the pathologic diagnosis of UC may not be reliable after the patient has been treated with anti-inflammatory drugs.

Intrarectal steroid therapy can produce even more dramatic effects on the reliability of diagnostic criteria.[26, 32] Steroid enemas can suppress active rectal inflammation in patients with UC, while leaving the more proximal colon unsuppressed. The therapy-induced pattern of relative rectal sparing may result in confusion of UC with CCD.

Effects of other forms of therapy may also lead to problems in diagnosis of colitis. Following abdominal colectomy with ileostomy for UC or CCD, active inflammation may develop in the rectal stump as a result of diversion colitis.[33] With antibiotic and azulfidine therapy, *Clostridium difficile* toxin-induced inflammatory disease may occur in patients with UC or CCD.[34] Patients with UC and CCD sometimes develop superimposed infectious colitis. These other forms of inflammatory disease in patients with underlying idiopathic IBD may be difficult to distinguish from UC and CCD. The effects of total parenteral nutrition on the reliability of diagnostic criteria are largely unknown. Thus, differentiation of UC and CCD after initiation of therapy may be difficult, leading to classification as colitis of indeterminate type.

INACTIVITY OF DISEASE

The most useful features for distinction between UC and CCD are generally found in active disease (see Table 1-3 and 1-5). When UC and CCD become inactive as a result of therapy or "burning out" during the natural history of the process, this distinction may become particularly difficult. This problem is accentuated in biopsy specimens owing to the lack of availability of the findings in the bowel wall.

FULMINANT COLITIS ("TOXIC MEGACOLON")

At the opposite extreme from inactivity of disease, fulminant colitis commonly leads to difficulty in the differential diagnosis between UC and CCD.[26] Fulminant colitis is the most common factor leading to categorization of a resection specimen as colitis of indeterminate type. Fulminant UC commonly shows severe active disease in the transverse or sometimes the sigmoid colon (Fig. 1-13). This distribution produces a pattern of proximal predominance with relative rectal sparing that suggests CCD (see Table 1-3). In addition, areas of fulminant activity can develop in association with inactive or low-grade active disease elsewhere in the colon. A discontinuous or segmental pattern of involvement can result, similar to that seen in CCD (Fig. 1-14).

In addition to atypical anatomic distribution, the character of the colonic mucosal and bowel wall abnormalities in fulminant UC may mimic CCD. Discrete, serpiginous, and fissuring ulcers

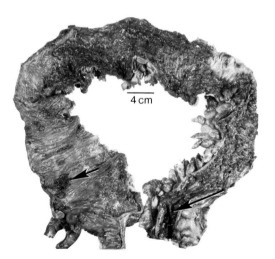

Fig. 1-13. Fulminant ulcerative colitis in a specimen from an abdominal colectomy. Discrete ulcers in the ascending colon (short arrow), severe involvement of the transverse colon, and linear ulcers (long arrow) and thickening of the wall in the sigmoid colon mimic Crohn's disease.

Fig. 1-14. Fulminant ulcerative colitis in colonoscopic biopsies from the same patient as in Figure 1-13. One fragment of tissue shows an area of deep ulceration (arrows) that extends into the muscularis propria (*MP*). The other fragment of tissue from a nearby site shows mucosa with only crypt distortion and chronic inflammation of the lamina propria. These findings suggest discontinuity of abnormality and mimic Crohn's disease. (H&E, × 30.)

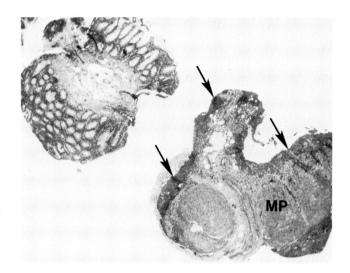

may occur. Inflammation extending to the serosal surface with peritonitis is frequent, and adhesions or perforation may result. In histopathologic sections from resection specimens, discrete ulcers surrounded by relatively uninflamed mucosa with maintained goblet cell mucin are common in fulminant UC. The submucosa is frequently widened due to edema associated with severe active inflammation. In addition, the ulcers usually extend into or through the muscularis propria, and may be fissuring, undermining and accompanied by transmural inflammation (Figs. 1-15 and 1-16). Vasculitis sometimes results from involvement of blood and lymphatic vessels by the severe inflammatory process in fulminant colitis.

The most common error in the interpretation of fulminant UC is misclassification as CCD, because of the mimicking features just described. Recognition of the inflammatory process as fulminant colitis is the first step in avoiding this error. In many cases, dilatation of the colon may not be apparent. For this reason, the term *fulminant colitis* is preferable to "toxic megacolon." Once the process is identified as severe active disease, the classification can be approached prudently.

Some characteristics, when present, may be

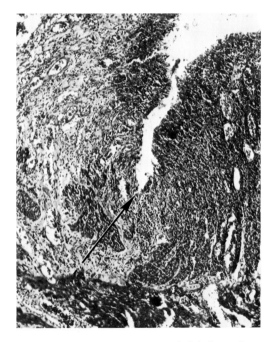

Fig. 1-15. Fissuring ulcer (arrow) in fulminant ulcerative colitis: same specimen as in Figure 1-13. The ulcer is lined by necrotic tissue, not granulation tissue as is usual in fissuring ulcers of Crohn's disease involving the colon. Blood vessel dilation nearby is striking. (H&E, × 90.)

Table 1-6. Comparison of Fulminant Ulcerative Colitis and Crohn's Disease Involving the Colon: Characteristics of Mimicking Features

Fulminant UC Feature Mimicking CCD	Fulminant Ulcerative Colitis	Colonic Crohn's Disease
Discontinuous proximal involvement with rectal sparing	Fulminant active disease	Active chronic disease
Discrete, serpiginous and fissuring ulcers	Acute necrotizing ulcers	Active chronic ulcers
Transmural inflammation	Associated with acute necrotizing ulcers	Lymphoid aggregates
Vasculitis	Associated with acute necrotizing inflammation	Separate from areas of active inflammation

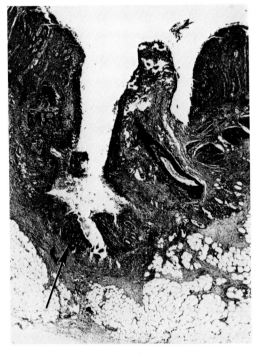

Fig. 1-16. Ulcer accompanied by transmural inflammation (arrow) extending through muscularis propria (*MP*) into pericolonic soft tissue in fulminant ulcerative colitis: same specimen as in Figure 1-13. These findings mimic Crohn's disease. (H&E, × 18.)

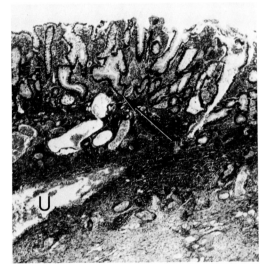

Fig. 1-17. Marked crypt distortion (arrow) in the mucosa of sigmoid colon with underlying ulcer (*U*) in fulminant ulcerative colitis: same specimen as that in Figure 1-13. Distal predominance of mucosal evidence of chronicity aids in recognition of the idiopathic IBD as ulcerative colitis. Vascular dilatation and congestion are striking and typical of active ulcerative colitis. (H&E, × 65.)

helpful in distinguishing typical fulminant UC from typical CCD (see Table 1-6). First, in fulminant UC the pattern of discontinuous proximal predominance with relative rectal sparing usually is present for severe active disease, but *not* for changes associated with chronicity. In chronic UC with superimposed fulminant colitis, evidence of chronicity is usually recognizable with a distal, continuous distribution (Fig. 1-17).

Second, the discrete, fissuring, and serpiginous ulcers in fulminant UC are usually acute lesions lined by necrotic tissue (Fig. 1-14). By contrast, the ulcers with these characteristics in patients with CCD are usually lined by granulation tissue. This point of distinction is lost, however, in the healing phases of fulminant UC. Third, the transmural inflammation in fulminant UC is usually associated with transmural ulceration (Fig. 1-15). Marked congestion, edema, and muscle fiber necrosis are frequent in the muscularis propria. These findings contrast with the transmural inflammation in CCD, which is characterized by prominent lymphoid aggregates, often with associated fibrosis. Finally, previous biopsy specimens, radiographic findings, and clinical history may be available and provide important information on the character of the disease prior to the fulminant phase.

Fulminant colitis does occur in CCD as well as in UC. As a result, differentiation between fulminant UC and fulminant CCD may not be possible in some specimens. The subsequent course of the patient's illness may then be the determining factor in differential diagnosis.[26]

FUTURE DIRECTIONS

The pathologic distinction between UC and CCD is currently based mainly on the application of gross pathology and histopathology. With the advent of newer methodologies, complementary techniques may become available for routine usage. Some possible future directions are summarized in Table 1-7.

A number of studies have examined differences in mucosal inflammatory cell populations

Table 1-7. Possible Future Directors for Distinguishing Ulcerative Colitis and Crohn's Disease Involving the Colon

Inflammatory cell populations
Inflammatory mediators
Neuropeptides
Mucus glycoproteins
Mucosal morphometry
Infectious agents

as potential distinguishing features for UC and CCD. Differences in the plasma cell populations have been reported by several groups of investigators. For example, in an immunohistochemical study, mucosal IgG1- and IgA1-containing cells were increased to a greater extent in UC than CCD, whereas mucosal IgG2 immunocytes were in higher proportion in CCD than in UC.[35, 36] Confirmatory results were obtained in an in vitro study.[37]

Inflammatory mediators have also drawn attention. An in vitro study showed that lamina propria mononuclear cells from CD patients included increased numbers of cells responsive to, or cells with exaggerated reactivity to, the lymphokine interleukin 2. By contrast, ulcerative colitis was characterized by loss of interleukin 2-responsive cells or hyporesponsiveness of the cell population.[38] In another study, leukotriene B4 levels in rectal dialysates were found to be higher in patients with UC than in CD.[39]

As described above (see Histopathology of Ulcerative Colitis and Crohn's Disease Involving the Colon), neural hyperplasia is a frequent feature of CD. The proliferated nerves are peptidergic, containing vasoactive intestinal peptide (VIP). Immunohistochemical assessment of VIP has been reported to be useful in distinguishing CCD from UC.[40]

Mucus glycoprotein differences between UC and CCD have been described. Patients with UC, even in the inactive phase, have been found to be deficient in a particular glycoprotein component.[41–43] This deficiency has been suggested to play an etiologic role in UC and is not found in patients with CD. Another study showed reduced in vitro mucus production in patients with inactive UC.[44]

Morphometric assessment of colonic mucosa has been reported to be useful in distinguishing idiopathic IBD from controls on the basis of increased lamina propria cellularity.[45] Application of this methodology[46] to distinguish UC and CCD has some potential.

Various infectious agents have been implicated over the years as the etiology of CD. The candidate organisms included viruses, cell wall deficient bacteria, and most recently an atypical mycobacterium. Identification of an infectious agent would provide a means of distinguishing CCD from UC.[47]

The clinical applicability of any or all of these findings is currently limited owing to a variety of factors. Some of the findings show considerable overlap between individual cases of UC and CCD and therefore may not be particularly helpful. The methodology used in some of the studies is currently complex and difficult, making it unsuitable for routine use. The findings in some of the studies are controversial because other investigators have not been able to replicate the results. As a consequence, these new techniques remain investigative at present.

SUMMARY

Distinguishing between UC and CCD is a frequent problem in gastrointestinal pathology. Useful criteria for differential diagnosis include features from gross pathology and histopathology of the mucosa and bowel wall, but no features are pathognomonic of either form of idiopathic IBD. Laboratory procedures can have a major impact on the ability to distinguish UC and CCD in resection specimens. Optimal interpretation of endoscopic biopsy specimens requires cooperation between endoscopists and pathologists, but biopsy interpretation is intrinsically difficult because only mucosal features are available for evaluation. In some patients, the inflammatory disease cannot be classified and is termed *colitis of indeterminate type*. New methodologies that may be helpful in diagnosis are under investigation, but pathology seems likely to be a mainstay in the differential diagnosis of UC and CCD for the forseeable future.

ACKNOWLEDGMENTS

The manuscript was typed by Mrs. Nancy Folker. The photomicrographs were taken by Mr. Raymond E. Lung, RBP.

Dr. Hamilton was supported by a Senior Fellow Award from the National Foundation for Ileitis and Colitis.

REFERENCES

1. Dozois RR, O'Rourke JS: Newer operations for ulcerative colitis and Crohn's disease. Surg Clin North Am 68:1339, 1988
2. Korelitz BI: Considerations of surveillance, dysplasia, and carcinoma of the colon in the management of ulcerative colitis and Crohn's disease. Med Clin North Am 74:189, 1990
3. Lennard-Jones JE: Classification of inflammatory bowel disease. Scand J Gastroenterol 24(suppl 170):2, 1989
4. Morson BC, Dawson IMP: Gastrointestinal Pathology. 2nd Ed. p. 781. Blackwell, Oxford, 1979
5. Rosai J: Ackerman's Surgical Pathology. 6th Ed. pp. 19, A46, A79. CV Mosby, St. Louis, 1981
6. Rowland R, Pounder DJ: Crohn's colitis. p. 267. In Sommers SC, Rosen PO (eds): Pathology Annual. Part 1, Vol. 17. Appleton-Century-Crofts, East Norwalk, CT, 1982
7. Price AB, Morson BC: Inflammatory bowel disease. The surgical pathology of Crohn's disease and ulcerative colitis. Human Pathol 6:7, 1975
8. Cook MG, Dixon MF: An analysis of the reliability of detection and diagnostic value of various pathological features in Crohn's disease and ulcerative colitis. Gut 14:255, 1973
9. Spiliadis CA, Spiliadis CA, Lennard-Jones JE: Ulcerative colitis with relative sparing of the rectum. Clinical features, histology, and prognosis. Dis Colon Rectum 30:334, 1987
10. Davison AM, Dixon MF: The appendix as a "skip lesion" in ulcerative colitis. Histopathology 16:93, 1990
11. Sarin SK, Malhotra V, Sen Gupta S, et al: Significance of eosinophil and mast cell counts in rectal mucosa in ulcerative colitis. A prospective controlled study. Dig Dis Sci 32:363, 1987
12. Bishop AE, Polak JM, Bryant MG, et al: Abnormalities of vasoactive intestinal polypeptide-containing nerves in Crohn's disease. Gastroenterology 79:853, 1980
13. Dvorak AM, Silen W: Differentiation between Crohn's disease and other inflammatory conditions by electron microscopy. Ann Surg 201:53, 1985
14. Goodman MJ, Kirsner JB, Riddell RH: Usefulness of rectal biopsy in inflammatory bowel disease. Gastroenterology 72:952, 1977
15. Yardley JH, Donowitz M: Colo-rectal biopsy in inflammatory bowel disease. p. 50. In Yardley

JH, Morson BC, Abell MR (eds): The Gastrointestinal Tract. International Academy of Pathology Monograph No. 18. Williams & Wilkins, Baltimore, 1977

16. Whitehead R: Mucosal Biopsy of the Gastrointestinal Tract. 3rd Ed. p. xi. Major Problems in Pathology. Vol. 3. WB Saunders, Philadephia, 1985

17. Mitros FA: The biopsy in evaluating patients with inflammatory bowel disease. In Symposium on Inflammatory Bowel Disease. Med Clin North Am 64:1037, 1980

18. Haggitt RC: Handling of gastrointestinal biopsies in the surgical pathology laboratory. Laboratory Med 13:273, 1982

19. Guinee DG Jr, Lee RG: Laboratory methods for processing and interpretation of endoscopic gastrointestinal biopsies. Laboratory Med 21:13, 1990

20. Skipper R, DeStephano DB: A rapid stain for *Campylobacter pylori* in gastrointestinal tissue sections using Diff-Quik®. J Histotechnol 12:303, 1989

21. Goodman MJ, Skinner JM, Truelove SC: Abnormalities in the apparently normal bowel mucosa in Crohn's disease. Lancet 1:275, 1976

22. Rotterdam H, Korelitz BI, Sommers SC: Microgranulomas in grossly normal rectal mucosa in Crohn's disease. Am J Clin Pathol 67:550, 1977

23. Korelitz BI, Summers SC: Rectal biopsy in patients with Crohn's disease. JAMA 237:2742, 1977

24. Iliffe GD, Owen DA: Rectal biopsy in Crohn's disease. Dig Dis Sci 26:321, 1981

25. Yardley JH, Hamilton SR: Focal non-specific inflammation in Crohn's disease. p. 62. In Pena AS, Waterman IT, Booth CC, Strober W (eds): Recent Advances in Crohn's Disease. Developments in Gastroenterology. Vol. 1. Martinus Nijhoff, The Hague, 1981

26. Price AB: Difficulties in the differential diagnosis of ulcerative colitis and Crohn's disease. p. 1. In Yardley JH, Morson BC, Abell MR (eds): The Gastrointestinal Tract. International Academy of Pathology Monograph No. 18. Williams & Wilkins, Baltimore, 1977

27. White CL III, Hamilton SR, Diamond MP, Cameron JL: Crohn's disease and ulcerative colitis in the same patient. Gut 24:857, 1983

28. Eyer S, Spadaccini C, Walker P, et al: Simultaneous ulcerative colitis and Crohn's disease. Am J Gastroenterol 73:345, 1980

29. Korelitz BI, Sommers SC: Responses to drug therapy in ulcerative colitis: Evaluation by rectal biopsy and histopathologic changes. Am J Gastroenterol 64:365, 1975

30. Korelitz BI, Sommers SC: Responses to drug therapy in ulcerative colitis: Evaluation by rectal biopsy and mucosal cell counts. Am J Dig Dis 21:441, 1976

31. Campbell AC, Skinner JM, Maclennan ICM, et al: Immunosuppression in treatment of inflammatory bowel disease. Part II. The effects of azathioprine in lymphoid cell populations in a double-blind trial in ulcerative colitis. Clin Exp Immunol 24:249, 1976

32. Schachter H, Goldstein MJ, Rappaport H, et al: Ulcerative and "granulomatous" colitis—validity of differential diagnostic criteria. A study of 100 patients treated by colectomy. Ann Intern Med 72:841, 1970

33. Glotzer DJ, Glick ME, Goldman H: Proctitis and colitis following diversion of the fecal stream. Gastroenterology 80:433, 1981

34. Bartlett JG: *Clostridium difficile* and inflammatory bowel disease. Gastroenterology 80:863, 1981

35. Kett K, Brandtzaeg P: Local IgA subclass alterations in ulcerative colitis and Crohn's disease of the colon. Gut 28:1013, 1987

36. Kett K, Rognum TO, Brandtzaeg P: Mucosal subclass distribution of immunoglobulin G-producing cells is different in ulcerative colitis and Crohn's disease of the colon. Gastroenterology 93:919, 1987

37. MacDermott RP, Nash GS, Nahm MH: Antibody secretion by human intestinal mononuclear cells from normal controls and inflammatory bowel disease patients. Immunol Invest 18:449, 1989

38. Kusugami K, Youngman KR, West GA, Fiocchi C: Intestinal immune reactivity to interleukin 2 differs among Crohn's disease, ulcerative colitis, and controls. Gastroenterology 97:1, 1989

39. Lauritsen K, Laursen LS, Bukhave K, Rask-Madsen J: In vivo profiles of eicosanoids in ulcerative colitis, Crohn's colitis, and Clostridium difficile colitis. Gastroenterology 95:11, 1988

40. O'Morain C, Bishop AE, McGregor GP, et al: Vasoactive intestinal peptide concentrations and immunohistochemical studies in rectal biopsies from patients with inflammatory bowel disease. Gut 25:57, 1984

41. Podolsky DK, Fournier DA: Emergence of antigenic glycoprotein structures in ulcerative colitis detected through monoclonal antibodies. Gastroenterology 95:371, 1988

42. Podolsky DK, Fournier DA: Alterations in mucosal content of colonic glycoconjugates in inflammatory bowel disease defined by monoclonal antibodies. Gastroenterology 95:379, 1988
43. Podolsky DK: The colonic goblet cell and glycoprotein heterogeneity. Immunol Invest 18:485, 1989
44. Cope GJ, Heatley RV, Kelleher JX, Axon AT: In vitro mucus glycoprotein production by colonic tissue from patients with ulcerative colitis. Gut 29:229, 1988
45. Jenkins D, Goodall A, Drew K, Scott BB: What is colitis? Statistical approach to distinguishing clinically important inflammatory change in rectal biopsy specimens. J Clin Pathol 41:72, 1988
46. Salzmann JL, Peltier-Koch F, Bloch F, et al: Morphometric study of colonic biopsies: A new method of estimating inflammatory diseases. Lab Invest 60:847, 1989
47. Kobayashi K, Blaser MJ, Brown WR: Immunohistochemical examination for mycobacteria in intestinal tissues from patients with Crohn's disease. Gastroenterology 96:1009, 1989

2

The Differential Diagnosis of Idiopathic Inflammatory Bowel Disease

Rodger C. Haggitt

The differential diagnosis of idiopathic inflammatory bowel disease (IBD) includes many conditions (Table 2-1), all of which must be excluded before the diagnosis of idiopathic IBD can be made. The pathologist plays an important role in the diagnosis of idiopathic IBD by excluding, insofar as possible, the other conditions shown in Table 2-1. Because some of these conditions produce a nonspecific tissue response, the pathologist frequently can only document the presence of disease and state that its histologic pattern suggests one or more of the disease categories listed, or that it has features consistent with idiopathic IBD. The final diagnosis may require microbiologic confirmation, clinical and roentgenographic data, or a response to specific therapy. Thus, all the available information concerning the patient must be considered before a final diagnosis is rendered.

In the ensuing discussion, the characteristic pathologic features that permit one to diagnose or to suspect a condition are dicussed, and brief comments about clinical features and differential diagnosis are made. The discussion is limited to the colon because the biopsy differential diagnosis of idiopathic IBD is essentially limited to colonic biopsies. Ischemic colitis is covered in a separate chapter and is not included here.

INFLAMMATION CAUSED BY INFECTIOUS AGENTS

VIRAL INFECTIONS

Acute viral gastroenteritis ranks as one of the most common illnesses affecting humans; in the United States, only the common cold is more frequent.[1] The causative viral agents were not discovered until the 1970s, when the advanced laboratory techniques necessary for their identification became available. Currently, two major groups of viruses are considered proven to be epidemiologically important causes of viral gastroenteritis: the Norwalk-like viruses and the rotaviruses.[2, 3] The site of human infection with these agents appears to be the small bowel; colonic involvement has not to date been convincingly documented.

Herpes Simplex Virus

Two members of the herpes group of viruses have been associated with gastrointestinal disease in man. These are the herpes simplex viruses and cytomegalovirus.[4] Herpes simplex virus may cause colitis in immunosuppressed individuals and in homosexual males with or

**Table 2-1. Classification of Inflammatory Disorders
of the Colon**

Idiopathic inflammatory bowel disease
    Ulcerative colitis
    Crohn's disease
    Colitis of indeterminate type

Inflammation caused by infectious agents
    Viruses
    Chlamydiae
    Bacteria
    Fungi
    Parasites

Inflammation associated with motor disorders
    Diverticulitis
    Solitary rectal ulcer syndrome

Inflammation secondary to vascular hypoperfusion
    Ischemic colitis
    Colitis complicating colonic obstruction

Colitis induced by therapeutic intervention
    Effects of enemas and laxatives
    Drug-induced
    Attributable to therapeutic radiation
    Graft-versus-host disease
    Following small intestinal bypass and diversion of fecal stream

Colitis associated with systemic disease
    Chronic granulomatous disease of childhood
    Immunodeficiency syndromes
    Hemolytic-uremic syndrome
    Behcet's disease

Miscellaneous types of colitis
    Collagenous colitis
    Nonspecific (idiopathic) ulcer
    Necrotizing enterocolitis in cancer patients
    Eosinophilic colitis and allergic proctitis

without AIDS.[5-8] The entire large intestine may contain well-defined, irregular ulcers in which herpesvirus can be demonstrated by electron microscopy and immunoperoxidase techniques. The colonic epithelium adjacent to the ulcers may contain multinucleated giant cells, but identifiable herpesvirus inclusion bodies are usually not present.[8] Goodell and colleagues isolated herpes simplex from 21 homosexual men with proctitis, 13 of whom had no other organism that could have explained the findings.[7] The presenting clinical signs and symptoms included severe anorectal pain, difficult urination, constipation, and an ulcerative process involving the distal rectum. Biopsies disclosed mucosal erosions with acute inflammation, decreased mucin production, crypt abscesses, and destruction of the crypt architecture. In addition, some biopsies showed perivascular lymphocytic infiltration in the submucosa, where occasional cells contained intranuclear inclusions. In order to exclude idiopathic IBD and to establish that herpesvirus is the cause of a proctitis or colitis, one must culture the organism from the tissue or identify multinucleated giant cells and intranuclear inclusion bodies that either displace the entire nucleoplasm to the periphery ("ground glass" inclusions) or are surrounded by a clear halo (Cowdry type A inclusions). Immunoperoxidase localization of antibodies or detection of virus-specific DNA sequences can also be used to document that herpes simplex virus is present.

Cytomegalovirus

Although cytomegalovirus (CMV) had been recognized in ulcerative lesions of the colon for many years, its etiologic relationship to the ulcers remained a point of controversy until recently.[9] What has become clear is that although CMV infection in adults is a regular feature of the immunosuppressed state[4, 9, 10] it may also rarely occur in immunocompetent individuals.[11] Prevalence rates of complement-fixing antibody to CMV in adults are influenced by socioeconomic conditions, ranging from 40 percent in industrialized nations to 100 percent in "developing" countries. The infection is presumably acquired during childhood, enters a latent phase, and then becomes active with immunosuppression of the host. Cytomegalovirus can behave as an opportunist that colonizes pre-existing colonic ulcers or may be the primary cause of the ulcers.[10, 12, 13] The most frequent clinical contexts in which colonic ulcers caused by CMV are seen are in renal transplant recipients and in patients with acquired immunodeficiency syndrome (AIDS).[10, 12] Cytomegalovirus infection of the colon has been recognized as a complication of ulcerative colitis for many years and may precipitate toxic megacolon.[14] Cooper and co-workers identified CMV in 5 of 7 patients with toxic dilatation,[14] whereas Goodman and colleagues found it in 2 of 13 cases.[12]

The ulcers of CMV colitis are often multiple, large, and usually not associated with ulcers in the ileum. One recognizes CMV infection by noting cytomegaly of the affected cells, which average 30 μm in diameter and which contain large, intranuclear, eosinophilic, oval to rectangular inclusion bodies surrounded by a clear halo. Cytoplasmic inclusion bodies may also be seen. Cytomegalovirus inclusion bodies

are most consistently identified in endothelial cells, fibroblasts, pericytes, and macrophages in the granulation tissue of ulcer bases; they are rarely found in epithelial cells. When present in intact mucosa, CMV colitis characteristically causes focal, perivascular mononuclear cell infiltration in the submucosa and base of the mucosa (Fig. 2-1). Single-cell necrosis and crypt abscess formation that resemble acute graft-versus-host disease may also be seen.[15] Immunocytochemistry and in situ hybridization using CMV-specific antibodies or DNA probes can be useful adjunctive techniques when the diagnosis of CMV inclusions is equivocal on hematoxylin and eosin (H&E)-stained sections.[16]

Chlamydiae

Microorganisms of the genus *Chlamydia*, formerly classed as viruses, are now recognized as a unique intermediate group of organisms whose obligate intracellular growth and sensitivity to physical inactivation are more like those of viruses, but whose chemistry, immunology, and morphology are more like bacteria.[17, 18] Two species are recognized, *Chlamydia psittaci*, which includes the agents of psittacosis and ornithosis, and *C. trachomatis*, which includes the agents responsible for trachoma, inclusion conjunctivitis, genital tract infections (nongonococcal urethritis, cervicitis, salpingitis), and lymphogranuloma venereum (LGV). Immunologic typing permits separation of *C. trachomatis* into LGV and non-LGV groups. Both may cause proctitis in homosexual men, but the LGV subgroups produce a more severe lesion.[19, 20] Clinical features include anorectal pain, tenesmus, and a bloody mucopurulent anal discharge. The sigmoidoscopic findings include friability of the rectal mucosa and discrete ulcers.[19, 21] The histologic appearance of the infection is nonspecific, but similar to idiopathic IBD, with inflammation of the lamina propria and crypt abscesses.[19, 21] Follicular lymphoid hyperplasia is particularly characteristic, and discrete granulomas may be present in as many as 20 percent of cases.[8, 22] The histologic picture may closely

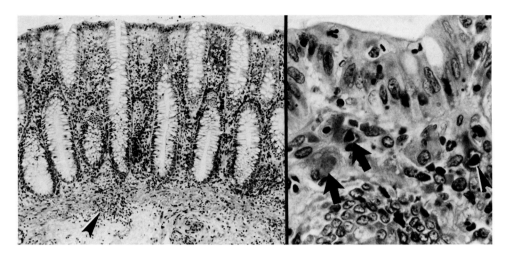

Fig. 2-1. CMV colitis in a patient with AIDS. The left panel illustrates mucosa that has normal crypt architecture and in which the only abnormality recognizable at this power is a focus of inflammation in the muscularis mucosae (arrow). Focal inflammation affecting the muscularis mucosae or submucosa, as shown here, is characteristic of CMV colitis in intact mucosa. In the right panel, two diagnostic CMV intranuclear inclusions are seen within mesenchymal cells (arrows). The arrowhead points to an infected cell, which is enlarged and which contains cytoplasmic inclusions but no diagnostic nuclear inclusion.

mimic rectal involvement by Crohn's disease. The necrotizing granulomatous inflammation typical in the inguinal nodes involved by LGV is not seen in extranodal lesions. Because of the nonspecific histologic picture, the diagnosis of proctitis attributable to lymphogranuloma venereum can be confirmed only by appropriate cultures or serologic tests.[19]

BACTERIAL INFECTIONS

Enteropathogenic bacteria produce disease by one of four mechanisms or combinations thereof: (1) elaboration of a preformed toxin that is then ingested (staphylococcal enterotoxins); (2) elaboration of enterotoxins following colonization of the gut and adherence of the organism to the mucosal surface (*Cholera*, *shigella*, *Salmonella*, *Yersinia*); (3) mucosal adherence and elaboration of cytotoxins that elicit tissue damage (*Shigella*, verotoxin-producing *Escherichia coli*, *Clostridium difficile*); and (4) invasion of and damage to the mucosa, with production of a bloody mucopurulent stool (*Shigella*, *Salmonella*, *Campylobacter*).[23, 24] The histologic changes depend in part on the pathogenetic mechanism involved in producing the injury. Thus, organisms that induce disease via the production of toxin tend to produce less severe morphologic change than do those that invade the mucosa. The former generally have a clinical picture dominated by diarrhea, whereas the latter tend to have a dysenteric syndrome with fever, abdominal pain, and numerous small-volume stools containing blood, mucus, and polymorphonuclear (PMN) leukocytes. The disease produced by any of these pathogenetic mechanisms may mimic idiopathic IBD clinically and pathologically; however, the invasive group accounts for most of the problems in differential diagnosis.

In order to establish the diagnosis of an infectious diarrhea, an organism must be identified in or cultured from the stool, or a rise in titer of a specific serum antibody must be demonstrated. The histologic appearance of colitis induced by enteric pathogens is nonspecific, but often has features suggesting an infection rather than idiopathic IBD when the biopsies have been

Table 2-2. Differential Diagnosis of Acute Self-Limited Colitis and Idiopathic Inflammatory Bowel Disease

Histologic Feature	ASLC[a]	UC	CDC
Distortion of crypt architecture[b]/atrophy	−	+ + +	+
Inflammation			
Neutrophils in lamina propria[c]	+ + +	+	+
Increased mononuclear cells	−/+	+ + +	+ +
Basal lymphoid aggregates	−	+ +	+
Epithelioid granulomas	−	−	+
"Granulomatous" inflammation	−/+	−/+	+ +
Basal giant cells	−	+	+

[a] ASLC includes culture-positive and -negative cases; about half will have negative cultures. Refers only to common infections such as *Salmonella*, *Shigella*, or *Campylobacter* and excludes tuberculosis and histoplasmosis.
[b] Defined as two or more branched crypts in a biopsy.
[c] Neutrophils in infectious colitis tend to concentrate in the lamina propria, whereas in ulcerative colitis (UC) and Crohn's disease of the colon (CDC) they accumulate predominantly in crypt epithelium and lumen.

taken early in the course of the infection (4 days or less).[25] When the stool culture is negative in a patient with a self-limited, and therefore presumably infectious, colitis, the term *acute self-limited colitis* (ASLC) is used. The percentage of patients with apparent infections who have negative cultures varies depending on how many different organisms are sought, but is typically in the range of 40 to 60 percent.[25, 26] Table 2-2 shows some general guidelines for differentiating infectious and idiopathic colitis. The most characteristic histologic feature of ASLC is the absence of features that suggest idiopathic IBD[26] (i.e., the absence of crypt architectural distortion as defined by the presence of two or more branched crypts, and dense lymphoplasmacytic infiltration extending to the base of the mucosa). Neutrophilic infiltration of the mucosa is a hallmark of acute infectious colitis. The neutrophilic infiltration is prominent within the lamina propria, as well as in the crypt epithelium and in crypt abscesses as in idiopathic IBD (Fig. 2-2). Thus, a biopsy from a patient with the acute onset of bloody diarrhea that showed an absence of crypt architectural distortion and dense lymphoplasmacystic infiltration, but that had marked neutrophilic infiltration of the lamina propria with less involvement of the crypt epithelium and few crypt abscesses would sug-

gest an infectious etiology. With the exception of tuberculosis, *Yersinia pseudotuberculosis*, syphilitic proctitis, and chlamydial proctitis, epithelioid granulomas, like those seen in Crohn's disease, are not found in patients with bacterial infections. Foci of ill-defined granulomatous inflammation formed by focal aggregation of macrophages may be seen in infections, especially with *Salmonella* and *Campylobacter* (Fig. 2-3). Such aggregates of macrophages differ from the epithelioid granuloma in that they are not as compact and discrete and lack giant cells.

A number of important points must be kept in mind when one interprets colonic and rectal biopsies. The effects of bowel preparation with hypertonic enemas or purgative laxatives can cause abnormalities of the surface epithelium and mild neutrophilic infiltration that may be mistaken for an acute infectious colitis (see Effects of Enemas and Laxatives, below). Infections may occasionally exactly mimic idiopathic IBD, especially if the biopsy is taken after the first 4 days of the infection. Such biopsies show the resolving phase of ASLC, in which there may be a focal cryptitis that mimics Crohn's disease.[25] The rectal biopsy may be normal or may show only nonspecific inflammation of the lamina propria in patients with culture-proven infectious diarrhea. Patients with idiopathic IBD

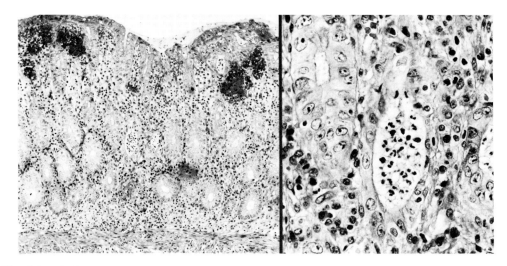

Fig. 2-2. ASLC attributable to *Shigella*. Note normal crypt architecture and depletion of goblet cell mucin with reactive hyperplasia of crypt epithelial nuclei, seen best at higher-power magnification in the right panel. The dark areas in the upper part of the mucosa in the left panel are extravasated red cells artifactually present as a result of the biopsy trauma. The lamina propria does not contain a significant increase in lymphocytes and plasma cells, a feature that in combination with the preserved crypt architecture is strongly suggestive of an ASLC.

appear to have an increased incidence of infectious diarrheas; in such patients, it is usually not possible to recognize the superimposed infection. Finally, it is important to reiterate that a biopsy can only suggest an infectious process; the diagnosis must be confirmed by culture, serologic tests, immunohistochemistry, or DNA probe technology.

Table 2-3 lists the enteric pathogens cultured during a 1-year, population-based study from the Puget Sound area of Washington State.[27] In this study, only the listed pathogens were sought. Table 2-4 shows data from a large British study in which a comprehensive attempt to identify most stool pathogens was made.[28] One notable exception from this study was *E. coli* 0157:H7. Thus, the spectrum of organisms identified in patients with infectious diarrhea very much depends on which organisms are sought.

Campylobacter fetus ss. jejuni

In several recent series of cases, *Campylobacter fetus* ss. *jejuni* has been the most frequently isolated enteric pathogen, accounting for 30 to 60 percent of all positive isolates from diarrheal stools.[29–32] The prevalence of *Campylobacter* isolates varies with geographic location. Within the United States, it is more common in the northern tier of states.[33]

Campylobacter enterocolitis affects all age groups, but is most common between ages 15 and 30.[30] Acute onset of fever, intermittent colicky abdominal pain, and diarrhea characterize the clinical picture.[34, 35] Frank blood typically appears in the stool a few days later. Significant vomiting and dehydration are usually not prominent. The small intestine or colon, or both, may be affected, and appendicitis and lymphadenitis have also been described.[36] Sigmoidoscopy typically discloses mucosal edema, hyperemia, granularity, and contact bleeding, as seen in ulcerative colitis, but the appearance may also be completely normal or mimic Crohn's disease. The infection is usually a mild to moderate self-limiting illness that resolves spontaneously without therapy within 1 week, but may persist for 6 weeks or longer. Hemolytic-uremic syndrome has been reported with *Campylobacter*.[37]

The rectal biopsy from patients with *Campylobacter* enterocolitis shows a nonspecific pic-

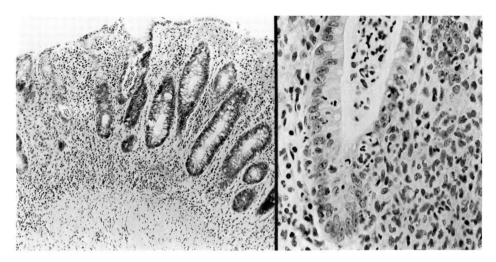

Fig. 2-3. ASLC attributable to *C. jejuni*. At low-power magnification this biopsy shows separation of crypts and failure of crypts to reach the muscularis mucosae, although their overall architecture is well preserved. Crypt abscesses are present, but limited primarily to the upper portions of crypts. The lamina propria contains only a minimal increase in lymphocytes and plasma cells. In the right panel, a crypt abscess with neutrophilic infiltration of the crypt epithelium (''cryptitis'') can be seen. An aggregate of macrophages adjacent to the lower right portion of the crypt gives the appearance of granulomatous inflammation, but without a discrete, compact granuloma.

Table 2-3. Enteric Pathogens Isolated from 4,500 Patients[a]

Organism	Number of Isolates
Campylobacter jejuni	165
Salmonellae	70
E. coli 0157:H7	25
Shigellae	23

[a] Only listed pathogens sought.
(From McDonald et al.,[27] with permission.)

Table 2-4. Enteric Pathogens Isolated from 423 Patients (Great Britain, 1983–1984)[a]

Organism	% of Positive Stools
Campylobacter jejuni	28
Rotavirus	20
Cryptosporidium	12
Salmonella	11
Adenovirus (by EM)	9
Enteropath *E. coli*	6
Giardia lamblia	6
Shigella sonnei	4
Other bacteria and viruses	5

[a] Data derived from 2,573 cultures (16 percent of total positive), mostly adult patients.
(From Casemore et al.,[28] with permission.)

ture that cannot be differentiated from other causes of infectious diarrhea; however, its appearance is usually sufficiently distinctive that one can recognize the strong possibility of an infectious agent.[32] The mucosa tends to be edematous and contains a patchy inflammatory infiltrate with focal neutrophilic infiltration of the lamina propria and crypt epithelium (Fig. 2-3). The scattered crypt abscesses tend to be located toward the surface of the mucosa and are associated with degeneration of the crypt epithelium. Aggregates of histiocytes forming microgranulomas and foci of "granulomatous" inflammation are not uncommon (Fig. 2-3) and make the appearance difficult to differentiate from Crohn's disease.

In view of the current frequency with which *Campylobacter* is being isolated from diarrheal stools, infections attributable to this organism undoubtedly went unrecognized in the past and the patient was probably considered to have "viral" gastroenteritis, or idiopathic IBD if the symptoms persisted for several weeks. Indeed, it is possible that some patients labeled as having idiopathic IBD on the basis of a single attack may well have had *Campylobacter* enterocolitis.[38] Another important point is that patients with well-documented idiopathic IBD appear to have an increased susceptibility to all the various enteric pathogens, including *Campylobacter*.[31] Infection with one of these agents in the IBD patient may provoke an acute exacerbation of the disease that will respond to appropriate antibiotic therapy.

Escherichia coli 0157:H7

As indicated in Table 2-3, *E. coli* 0157:H7 was the third most common organism isolated in a 1-year, prospective population-based study.[27] First described in 1983,[39] this organism is being recognized with increasing frequency in the United States and Canada. Enteric infection with *E. coli* 0157:H7 produces a spectrum of illness that includes asymptomatic infection, nonbloody diarrhea, bloody diarrhea, hemolytic-uremic syndrome, and thrombotic thrombocytopenic purpura.[27, 39] Bloody diarrhea was present in 95 percent and hemolytic-uremic syndrome in 12 percent of cases in one report.[40] The clinical picture differs from that of the bloody diarrhea or dysentery described in shigellosis, campylobacteriosis, and invasive *E. coli* by the lack of fever and the bloody discharge resembling lower gastrointestinal bleeding.[39] *E. coli* 1057:H7 is not invasive and produces neither a heat-labile nor a heat-stable enterotoxin. It produces a cytotoxin active against Vero cells that is known as *verotoxin*.[41]

The histologic appearance of the colon infected by *E. coli* 0157:H7 varies depending on the severity of the clinical illness. In patients with nonbloody or bloody diarrhea, the biopsy appearance ranges from normal to a mild and patchy neutrophilic infiltration of the lamina propria and crypts, whereas others show the characteristic appearance of ASLC.[41] In more severe infections that result in colonic resection or death, the colitis is characterized by marked edema, fibrin deposition, and mucosal and submucosal hemorrhage.[42] Microvascular thrombi are prominent, and pseudomembranous colitis similar to that induced by *C. difficile* may be seen.[42]

Clostridium difficile

Overgrowth of *C. difficile* with production of its toxin is well documented as the cause of most cases of antibiotic-associated diarrhea (AAD).[43, 44] Many antimicrobial agents have been implicated, but most cases are associated with clindamycin, ampicillin, and the cephalosporins.[45, 46] The reported prevalence of AAD ranges from 10 to 20 percent of patients taking antibiotics, whereas that for pseudomembranous colitis varies from 1 to 10 percent.[45–47] The type of antibiotic may influence the prevalence. More cases appear to be associated with oral, rather than parenteral, administration of the agents. Diarrhea is the most prominent clinical symptom and usually begins during the course of antibiotic therapy, but it occasionally begins later, and toxin-positive cases developing

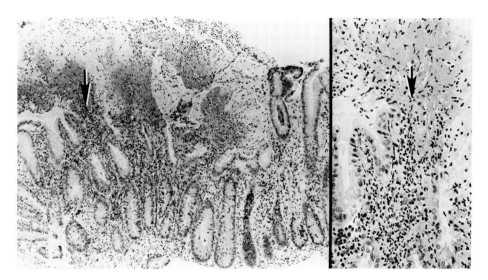

Fig. 2-4. Pseudomembranous colitis owing to *C. difficile*. An eruption of purulent exudate escapes from the lamina propria in areas of surface epithelial erosion (arrow). Well-preserved crypt architecture, generalized depletion of goblet cell mucin, and inflammation of lamina propria may be noted. The higher-power view in the right panel shows exudate escaping from the lamina propria in the region of a surface epithelial erosion (arrow).

as long as 8 weeks after a course of antibiotics are documented.[47] The endoscopic and biopsy appearance of the colonic mucosa in patients with AAD shows a spectrum of changes ranging from normal to pseudomembranous colitis (PMC), the latter representing the most severe form of AAD. The rectal biopsy may show pseudomembranes composed of mucopurulent, fibrin-rich exudate adherent to the mucosal surface but is otherwise similar to that of the other forms of ASLC (Fig. 2-4). Because PMC may spare the rectum and left colon, proctosigmoidoscopy may show only normal mucosa.[48] Price and Davies divided the histologic appearance of PMC into three patterns representing various stages in the evolution of the lesions.[49] Early lesions have only disruption of the surface epithelium with adherent plaques of exudate, whereas more advanced lesions show progressively greater degrees of necrosis and ulceration. Progression of the lesions to toxic megacolon may occur.[50]

Stool cultures and assays for *C. difficile* toxin

are positive in over 95 percent of patients with antibiotic-associated PMC and in approximately 25 percent of patients with AAD, but with no recognizable pseudomembranes.[45, 47] A significant positive correlation between the titer of toxin and the presence of pseudomembranes has been reported.[44] *C. difficile* and its toxin are not infrequently found in healthy neonates who have never received antibiotics, indicating that these individuals are not susceptible to the effects of the organism.[47]

Assay for the toxin is the preferred method for establishing the diagnosis of *C. difficile*, because the techniques for culturing the organism are difficult.[45] In addition, the presence of toxin correlates best with symptomatic disease.

Several studies implicate *C. difficile* as a cause of relapses of idiopathic IBD, primarily in patients taking antibiotics, but also in those not receiving these drugs.[51–53] Other studies have failed to confirm this association, a fact that may be explained by epidemiologic factors, since there is good evidence that *C. difficile* may be acquired as a nosocomial infection.[54–56] Colitis attributable to *C. difficile* in the absence of antibiotic therapy has also been reported in patients who are immunosuppressed[57] as well as in otherwise healthy adults.[58, 59]

Yersinia

The gram-negative rods *Y. enterocolitica* and *Y. pseudotuberculosis* belong to the family Enterobacteriaceae and resemble non-lactose-fermenting *E. coli.* Both organisms are human pathogens responsible for a variety of clinical syndromes that are most often seen in children and infants. Affected infants tend to have an acute gastroenteritis, with fever, vomiting, and diarrhea, whereas older children and adults usually have an appendicitis-like syndrome with fever, abdominal pain, and diarrhea. Laparotomy, done because of the clinical impression of appendicitis, discloses mesenteric adenitis and terminal ileitis with variable involvement of the appendix and colon. Less common manifestations of yersinosis include a typhoid-like septicemic illness,[60] or erythema nodosum and arthritis that may suggest a rheumatic disease.[61] Epidemiologic investigations indicate that many infections are self-limited and produce such a mild disease that they go unrecognized.[62] Cases of yersinosis have been documented most frequently in Scandinavia and Western Europe.[62] In Belgium, Canada, Australia, and the Netherlands, *Y. enterocolitica* causes acute gastroenteritis almost as frequently as *Salmonella* and *Campylobacter.*[63] The incidence in the United States appears to be increasing, probably because of increased recognition of the disease.[64] Animals, both wild and domestic, are reservoirs of the organism, and the infection is usually acquired via the oral route.[65] An outbreak related to household preparation of chitterlings has been reported.[66] The organisms can be cultured from the stool and affected tissues, but false-negative cultures are not infrequent. Serum antibody titers can also establish the diagnosis, but are not generally available except for epidemiologic and research studies. Serotyping permits subdivision of both species into a number of groups.[62, 65, 67]

Most of the pathologic descriptions of yersinosis are based on material derived from surgically resected specimens or autopsies rather than from biopsies.[65, 67] The affected bowel may show congestion, edema, massively enlarged lymphoid follicles, and mucosal ulceration. The enlarged mesenteric lymph nodes may be matted; sectioning them reveals yellowish microabscesses. Microscopically, the characteristic picture in *Y. enterocolitica* infections is a necrotizing process, with microabscesses involving the lymphoid tissues of the bowel wall and mesenteric lymph nodes. Mononuclear phagocytes are prominent components of the inflammatory infiltrate, particularly around the edges of the microabscesses, but discrete granulomas are not found in the usual case.[62, 67] Involvement of individual lymphoid follicles in the colon may produce aphthoid lesions indistinguishable from those seen in Crohn's disease (Fig. 2-5).[62] The microscopic appearance of *Y. pseudotuberculosis* infections may be similar to that seen with *Y. enterocolitica*[68]; however, granulomatous inflammation was identified in the majority of cases reported by El-Maraghi and colleagues.[65] Epithelioid granulomas with central necrosis and/or microabscesses occur in the mesenteric lymph nodes, terminal ileum, and appendix. Most of the intestinal granulomas are in the mucosa and submucosa, but they also may occur in the serosa, and may be accompanied by diffuse lymphoid hyperplasia and histiocytic proliferation.[65]

Other Bacterial Infections

The preceding discussion reviews some of the newer developments in colitis attributable to bacterial infections. In addition to the organisms described therein, *Salmonella*, *Shigella*, *Treponema pallidum*, *Neisserra gonorrhea*, *E. coli* and *Edwardsiella tarda* also may cause an infectious diarrhea that produces a nonspecific histologic picture.[69–75] Biopsies from *Salmonella* colitis may show microgranulomas[69, 71]

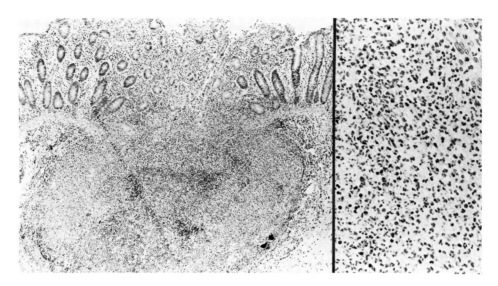

Fig. 2-5. Colonic involvement by *Y. enterocolitica*. Section from an apthoid lesion. The mucosa overlying the prominent lymphoid shows a fissure that extends into the follicle. The center of the follicle has been converted into a microabscess filled with neutrophilic exudate (right panel).

but these are not distinctive enough to permit a specific diagnosis. The biopsy appearance produced by all of these agents, although nonspecific, often has features that suggest an infectious agent (Table 2-2).

Several studies document a high incidence of infectious proctitis in homosexual males.[20, 76] The agents isolated include the gonococcus, herpes simplex virus, *T. pallidum*, *Giardia lamblia*, *Entamoeba histolytica*, *C. trachomatis*, and *Campylobacter*.[20, 76] The light microscopic appearance of the proctitis produced by these organisms does not permit a specific diagnosis. Although all of the above organisms may also produce infection in patients with AIDS, a different spectrum of pathogens predominates in this group, as is shown below.

Tuberculosis is not currently an important cause of infectious diarrhea in the United States. One can differentiate tuberculosis from Crohn's disease by noting the much larger and more numerous granulomas in tuberculosis. In addition, caseation necrosis is prominent in tuberculosis granulomas, and one can identify the organism with appropriate stains.[77]

FUNGAL INFECTIONS

Primary fungal infections of the gastrointestinal tract caused by organisms that elicit a granulomatous inflammatory response mimicking idiopathic IBD are rare. Secondary gastrointestinal involvement in patients with disseminated fungal infections is more common; most such cases seen in the United States are due to histoplasmosis. Primary and secondary gastrointestinal infections caused by opportunistic fungi that do not characteristically incite a granulomatous host reaction are quite common in immunosuppressed patients, but because of the clinical context they are not usually confused with idiopathic IBD.

The two principal fungi that produce disease that can be mistaken for idiopathic IBD are paracoccidioidomycosis (South American blastomycosis) and histoplasmosis. The former is a chronic myosis caused by the dimorphic fungus *Paracoccidioides brasiliensis*.[78] Paracoccidioidomycosis, an important public health problem in Brazil, is also seen in most South American countries, but does not extend beyond

Central America and Mexico; thus, the only cases seen in the United States are imported cases. The organism is thought to spread to the intestine through deposition in the submucosal lymphoid tissue with subsequent erosion into the mucosa and lumen.[78] Although skin and serologic tests are available, microscopic demonstration of the fungus in pus from the primary lesion is the most useful diagnostic test. Histologically, the typical picture consists of a granulomatous reaction combined with pyogenic inflammation. In lesions without secondary infection, epithelioid granulomas like those of sarcoid may be seen. A case has been reported in which the clinical presentation mimicked ulcerative colitis, and biopsy showed a diffuse infiltrate of inflammatory cells and organisms in the mucosa.[79] The organism is a yeast that varies in size from 5 to 15 μm, and can often be found in giant cells. The differential diagnosis is relatively limited because so few fungi with granulomatous inflammation produce intestinal disease. Histoplasma organisms are smaller, North American blastomycosis does not involve the gut, and cryptococci have a mucicarminophilic capsule.

Histoplasma capsulatum also produces intestinal disease that can be mistaken for idiopathic IBD.[78] The infection usually originates in the respiratory tract and is often asymptomatic, but may produce a benign acute or chronic pulmonary disease that can disseminate widely. Disseminated disease affects the small bowel and colon in as many as one third of the cases.[80] The histologic appearance of the lesion depends to a certain extent on whether the sections studied are from fatal disseminated disease or from the localized, nonfatal form.[81, 82] In the former, there is marked proliferation of macrophages whose cytoplasm contains the organism, whereas in the localized form a granulomatous inflammatory reaction resembling tuberculosis occurs. The diagnosis is established by recognizing the organism in the tissues or by culture. It is a small yeast averaging 3 μm in diameter in which a single nucleus may be identifiable. We have encountered several cases of disseminated histoplasmosis involving the gastrointestinal tract in AIDS patients.

PARASITIC INFECTIONS

Amebiasis

The clinical and sigmoidoscopic picture produced by amebiasis may be confused with ulcerative colitis or Crohn's disease; thus, some effort must be made to exclude amebiasis during the initial diagnostic evaluation of all patients with colitis.[83] Long duration of the colitis does not exclude amebiasis because it may persist for years.[83] I have seen one patient with amebiasis of 17 years' duration.

Prathap and Gilman recognized five different morphologic patterns in rectal biopsies from patients with acute amebiasis: nonspecific lesions, mucopenic depression with microulceration, early invasive lesion with superficial ulceration, late invasion lesion with deep ulceration, and granulating ulcer.[84] The appearance of the nonspecific lesion does not suggest the diagnosis of amebiasis.[85] The mucopenic depression results from a combination of erosion, with thinning of the mucosa at the depression, and hyperplasia of the adjacent crypts (Fig. 2-6). Goblet cell mucin is depleted in the crypts under the depression, but is normal or even increased in the adjacent mucosa. Within the exudate adherent to the mucosal depressions, organisms diagnostic of *E. histolytica* can usually be identified (Fig. 2-6). The amoebae are large cells that measure 15 to 30 μm in diameter and contain nuclei that are small in relation to the cytoplasmic volume. The nuclei are round and contain chromatin arranged as a rim about the nuclear membrane and as a central dot. The cytoplasm contains phagocytized red cells and stains pale gray-blue with H&E, but is intensely fuchsinophilic with periodic acid-Schiff (PAS) staining. Some sections may show a rare organism within the most superficial part of the lamina propria, but unless ulcers are present, they are usually seen only in the adherent exudate and not in the tissue. Rectal biopsy is not a sensitive method for establishing the diagnosis of amebiasis because the organism may not be identified in as many as 50 to 60 percent of proven cases.[86, 87] Gilman and colleagues increased the diagnostic yield of biopsies to 84 and 74 percent,

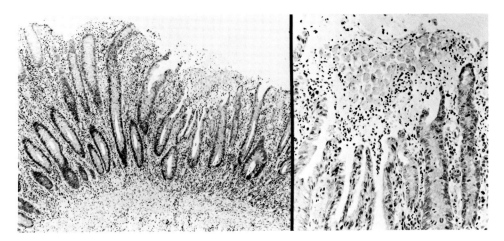

Fig. 2-6. Amoebic colitis with mucopenic depression. The depression, seen in the right portion of the left panel, is due to a combination of erosion of the mucosa to the right and elongation of the adjacent crypts to the left. Well-preserved crypt architecture and minimal inflammation of the lamina propria may be noted. The higher-power view in the right panel shows erosion of the surface epithelium with overlying exudate. The organisms within the exudate average approximately 30 μm in diameter. The depletion of goblet cell mucin and mild inflammation of the lamina propria are seen in this panel.

respectively, by performing immunofluorescence and PAS stains on alcohol-fixed specimens.[86] Formalin fixation was less satisfactory because of background fluorescence and apparent dissolution of glycogen, resulting in some loss of PAS positivity. The diagnostic method of choice for amebiasis is the examination of fresh aspirated exudate and fresh, warm stool specimens for hemophagocytic motile trophozoites.[86] This must be done prior to cleansing enemas, barium enemas, or therapy, because these procedures markedly diminish the positive yield.[83] Because the diagnosis of amebiasis is often not considered by the clinician, probably because of its relatively low incidence in most areas of the country, preparations of exudate and stool are not often made, and the biopsy may be the only means of establishing the diagnosis. For this reason, all biopsies that contain exudate adherent to the mucosal surface should be searched for amoebae. In the absence of morphologic confirmation the diagnosis can be established by serologic testing.[88]

As with the bacterial infections mentioned above, the male homosexual population in this country has been shown to have a high incidence of amebiasis, and the practicing pathologist is likely to encounter an occasional case in biopsy material.[89] Nonpathogenic strains of *E. histolytica* may be commonly encountered as commensal organisms in homosexuals.[90]

The pathogenetic mechanism by which amoebae produce colitis has yet to be elucidated.[91] Because definite evidence of tissue injury occurs in the absence of recognizable tissue invasion, it has been postulated that the organisms elaborate a toxic substance.[85, 91] This putative substance damages the mucosa, and tissue invasion then occurs.

Cryptosporidium

Cryptosporidia are protozoan parasites currently classified within the subphylum Sporozoa and the subclass Coccidia.[92] Although a large number of different species of Coccidia produce disease in animals, most are highly specific to the host and are not involved in human infection. Only *Isospora belli*, *I. natalensis*, and *Cryptosporidium* have been implicated in human dis-

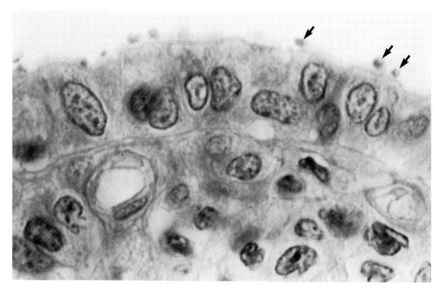

Fig. 2-7. Cryptosporidiosis. The organism can be seen as a small grey sphere attached to the striate border of the surface epithelial cells (arrows).

ease. All are common causes of diarrhea in AIDS patients, but *Cryptosporidium* is highly prevalent in immunocompetent individuals and has been implicated as a cause of traveler's diarrhea.[93–95] The small bowel is the most prominent site of involvement in cryptosporidiosis, but patients with colonic disease resembling Crohn's disease have been described.[96, 97] The mucosa shows a nonspecific inflammatory process with ulceration, depletion of goblet cell mucin, and neutrophilic infiltration of the crypt epithelium. The biopsy diagnosis is made by finding the organism attached to the striate border of surface epithelial cells (Fig. 2-7). Cryptosporidia are approximately 2 μm in diameter, oval, basophilic, and gram negative. Careful electron microscopic studies in guinea pigs have shown that the organism becomes internalized in absorptive cells.[98] *I. belli* also has an intracytoplasmic life cycle. The source of human infections with cryptosporidia has not been established. Since the organisms are common in animals, transmission from them is a possibility, but remains unproven.

Schistosoma

Schistosomiasis is an infestation by trematodes or flukes of the genus *Schistosoma*. The disease probably affects 200 million people worldwide, making it second only to malaria as a cause of serious morbidity and mortality on a global basis.[99] The practicing pathologist in the United States rarely sees schistosomiasis. Three species of *Schistosoma* cause most human infestations: *S. mansoni*, *S. japonicum*, and *S. hematobium*. Humans become infected by schistosomes when the cercarial stage of the organism emerges from a freshwater snail and penetrates the skin. The organisms migrate to the lungs, and then to the liver, where they mature into adult worms within the portal venous system. *S. mansoni* and *S. japonicum* inhabit veins of the mesenteric circulation, whereas *S. hematobium* prefers the vesicle plexus.[99] Adult worms do not cause clinical disease but produce myriads of ova that migrate through venous walls into the tissues of the bowel and then into the lumen. They are then passed with the feces to reinitiate the life cycle.[100] The ova, in their course through the tissues, elicit a cell-mediated immune response of the delayed hypersensitivity type.[101] The granulomas thus produced secrete a fibroblast-stimulating factor that may cause extensive fibrosis.[102] The gross lesions of schistosomiasis include single or multiple intestinal polyps, most often in the rectum and left colon, that may resemble familial polyposis. In other cases, ulceration of the mucosa and thickening of the bowel wall produce a picture similar to Crohn's disease.[103] The lesions may also be mistaken for carcinomas. Microscopically there may be a diffuse cellular infiltrate or circumoval granulomas. The diffuse infiltrate, which presumably occurs early in the eggs' migration, includes numerous eosinophils and neutrophils. The appearance of the granulomas varies with their age: early ones have a zone of epithelioid macrophages surrounding the ovum, often with an associated intense eosinophilia. As the granuloma matures, fibrous tissue accumulates about the periphery and forms concentric rings around late granulomas. Dense hyalin connective tissue that may produce a fibrous stricture develops about affected ova. The diagnosis is established by identifying the ova within granulomas in tissue sections, or by rectal biopsy crush preparations.[104]

Anisakidae

Anisakiasis is an infestation of humans caused by larval nematodes of the family Anisakidae. The adult worm is an ascarid usually found in marine mammals. The life cycle involves three larval stages, the third of which resides in the somatic muscles of certain saltwater fish such as cod, herring, and salmon. When a person eats inadequately prepared fish that contain larvae, they attach to the mucosa of the stomach, small bowel, or colon, causing local ulceration; penetration and perforation of the wall may ensue. The stomach is most frequently involved, the small bowel less commonly, and the colon least commonly.[105, 106]

Grossly, the affected bowel is edematous and diffusely thickened so that it resembles Crohn's disease.[107] Acute lesions contain an inflammatory infiltrate with numerous neutrophils and eosinophils, whereas more advanced lesions have granulomas with central eosinophilic necrosis, a peripheral zone of macrophages, and occasional multinucleated giant cells.[107, 108] The granulomas probably represent a hypersensitivity phenomenon and resemble those of allergic granulomatosis. Identification of fragments of the larval nematode in the lesions establishes the diagnosis; however, in the later stages the parasite may be destroyed, leaving only remnants of granulomatous inflammation. When the parasite cannot be identified, the diagnosis depends on the clinical history of symptoms following consumption of raw or undercooked fish.

Although most cases of anisakiasis have been reported from Japan and Scandinavia, the disease has been seen in the United States.[107, 108] Infected fish are commonly marketed in this country; anisakine larvae were found in fish obtained from the market where the patient reported by Valdiserri did her shopping,[108] and were found in all samples of marketed salmon examined in Michigan by Rosset and colleagues.[109]

COLITIS ASSOCIATED WITH MOTOR DISORDERS

DIVERTICULITIS

Estimates suggest that nearly 50 percent of the aged in the United States will develop colonic diverticula.[110] Since ulcerative colitis and Crohn's disease are not uncommon conditions, one would expect them occasionally to coexist with diverticular disease. This combination has been documented in Crohn's disease,[111, 112] but the coexistence of ulcerative colitis and diverticulitis is very rare.[113] Perhaps the pathophysiologic mechanisms in ulcerative colitis preclude the development of diverticular disease. Several problems arise in the clinical differential diagno-

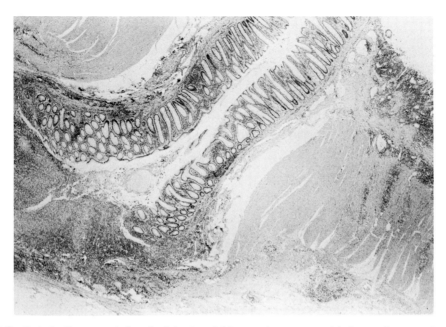

Fig. 2-8. Crohn's disease and diverticulitis. In addition to the extramural inflammation associated with the erosion at the base of the diverticulum, the mucosa and muscularis propria adjacent to the diverticulum are also inflamed. This serves to identify the process as Crohn's disease rather than uncomplicated diverticulitis.

sis of diverticulitis and Crohn's disease. First, some patients with documented diverticulosis present with an apparent episode of diverticulitis that subsequently proves to be Crohn's disease. Second, in some patients the diagnosis of diverticulitis is made, but the patient is subsequently shown to have Crohn's disease and no evidence of diverticulosis.[112] This is an important distinction, because individuals with diverticulitis have a much better postoperative course than do those with Crohn's disease. Finally, individuals with diverticulosis appear to have an increased incidence of diverticulitis and its complications when they also have Crohn's disease.[111] Clinically, the patient with coexisting Crohn's disease and diverticulitis is likely to have diarrhea, rectal bleeding, anal lesions, and an abnormal sigmoidoscopic appearance. In contrast, patients with diverticulitis without Crohn's disease more often have abdominal pain and constipation.[112] Pathologically, if the noncaseating granulomas of Crohn's disease are present, they resolve the diagnostic problem. Since foreign body granulomas attributable to injection of fecal material through ulcerated mucosa are frequently present, the pathologist must be careful not to mistake them for the sarcoid-like granulomas of Crohn's disease. The inflammation in diverticulitis is typically extramural, that is, related to ulceration and perforation of diverticula with pericolonic inflammation and/or abscess formation. The mucosa between diverticula is usually normal, whereas in Crohn's disease the inflammatory process may involve the mucosa between diverticula (Fig. 2-8). The narrow, deeply penetrating ulcers (fissures) characteristic of Crohn's disease do not occur in diverticulitis; however, the potential for confusion occurs when the entire mucosal lining of a diverticulum becomes ulcerated, leaving a structure that resembles a fissure but that is much broader. Long paracolic fistulous tracts, once thought to be characteristic of Crohn's disease, may also be seen in diverticulitis regardless of whether it is complicated by Crohn's disease.[114, 115]

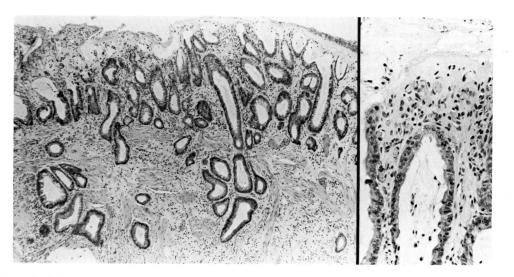

Fig. 2-9. Solitary rectal ulcer syndrome. Erosion of the surface epithelium and marked distortion of the crypt architecture with portions of crypts extending below the muscularis mucosae may be noted. There is marked disarray of the muscularis mucosae, and bundles of smooth muscle surround individual crypts in the lower portion of the illustration. At higher-power magnification in the right panel, erosion of the surface epithelium and replacement of the lamina propria by granulation tissue and a mild chronic inflammatory infiltrate may be noted. The crypt epithelium shows depletion of goblet cell mucin and hyperplasia that can occasionally be mistaken for an adenoma.

SOLITARY RECTAL ULCER SYNDROME

The solitary rectal ulcer syndrome has become recognized as a distinct clinical entity with a characteristic, but nonspecific, histologic appearance.[116–118] The term is a misnomer because the lesions may be multiple, they may involve the sigmoid as well as the rectum (personal observations), they are usually erosions rather than ulcers, and they are preceded by a pre-erosive or preulcerative phase.[118] The condition is caused by prolapse of the rectal mucosa, which is secondary to a motor disorder affecting the puborectalis and external sphincter muscles.[116, 119, 120] The syndrome is more common in younger people, as the mean age is about 35 years; it is slightly more common in women, with a female:male ratio of 1.35 in one study.[116] The most common clinical symptoms are the passage of fresh blood and mucus with the stool, alteration in bowel habit, tenesmus, a persistent feeling of anal obstruction, and anorectal pain that is usually slight but may be disabling.[116, 117] About half of the patients complain of irregular bowel habits, with either constipation or diarrhea. Difficult defecation requiring considerable straining is frequently present and may reflect the underlying motor disorder documented in some patients. At proctoscopy, erosions or ulcers ranging up to 3 cm in diameter are present in about two-thirds of patients, while the remainder have polyps, sessile plaques, or hyperemia alone. When palpated on digital rectal exam, the lesion is often mistaken for a neoplasm, and the endoscopist not infrequently suspects a neoplasm or Crohn's disease. A large majority of the lesions are located on the anterior rectal wall; about one-third of patients have more than one lesion.[116]

Histologically there is gross distortion of the crypt architecture and erosion of the surface epithelium with adherent exudate producing a "pseudomembrane." Granulation tissue obliterates the upper lamina propria, whereas the lower portion is replaced by fibroblasts and smooth muscle cells (Fig. 2-9). There may be diffuse fibrosis of the lamina propria.[121] The muscularis mucosae is markedly hypertrophic and disorganized, and bundles of smooth muscle extend high into the lamina propria around crypts. In a minority of cases, glands are displaced into the submucosa, where they may become cystically dilated to produce so-called colitis cystica profunda. The epithelium may appear quite hyperplastic, a finding that has led to the erroneous interpretation of some cases as adenomas or, when submucosal cysts are present, as invasive carcinoma. Careful inspection of the epithelium reveals that the cytologic features of neoplasia, including crowded, stratified, elongated nuclei, and diminished mucin production are either not present or not well-developed, and the submucosal component lacks the desmoplastic reaction that almost universally accompanies invasive carcinoma of the rectum.[122] I have seen one convincing example of an adenocarcinoma arising within the displaced epithelium in solitary rectal ulcer syndrome, but this was probably a coincidence.

Although the etiology of solitary rectal ulcer syndrome is not completely established, about 85 to 95 percent of the patients have a demonstrable rectal prolapse that is often internal and occult, so that the patient may be unaware of it.[116, 119, 120] The endoscopist likewise may not recognize the prolapse unless the patient is asked to perform a Valsalva maneuver as the mucosa is examined proctoscopically or unless defecatory radiographic studies are obtained. Electromyographic studies, proctography, and manometry show that most of the patients have faulty motility of the puborectalis and/or external sphincter muscles, causing them to contract when they should relax.[118, 120] This raises voiding pressure and causes the patient to have to strain to defecate, with internal prolapse as the ultimate result.[120] Additional support for prolapse as the underlying problem comes from the fact that the entire spectrum of histologic changes seen in solitary rectal ulcer syndrome is duplicated in cases of overt rectal prolapse and in prolapsed hemorrhoids and ileostomy stomas. The mechanism by which prolapse results in the changes of solitary rectal ulcer syndrome is unclear, but trauma to the mucosa and ischemia from stretching of the vessels are probably important factors. Some investigators

postulate that the submucosal displacement of glands (colitis cystica profunda) found in 10 to 15 percent of patients with the syndrome is caused by re-epithelialization of deep ulcers or abscesses that communicate with the mucosa.[123] An alternative mechanism, suggested by the presence of submucosal cysts underlying intact mucosa and muscularis mucosae, is that pressure generated by the hypertrophic muscularis mucosae forces glands to herniate into the submucosa. Patients with solitary rectal ulcer syndrome have a localized form of colitis cystica profunda that must be differentiated from the diffuse form that may complicate ulcerative colitis or Crohn's disease, and that involves longer segments of the colon.[123, 124]

Patients with a histologic picture similar to that of solitary rectal ulcer syndrome, but affecting mucosa of the transitional zone of the anus, have been described; some of these patients have had characteristic clinical features of the solitary rectal ulcer syndrome.[125, 126] Whether these patients develop their lesion through the same pathologic mechanism as solitary rectal ulcer syndrome has not been established. Lesions that resemble solitary rectal ulcer, but which are located in the anal canal, must be interpreted with caution, as hemorrhoids and the anal lesions of Crohn's disease may also be associated with such changes.[126]

COLITIS SECONDARY TO A VASCULAR HYPOPERFUSION

Ischemia

Ischemic colitis is covered in Chapter 5 and is not discussed here.

Colitis Complicating Colonic Obstruction

Patients with obstructing lesions of the colon from any cause may develop a colitis, usually proximal to the obstruction, but occasionally distal as well.[127, 128] This is now recognized as ischemic in origin and is thought to be due to one or a combination of factors, including decreased colonic blood flow from increased intraluminal pressure, decreased perfusion secondary to hyperperistalsis, and muscular spasm in the colon. The most common obstructing lesion producing the colitis is carcinoma. Ten percent of all cases with ischemic colitis in the series of Boley were caused by obstructing carcinomas, whereas another 10 percent were due to other obstructing lesions, including diverticulitis, volvulus, Hirschsprung's disease, fecal impaction, and so on.[127] As noted previously, the ischemic damage may occur below the obstructing lesion as well as above it, and there may be a short segment of normal colon between the obstructing lesion and the proximal ischemic colitis.

Because the appearance of ischemic colitis complicating obstructing lesions is identical in every respect to the other types of ischemic colitis, the reader is referred to Chapter 5, Reexamination of the Spectrum of Ischemic Bowel Disease, for a discussion of its appearance.

COLITIS INDUCED BY THERAPEUTIC INTERVENTION

Effects of Enemas and Laxatives

The various agents used to prepare the colon for endoscopic examination may induce changes in the mucosa that can be mistaken for mild colitis. The administration of hypertonic phosphate enemas (Fleets Phospho-Soda) may induce vacuolization of the surface epithelial cells, with detachment of the surface epithelium from the basal lamina, subepithelial infiltration by a few neutrophils, and edema of the lamina propria.[129, 130] Bisacodyl (Dulcolax) may induce more severe changes, with pale, vacuolated surface and crypt epithelium extending deep into the mucosa and neutrophilic infiltration of the epithelium and lamina propria[129, 131] (Fig. 2-10). Clinically, both agents produce proctoscopic abnormalities that can be mistaken for mild colitis, including obliteration of the vascular pattern by mucosal hyperemia and mucosal

friability. Inflammation induced by bisacodyl can resemble mild idiopathic ulcerative proctitis.[129] Prolonged consumption of bisacodyl has been associated with marked abnormalities of the colon referred to as the *cathartic colon syndrome*.[132] Characteristic findings include marked shortening of the colon, atrophic mucosa, fibrosis and inflammation of the muscularis mucosae, and marked fatty infiltration of the submucosa.[132, 133] Other laxatives implicated in the cathartic colon syndrome include anthraquinone purgatives (senna), phenolphthalein, castor oil, and others. The anthraquinone group of purgatives produces damage and loss of the intrinsic innervation, atrophy of the muscularis propria, and melanosis coli. Changes in the myenteric plexus include loss of neurons and replacement of the ganglia by Schwann cells; this may require silver stains for detection.[133]

Other agents that may cause colitis include the water-soluble contrast media used in radiography.[134] Gastrografin has been shown experimentally to produce a severe colitis, probably due to its content of the wetting agent Tween-80.[134] The administration of soap may also induce a severe colitis with mucosal edema; the histologic appearance of this lesion is not well described.[135] Hydrogen peroxide administered as an enema has been implicated as a cause of colitis that resembled ischemic colitis.[136] A more likely possibility is that the hydrogen peroxide injury actually caused ischemia. Hydrogen peroxide used as a cleaning agent for colonoscopes can cause a distinctive lesion referred to as *pseudolipomatosis*, in which gas bubbles are present in the lamina propria, presumably owing to release of nascent oxygen by the peroxide.[137–140]

Drug-Induced Colitis

Therapeutic agents may cause colitis. Most of these produce a nonspecific histologic picture that could be confused with either ulcerative colitis or Crohn's disease, depending on the distribution of the lesions and the clinical presentation. For example, methyldopa, isoretinoin,

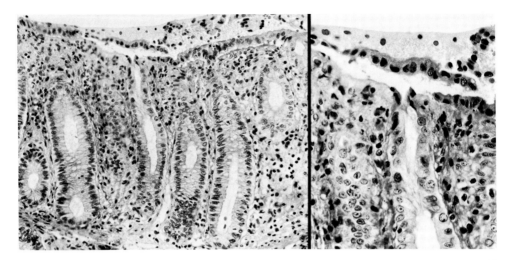

Fig. 2-10. Laxative effect owing to bisacodyl. The goblet cell mucin is depleted and the surface epithelium focally detached. Neutrophils are focally present within the crypt epithelium and upper lamina propria. At higher-power magnification in the right panel, abnormal surface epithelium, which has assumed a cuboidal rather than columnar appearance, and which has marked irregularity of the nuclei is seen. These changes should not be mistaken for mild colitis.

and nonsteroidal anti-inflammatory drugs have been documented as causes of acute colitis in small numbers of patients.[141–144] Insufficient information has been published to determine how closely the colitis induced by these agents mimics ulcerative colitis or Crohn's disease.

Enterocolitis may rarely complicate gold salt therapy for rheumatoid arthritis.[145, 146] The non-specific histologic picture consists principally of an inflammatory infiltrate in the lamina propria. Interestingly, tissue eosinophilia appears to be a prominent component of the inflammatory infiltrate in these cases.

An acute hemorrhagic right-sided colitis has been attributed to penicillin and ampicillin; this differs from the antibiotic-associated colitis attributable to *C. difficile*.[147, 148] The patients described have developed the acute onset of bloody diarrhea 2 to 7 days following the onset of therapy. The histologic appearance has not been described well enough to determine its resemblance to idiopathic IBD. The condition resolves spontaneously following cessation of antibiotic therapy. A hypersensitivity mechanism producing ischemia of the colonic mucosa has been

postulated as the mechanism responsible for the colitis.[147]

Perhaps the most severe colitis induced by drugs is that seen in patients given chemotherapeutic agents for the treatment of malignant tumors. Although a number of different drugs have been implicated,[149] the best documented is 5-fluorouracil.[150, 151] The lesions usually develop between 4 and 9 days after the beginning of therapy. The earliest recognizable change affects the crypt bases, where the nuclei undergo pyknosis, loss of polarity, and karyorrhexis.[151] The lesions may progress to necrosis of the upper part of the mucosa, with inflammation in the crypt epithelium and lamina propria. During the resolving phase the crypt epithelium may become hyperplastic, or there may be cystic dilatation of crypts that are lined by bizarre epithelial cells (Fig. 2-11). Since there is destruction of crypts, the architecture of the mucosa following regeneration may be abnormal and resemble healed ulcerative colitis.[151]

A comprehensive review of drugs that have been implicated as causes of colitis has appeared.[149]

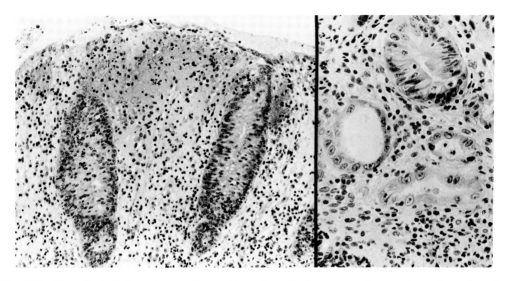

Fig. 2-11. The effect of chemotherapeutic agents on the colonic mucosa. Decreased numbers of crypts, edema of the lamina propria, acute and chronic inflammation, and marked hyperplasia of the crypt epithelium are seen. Temporal data indicated a relationship to COPP therapy for Hodgkin's disease. All other etiologies of colitis were excluded; the patient spontaneously recovered following chemotherapy. The right panel shows another area from the same biopsy. Marked distortion of the crypts, the focal flattening of the crypt epithelial cells, and the marked nuclear atypism may be noted. These changes are not diagnostic of chemotherapeutic effect and may also be seen in radiation colitis, graft-versus-host disease, and occasionally in infectious or ischemic colitis.

COLITIS ATTRIBUTABLE TO THERAPEUTIC RADIATION

The colon is the most frequently injured site in the gastrointestinal tract during and following radiation therapy to the abdomen and pelvis.[152] Since the most frequent indication for radiation to these sites is carcinoma of the uterine cervix or corpus, radiation damage to the colon predominantly affects women, who accounted for 95 percent of cases of radiation injury in the gastrointestinal tract in one study.[153] Radiation injuries can be divided into acute effects, beginning during the course of radiation therapy, and delayed effects, beginning from several weeks to 30 years following therapy.[154] Most chronic injuries develop within 1 year. Depending on the total dose of radiation delivered,[154] about 10 to 12 percent of patients develop gastrointestinal complications.[153] Acute injury may occur with doses as small as 150 rads, but clinically significant complications do not become frequent until the dose reaches 4,500 rads or above. At doses of 5,000 to 6,000 rads, 25 to 50 percent of patients have some clinically significant lesion.[154]

The effects of acute radiation injury to the rectal mucosa have been well studied.[155, 156] During the course of radiation therapy, three-fourths of patients develop clinical symptoms, usually by the middle of the second week. These symptoms include diarrhea, mucoid rectal discharge, tenesmus, abdominal distention, and cramping abdominal pain. About half of patients will have sigmoidoscopic abnormalities, including moderate edema, duskiness of the mucosa, and loss of vascular pattern. Experimental data show that histologic abnormalities occur within hours of radiation.[154] The earliest recognizable lesions include nuclear pyknosis and karyorrhexis, conversion of cells from a columnar to a cuboidal shape, loss of nuclear polarity, en-

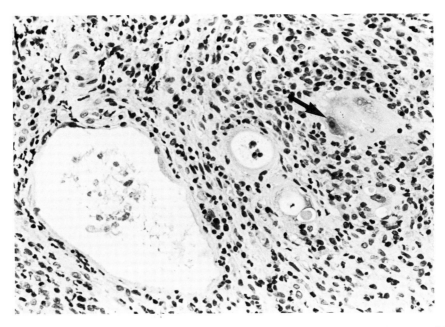

Fig. 2-12. Acute radiation proctitis. Marked dilatation of the crypt at left may be noted. The crypt epithelium is markedly attenuated, apparently in an effort to cover the basement membrane. Marked atypism of the nucleus in one of the residual epithelial cells that no longer forms part of a recognizable crypt (arrow) can be seen.

largement of nuclei, decreased numbers of mitoses, and diminished mucin content.[155] The decrease in mitotic activity indicates defective cellular replication, so that as cells are lost from the mucosal surface, they are not replaced by cells migrating up from the base of the crypt. This results in denudation of the surface and upper crypt, with a flattening-out of remaining crypt epithelial cells in an apparent effort to cover the basement membrane of the crypt (Fig. 2-12). With higher doses, superficial erosions occur. Inflammation of the lamina propria with prominent eosinophilia and eosinophilic crypt abscesses is characteristic but not diagnostic.[155] Marked cellular atypia may occur after doses as small as 150 rads but is usually not seen until the cumulative dose reaches 1,000 to 2,500 rads.[156] Complete reversal of the acute changes requires from 4 to 8 weeks.[155, 156]

Novak and colleagues described a radiation-associated pancolitis, which clinically simulated ulcerative colitis, in two patients who had not received radiation to the entire colon.[152] The etiology of this unusual complication is not clear.

The delayed effects of radiation may begin a few weeks to months following radiation therapy, or they may not become apparent until as long as 30 years postradiation.[152] Symptoms include diarrhea, which is often bloody, and cramping abdominal pain accompanied by nausea and vomiting. In decreasing order of frequency, the lesions produced by abdominal and pelvic radiation in the series of DeCosse and co-workers included proctitis, rectal ulcer, rectal stricture, rectovaginal fistula, colitis, and enteritis.[153] Thus, the rectum is the most frequently involved site of chronic complications following radiation therapy. Factors that increase the incidence of radiation injury to the colon and rectum include previous abdominal surgery,[157] hypertension, diabetes, and cardiovascular disease.[153] Histologically, in the chronic phase mesenchymal changes dominate the picture (Fig. 2-13).[158, 159] The most characteristic and consistent lesions include hyalinization of connective tissue, especially in the submucosal and subserosal regions; atypical fibroblasts; telangiectasis; and intimal fibrosis and hyaline degeneration of vessel walls.[159, 160] Other changes include swelling of endothelial cells, phlebosclerosis, and atrophy of fibers of the muscularis propria with interstitial fibrosis (Fig. 2-14). To what extent these changes represent the effects of ischemia from damaged vessels, rather than primary radiation damage to the connective tissues of the bowel wall, is enigmatic. Haselton and colleagues believe that the blood vessels are the main site of injury and that the endothelial cell is the initial target for radiation damage.[160] The accumulation of foam cells in the subendothelial region of vessels is highly characteristic of radiation injury,[161] but not diagnostic.[158] Vaso-occlusive lesions developing secondary to radiation cause ischemic ulcers and strictures that exactly mimic those seen in patients with arteriosclerotic occlusive disease who have not been exposed to radiation. The effects of radiation injury are progressive with time and represent an ongoing process.[160]

Women who have been irradiated for gynecologic malignancies have a relative risk for subsequent colorectal cancer that is 2.0 to 3.6 times normal.[162] Such women are therefore appropriate candidates for careful surveillance for colorectal cancer.

COLITIS IN GRAFT-VERSUS-HOST-DISEASE

Recipients of allogeneic bone marrow transplantation as part of their treatment for leukemia, lymphoma, or aplastic anemia are prone to develop a syndrome known as graft-versus-host disease (GVHD) that comprises skin rash, hepatocellular dysfunction, and diarrhea.[163, 164, 165, 166] The graft-versus-host reaction affects the ileal and colonic mucosa and can be difficult to recognize because of other complications of bone marrow transplantation,

such as the effects of chemotherapy, total-body irradiation, and infections resulting from the immunosuppressed state. The earliest changes of GVHD in the rectal mucosa can be recognized only after the effects of the conditioning dose of chemotherapy and radiation have resolved. This requires about 20 days, after which GVHD can be identified by the presence of crypt cell degeneration.[163] This occurs focally near the base of the crypt as a vacuole containing karyolytic debris (''apoptotic'' body). Progression to the formation of crypt abscesses with ultimate destruction of crypts may leave mucosa with long stretches devoid of crypts. If ulceration occurs, superimposed infection complicates the histologic picture.

The major concern in diagnosing GVHD is to rule out the effects of chemotherapy, total-body irradiation, and superimposed infections. As stated above, the biopsy cannot be interpreted for evidence of GVHD until after 20 days following conditioning. Infections can be ruled out only by appropriate cultures and special techniques, including those for viruses. It is important to exclude CMV infection, as it may be associated with GVHD-like changes.[167] The histologic picture most closely simulates the effects of chemotherapy and radiation. A GVHD-like picture has been described in patients with severe T-cell deficiencies.[168]

COLITIS FOLLOWING SMALL INTESTINAL BYPASS AND DIVERSION OF THE FECAL STREAM

A clinical syndrome comprising a sudden increase in diarrhea, abdominal pain, tenderness, nausea, fever, leukocytosis, and in some patients arthralgias and skin lesions has been described following small intestinal bypass as a treatment for obesity.[169] The bypassed loops of small bowel contain a bacterial flora resembling that in the colon, whereas the mucosa demonstrates nonspecific chronic inflammation. Improvement in the clinical condition following

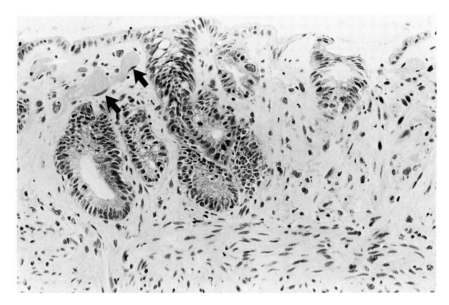

Fig. 2-13. Effect of chronic radiation on rectal mucosa. The predominant changes are in the mesenchymal cells of the lamina propria. Fibrosis and enlarged nuclei of all the mesenchymal cells, including the capillary endothelial cells (arrows) are seen. The crypts have distorted architecture and are lined by hyperplastic epithelial cells with nuclear atypism.

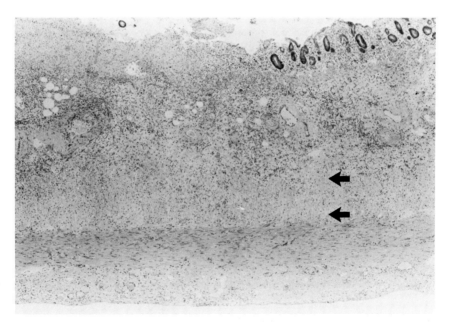

Fig. 2-14. Effect of chronic radiation on colon. Necrosis and ulceration of the mucosa, marked thickening of the vascular walls, and fibrosis of the submucosa are seen. The inner circular layer of the muscularis propria (arrows) has been completely replaced by hyalinized fibrous tissue.

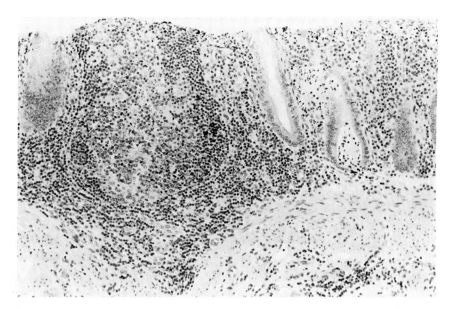

Fig. 2-15. Proctitis following diversion of the fecal stream. This patient underwent subtotal colectomy with ileostomy for toxic megacolon complicating pseudomembranous colitis, and subsequently developed a mild proctitis. A hyperplastic lymphoid follicle and crypt abscess are present.

treatment with various antibiotics or dismantling of the bypass suggests that bacterial by-products originating in the excluded gut cause the syndrome. Most of the affected individuals have had lesions restricted to the small intestine; however, a few cases mimicking Crohn's disease of the colon or ulcerative colitis have been described.[170, 171] In one patient, the ileum and colon were affected by a granulomatous inflammatory process resembling Crohn's disease.[170] Another patient developed transmural colitis with sinus tracts and fissures.[171] While it is possible that the rare examples of colonic inflammation after small-bowel bypass represent coincidental development of idiopathic IBD, the possibility remains that they are causally related to the bypass.

In 1980, Glotzer and colleagues described a proctitis and/or colitis that developed following diversion of the fecal stream.[172] Affected individuals have an inflammatory process limited to the distal excluded segment of the colon. The original indication for the colostomy or ileostomy is variable. Clinical symptoms are usually absent, and the barium enema shows normal mucosa, but proctoscopy discloses mucosal erythema and friability, with petechiae and granularity in some patients. Biopsies usually reveal a mild colitis with focal crypt abscesses (Fig. 2-15). Degeneration of the surface epithelium is variably present, there is moderate inflammation in the lamina propria, and lymphoid hyperplasia is commonly observed. Occasionally, however, the inflammation is more marked and may be associated with distortion of the crypt architecture and ulceration.[173, 174] In such cases, differentiation from ulcerative colitis and Crohn's disease may not be possible, and close attention to the original indication for the diversion and follow-up data are necessary to exclude idiopathic IBD. The lesion may persist for years but subsides following closure of the colostomy. The etiology of this condition is unknown; however, Harig and colleagues hypothesized that it was due to a deficiency of short-chain fatty acids in the excluded lumen and were able to reverse the inflammation by instilling these substances into the lumen.[175]

COLITIS ASSOCIATED WITH SYSTEMIC DISEASES

CHRONIC GRANULOMATOUS DISEASE OF CHILDHOOD

Chronic granulomatous disease is a recessively inherited disorder in which PMN leukocytes and mononuclear phagocytes are unable to destroy certain phagocytized microorganisms. The defect in microbicidal acitivity is due to an inadequate phagocytosis-induced metabolic burst that is partially related to inadequate hydrogen peroxide production.[176] The microorganisms most commonly found in the lesions are catalase-positive and do not form hydrogen peroxide. These include staphylococci, gram-negative enteric bacilli, and certain fungi.[176, 177] Repeated, severe infections involving the lungs, lymph nodes, liver, skin, and bone begin in infancy or childhood. Histologically, there are multiple abscesses, lipid-filled macrophages, and granulomas in the affected organs. The diagnosis can be established by a variety of neutrophil function tests, all of which are designed to detect the defective phagocytosis-induced metabolic burst.[176] The gastrointestinal tract is frequently involved in chronic granulomatous disease.[177] Chronic diarrhea and anal fistulas are the most prominent signs. Laboratory investigation may disclose steatorrhea and vitamin B_{12} malabsorption in some of the patients.[177] Ament and Ochs demonstrated yellowish-brown pigmented macrophages in the lamina propria of the small bowel and rectum in all of eight biopsied patients.[177] The macrophages, which occurred even in patients without gastrointestinal symptoms, had staining characteristics suggesting that they contained lipofuscin. Although granulomas were not found in any of the small bowel biopsies, they were present in rectal biopsies taken from five of eight patients. One of these patients had colitis and roentgenographic evidence of bowel disease that was morphologically indistinguishable from Crohn's disease. Subsequently, additional cases very closely simulating Crohn's disease, clinically, roentgeno-graphically, and pathologically have been reported.[178–180] The major feature of chronic granulomatous disease that is not a component of Crohn's disease is the infiltration of the affected tissues by pigmented, lipid-filled histiocytes within the mucosa and submucosa. The clinical presentation and leukocyte function studies readily differentiate patients with Crohn's disease from those with chronic granulomatous disease with gastrointestinal involvement, since the former have normal leukocyte bactericidal activity.[181]

IMMUNODEFICIENCY SYNDROMES

Patients with immunodeficiency syndromes frequently develop gastrointestinal disorders, including atrophic gastritis, diarrhea with malabsorption, disaccharidase deficiency, protein-losing enteropathy, nodular lymphoid hyperplasia, lymphoma, and carcinoma.[182] In addition, both ulcerative colitis and Crohn's disease occur in individuals with immunodeficiency, usually of the common variable type.[183] Rectal biopsies from patients with one of the syndromes but without gastrointestinal symptoms demonstrate a range of findings that includes normal mucosa; crypt abscesses; presence, absence, or increased numbers of plasma cells; large or small lymphoid follicles; absence of lymphoid follicles; and presence of PMN leukocytes in the lamina propria and surface epithelium.[183] At least some of these findings probably represent complications of the underlying immunodeficiency syndrome; however, a patient with an unusual type of colitis with bloody diarrhea that was confined to the rectosigmoid region was described by Strauss and colleagues.[182] The colitis did not resemble ulcerative colitis because it was segmental, transmural, and had an inflammatory infiltrate that included numerous macrophages but no discrete granulomas. The investigators did not consider this inflammatory process typical of Crohn's disease either and interpreted the colitis as a distinctive lesion of the immunodeficient state. They pointed out that it was difficult to exclude the possibility that this collitis was not an expression of a known disorder modified by the patient's altered immunity. Clearly, additional cases will need to be described before this can be considered a distinct entity.

The above discussion focuses on patients with hereditary immunodeficiency syndromes. Patients with AIDS develop a wide variety of intestinal infections, most of which have been covered in preceding sections. Infection of lamina propria lymphocytes, macrophages, dendritic reticulum cells, and, rarely, crypt epithelium in these patients has been described.[184–186] Whether infection of the intestine with human immunodeficiency virus (HIV) alone causes a clinically symptomatic primary enteropathy is unsettled.

HEMOLYTIC-UREMIC SYNDROME

The hemolytic-uremic syndrome consists of acute renal failure, microangiopathic hemolytic anemia, and thrombocytopenia. Gastrointestinal complaints constitute the most frequent presenting symptoms and signs; these include bloody diarrhea, vomiting, and cramping abdominal pain.[187–189] Because the barium enema may show evidence of diffuse colitis, and proctoscopy may reveal hyperemia, friable mucosa, and ulceration, the clinical diagnosis of ulcerative colitis is frequently made, thereby delaying the establishment of the correct diagnosis. The published reports of the colitis of hemolytic-uremic syndrome contain little information regarding the histopathology of the colonic mucosa; microthrombi within vessels, combined with necrosis of the mucosa, suggest an ischemic etiology for the syndrome.[188, 189] The intestinal symptoms respond rapidly to appropriate medical management of the renal failure but, if the correct diagnosis is not established and appropriate management is delayed, full-thickness necrosis of the colonic wall with its attendant complications may supervene.[188, 189] As indicated previously, hemolytic-uremic syndrome may develop during the course of Campylobacter and *E. coli* 0157:H7 colitis.[37, 40]

BEHCET'S DISEASE

Behcet's disease is a systemic condition characterized by the clinical triad of relapsing iritis and ulcers of the oral mucosa and genitalia.[190, 191] Other important clinical manifestations include the development of a variety of cutaneous lesions, arthritis, thrombophlebitis, and neurologic lesions.[192] The common pathologic changes consist of ulcers, perivascular lymphoid infiltrates, vasculitis, and, occasionally, granulomas.[191, 193] Although gastrointestinal symptoms are not uncommon, documented lesions in the intestinal tract are infrequent. Any part of the gut may be involved; the described colonic lesions have been discrete ulcers resembling the aphthoid ulcers of Crohn's disease and granulomas. Whether these simply represent a manifestation of vasculitis affecting the intestinal vasculature is not clear. Whether the colitis of Behcet's disease is a specific entity or may represent coexistent ulcerative colitis or Crohn's disease is controversial.[191] The diagnosis of Behcet's disease is not a histologic one but rather is made by careful clinicopathologic correlation. James has devised a useful scoring system for establishing the diagnosis.[192]

MISCELLANEOUS TYPES OF COLITIS

COLLAGENOUS COLITIS

A condition characterized clinically by watery diarrhea and pathologically by subepithelial deposition of collagen beneath the surface epithelium of the colonic mucosa was described and named *collagenous colitis* by Lindstrom in 1976.[194] Since then, several series of cases have been reported, and the entity has become better defined.[195–198] Collagenous colitis occurs predominantly in middle-aged to older patients and is more frequent in females. The affected individuals have watery diarrhea that can be continuous or intermittent and that has been known to persist for up to 15 years.[196, 198] Endoscopy

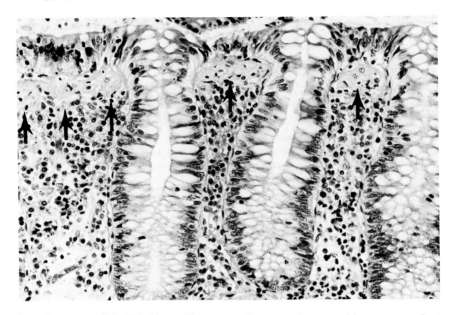

Fig. 2-16. Collagenous colitis. This biopsy illustrates well-preserved crypt architecture, a moderate chronic inflammatory infiltrate with a predominance of plasma cells in the lamina propria, and lymphocytic infiltration of the surface epithelium. The subepithelial collagen table located between the base of the surface epithelial cells and the arrows is markedly thickened and has a lacy appearance. The subepithelial collagen table in this biopsy ranges from 20 to 30 μm thick.

usually shows either normal mucosa or mild congestion and contact bleeding.[199] Microscopically, the collagen table beneath the surface epithelium, but not around the crypts, is increased to a mean thickness of approximately 15 μm. The amount of thickening of the collagen table required to establish the diagnosis of collagenous colitis has not been established with certainty. The normal basement membrane is 3 μm or less in thickness, whereas in most patients with the characteristic clinical syndrome the membrane and subepithelial collagen complex have been over 10 μm thick. Wang and colleagues found that subepithelial collagen deposition correlated with watery diarrhea only when it exceeded 15 μm in thickness, involved more than 30 percent of the surface of a biopsy, and was proximal to the rectum and sigmoid.[200]

The collagen deposition may be diffuse or patchy and tends to be less prominent in the distal sigmoid and rectum. Several patients in whom the rectal mucosa was not affected have been reported, indicating the necessity for colo-noscopy with biopsies of the more proximal colon to confirm the diagnosis.[201] The crypt architecture is usually well preserved, and the lamina propria typically contains a mild to moderate infiltrate of lymphocytes, plasma cells and scattered eosinophils (Fig. 2-16). Neutrophilic infiltration of the crypt epithelium is present in about one-half of the patients, but this is focal, mild, and more likely to be observed early in the course of the disease than later. The surface epithelium becomes flat or cuboidal, the nuclei become irregular, and increased numbers of lymphocytes can be seen within it. This injury and lymphocytic infiltration to the surface epithelium resemble the lesion seen in the surface epithelium of the small bowel in celiac sprue. This observation, along with a high prevalence of associated thyroid disease and arthritis, have led to the suggestion that the condition has an autoimmune etiology or pathogenesis.[196] The thickened subepithelial collagen table typically has a "lacy" appearance rather than being a homogeneous band, and capillaries, fibroblasts, and lymphocytes may be seen within it (Fig. 2-16).

Electron microscopic examination has disclosed separation of the pericryptal fibroblast sheath from the epithelium and transformation of the pericryptal fibroblasts to myofibroblasts.[195] The basal lamina was focally deficient, and the surface epithelial cells rested directly on a thickened collagen table. The excess collagen appeared to be secreted by activated myofibroblasts derived from the pericryptal sheath.[195] The diarrhea in collagenous colitis results from net water and electrolyte secretion and has been postulated to be attributable to "malabsorption" caused by the thickened subepithelial collagen table.[196]

Apart from the absence of the increased thickness of the subepithelial collagen table, a condition described under the name *microscopic colitis* appears clinically and histologically similar to collagenous colitis, leading to the suggestion that microscopic colitis and collagenous colitis may be part of the same spectrum of disease.[202, 203] The development of colitis in sequential biopsies beginning with a mild, nonspecific inflammatory process and ending with collagenous colitis, has been described in a number of patients.[198, 203] Lazenby and associates have found that lymphocytic infiltration of the crypt and surface epithelium is prominent in patients with "microscopic" colitis and have proposed the name *lymphocytic colitis*.[204]

About 50 percent of patients with collagenous colitis who were treated with corticosteroids, sulfasalazine, or 5-aminosalicylic acid orally have had resolution of their diarrhea, but this must be interpreted with caution, as in other patients the diarrhea resolved spontaneously.[205] In most of the patients whose diarrhea stopped, the collagen band remained, but in a few, the collagen has decreased or disappeared.[201] I have seen one patient in whom the diarrhea and collagen disappeared spontaneously over a period of 3 months.

Because the mucosal architecture is largely preserved and there is only a slight chronic inflammatory infiltrate within the lamina propria, collagenous colitis does not resemble the more common inflammatory conditions that affect the colon, especially idiopathic IBD. However, collagenous thickening of the basement membrane may occasionally be seen in idiopathic IBD, ischemic colitis, and in other conditions as well, so the entire histologic picture and clinical context must be considered before the diagnosis is made.

NONSPECIFIC (IDIOPATHIC) ULCER

Nonspecific ulcers of the colon may present as acute perforating lesions or as a chronic syndrome with abdominal pain, intractable diarrhea, and a tender right lower quadrant mass.[206, 207] Any site in the colon may be involved, but the cecum and right colon account for 65 to 75 percent of cases.[208, 209] When the lesion involves the cecum, the clinical presentation mimics acute perforating appendicitis. Solitary ulcers predominate, but multiple lesions are present in up to 12 percent of patients.[209] Roentgenograms disclose ulcers, constricting lesions, or annular masses.[206] Pathologically, the lesions consist of discrete, sharply punched-out ulcers extending for variable depths into the bowel wall. Acute cases have necrosis and perforation, whereas chronic cases have ulcer beds composed of granulation tissue with fibrosis. Fibrin thrombi within the small vessels at the base of the ulcer or adjacent to it can sometimes be identified. The ulcers are typically located on the antimesenteric aspect of the colon; those in the cecum are usually anterior.[206]

Although nonspecific ulcers occur in otherwise healthy young adults, most develop in individuals with some underlying condition, especially if steroid therapy has been given.[210] A particularly high incidence is seen following renal transplantation.[211, 212] Other clinical settings associated with nonspecific ulcer include trauma, nonspecific stress, hypoperfusion of the viscera, oral contraceptive therapy, and phenylbutazone and oxyphenbutazone therapy.[213–215]

The eitology of nonspecific ulcer of the colon remains undetermined. The numerous associated conditions lead one to suspect more than one etiology, perhaps with ischemia as a final common pathway leading to the ulcer. Sutherland and colleagues identified CMV inclusion bodies associated with capillary destruction and breakdown of the mucosa in seven of nine nonspecific ulcers.[211] They attributed the ulcers to CMV, but assigning an etiologic role to CMV is difficult because of its known role as a secondary invader in other ulcerative conditions of the colon.

Nonspecific colonic ulcers must be differentiated from diverticulitis of the cecum and ascending colon.[216] Diverticula in the right colon are frequently solitary and, if inflamed and ulcerated, can be mistaken for nonspecific ulcer. If no remnants of mucosa are left in the diverticulum, it may be impossible to differentiate these two conditions.

NECROTIZING ENTEROCOLITIS IN CANCER PATIENTS

Necrotizing enterocolitis complicating chemotherapy of cancer develops as a fulminating segmental colitis or enteritis in individuals who are immunosuppressed, granulocytopenic, and, most often, have leukemia or lymphoma.[217–220] Twelve percent of an unselected autopsy series of leukemic patients studied by Steinberg and colleagues were affected.[218] The condition most commonly affects the cecum (*typhlitis*, from the Greek *typhlon*, meaning cecum) and right colon, but other regions of the colon and the distal ileum may be involved as well. Examples have been reported under a variety of synonyms, including neutropenic enterocolitis,[221] typhlitis,[222, 223] agranulocytic colitis, and the ileocecal syndrome.[221, 224]

Some of the cases described as necrotizing enterocolitis appear to represent antibiotic-associated pseudomembranous colitis, probably secondary to *C. difficile*. Freeman and colleagues reported a patient with necrotizing enterocolitis who improved after oral vancomycin therapy; however, the stools were consistently negative when examined for *C. difficile* toxin.[225] In cases that do not resemble pseudomembranous colitis, the predominant lesion has been hemorrhage, with marked edema, necrosis, and ulceration of the mucosa. Colonies of bacteria and submucosal gas cysts are often present.[218] Because the patients are usually granulocytopenic, inflammation is minimal or absent.

Necrotizing enterocolitis does not constitute a diagnostic problem in terms of separating it from the other forms of colitis because of the distinctive clinical setting and necrotizing, hemorrhagic nature of the process.

EOSINOPHILIC COLITIS AND ALLERGIC PROCTITIS

Eosinophilic gastroenteritis is defined as eosinophilic infiltration of the gastric or small intestinal wall accompanied by peripheral blood eosinophilia.[226] Recently, a number of patients with colonic involvement, usually as a part of ileocolitis, have been described.[227–230] Some patients with eosinophilic gastroenteritis develop symptoms following ingestion of specific foods, suggesting that food allergy plays a role in the pathogenesis of the condition.[231, 232] The clinical presentation depends on the part of the gastric or intestinal wall that is most severely affected. Those with predominantly mucosal involvement tend to have malabsorption (owing to small bowel disease), with iron-deficiency anemia and protein loss from the gut.[232] When the muscularis is the predominant site of involvement, obstructive symptoms are the major clinical problems. Rarely, eosinophlic ascites occurs in patients with predominantly serosal disease. In the cases reported to involve the colon, the symptoms have included diarrhea, bright red rectal bleeding, abdominal pain, and fever. Barium enema and colonoscopy disclose changes indistinguishable from Crohn's disease, usually confined to the ileum and right colon. Histologically, the mucosa shows marked infiltration by eosinophilic leukocytes; however, because eosinophilic infiltration of the gut occurs commonly in a variety of different inflammatory conditions, including both ulcerative colitis and Crohn's disease, it is nonspecific. For this reason, the diagnosis of eosinophilic gastroenteritis should not be made in the absence of an appropriate clinical history and peripheral blood eosinophilia. Peripheral blood eosinophil counts may be elevated in Crohn's disease, but not to the marked levels seen in eosinophilic gastroenteritis involving the colon.[230]

Rosekrans and colleagues described an entity they designated *allergic proctitis*.[233] Affected individuals constituted a subgroup of patients with ulcerative proctitis in whom increased numbers of IgE-containing cells in the rectal lamina propria predicted a response to disodium cromoglycate therapy. This group of patients did not otherwise differ from those with typical ulcerative proctitis, a condition distinguished from ulcerative colitis by its intermittent, benign course and limitation to the rectum. The patients with alleged allergic proctitis did not differ from those with ulcerative proctitis histologically, apart from the increased numbers of IgE-containing cells demonstrated by immunoperoxidase staining.[233]

Food allergy has been alleged to be the most common cause of colitis in infants,[234] and rectal biopsy has been proposed as a useful adjunct in diagnosing it.[235] Winter and colleagues suggest that rectal biopsies from infants in which there are more than 60 eosinophils per high-power field and in which eosinophils are found in the muscularis mucosae or as the predominant cell in crypt abcesses correlate with allergy-related disease.[235] Allergic proctitis has been said to respond well to dietary change, in contrast to allergic gastroenteritis, in which multiple relapses and a requirement for corticosteroid therapy are characteristic.[236]

ACKNOWLEDGMENT

I am indebted to Cyrus E. Rubin for his help with the photomicrographs and to Stephanie Scholl and Sheila Ojendyk for their expert assistance with the manuscript.

REFERENCES

1. Blacklow NR, Cukor G: Viral gastroenteritis. N Engl J Med 304:397, 1981
2. Plotkin GR, Kluge RM, Waldman RH: Gastroenteritis: etiology pathophysiology and clinical manifestations. Medicine 58:95, 1979
3. Dolin R, Treanor JJ, Madore HP: Novel agents of viral enteritis in humans. J Infect Dis 155:365, 1987
4. Timbury MC, Edmond E: Herpesviruses. J Clin Pathol 32:859, 1979
5. Buss DH, Scharyj M: Herpesvirus infection of the esophagus and other visceral organs in adults. Incidence and clinical significance. Am J Med 66:457, 1979
6. Boulton AJM, Slater DN, Hancock BW: Herpesvirus colitis: a new cause of diarrhoea in a patient with Hodgkin's disease. Gut 23:247, 1982
7. Goodell SE, Quinn TC, Mkrtichian EE, et al: Herpes simplex virus: an important cause of acute proctitis in homosexual men. Gastroenterology 80:1159, 1981
8. Surawicz CM, Goodell SE, Quinn TC, et al: Spectrum of rectal biopsy abnormalities in homosexual men with intestinal symptoms. Gastroenterology 91:651, 1986
9. Levine RS, Warner NE, Johnson CF: Cytomegalic inclusion disease in the gastro-intestinal tract of adults. Ann Surg 159:37, 1964
10. Rene E. Marche C, Chevalier T, et al: Cytomegalovirus colitis in patients with acquired immunodeficiency syndrome. Dig. Dis Sci 33:741, 1988
11. Surawicz CM, Myerson D: Self-limited cytomegalovirus colitis in immunocompetent individuals. Gastroenterology 94:194, 1988
12. Goodman ZD, Boitnott JK, Yardley JH: Perforation of the colon associated with cytomegalovirus infection. Dig Dis Sci 24:376, 1979
13. Foucar E, Kiyoshi M, Foucar K, et al: Colon ulceration in lethal cytomegalovirus infection. Am J Clin Pathol 76:788, 1981
14. Cooper HS, Raffensperger ED, Jonas L, et al: Cytomegalovirus inclusions in patients with ulcerative colitis and toxic dilation requiring colonic resection. Gastroenterology 72:1253, 1977
15. Snover DC: Mucosal damage simulating acute graft-versus-host reaction in cytomegalovirus colitis. Transplantation 39:669, 1985

16. Robey SS, Gage WR, Kuhajda FP: Comparison of immunoperoxidase and DNA in situ hybridization techniques in the diagnosis of cytomegalovirus colitis. Am J Clin Pathol 9:666, 1988

17. Grayston JT, Want SP: New knowledge of Chlamydiae and the diseases they cause. J Infect Dis 132:87, 1975

18. Taylor-Robinson D, Thomas BJ: The role of *Chlamydia trachomatis* in genital tract and associated diseases. J Clin Pathol 33:205, 1980

19. Quinn TC, Goodell SE, Mkrtichian E, et al: *Chlamydia trachomatis* proctitis. N Engl J Med 305:195, 1981

20. Quinn RC, Corey L, Chaffee RG, et al: The etiology of anorectal infections in homosexual men. Am J Med 71:395, 1981

21. Levine JS, Smith PD, Brugge WR: Chronic proctitis in male homosexuals due to lymphogranuloma venereum. Gastroenterology 79:563, 1980

22. De La Monte SM, Hutchins GM: Follicular proctocolitis and neuromatous hyperplasia with lymphogranuloma venereum. Hum Pathol 16:1025, 1985

23. Evans N: Pathogenic mechanisms in bacterial diarrhoea. Clin Gastroenterol 8:599, 1979

24. Abrams GD: Pathogenesis of gastrointestinal infections. Am J Surg Pathol 12:76, 1988

25. Nostrant TT, Kumar NB, Appelman HD: Histopathology differentiates acute self-limited colitis from ulcerative colitis. Gastroenterology 92:318, 1987

26. Surawicz CM, Belic L: Rectal biopsy helps to distinguish acute self-limited colitis from idiopathic inflammatory bowel disease. Gastroenterology 86:104, 1984

27. MacDonald KL, O'Leary MJ, Cohen ML, et al: *Escherichia coli* 1057:H7, an emerging gastrointestinal pathogen. JAMA 256:3567, 1988

28. Casemore DP, Armstrong M, Sands RL: Laboratory diagnosis of cryptosporidiosis. J Clin Pathol 38:1337, 1985

29. Skirrow MB: *Campylobacter* enteritis: a "new" disease. Br Med J 2:9, 1977

30. Blaser MJ, Berkowitz ID, LaForce M: *Campylobacter* enteritis: clinical and epidemiologic features. Ann Intern Med 91:179, 1979

31. Colgan T, Lambert JR, Newman A: *Campylobacter jejuni* enterocolitis. A clinicopathologic study. Arch Pathol Lab Med 104:571, 1980

32. Price AB, Jewkes J, Sanderson PJ: Acute diarrhoea: *Campylobacter* colitis and the role of rectal biopsy. J Clin Pathol 32:990, 1979

33. Blaser MJ, Wells JG, Feldman RA, et al: *Campylobacter* enteritis in the United States. Ann Intern Med 98:360, 1983

34. Blaser MJ, Reller LB: *Campylobacter* enteritis. N Engl J Med 305:1442, 1981

35. Drake AA, Gilchrist MJR, Washington JA, et al: Diarrhea due to *Campylobacter fetus* subspecies *jejuni*. A clinical review of 63 cases. Mayo Clin Proc 56:414, 1981

36. Karmali MA, Fleming PC: *Campylobacter* enteritis. Can Med Assoc J 120:1525, 1979

37. Chamovitz BN, Hartstein AI, Alexander SR, et al: Campylobacter jejuni-associated hemolytic-uremic syndrome in a mother and daughter. Pediatrics 71:253, 1983

38. Blaser MJ, Parsons RB, Want WLL: Acute colitis by *Campylobacter fetus* ss. *jejuni*. Gastroenterology 78:448, 1980

39. Riley LW, Remis RS, Helgerson SD et al: Hemorrhagic colitis associated with a rare *Escherichia coli* serotype. N Engl J Med 308:681–685, 1983

40. Ostroff SM, Kobayashi JM, Lewis JH: Infections with *Escherichia coli* 0157:H7 in Washington state. JAMA 262:355, 1989

41. Kelly JK, Pai CH, Inderman HJ, et al: The histopathology of rectosigmoid biopsies from adults with bloody diarrhea due to verotoxin-producing *Escherichia coli*. Am J Clin Pathol 88:78, 1987

42. Kelly J, Oryshak A, Wenetsek M, et al: The colonic pathology of *Escherichia coli* 0157:H7 infection. Am J Surg Pathol 14:87, 1990

43. Bartlett JG, Moon N, Chang TW, et al: Role of *Clostridium difficile* in antibiotic-associated pseudomembranous colitis. Gastroenterology 75:778, 1978

44. Burdon DW, George RH, Mogg GAG, et al: Faecal toxin and severity of antibiotic-associated pseudomembranous colitis. J Clin Pathol 34:548, 1981

45. Bartlett JG: Laboratory diagnosis of antibiotic-associated colitis. Lab Med 12:347, 1981

46. Robertson MB, Breen JK, Desmond PV, et al: Incidence of antibiotic-related diarrhoea and pseudomembranous colitis. A prospective study of lincomycin, clindamycin and ampicillin. Med J Aust 1:243, 1977

47. Viscidi R, Willey S, Bartlett JG: Isolation rates and toxigenic potential of *clostridium difficile* isolates from various patient populations. Gastroenterology 81:5, 1981

48. Tedesco FJ, Corless JK, Brownstein RE: Rectal

sparing in antibiotic-associated pseudomembranous colitis: a prospective study. Gastroenterology 83:1259, 1982

49. Price AB, Davies DR: Pseudomembranous colitis. J Clin Pathol 30:1, 1977

50. Hoogland T, Cooperman AM, Farmer RG, et al: Toxic megacolon-unusual complication of pseudomembranous colitis. Cleveland Clin Q 44:149, 1977

51. Bartlett JG: *Clostridium difficile* and inflammatory bowel disease. Gastroenterology 80:863, 1981

52. Bolton RP, Sherriff RJ, Read AE: *Clostridium difficile* associated diarrhoea: a role in inflammatory bowel disease. Lancet 1:383, 1980

53. Trnka YM, Lamont JT: Association of *Clostridium difficile* toxin with symptomatic relapse of chronic inflammatory bowel disease. Gastroenterology 80:693, 1981

54. Keighley MRB, Youngs D, Johnson M, et al: *Clostridium difficile* toxin in acute diarrhea complicating inflammatory bowel disease. Gut 23:410, 1982

55. Meyers S, Mayer L, Bottone E, et al: Occurrence of *Clostridium difficile* toxin during the course of inflammatory bowel disease. Gastroenterology 80:697, 1981

56. McFarland LV, Mulligan ME, Kwok RYY, Stamm WE: Nosocomial acquisition of *clostridium difficile* infection. N Engl J Med 320:204, 1989

57. Cudmore MA, Silva J, Fekety R, et al: *Clostridium difficile* colitis associated with cancer chemotherapy. Arch Intern Med 142:333, 1982

58. Peikin SR, Galdibini J, Bartlett JG: Role of *Clostridium difficile* in a case of nonantibiotic-associated pseudomembranous colitis. Gastroenterology 79:948, 1980

59. Wald A, Mendelow H, Bartlett JG: Non-antibiotic-associated pseudomembranous colitis due to toxin-producing clostridia. Ann Intern Med 92:798, 1980

60. Caplan LMK, Dobson ML, Dorkin H: *Yersinia enterocolitica* septicemia. Am J Clin Pathol 69:189, 1978

61. Leino R, Kalliomaki JL: Yersiniosis as an internal disease. Ann Intern Med 81:458, 1974

62. Vantrappen G, Agg HO, Ponette E, et al: Yersinia enteritis and enterocolitis: gastroenterological aspects. Gastroenterology 72:220, 1977

63. Cover TL, Aber RC: *Yersinia entercolitica.* N Engl J Med 321:16, 1989

64. Rodriguez WJ, Controni G, Cohen J, et al: *Yersinia enterocolitica* enteritis in children. JAMA 242:1978, 1979

65. El-Maraghi NRH, Mair NS: The histopathology of enteric infection with *Yersinia pseudotuberculosis.* Am J Clin Pathol 71:631, 1979

66. Lee LA, Gerber AR, Lonsway DR, et al: *Yersinia enterocolitica* 0:3 infections in infants and children, associated with the household preparation of chitterlings. N Engl J Med 322:984, 1990

67. Bradford WD, Noce PS, Gutman LT: Pathologic features of enteric infection with *Yersinia enterocolitica.* Arch Pathol 98:17, 1974

68. Bohm N, Wybitul K: Different histologic types of mesenteric lymphadenitis in *Yersinia pseudotuberculosis* type I and type II infection. Pathol Res Pract 162:301, 1978

69. Day DW, Mandal BK, Morson BC: The rectal biopsy appearances in salmonella colitis. Histopathology 2:117, 1978

70. McGovern VJ, Slavutin LJ: Pathology of salmonella colitis. Am J Surg Pathol 3:483, 1979

71. Dickinson RJ, Gilmour HM, McClelland DBL: Rectal biopsy in patients presenting to an infectious disease unit with diarrhoeal disease. Gut 20:141, 1979

72. Jewkes J, Larson HE, Price AB, et al: Aetiology of acute diarrhoea in adults. Gut 22:38, 1981

73. Nagel PH, Serritella A, Layden TJ: *Edwardsiella tarda* gastroenteritis associated with a pet turtle. Gastroenterology 82:1436, 1982

74. Marsh PK, Gorbach SL: Invasive enterocolitis caused by *Edwardsiella tarda.* Gastroenterology 82:336, 1982

75. Kilpatrick AM: Gonorrheal proctitis. N Engl J Med 287:967, 1972

76. McMillan A, Lee FD: Sigmoidoscopic and microscopic appearance of the rectal mucosa in homosexual men. Gut 22:1035, 1981

77. Haggitt RC: Granulomatous diseases of the gastrointestinal tract. p. 257. In Ioachim, HL (ed): The Pathology of Granulomas. Raven Press, New York, 1982

78. Smith JMB: Mycoses of the alimentary tract. Gut 10:1035, 1969

79. Penna FJ: Blastomycosis of the colon resembling clinically ulcerative colitis. Gut 20:896, 1979

80. Schulz DM: Histoplasmosis: a statistical morphologic study. Am J Clin Pathol 24:11, 1954

81. Miller DP, Everett ED: Gastrointestinal histoplasmosis. J Clin Gastroenterol 1:233, 1979

82. Goodwin RA, Shapiro JL, Thurman GH, et

al: Disseminated histoplasmosis: clinical and pathologic correlations. Medicine 59:1, 1980

83. Pittman FE, El-Hashimi WK, Pittman JC: Studies of human amebiasis. I. clinical and laboratory findings in eight cases of acute amebic colitis. Gastroenterology 65:581, 1973

84. Prathap K, Gilman R: The histopathology of acute intestinal amebiasis. a rectal biopsy study. Am J Pathol 60:229, 1970

85. Pittman FE, El-Hashimi WK, Pittman JC: Studies of human amebiasis. II. Light and electron-microscope observations of colonic mucosa and exudate in acute amebic colitis. Gastroenterology 65:588, 1973

86. Gilman R, Islam M, Paschi S, et al: Comparison of conventional and immunofluorescent techniques for the detection of *Entamoeba histolytica* in rectal biopsies. Gastroenterology 78:435, 1980

87. Pittman FE, Hennigar GR: Sigmoidoscopic and colonic mucosal biopsy findings in amebic colitis. Arch Pathol 97:155, 1974

88. Patterson M, Healy GR, Shabot JM: Serologic testing for amoebiasis. Gastroenterology 78:136, 1980

89. Phillips SC, Mildvan D, William DC, et al: Sexual transmission of enteric protozoa and helminths in a veneral-disease-clinic population. N Engl J Med 305:603, 1981

90. Allason-Jones E, Mindel A, Sargeaunt P, Williams P: Entamoeba histolytica as a commensal intestinal parasite in homosexual men. N Engl J Med 315:353, 1986

91. Brandt H, Tamayo RP: Pathology of human amebiasis. Hum Pathol 1:351, 1970

92. Meisel JL, Perera DR, Meligro BS, et al: Overwhelming watery diarrhea associated with a cryptosporidium in an immunosuppressed patient. Gastroenterology 70:1156, 1976

93. Wolfson JS, Richter JM, Waldron MA, et al: Cryptosporidiosis in immunocompetent patients. N Eng J Med 312:1278, 1985

94. Casemore DP, Sands RL, Curry A: Cryptosporidium species a "new" human pathogen. J Clin Pathol 38:1321, 1985

95. Jokipii L, Pohjola S, Jokipii AMM: Cryptosporidiosis associated with traveling and giardiasis. Gastroenterology 89:838, 1985

96. Weinstein L, Edelstein SM, Madara JL, et al: Intestinal cryptosporidiosis complicated by disseminated cytomegalovirus infection. Gastroenterology 81:584, 1981

97. Nime FA, Burek JD, Page DL, et al: Acute enterocolitis in a human being infected with the protozoan cryptosporidium. Gastroenterology 70:592, 1976

98. Marcial MA, Madara JL: Cryptosporidium: cellular localization, structural analysis of absorptive cell-parasite membrane-membrane interactions in guinea pigs, and suggestion of protozoan transport by M cells. Gastroenterology 90:583, 1986

99. Mahmoud AA: Schistosomiasis. N Engl J Med 297:1329, 1977

100. McCully RM, Barron CN, Cheever AW: Diseases caused by trematodes. p. 482. In Binford CH, Connor DH (eds): Pathology of Tropical and Extraordinary Diseases. Armed Forces Institute of Pathology, Washington, D.C., 1976

101. Warren KS: The pathology, pathobiology and pathogenesis of schistosomiasis. Nature 273:609, 1978

102. Warren KS: The relavance of schistosomiasis. N Engl J Med 303:203, 1980

103. Chen M, Wang SC, Chang PY, et al: Granulomatous disease of the large intestine secondary to schistosome infestation. Chinese Med J 4:371, 1978

104. Kruatrachue M, Bhaibulaya M, Harinasuta C: Evaluation of rectal biopsy as a diagnostic method in *Schistosoma japonicum* infection in man in Thailand. Ann Trop Med Parasitol 48:276, 1964

105. Yokogawa M, Yoshimura H: Clinicopathologic studies on larval anisakiasis in Japan. Am J Trop Med Hygiene 16:723, 1967

106. Ashby BS, Appleton PJ, Dawson I: Eosinophilic granuloma of gastrointestinal tract caused by herring parasite *Eustoma rotundatum*. Br Med J 1:1141, 1964

107. Pinkus GS, Coolidge C, Little MD: Intestinal anisakiasis. First case report from North America. Am J Med 59:114, 1975

108. Valdiserri RO: Intestinal anisakiasis. Report of a case and recovery of larvae from market fish. Am J Clin Pathol 76:319, 1981

109. Rosset JS, McClatchey KD, Higashi GI, et al: Anisakis larval type I in fresh salmon. Am J Clin Pathol 78:54, 1982

110. Almy TP, Howell DA: Diverticular disease of the colon. N Engl J Med 302:324, 1980

111. Meyers MA, Alonso DR, Morson BC, et al: Pathogenesis of diverticulitis complicating

granulomatous colitis. Gastroenterology 74:24, 1978

112. Schmidt GT, Lennard-Jones JE, Morson BC, et al: Crohn's disease of the colon and its distinction from diverticulitis. Gut 9:7, 1968

113. Morson BC: Pathology of diverticular disease of the colon. Clin Gastroenterol 4:37, 1975

114. Marshak RH, Janowitz HD, Present DH: Granulomatous colitis in association with diverticula. N Engl J Med 283:1080, 1970

115. Marshak RH, Lindner AE, Maklansky D: Paracolic fistulous tracts in diverticulitis and granulomatous colitis. JAMA 243:1943, 1980

116. Ford MJ, Anderson JR, Gilmour HM, et al: Clinical spectrum of "solitary ulcer" of the rectum. Gastroenterology 84:1533, 1983

117. Madigan MR, Morson BC: Solitary ulcer of the rectum. Gut 10:871, 1969

118. Rutter KRP, Riddell RH: The solitary ulcer syndrome of the rectum. Clin Gastroenterol 4:505, 1975

119. Levine DS: "Solitary" rectal ulcer syndrome: are "solitary" rectal ulcer syndrome and "localized" colitis cystica profunda analogous syndromes caused by rectal prolapse? Gastroenterology 92:243, 1987

120. Womack NR, Williams NS, Holmfield JHM, Morrison JFB: Pressure and prolapse—the cause of solitary rectal ulceration. Gut 28:1228, 1987

121. Levine DS, Surawicz CM, Ajer TN, et al: Diffuse excess mucosal collagen in rectal biopsies facilitates differential diagnosis of solitary rectal ulcer syndrome from other inflammatory bowel diseases. Dig Dis Sci 33:1345, 1988

122. Silver H, Stolar J: Distinguishing features of well differentiated mucinous adenocarcinoma of the rectum and colitis cystica profunda. Am J Clin Pathol 51:493, 1969

123. Wayte DM, Helwig EB: Colitis cystica profunda. Am J Clin Pathol 48:159, 1967

124. Epstein SE, Ascari WQ, Ablow RC, et al: Colitis cystica profunda. Am J Clin Pathol 45:186, 1966

125. Lobert PF, Appelman HD: Inflammatory cloacagenic polyp: a unique inflammatory lesion of the anal transitional zone. Am J Surg Pathol 5:761, 1981

126. Saul SH: Inflammatory cloacagenic polyp: relationship to solitary rectal ulcer syndrome/mucosal prolapse and other bowel disorders. Hum Pathol 18:1120, 1987

127. Boley SJ, Brandt LJ, Veith FJ: Ischemic disorders of the intestines. Curr Prob Surg 15:1, 1978

128. Saegesser F, Sandblom P: Ischemic lesions of the distended colon. A complication of obstructive colorectal cancer. Am J Surg 129:309, 1975

129. Meisel JL, Bergman D, Graney D, et al: Human rectal mucosa: proctoscopic and morphological changes caused by laxatives. Gastroenterology 72:1274, 1977

130. Leriche M, Devroede G, Sanchez G, et al: Changes in the rectal mucosa induced by hypertonic enemas. Dis Colon Rectum 21:227, 1978

131. Saunders DR, Haggitt RC, Kimmey MB, Silverstein FE: Morphological consequences of bisacodyl on normal rectal mucosa: effect of a prostaglandin E1 analog on mucosal injury. Gastrointest Endosc 36:101, 1990

132. Urso FP, Urso MJ, Lee CH: The cathartic colon: pathological findings and radiological pathological correlation. Radiology 116:557, 1975

133. Smith B: Pathologic changes in the colon produced by anthraquinone purgatives. Dis Colon Rectum 16:455, 1973

134. Lutzger LG, Factor SM: Effects of some water-soluble contrast media on the colonic mucosa. Diag Radiol 118:545, 1976

135. Pike BF, Phillippi PJ, Lawson EH: Soap colitis. N Engl J Med 285:217, 1971

136. Meyer CT, Brand M, DeLuca VA, Spiro HM: Hydrogen peroxide colitis: a report of three patients. J Clin Gastroenterol 3:31, 1981

137. Jonas G, Mahoney A, Murray J, Gertler S: Chemical colitis due to endoscope cleaning solutions: a mimic of pseudomembranous colitis. Gastroenterology 95:1403, 1988

138. Snover DC, Sandstad J, Hutton S: Mucosal pseudolipomatosis of the colon. Am J Clin Pathol 84:575, 1985

139. Snover DC, Bond J: Mucosal plaques seen at colonoscopy: chemical colitis or mucosal pseudolipomatosis? Gastroenterology 96:1626, 1989

140. Bilotta JJ, Waye JD: Hydrogen peroxide enteritis: the "snow white" sign. Gastrointest Endosc 35:428, 1989

141. Bonkowsky HL, Brisbane J: Colitis and hepatitis caused by methyldopa. JAMA 236:1602, 1976

142. Ingle JN: Acute colitis with methyldopa. N Engl J Med 304:1044, 1981

143. Martin P, Manley PN, Depew WT, Blakeman

JM: Isotretinoin-associated proctosigmoiditis. Gastroenterology 93:606, 1987

144. Uribe A, Johansson C, Slezak P, Rubio C: Ulcerations of the colon associated with naproxen and acetylsalicylic acid treatment. Gastrointest Endosc 32:242, 1986

145. Martin DM, Goldman JA, Gilliam J, et al: Gold-induced eosinophilic enterocolitis: response to oral cromolyn sodium. Gastroenterology 80:1567, 1981

146. Michet CJ, Jr, Rakela J, Luthra HS: Auranofin-associated colitis and eosinophilia. Mayo Clin Proc 62:142, 1987

147. Toffler RB, Pingoud EG, Burrell MI: Acute colitis related to penicillin and penicillin derivatives. Lancet 2:707, 1978

148. Sakurai Y, Tsuchiya H, Ikegami F, et al: Acute right-sided hemorrhagic colitis associated with oral administration of ampicillin. Dig Dis Sci 24:910, 1979

149. Riddell RH: The gastrointestinal tract. p. 523. In Riddell RH (ed): The Pathology of Drug-Induced and Toxic Diseases. Churchill Livingstone, New York, 1982

150. Milles SS, Muggia AL, Spiro HM: Colonic histologic changes induced by 5-fluorouracil. Gastroenterology 43:391, 1962

151. Floch MH, Hellman L: The effect of five-fluorouracil on rectal mucosa. Gastroenterology 48:430, 1964

152. Novak JM, Collins JT, Donowitz M, et al: Effects of radiation on the human gastrointestinal tract. J Clin Gastroenterol 1:9, 1979

153. DeCosse JJ, Rhodes RS, Wentz WB, et al: The natural history and management of radiation induced injury of the gastrointestinal tract. Ann Surg 170, 369, 1969

154. Berthrong M, Fajardo LF: Radiation injury in surgical pathology. II. Alimentary tract. Am J Surg Patho 5:153, 1981

155. Gelfand MD, Tepper M, Katz L, et al: Acute irradiation proctitis in man. development of eosinophilic crypt abscesses. Gastroenterology 54:401, 1968

156. Weisbrot IM, Liber AF, Gordon BS: The effects of therapeutic radiation on colonic mucosa. Cancer 36:931, 1975

157. LoIudice T, Baxter D, Balint J: Effects of abdominal surgery on the development of radiation enteropathy. Gastroenterology 73:1093, 1977

158. Fajardo LF, Berthrong M: Radiation injury in surgical pathology, I. Am J Surg Pathol 2:159, 1978

159. Warren S, Friedman NB: Pathology and pathologic diagnosis of radiation lesions in the gastrointestinal tract. Am J Pathol 18:499, 1942

160. Hasleton PS, Carr N, Schofield PF: Vascular changes in radiation bowel disease. Histopathology 9:517, 1985

161. Ackerman LV: The pathology of radiation effect of normal and neoplastic tissue. Am J Roentgenol 114:447, 1972

162. Sandler RS, Sandler DP: Radiation-induced cancers of the colon and rectum: assessing the risk. Gastroenterology 84:51, 1983

163. Epstein RJ, McDonald GB, Sale GE, et al: The diagnostic accuracy of the rectal biopsy in acute graft-versus-host disease: a prospective study of thirteen patients Gastroenterology 78:764, 1980

164. Sale GE, McDonald GB, Shulman HM, et al: Gastrointestinal graft-versus-host disease in man. A clinicopathologic study of the rectal biopsy. Am J Surg Pathol 3:291, 1979

165. McDonald GB, Shulman HM, Sullivan KM, Spencer GD: Intestinal and hepatic complications of human bone marrow transplantation, Part 1. Gastroenterology 90:460, 1986

166. McDonald GB, Shulman HM, Sullivan KM, Spencer GD: Intestinal and hepatic complications of human bone marrow transplantation, Part 2. Gastroenterology 90:770, 1986

167. Snover DC: Graft-versus-host disease of the gastrointestinal tract. Am J Surg Pathol 14(Suppl 1):101, 1990

168. Snover DC, Filipovich AH, Ramsay NKC, et al: Graft-versus-host-like histopathological findings in pre-bone-marrow transplantation biopsies of patients with severe T cell deficiency. Transplantation 39:95, 1985

169. Drenick EJ, Ament ME, Finegold SM, et al: Bypass enteropathy. Intestinal and systemic manifestations following small-bowel bypass. JAMA 236:269, 1967

170. Causey JQ: Granulomatous colitis and ileitis complicating jejunoileal bypass. Arch Intern Med 138:1727, 1978

171. Francis WW, Iannuccilli E: Acute fulminating transmural ileocolitis after small bowel bypass for morbid obesity. Am J Surg 135:524, 1978

172. Glotzer DJ, Glick ME, Goldman H: Proctitis and colitis following diversion of the fecal stream. Gastroentrology 80:438, 1981

173. Ma CK, Gottlieb C, Haas PA: Diversion colitis: a clinicopathologic study of 21 cases. Hum Pathol 21:429, 1990

174. Komorowski RA: Histologic spectrum of diversion colitis. Am J Surg Pathol 14:548, 1990

175. Harig JM, Soergel KH, Komorowski RA, Wood CM: Treatment of diversion colitis with short-chain-fatty acid irrigation. N Engl J Med 320:23, 1989

176. Babior BM: Disorders of neutrophil function. p. 950. In Wyngaarden JB, Smith LH (eds): Cecil Textbook of Medicine. 17th Ed. WB Saunders, Philadelphia, 1985

177. Ament ME, Ochs HD: Gastrointestinal manifestations of chronic granulomatous disease. N Engl J Med 288:382, 1973

178. Sty JR, Chusid MJ, Babbitt DP, et al: Involvement of the colon in chronic granulomatous disease of childhood. Radiology 132:681, 1979

179. Werlin SL, Chusid MJ, Caya J, et al: Colitis in chronic granulomatous disease. Gastroenterology 82:328, 1982

180. Harris BH, Boles ET: Intestinal lesions in chronic granulomatous disease of childhood. J Pediatr Surg 8:955, 1973

181. Yogman MW, Touloukian RJ, Gallagher R: Intestinal granulomatosis in chronic granulomatous disease and in Crohn's disease. N Engl J Med 290:228, 1974

182. Strauss RG, Ghishan F, Mitros F, et al: Rectosigmoidal colitis in common variable immunodeficiency disease. Dig Dis Sci 25:798, 1980

183. Ament ME: Immunodeficiency syndromes and gastrointestinal disease. Pediatr Clin North Am 22:807, 1975

184. Jarry A, Cortez A, Rene E, et al: Infected cells and immune cells in the gastrointestinal tract of AIDS patients. An immunohistochemical study of 127 cases. Histopathology 16:133, 1990

185. Madea B, Roewert HJ, Krueger GRF, et al: Search for early lesions following human immunodeficiency virus type 1 infection. Arch Pathol Lab Med 114:379, 1990

186. Kotler DP, Gaetz HP, Lange M, et al: Enteropathy associated with the acquired immunodeficiency syndrome. Ann Intern Med 101:421, 1984

187. Crancer GE, Burdick GE: Acute colitis resembling ulcerative colitis in the hemolytic-uremic syndrome. Dig Dis 21:74, 1976

188. Whitington PF, Friedman AL, Chesney RW: Gastrointestinal disease in the hemolytic-uremic syndrome. Gastroenterology 76:728, 1979

189. Yates RS, Osterholm RK: Hemolytic-uremic syndrome colitis. J Clin Gastroenterol 2:359, 1980

190. Lakhanpal S, Tani K, Lie JT, et al: Pathologic features of Behcet's syndrome: a review of Japanese autopsy registry data. Hum Pathol 16:790, 1985

191. Lee RG: The colitis of Behcet's syndrome. Am J Surg Pathol 10:888, 1986

192. James DG: "Silk route disease" (Behcet's disease). West J Med 148:433, 1988

193. O'Connell DJ, Courtney JV, Riddell RH: Colitis of Behcet's syndrome—radiologic and pathologic features. Gastrointest Radiol 5:173, 1980

194. Lindstrom CG: "Collagenous colitis" with watery diarrhoea—a new entity? Pathol Eur 11:87, 1976

195. Hwang WS, Kelly JK, Shaffer EA, Hershfield NB: Collagenous colitis: a disease of pericryptal fibroblast sheath? J Pathol 149:33, 1986

196. Jessurun J, Yardley JH, Giardiello FM, et al: Chronic colitis with thickening of the subepithelial collagen layer (collagenous colitis): histopathologic findings in 15 patients. Hum Pathol 18:839, 1987

197. Kingham JGC, Levison DA, Morson BC, Dawson AM: Collagneous colitis. Gut 27:570, 1986

198. Teglbjaerg PS, Thaysen EH: Collagenous colitis: an ultrastructural study of a case. Gastroenterology 82:561, 1982

199. Bogomoletz WV, Adnet JJ, Birembaut P, et al: Collagenous colitis an unrecognized entity. Gut 21:164, 1980

200. Wang HH, Owings DV, Antonioli DA, Goldman H: Increased subepithelial collagen deposition is not specific for collagenous colitis. Mod Pathol 1:329, 1988

201. Giardiello FM, Bayless TM, Jessurun J, et al: Collagenous colitis: physiologic and histopathologic studies in seven patients. Ann Intern Med 106:46, 1987

202. Bo-Linn GW, Vendrell DD, Lee E., Fordtran JS: An evaluation of the significance of microscopic colitis in patients with chronic diarrhea. J Clin Invest 75:1559, 1985

203. Jessurun J, Yardley JH, Lee EL, et al: Letter. Gastroenterology 91:1584, 1986

204. Lazenby AJ, Yardley JH, Giardiello FM, et al: Lymphocytic ("microscopic") colitis: a

comparative histopathologic study with particular reference to collagenous colitis. Hum Pathol 20:18, 1989

205. Wang KK, Perrault J, Carpenter HA, et al: Collagenous colitis: a clinicopathologic correlation. Mayo Clin Proc 62:665, 1987

206. Butsch JL, Dockerty MB, McGill DB, et al: "Solitary" nonspecific ulcers of the colon. Arch Surg 98:171, 1969

207. Blundell CR, Earnes DL: Idiopathic cecal ulcer. Diagnosis by colonoscopy followed by nonoperative management. Digest Dis Sci 25:494, 1980

208. Mahoney TJ, Bubrick MP, Hitchcock CR: Nonspecific ulcers of the colon. Dis Colon Rectum 21:623, 1978

209. Smithwick W, Anderson RP, Ballinger WF: Nonspecific ulcer of the colon. Arch Surg 97:133, 1968

210. Warshaw AL, Welch JP, Ottinger LW: Acute perforation of the colon associated with chronic corticosteroid therapy. Am J Surg 131:442, 1976

211. Sutherland DER, Chan FY, Foucar E, et al: The bleeding cecal ulcer in transplant patients. Surgery 86:386, 1979

212. Komorowski RA, Cohen EB, Kauffman HM, Adams MB: Gastrointestinal complications in renal transplant recipients. Am J Clin Pathol 86:161, 1986

213. Bernardino ME, Lawson TL: Discrete colonic ulcers associated with oral contraceptives. Dig Dis 21:503, 1976

214. Debenham GP: Ulcer of the cecum during oxyphenbutazone (Tandearil) therapy. Can Med Assoc J 28:1182, 1976

215. Bravo AJ, Lowman RM: Benign ulcer of the sigmoid colon. Radiology 90:113, 1968

216. Williams KL: Acute solitary ulcers and acute diverticulitis of the cecum and ascending colon. Br J Surg 47:351, 1960

217. Dosik GM, Luna M, Valdivieso M, et al: Necrotizing colitis in patients with cancer. Am J Med 67:646, 1979

218. Steinberg D, Gold J, Brodin A: Necrotizing enterocolitis in leukemia. Arch Intern Med 131:528, 1973

219. Katz JA, Wagner ML, Gresik MV, et al: Typhlitis—an 18-year experience and postmortem review. Cancer 65:1041, 1990

220. Starnes HF, Jr, Moore FD, Jr, Mentzer S, et al: Abdominal pain in neutropenic cancer patients. Cancer 57:616, 1986

221. Kies MS, Luedke DW, Boyd JF, et al: Neutropenic enterocolitis. Two case reports of long-term survival following surgery. Cancer 43:730, 1979

222. Varki AP, Armitage JO, Feagler JR: Typhlitis in acute leukemia. Successful treatment by early surgical intervention. Cancer 43:695, 1979

223. Pokorney BH, Jones JM, Shaikh BS, et al: Typhlitis. A treatable cause of recurrent septicemia. JAMA 243:682, 1980

224. Sherman NJ, Woolley MM: The ileocecal syndrome in acute childhood leukemia. Arch Surg 107:39, 1973

225. Freeman JH, Rabeneck L, Owen D: Survival after necrotizing enterocolitis of leukemia treated with oral vancomycin. Gastroenterology 81:791, 1981

226. Caldwell JH, Mekhjian HS, Hurtubise PE, et al: Eosinophilic gastroenteritis with obstruction. Immunological studies of seven patients. Gastroenterology 74:825, 1978

227. Haberkern CM, Christie DL, Haas JE: Eosinophilic gastroenteritis presenting as ileocolitis. Gastroenterology 74:896, 1978

228. Partyka EK, Sanowski RA, Kozarek RA: Colonoscopic features of eosinophilic gastroenteritis. Dis Colon Rectum 23:353, 1980

229. Schulze K, Mitros FA: Eosinophilic gastroenteritis involving the ileocecal area. Dis Col Rect 47, 1979

230. Tedesco FJ, Huckaby CB, Hamby-Allen M, et al: Eosinophilic ileocolitis. expanding spectrum of eosinophilic gastroenteritis. Dig Dis Sci 26:943, 1981

231. Johnstone JM, Morson BC: Eosinophilic gastroenteritis. Histopathology 2:335, 1978

232. Klein NC, Hargrove RL, Sleisenger MH, et al: Eosinophilic gastritis. Medicine 49:299, 1970

233. Rosekrans PCM, Meijer CJLM, Van Der Wal AM, et al: Allergic proctitis, a clinical and immunopathological entity. Gut 21:1017, 1980

234. Jenkins HR, Pincott JR, Soothill JF et al: Food allergy: the major cause of infantile colitis. Arch Dis Child 59:326, 1984

235. Winter HS, Antonioli DA, Fukagawa N, et al: Allergy-related proctocolitis in infants: diagnostic usefulness of rectal biopsy. Mod Pathol 3:5, 1990

236. Goldman H, Proujansky R: Allergic proctitis and gastroenteritis in children: clinical and mucosal biopsy features in 53 cases. Am J Surg Pathol 10:75, 1986

3

Immunopathogenesis of Inflammatory Bowel Disease

David F. Keren

ETIOLOGIC AGENTS

The cause of Crohn's disease and ulcerative colitis is unknown. Consequently, the term *idiopathic* inflammatory bowel disease (IBD) aptly describes our present state of knowledge.

Several microorganisms have been suggested as possible etiologic agents in idiopathic IBD. However, there has been no *consistent* demonstration that these candidate microorganisms could be cultured reproducibly from diseased tissues or that the disease itself could be consistently passed by injecting tissue extracts into experimental animals.

Some earlier workers succeeded in producing lesions resembling IBD by injecting tissue extracts from patients with Crohn's disease into experimental animals and examining the lesions produced, both at the injection site and in the bowel.[1-6] More recent attempts by other workers failed to reproduce these lesions.[7-9] Further, independent study of the actual tissue sections purportedly displaying granulomas disclosed that some of the lesions from the earlier studies were not granulomas.[10, 11]

Whereas earlier studies on etiologic agents concentrated on uncommon or unusual bacteria, some recent studies have explored the possibility that an association may exist between more common microorganisms and IBD. Although several studies conflicting reports have appeared as to whether *Escherichia coli* were associated with IBD, a recent study by Burke and Axon found that patients with IBD were much more likely to possess adhesive *E. coli* in their stool than were patients with infectious diarrhea or in stool from control individuals.[12] There are also some parallels between the occurrence of *Campylobacter jejuni* colitis and IBD. These conditions share the pathologic features of acute colitis and a similarity in age of occurrence (second and third decades of life). However, no relationship was found in microbiologic, serologic, and immunohistochemical study of the occurrence of *C. jejuni* to implicate these bacteria in the pathogenesis of IBD.[13] The role of microbiologic agents in IBD is still problematic. At this point in time, no exceptionally attractive candidate has been demonstrated. A review of proposed agents by Beeken provides a good overview of this area.[14]

CLASSIC INFLAMMATORY REACTIONS

In the past 15 years, numerous experimental models for IBD have been produced. Many of these models have as their basis an immune-mediated mechanism. Indeed, many histopathologic features of IBD could be explained by invoking already-known immunologic mechanisms.

The classic acute inflammation and cryptitis seen in active IBD is consistent with features known to result from the Arthus reaction (Fig. 3-1). In the Arthus reaction, pre-existing antibodies react with antigen when it is injected

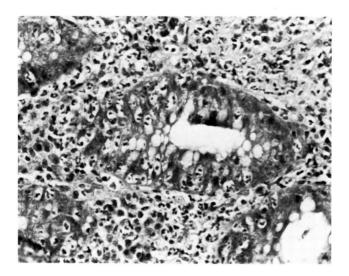

Fig. 3-1. Photomicrograph of active IBD with neutrophils invading surface epithelium. (H&E, ×330.)

locally; usually this occurs in vessel walls. The antigen-antibody complexes deposit in the vessel walls and activate complement locally. There is some evidence that in IBD, the initial complement activation may be related to immune complex deposition or damage to the surface epithelial cells (see below). The complement activation sets up a chemotactic gradient, which encourages granulocytes to enter this region. While the granulocytes phagocytose the immune complexes, they release superoxide radicals and digestive enzymes that damage the epithelial surface and lamina propria. Such a mechanism is already well documented in renal disease. Another mechanism for acute injury in IBD involves cytotoxic antibodies directed against surface epithelial cells. This would result in complement activation at that site with damage to the integrity of the epithelial barrier. Such a direct antiepithelial cell phenomenon is key to the pathogenesis of glomerular destruction in patients with Goodpasture's disease.

In patients with ulcerative colitis and Crohn's disease of the colon, it has been difficult to demonstrate immune complexes beneath the epithelium. However, recent studies have shown significantly more deposition of terminal complement components (C5b-9) in patients with IBD than in controls. This suggests that, although the changes may be subtle, there is excessive complement activation locally in patients with IBD[15] (Fig. 3-2).

Other evidence of increased acute inflammatory mediator activity in IBD includes the presence of significantly raised fecal concentrations of the serum protease prohibitor (serpin) α_1-antitrypsin in patients with IBD. Fecal α_1-antitrypsin levels have been recommended to assess disease activity. The clinical disease activity in IBD also correlates with the sedimentation rate and acute phase reactants.[16]

Another important protein involved in inflammation and repair processes is fibronectin. This large glycoprotein is known to bind to fibroblasts and to interact with connective tissue during inflammation and repair. Lower concentrations of plasma fibronectin are found in patients with Crohn's disease than in healthy controls. Indeed, individuals with more extensive disease had significantly lower levels of plasma fibronectin than those with disease confined to only one segment of the bowel (Crohn's disease). Allan and coworkers suggest that extent of disease is more important than severity in determining the plasma fibronectin concentration. Interestingly, higher plasma fibronectin levels are also positively related to the presence of strictures.[17]

Other inflammatory mediators that are better understood in IBD are the leukotrienes. Leukotrienes are products of arachidonic acid metabo-

Fig. 3-2. Staining for terminal complement complex in a colon specimen from a patient with ulcerative colitis. Intense fluorescence staining is seen in the submucosal vessel walls (arrows). (From Halstensen et al.,[15] with permission.)

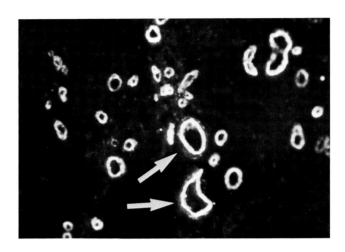

lism that have been shown to be important inflammatory mediators with regard to their chemotactic potential. They are especially effective in increasing vascular permeability. Patients with IBD have increased levels of leukotriene B_4 (LTB$_4$), which is released into the rectal fluids in considerably greater amounts than in controls.[18, 19] In a recent study, Wallace and colleagues determined that suppression of LTB$_4$ synthesis significantly improved healing following administration of an intracolonic irritant in their rat model of IBD. These findings indicate that leukotrienes play a key role in the pathogenesis of injury in IBD. Furthermore, use of agents that inhibit LTB$_4$ are a logical approach for future therapy.[20]

Indeed, patients with IBD have been shown to have increased neutrophil receptors for the proinflammatory bacterial peptide formylmethionyl-leucyl-phenylalanine (FMLP), as well as an enhanced response when this chemotactic peptide is presented in vitro.[21] Some workers have been so impressed by the potential role of acute inflammation in IBD that they have employed extreme measures, such as methotrexate therapy, as both an antimetabolite and an anti-inflammatory agent.[22]

The potent inflammatory factor bacterial FMLP has several effects in vitro, including promoting chemotaxis, adhesion, and release of damaging enzymes and superoxide radicals from leukocytes. Several different species of intestinal bacteria produce these peptides.[23, 24] In one model system for acute colitis, colonic inflammation was produced in rodents by instillation of FMLP into the colon. This resulted in edema and an acute inflammatory infiltrate within 2 hours. Thus, classic acute inflammatory reactions in IBD may relate to a change in mucosa that allows bacterial products such as FMLP to initiate chemotaxis of granulocytes.[25]

The chronic changes in IBD show crypt distortion, increased numbers of plasma cells, and increased numbers of lymphocytes in the lamina propria (Fig. 3-3). The distorted crypts clearly relate to a repair process that follows acute cryptitis. The increased numbers of plasma cells in the lamina propria of patients with IBD could have at least two possible meanings. They may increase secondarily to enhanced local antigenic stimulation following damage to the surface epithelium, which allows numerous intraluminal products to gain access to the gut mucosa. Alternatively, these plasma cells may produce antibodies that mediate local tissue damage. These lymphocytic accumulations and granulomas seen in IBD parallel the classic picture seen in chronic delayed-type hypersensitivity reactions. It is not clear whether this reflects ongoing antigenic stimulation (producing chronicity) or poor antigen processing owing to altered or inefficient immune reactivity. The latter would result in

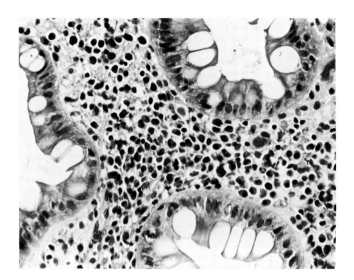

Fig. 3-3. Chronic IBD with large numbers of plasma cells and lymphocytes in lamina propria. (H&E, ×330.)

a chronic inflammatory response even though the antigen was present only occasionally along the gut mucosa.

Experimental evidence has been gathered that invokes all of these mechanisms and explores other newly described mechanisms for immunologically mediated injury for surface epithelial damage in IBD. These ideas are discussed in the next sections. There are no easy answers offered here. The many studies of the immunopathologic mechanisms in IBD frequently present conflicting information owing to the complexity of the disease and the subtle differences of the methods used to examine the different aspects of the mucosal immune response.

ROLE OF IMMUNE COMPLEXES

In some studies, circulating immune complexes have been detected in the sera of patients with IBD.[26, 27] It is possible that these circulating immune complexes relate to the pathogenesis of IBD by depositing in the gut epithelial basement membrane, thereby initiating a local Arthus-type reaction, as discussed above. Indeed, an ultrastructural study by Otto[28] indicates that both IgG and complement can be found beneath the epithelium in the colon of patients with IBD.

Experimental models have demonstrated that immune complexes can play a role in producing a histopathologic lesion that resembles IBD. For example, Hodgson and co-workers[29] and Mee and co-workers[30] found that when preformed immune complexes were injected intravenously into rabbits and a nonspecific irritation was simultaneously created by a dilute formalin enema, a severe colitis that histologically resembled acute IBD resulted. In other studies, Rhodes and co-workers[31] found that hydroxychloroquine administration prevented the experimental immune complex-mediated colitis in rabbits. The mechanism of hydroxychloroquine is ascribed to inhibition of leukocyte motility, presumably interrupting this effector arm of the acute inflammatory response.

However, studies that question the role of immune complexes in IBD have also been reported. Notably, a study by Kemler and Alpert[32] found that most patients with chronic IBD had no circulating immune complexes when assayed by a sensitive Raji cell technique. In addition, Kemler and Alpert reported that the immune complexes detected did not correlate with disease severity, type, or location. This correlation would be of key importance if immune complexes played a role in initiating IBD. Soltis and co-workers[33] have suggested that aggregated immunoglobulins may have erroneously been interpreted as immune complexes in patients with IBD. They found no significant difference between IBD patients and controls when immune complexes were assayed using the C1q precipitation technique.

Another interesting, although poorly understood, phenomenon has been described by Leroux-Roels and colleagues[34] in serum samples from patients with IBD. Among the 20 patients with IBD that they studied, alkaline phosphatase-immunoglobulin complexes were found in three patients and lactic dehydrogenase-immunoglobulin complexes were found in two others. Such formation of complexes between immunoglobulins and enzymes is not unique to IBD.[35] However, it is unusual for such enzyme-immunoglobulin complexes to be associated with a particular disease.

INFLAMMATORY MEDIATORS

Whether or not immune complexes are initiating epithelial injury in IBD, it is clear that local inflammation is involved in the mucosal damage. There is strong evidence that components of complement and prostaglandins are activated in patients with IBD. For instance, these individuals have an increased synthesis and catabolism of C3 in the serum.[36, 37] In addition, decreased serum concentrations of the complement alternative pathway components properdin and properdin convertase were found by Lake and colleagues.[38] Potter and co-workers[39] found that catabolism and synthesis of C1q are increased in patients with IBD. These findings of activation of C1q, C3, and properdin factors suggest that both the classic and alternative pathways of complement may be part of the inflammatory process in IBD. Unfortunately, conflicting information makes a simple interpretation of this information impossible. In other studies, Lake and co-workers[40] were not able to detect abnormalities of the classic complement pathway components, and Ward and Eastwood[41] found normal levels of C2 in patients with active IBD.

Inhibitors of the complement system include C1 INH (C1 esterase inhibitor) and C3b INA (C3b inactivator). These inhibitors act as a negative balance to prevent overactivation of complement by trivial stimuli. Studies by Potter and coworkers demonstrated increased concentrations of both inhibitors in patients with active IBD.[42] Such increased levels of inhibitor are consistent with the increased synthesis and catabolism of both the C3 and C1q described above.

In addition to complement, it is clear that prostaglandins play an important role in mediating inflammatory reactions. High serum levels of prostaglandin have been reported in patients with ulcerative colitis.[43] This increase in prostaglandins in patients with ulcerative colitis may be due to a rate of synthesis of prostaglandin E_2 that is twice normal.[44] Further, in vivo studies by Rampton and co-workers[45] indicated that prostaglandin E_2-like material obtained by rectal dialysis was increased significantly in patients with both active and inactive ulcerative colitis. The levels were increased 3-fold in patients with ulcerative colitis in remission, but 13-fold in those patients with active disease.

Using an in vitro organ culture system, Hawkey and Truelove[46] found that the mean synthesis of prostaglandin E_2 by inflamed IBD tissues was significantly greater than that of noninflamed tissues (Fig. 3-4). By incubating these tissues with prednisolone, this increased synthesis of prostaglandin E_2 could be inhibited. The source of the prostaglandin E_2 was traced to the peripheral blood mononuclear cells in patients with active Crohn's disease.[47] These patients had peripheral blood mononuclear cells with 2 to 3 times the level of prostaglandin E_2 synthesis compared to control cells. In addition, the peripheral blood mononuclear cells from patients with Crohn's disease had an increased synthesis of thromboxane B2.

The increased synthesis of prostaglandins could be inhibited in vitro by sulfasalazine.[48] However, when 14 patients with active ulcerative colitis were treated with flurbiprofen or prednisolone enemas and/or sulfasalazine, no evidence was found for efficacy of the prostaglandin inhibitor in decreasing symptoms; but prostaglandin E_2 in rectal dialysis fluids de-

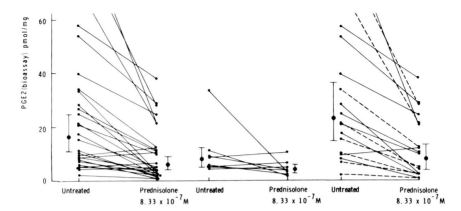

Fig. 3-4. Prostaglandin E_2 levels produced in organ culture from all biopsies (left), uninflamed (center), and inflamed (right) tissues from patients with IBD. Note the effect of prednisolone to decrease prostaglandin E_2 production, especially in inflamed tissue (right). (From Hawkey & Truelove,[46] with permission.)

creased when either conventional therapy (prednisolone with or without sulfasalazine) or flurbiprofen therapy was initiated.[49] Indeed, flurbiprofen alone may have had a deleterious effect on rectal mucosal electrical potential difference, perhaps because of its action as a cyclooxygenase inhibitor. When respect to the altered immunologic reactivity demonstrated in patients with IBD, it is not clear whether the increased prostaglandin synthesis is causing such reactions or whether the increased synthesis is merely the result of mucosal injury.[50]

PHAGOCYTE FUNCTION

Despite the evidence of systemic activation of complement components in patients with IBD, studies of leukocyte function in these patients indicate that their directed migration into experimentally induced areas of injury is retarded compared to controls.[51] By using the skin window technique, Morain and colleagues[52] and, independently, Wandall and Binder[53] found that neutrophils in vivo from patients with Crohn's disease have a decreased ability to migrate into these chambers. The impaired migration was correlated neither with disease severity nor with drug therapy. Studies by Rhodes and colleagues[54] implicated a 7S

serum inhibitor, precipitable by 40 percent ammonium sulfate in the inhibition of neutrophil migration into skin windows. Furthermore, these serum chemotactic factor inhibitors are nonspecific in that similar inhibitory activity was present, albeit to a lesser extent in the 7S fraction of normal serum.[55] Yet, when monocytes and neutrophils from patients with IBD were studied in vitro, they had increased random motility and chemotaxis compared to control phagocytes.[56] This implied that although the cells were able to respond properly, a defective signal for chemotaxis was likely responsible for the impaired ability of leukocytes to migrate into the skin window. The defect has been shown to be related to a decreased release of the important chemotactic factor C5a during inflammation rather than due to a defect in the neutrophils themselves.[57] Of course, it may merely reflect the fact that so much complement is being activated owing to the acute injury in the bowel that there is insufficient circulating C5 to deal with other stimuli in some of these patients.

In addition to poor chemotaxis in vivo, there is good evidence that neutrophils from patients with IBD are not effective in phagocytosing and destroying ingested microorganisms. Mahida and colleagues[58] reported that populations of phagocytic cells are different in IBD colon compared with control tissues. They used monoclonal antibody RFD9 (which reacts with epithe-lioid cells and tingible body macrophages) and 3G8 (which labels the Fc gamma receptor on polymorphonuclear neutrophils, natural killer cells, and some macrophages) in immunohisto-chemical studies of tissues from patients with IBD. They found that the pattern of staining with these monoclonal antibodies in IBD tissues was different from that which is seen in infec-tious colitis. These different proportions of phagocytes in patients with untreated Crohn's disease may explain why they have a deficient production of hydrogen peroxide and why pa-tients with both ulcerative colitis and Crohn's disease have a significantly reduced production of superoxide anion as well as a decreased amount of the cytoprotective enzyme superoxide dismutase.[59, 60] Taken together, one can specu-late that the poor chemotaxis of leukocytes to areas where foreign material accumulates offers one explanation for the chronic granulomatous inflammation in Crohn's disease. This ineffec-tual effort by the acute inflammatory response may account for the persistent antigen and in-creased numbers of macrophages and chronic inflammatory cells in the lamina propria of these patients.

AUTOCYTOTOXIC PHENOMENA

HUMORAL PHENOMENA

Twenty-five years ago, anticolon antibodies were detected in the serum of IBD patients by Broberger and Perlman.[61] Later, Carlsson and co-workers documented an increased titer of anticolon antibodies in 60 percent of patients with Crohn's disease, but only in 13 percent of control individuals.[62] Nonetheless, 13 percent is far too high a number in the controls to make this a useful screening test for diagnosis. The specificity of this antibody is far from clear because the greatest prevalence of this antibody was found among patients who had urinary tract infection or cirrhosis (69 and 62 percent respec-tively). More recent studies of serum from pa-tients with IBD have revealed other antibodies directed at colonic epithelial antigens that appear to be more specific for IBD. Auer and co-work-ers found that specific cytotoxic IgG antibodies against the colon cancer cell line RPMI 4788 could be detected in the serum of 29 percent of patients with ulcerative colitis, 3 percent of patients with Crohn's disease, and in none of the healthy controls when a 4-hour cytotoxicity assay was used. The nature of the antigen is not yet known, however, by absorption studies it was found to be particularly prevalent in co-lonic tissue from patients with ulcerative colitis, although it is also present in normal bowel, liver, and kidney.[63] There is other evidence for altered antigen expression in mucosa from pa-tients with IBD. Haviland and colleagues found that colonic mucosa from patients with ulcer-ative colitis had increased expression of anti-genic determinants recognized by monoclonal antibodies to mucin-like glycoproteins uniquely associated with tumor cells.[64] It is not known if these unique determinants are related to the cytotoxic antibodies against colonic epithelium, which preferentially occurs in IBD patients.

Roche and colleagues found that there was a high incidence of humoral immunity against an epithelial cell-associated component (ECAC) (macromolecule) from human intestinal epithe-lium in patients with IBD.[65] Further, there was evidence for genetic linkage of the disease, since 57 percent of first-degree relatives of patients with IBD had titers of antibodies against ECAC two standard deviations greater than control lev-els when assayed by an antibody-dependent cell-mediated cytotoxicity (ADCC) (see below) reac-tion, whereas 73 percent of IBD patients had this level of reactivity. Nonetheless, the phe-nomenon is not specific enough to be used for diagnosis because 27 percent of patients with other gastrointestinal inflammations and 10 per-cent of patients with autoimmune disease were positive.[66] Another candidate antibody for mu-cosal damage in IBD is antienterobacterial com-mon antigen, which, as shown by Bull,[67] has acitivity against gut epithelium. Despite their lack of proven specificity for IBD, these antibod-ies add support to the notion that a cytotoxic mechanism for IBD involving humoral immu-

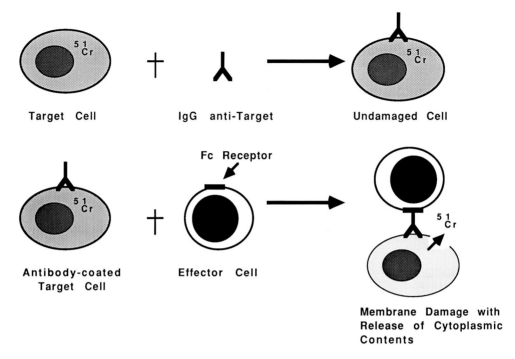

Fig. 3-5. Schematic representation of ADCC.

nity would be a plausible explanation for mucosal damage in patients with IBD.

CELLULAR PHENOMENA

Although humoral immunity directed against colonic epithelial components has been found repeatedly in patients with IBD, the mechanism by which these antibodies cause damage is obscure. One possible mechanism for this injury is ADCC. This mechanism is defined by an in vitro test involving mixing specific antibodies against target cells that contain cromium 51 (^{51}Cr) in the cytoplasm (Fig. 3-5). The specificity of the cytotoxicity is due to the recognition of antigenic determinants on the target cell by the antibody. However, no damage occurs to the cell (no ^{51}Cr is released) assuming that complement has not been added to the system. When effector cells, which include null lymphocytes, macrophages, neutrophils, or eosinophils, are added, they are able to attach to the antibody and mediate damage to the cytoplasmic membrane measured by the release of ^{51}Cr.

Fanger and co-workers[68] found that peripheral blood monocytes and polymorphonuclear leukocytes bear surface receptors for IgA. Further, there is some evidence that IgA can mediate ADCC.[69–72] Interepithelial lymphocytes (see below) can effect this form of cytotoxicity in experimental animals.[73] Eosinophils may be important in host defense using an ADCC mechanism with parasites.[74] This indicates that there is the potential for this type of mechanism in inflammatory conditions along the bowel.

There is evidence that some type of cell-mediated tissue damage occurs in IBD. Several years ago, Shorter and colleagues[75] demonstrated that mononuclear cells from the peripheral blood of patients with IBD, in the absence of complement, were able to kill in vitro cultured colonic epithelial cells. Furthermore, since the cytotoxic ability of peripheral blood mononuclear cells from these patients could no longer be demonstrated 10 days following colectomy, it was assumed to be related to the disease. However, no specific antibodies were detected in these studies. The effector cells for this phenomenon were null lymphocytes (neither T nor B cells) and are especially prevalent in mesenteric lymph nodes from patients with Crohn's disease, compared to control lymph nodes. It has been suggested that this may be a form of ADCC in which the effector cells carry the antibody to the target.[76]

Although these processes are still poorly understood, since many IBD patients have circulating antibodes that react with colonic epithelium and effector cells exist in the colon that can mediate ADCC, one can envision how ADCC provides a plausible explanation for mucosal damage in patients with IBD. However, a direct connection between the possible local production of cytotoxic antibodies for colonic epithelium and possible mucosal ADCC has not been made. Perhaps these studies will require the use of effector cells and secretory antibodies isolated directly from the intestinal epithelial layer and lamina propria.

LOCAL ANTIBODY PRODUCTION

Antibodies along the mucosal surface of the bowel are mainly secretory IgA produced by plasma cells in the lamina propria. The number of plasma cells in the lamina propria of the bowel is directly proportional to the degree of antigenic stimulation.[77] The number of immunoglobulin-containing cells in the lamina propria of colonic mucosa from patients with IBD may relate to the pathogenesis of IBD and has been studied by several groups.

By using immunohistochemistry on frozen sections of bowel from patients with either acute or chronic IBD, most workers have found increased numbers of all types of plasma cells in the lamina propria as compared to control bowel.[78–85] There have been some conflicting data in these studies owing to the fact that most studies examined relatively few samples and most examined only the extreme examples of

disease activity. In a recent descriptive study, MacDermott and co-workers found that there was a quantitative difference in the subclasses that are present in the serum of patients with IBD compared to controls, and to serum from patients with systemic lupus erythematosus. Patients with ulcerative colitis had a significantly increased IgG1 levels.[86] This is interesting because mononuclear cells isolated from the colonic specimens of patients with ulcerative colitis and Crohn's disease spontaneously secrete more IgG1 and IgG2, respectively, than control colon.[87] The same increase in IgG1 and IgG2 has been demonstrated by immunohistochemistry.[88]

Studies that related immunohistochemical findings to disease activity consistently have found a positive correlation between the histopathologic index of activity and the number of immunoglobulin-containing cells in the lamina propria.[83, 89] Most of the cases in which there was an increase in the number of IgG-containing plasma cells had focal proliferations of these cells. In contrast, the increase in IgA- and IgM-containing plasma cells was diffuse. This implies that a different mode of antigenic stimulation may occur in different parts of the bowel from patients with IBD.

The numbers of immunoglobulin-containing cells in the lamina propria also may be a useful parameter in distinguishing acute self-limited colitis (ASLC) from active IBD. Today, ASLC is thought to be due to various infectious agents. It has some features that are reminiscent of active IBD, including cryptitis, crypt abscesses, and regenerative surface epithelium. However, it lacks crypt distortion, has relatively normal numbers of plasma cells in the lamina propria, and does not have granulomas, crypt atrophy, or basal lymphoid aggregates often seen in IBD.[90] Nostrant and colleagues emphasized the importance of plasmacytosis extending to the base of the mucosa with mucosal distortion in ulcerative colitis. These features were absent in ASLC.[91] The morphologic differences are due to the fact that ASLC is an acute process where, prior to the present episode, the crypt epithelium had not been injured and, conse-

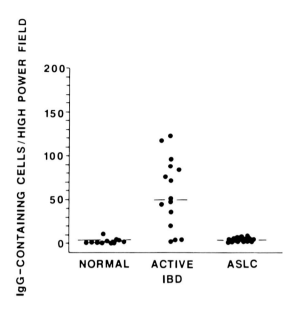

Fig. 3-6. IgG-containing plasma cells were compared in colon from patients with no histologic abnormality (normal), patients with active chronic IBD disease (active IBD) and acute self-limited colitis (ASLC). The presence of increased numbers of plasma cells highly favored a diagnosis of active IBD. (From Keren et al.[93] with permission.)

quently, had not undergone the regenerative and repair changes that lead to crypt distortion.

Van Spreeuwel and co-workers found significantly fewer IgG-containing plasma cells in the bowel from patients with ASLC compared to the active IBD.[92] Similarly, in our studies on formalin-fixed, paraffin-embedded bowel, we found that quantification of the numbers of IgG, IgA, and IgM plasma cells in the lamina propria was useful in providing quantitative information to help in the differential diagnosis of difficult cases[93] (Fig. 3-6). The difference in the plasma cell content between IBD and ASLC reflects the time required for stimulation of a mucosal immune response. In IBD there has been considerable antigenic stimulation in the past, thus there is an ongoing inflammation with a rapid mucosal memory response. With mucosal memory responses, after local stimulation in the gastrointestinal tract, it takes 2 to 4 days before large numbers of plasma cells reactive to this antigen can home to the lamina propria. The initial (primary) mucosal immune response to an antigen is relatively weak and doesn't peak

until about 2 weeks after stimulation. This is why when plasma cell content is examined late in the course of ASLC, it is more likely to be confused with an acute exacerbation of IBD. The patchy or focal nature of the ASLC response causes it to resemble Crohn's disease, especially in the later stages of ASLC.

There has been disagreement as to whether the number of IgE-containing plasma cells are increased in the colon from patients with IBD. The first studies published by Lloyd and colleagues[94] demonstrated a slight decrease in the number of IgE-containing cells in the colon specimens from patients with Crohn's colitis as compared to control colon. However, O'Donoghue and Kumar[95] found a markedly increased number of IgE-containing plasma cells in rectal biopsy specimens from patients with IBD. This discrepancy can be resolved if allergic proctitis is considered to be a distinct entity from ulcerative proctitis. Heatley and colleagues[96] first suggested this possibility. Rosekrans and co-workers[97] demonstrated a marked increase in the number of IgE-containing

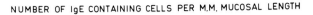

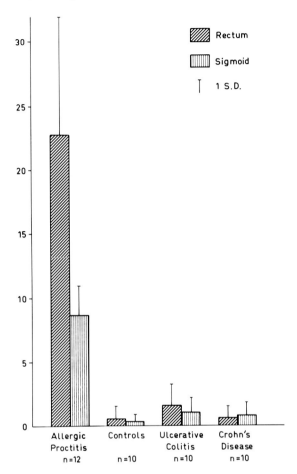

Fig. 3-7. IgE-containing cells are increased in the bowel of patients with allergic proctitis. (Data from Rosekrans et al.[83])

cells in the lamina propria of rectal biopsies from 8 to 12 patients with allergic proctitis but not in patients with ulcerative colitis or Crohn's disease (Fig. 3-7). Their findings were confirmed by Murdoch and Piris, who used monoclonal antibodies against IgE to demonstrate that positively stained cells were rarely found in either patients with ulcerative colitis or controls.[98] All of the patients with allergic proctitis responded to therapy with disodium chromoglycate.[99] It seems likely that earlier reports of increased numbers of IgE-containing plasma cells in patients with IBD were really cases of allergic proctitis. This information may also explain the earlier suggestions that some

cases of ulcerative colitis may be related to allergy.[99, 100]

Another feature found using immunohistochemical studies of the secretory immune system in patients with IBD relates to the immunoglobulins in the intestinal epithelium and the J chain in the plasma cells. Normally, IgA is secreted as a dimer by the plasma cells in the lamina propria. J chain is a small, 12,000-dalton polypeptide made by these plasma cells that binds the IgA together as dimers. It also serves to link pentameric IgM. Interestingly, both secretory component in the surface epithelial cells and J-chain expression in colonic plasma cells are decreased in patients with IBD, perhaps reflecting a rapid synthesis and secretion of IgA using up both the J chain in the plasma cell cytoplasm and the secretory component in the epithelium.[101]

The functional significance of these immunohistochemical studies is unclear. There is no information presently available that conclusively states that the increased numbers of plasma cells or that the alterations in plasma cell subclass populations in ulcerative colitis and Crohn's disease relate to the pathogenesis of the histologic lesions observed, or to the clinical picture in IBD. It is this author's view that the increased numbers of immunoglobulin-containing cells in the lamina propria of patients with IBD mainly reflect the result of IBD injury rather than the cause of it. That is, after injury has occurred to the surface epithelium, large numbers of antigens become readily available to the gut lamina propria. A tremendous immune response of both a local and systemic nature results in the large numbers of plasma cells that are seen. It is possible that a few of the plasma cells in the gut lamina propria are making either anticolon antibodies, as described earlier, or other antibodies reacting with the gut epithelium. Indeed, the disparity in the IgG subclasses that are found in controls, ulcerative colitis, and Crohn's disease suggests a differential effect that may be due to specific subisotype expansion to particular stimuli (which are as yet unknown). As better tools, such as monoclonal antibodies, which can react with specific anti-idiotype specificities of the antibodies being produced by the plasma cells, become available, we may be able to determine whether or not such anticolon epithelial antibodies are indeed initiating mucosal injury in IBD.

CELL-MEDIATED IMMUNITY

Because we have not yet identified the microorganism or antigen common to IBD, we have expanded considerable efforts searching through the maze of immunoregulatory cells to find abnormalities that may point to the pathogenesis or that may give further clues for treatment of IBD. Unfortunately, since these patients often have severe acute inflammatory reactions owing to their disease (see above), or are being treated with immunosuppressive therapy to allay their symptoms, there is considerable background noise with which investigators must contend.

Looking at the published data for an etiologic agent is like trying to hear a particular note played by a piccolo at the height of Beethoven's Fifth Symphony. Nonetheless, some of the observations on cell-mediated immunity help us to explain the humoral events described above. For instance, increased immunoglobulin synthesis in IBD may be partly due to disordered regulation of synthesis by lamina propria lymphocytes from patients with IBD. Verspaget and co-workers found that lamina propria mononuclear cells from patients with Crohn's disease differed greatly from control lamina propria mononuclear cells in their regulation of immunoglobulin synthesis in vitro.[102]

Part of the disordered regulation may relate to increased antigen processing cells in the lamina propria of patients with IBD. It is known that dendritic macrophages that bear class II major histocompatability complex (MHC) antigens are involved in presenting antigens to lymphocytes.[103] Using two monoclonal antibodies that react with these dendritic cells, Seldenrijk and colleagues found that the locations of dendritic cells and scavenger macrophages differ.[104] Normally, scavenger macrophages are found beneath the colonic epithelium. However, in both Crohn's disease and ulcerative colitis, these scavenger macrophages were found lining the bottom of ulcerated areas. In contrast, normal gut dendritic cells were present just above the muscularis mucosae or in T-cell regions of lymphoid follicles, whereas in IBC, these were usually seen together with accumulations of T lymphocytes outside of the scavenger macrophages at the base of ulcerations. These scavenger macrophages are likely presenting antigen to the associated T lymphocytes. The T lymphocytes would then function to enhance or suppress the immunologic response depending on their genetic predisposition.

In IBD there is evidence for defective suppression in the ability of T lymphocytes to inhibit self-reactivity. Kelleher and colleagues found that the autologous mixed lymphocyte reaction (an in vitro test for the ability of T cells to respond to self-antigens) demonstrated a marked defect in suppressor T-cell function to inhibit IgG, IgA, and IgM production in patients with IBD.[105] Irradiated T lymphocytes from patients with Crohn's disease effected a significantly greater increase in IgA production in vitro than control T lymphocytes.[105.] Again, this may relate to the eventual production of antibodies directed against epithelial antigens. Occasionally, however, patients with excessive suppressor T-cell functions resulting in hypogammaglobulinemia have been described.[106] This suggests that a nonsystematic alteration in T-cell activity exists in these individuals. Nonsystematic processes are always more difficult to make sense of than systematic ones, and may help us to understand the diverse, occasionally conflicting information that has been produced on samples from patients with IBD.

In addition to the altered humoral immune status in patients with IBD, the delayed-type hypersensitivity response is poor in patients with IBD. Impaired skin test responses to paraphenylenediamine (PPD) have been recorded, and cutaneous anergy to dinitrochlorobenzene (DNCB) has been found in patients with IBD.[107] As confirmation of these in vivo events, in vitro studies have demonstrated poor reactivity in lymphocytes from the peripheral blood of patients with IBD when these lymphocytes were mixed with normal lymphocytes.[108]

Attempts to explain the altered cellular responses included earlier studies on peripheral blood T and B lymphocytes that provided only marginally useful information. Differences in helper and suppressor populations were determined first with crude labels such as Fc receptors for IgM and later with monoclonal antibodies specific for various lymphocyte subpopulations. Other studies on the T-cell responses in IBD

patients who were either clinically well or only moderately ill (not requiring high doses of steroids to control their symptoms) found no significant decreased responsiveness in the allogeneic and autologous mixed lymphocyte reaction or in cytotoxic capabilities in cell-mediated lympholysis studies.[109] Even studies enumerating T-cell subpopulations in the peripheral blood have found little evidence of grossly altered populations.[110] However, functional studies using monoclonal antibodies to the CD3 component of T lymphocyte surface membrane to bypass the requirement for antigen triggering in T-cell cytotoxicity studies have found significantly increased levels of T-cell cytotoxicity in patients with IBD. Even more interesting, this increased T-cell cytotoxicity persisted postcolectomy in patients with ulcerative colitis, suggesting that there may be a fundamental hyperresponsiveness associated with the disease.[111]

Similar to studies on the capabilities of T lymphocytes, studies of natural killer cell activity in the peripheral blood yield controversy and conflicting data. Natural killer lymphocytes are thought to be part of host defense against virally infected cells and against neoplastic transformation.[112] Although the numbers of circulating natural killer cells have been found to be normal when using surface marker techniques, their functional activity has been found to be impaired[113] in one study, whereas another with similar methodology found a wide variation in activity with no significant difference from controls.[114] A decrease in natural killer lymphocyte activity would be consistent with the proclivity of these patients to develop colon cancer.

Another functional capability of lymphocytes is to suppress production of antibody by B cells or to suppress the cytotoxic activities of antigen-specific killer T lymphocytes. Once again, we must sort through conflicting evidence for a defect in the activities of suppressor T lymphocytes in patients with IBD. On the one hand, in 1978 Hodgson and colleagues found that suppressor T-cell activity was decreased in 7 of 11 patients with IBD. Since suppressor T cells are important in preventing autoimmune disease in some experimental animal models of systemic lupus erythematosus,[115] the decreased numbers of suppressor T cells may be related to the development of autoreactive phenomena such as the anticolon epithelial cell antibodies and lymphocytotoxic antibodies described above. In addition, studies by Ginsburg and Falchuk found that the activation of suppressor T cells from the peripheral blood of patients with IBD was diminished in 44 of the 51 patients with IBD that they examined. Their finding was independent of disease type, activity, or steroid therapy.[116]

Decrease in suppressor cell activity, however, may only be relative to the techniques used to assess it. Elson and colleagues[117] used a technique that involved separating the suppressor cell population in vitro, and found that the suppressor T-cell activity was not impaired by this technique in patients with IBD. Further, other workers used cell mixing studies to demonstrate that the lamina propria lymphocytes from patients with IBD markedly suppressed the mitogen responses of their autologous peripheral blood lymphocytes.[118]

Holdstock and co-workers[119] found that patients with IBD have increased numbers of indomethecin-sensitive prostaglandi-producing supressor T cells in the peripheral blood, whether or not patients had active disease. These findings may explain the increased levels of prostaglandin in the dialysates of the colon described above. Since the system that Holdstock and colleagues used to measure suppressor T-cell activity[119] is different from that used by Victorino and Hodgson,[120] it is not clear if the same cell populations were being studied. More recently, both Kelleher and colleagues and Ginsburg and Falchuk found decreased suppression of allogeneic mixed lymphocyte responses in these patients.[105, 121]

It is very difficult to sort out the significance of the suppressor cell studies. These studies use different techniques to isolate the cells for study, and have different assay systems for suppression. Perhaps one can only safely conclude that a dysregulation of mucosal immune function exists.

LOCAL LYMPHOCYTE FUNCTION IN THE GUT

One difficulty with the above studies of peripheral blood lymphocytes and monocytes in patients with IBD is that they may not be relevant to events occurring at the mucosal surface. Recent studies have begun to examine the cells in the mucosa itself, which may be more likely to provide us with useful information about mechanisms of damage at the gut surface epithelium. For many years it has been known that lymphocytes existed both within the lamina propria and also within the epithelium (Fig. 3-8). Today, it is clear that these are viable, active cells.

Studies by several groups have documented that the interepithelial lymphocytes and the lamina propria lymphocytes are different populations of cells with different activities. While both populations of cells are overwhelmingly T lymphocytes, the interepithelial lymphocytes are mainly CD8 positive suppressor/cytotoxic cells and the lamina propria lymphocytes are mainly CD4 positive helper T lymphocytes.[122] Although interepithelial lymphocytes are in close proximity to the surrounding absorptive epithelial and goblet cells, ultrastructural studies indicate that there is no attachment to the latter. By using immunohistochemistry, Selby and colleagues found that the ratio of CD4 (T helper) to CD8 (T suppressor) lymphocytes in the intraepithelial and lamina propria layers of the bowel were the same as in control samples.[123]

Both of these mucosal lymphocyte populations contain cytotoxic lymphocytes. Some of these may have relevance for IBD. For instance, a report by Roche and co-workers indicates that cytotoxic T lymphocytes also exist in the lamina propria from patients with IBD and react with purified ECAC in vitro.[124]

The functions of the lymphoid cells are controlled by the intercellular communication mechanism using lymphokines. Interleukin 1 (IL-1) is secreted by macrophages and serves as endogenous pyrogen, elicits production of acute phase proteins such as α_1-antitrypsin and haptoglobin from the liver, and activates T

Fig. 3-8. Intraepithelial lymphocyte (arrows) be tween epithelial cells. (H&E, ×825.)

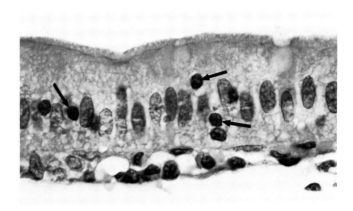

lymphocytes.[125] Mahida and colleagues looked at the production of IL-1 by monocytes in normal and IBD mucosa with active disease. They found that the IL-1 level was much greater in the cultures from IBD patients than from controls.[126] This difference was not accounted for by increased numbers of macrophages in the population, since they found similar numbers of macrophages from normal and inflamed colonic mucosa.

Interleukin 2 (IL-2) is another lymphokine that is altered in the gut mucosa of patients with IBD. IL-2 is a soluble product of activated T lymphocytes, which stimulates proliferation, and clonal expansion of T cell populations. Fiocchi and colleagues found that the lamina propria mononuclear cells from patients with IBD had significantly decreased release of IL-2 in vitro than mononuclear cells from control lamina propria.[127] This inability to respond appropriately to an antigen could result in the chronicity of inflammation that see in IBD. Lymphokines are important to activate some cytotoxic function. As with natural killer cells, the so-called lymphokine-activated killer cells have been thought to play a role in resistance to neoplasia.[128]

However, natural killer cell activity in the human intestine may not be of paramount importance owing to its low level of activity. However, lymphokine-activated killing is present at a considerably greater level than natural killer activity and may be a key factor in host defense

in the mucosa.[129] Kusuami and co-workers looked at the lymphokine-activated killer cell activity in the mononuclear cells isolated from the lamina propria of patients with IBD. They found that when exogenous IL-2 was added to cultures the mononuclear populations from patients with IBD had equivalent activity to controls. However, as seen by Roche and colleagues (above), the IBD cells produced considerably less IL-2 in culture than did control cells.[130] When the isolated lamina propria cells were first stimulated to produce endogenous IL-2, the Crohn's disease cells showed comparable levels of cytotoxicity compared to the controls, while the ulcerative colitis cells were significantly lower in activity (Table 3-1). These results suggest that in Crohn's disease, although a decreased level of IL-2 is produced, there is a potential for increased lymphokine-activated killer cells after appropriate IL-2 stimulation,

Table 3-1. Cytotoxic Activities of Lamina Propria Cells After IL-2 Activation[a]

	% Cytotoxicity
Crohn's disease	35
Ulcerative colitis	8
Control	34

[a] Endogenous IL-2 was generated by lamina propria mononuclear cells incubated for 4 days with 30 percent culture supernatant of autologous cells stimulated by OKT3 and phorbol myristate acetate.
(Data from Kusugami et al.[130])

whereas in ulcerative colitis, a hyporesponsive state to IL-2 exists locally in the gut.

In these studies, a common theme is dysfunctional regulation of the immune response by T cells or their lymphokine products. This does correlate with what we know about IBD and response to therapy. Immunosuppressive drugs, especially corticosteroids, have been key to treatment of this disease for many years. Recently, the immunosuppressive drug used for transplant patients, cyclosporine, has been found to help patients with active Crohn's disease[131] (Table 3-2). This is important in understanding pathogenesis because while corticosteroids have a suppressive effect both on specific lymphocyte-mediated immune responses and on acute inflammation, cyclosporine has a selective suppressive effect on T-lymphocyte-mediated immunity.

Lastly, James published a case report of a patient with an 18-year history of Crohn's disease of the colon who had a complete remission of symptoms following development of acquired immunodeficiency syndrome (AIDS).[132] The most impressive feature of this case was that the patient had well-documented regular attacks of severe Crohn's disease until after diagnosis of human immunovirus infection. This single case is the strongest evidence to date that cellular immunity, specifically CD4 positive T-helper lymphocytes, plays a key role in the pathogenesis of Crohn's disease.

CELL-MEDIATED HYPERSENSITIVITY MODEL

Although much of the above information is confusing, and some conflicting, a consistent theme is that cellular immunity is, in some way, important in the pathogenesis of IBD. A cell-mediated hypersensitivity model proposed by Rabin and Rogers[133] involved sensitizing rabbits with dinitrochlorobenzene (DNCB). Later, these animals were challenged with an intracolonic dose of DNCB. This procedure resulted in a histologic appearance in the colon that resembled IBD, but which would regress and then

Table 3-2. Response of Patients with Active Crohn's Disease to Cyclosporine Therapy

Time after Therapy	Cyclosporine (%)	Placebo (%)
2 weeks	51	21
1 month	51	24
3 months	59	32

%, percentage with improvement.
(Data from Brynskov et al.[131])

reappear when DNCB was reapplied to the mucosal surface of the bowel. Glick and Falchuck confirmed this model using a guinea pig system.[134] They found that there were increased percentages of T lymphocytes with a greater capacity to mediate mitogen-induced cellular cytotoxicity than lymphocytes from the mucosa of control animals. More recently, Morris and co-workers developed a rat model of chronic colonic inflammation that may be of use in studying IBD.[135] They administered the hapten 2,4,6-trinitrobenzenesulfonic acid in 50 percent ethanol as an enema. The ethanol damaged the epithelium enough to permit ready passage of the hapten. Granulomas were found in 57 percent of the rats. This type of study using carefully controlled antigen doses in an animal model system are likely to be very helpful in understanding the mechanisms involved in colonic inflammation. This type of understanding will be a key to determining the relevance of the many human studies under the confusing conditions of bowel inflammation and immunosuppressive therapy in a population where diet and living conditions cannot be strictly controlled.

GENETIC LINKAGE

The MHC in humans has provided considerable information about genetic linkage of certain diseases. The molecules of MHC are involved in communications between lymphocyte subpopulations. There are two types of molecules that control the interactions of cells in the immune system: class I and class II. This system is quite complex with many alleles in the gene pool that may be present at each locus. This reflects the fact that these are the molecules that need to interact with the array of foreign antigens to which the body is exposed.

Class I molecules are found on the surface of nucleated cells and platelets. They present the foreign material, such as viral antigen, to T lymphocytes that can mediate cytotoxic functions (CD8). In contrast, the class II molecules are involved in presentation of the antigen to helper T cells (CD4). These molecules are found mainly on cells of the immune system: B lymphocytes, T lymphocytes, and macrophages (although they have been reported on epithelial cells). In looking at the gut epithelium, patients with Crohn's disease have an increased expression of the MHC class II antigens on their surface compared to control epithelium.[136] Indeed, these epithelial cells can present antigen to T lymphocytes (especially suppressor lymphocytes).[137] The class II molecules are DP, DQ, and DR. The antigen is thought to require interaction with the class II molecule, which then, together with the antigen, is presented to the CD4-bearing T lymphocyte.[138, 139]

While early workers found no significant association between HLA antigens and IBD,[140] more recent studies using more precisely defined genetic populations of individuals have found some interesting associations. Smolen and colleagues[141] found a highly significant association of HLA-B12 in patients with Crohn's disease compared with control individuals or with patients with ulcerative colitis, when they looked at a population of 27 Vietnamese with Crohn's disease. Delpre and co-workers demonstrated a significant association of HLA-BW35 and HLA-AW24 with ulcerative colitis in European-born Jews. Further, they found that HLA-AW24 was associated with an early onset of the disease.[142] Purrmann and colleagues looked at 231 patients with Crohn's disease for the presence of anklylosing spondylitis and their HLA associated antigens. They found that individuals who were positive for HLA-B27, B44 were highly at risk for developing both Crohn's disease and ankylosing spondylitis.[143] Note,

however, that in their study, Crohn's disease patients had a normal frequency of B44 compared to controls. However, the phenotype B27, B44 was rare in both controls and individuals with only Crohn's disease without ankylosing spondylitis. Only when ankylosing spondylitis and Crohn's disease were considered together did the association become obvious. Genetic linkage has also been found with immunoglobulin genes. Patients with Crohn's disease have been associated with immunoglobulin heavy chain (Gm) allotypes.[144]

The implication of these Gm and HLA associations with IBD is that there is some linkage between the occurrence of IBD with genes regulating the immune response. The HLA antigens themselves may be the cell surface receptors for antigens or microorganisms involved in initiating IBD. It is possible that the causative antigens or microorganisms may contain HLA-like surface antigens and may result in a poor immune response, allowing the antigen to dwell longer in affected tissues, and thereby to initiate the chronic inflammation so characteristic of IBD.

OVERVIEW

The studies described in this chapter are in many ways exciting, but also frustrating. Through studies of the immune function in IBD, we have learned a considerable amount about the mucosal immune system, under unusual and confusing circumstances. However, it is not clear if this information has placed us closer to a real understanding of the etiology of IBD. Immune studies directed at the peripheral blood antibodies or mononuclear cells, or cellular events in the mucosa of patients with IBD, have shown a wide variety of nonspecific, and often conflicting phenomena, which may be related to the causative agent of IBD, but which more likely are related to the fact that these are sick patients with a tremendous antigen load at the damaged intestinal mucosal barrier. Perhaps the future focus in research on IBD should not be on IBD patients, with their complex interplay of a primary gastrointestinal disease, secondary inflammation from the myriads of antigens exposed to their damaged intestinal surface epithelium, and varying amounts of immunosuppressive drugs which they receive. The focus should turn to a better understanding of host defense mechanisms against microorganisms and discrete antigens under normal or controlled circumstances with consistent defined techniques. For the diagnostic pathologist there are few take-home lessons from the past 15 years of work on the immunopathogenesis of IBD. The presence of large numbers of plasma cells in the lamina propria can provide the pathologist with supportive evidence for IBD versus acute self-limited colitis. However, the newer technologies of flow cytometry, monoclonal antibodies, and cellular immunology are still far from having any useful application to the diagnosis of IBD. Yet, we must keep ourselves attuned to new developments in this field. The striking observation that a patient with Crohn's disease had a prolonged remission during development of AIDS shows that the T-helper lymphocyte plays some role in the overt manifestations of this disease. Perhaps we await another serendipitous association for which the many studies during the past few years have prepared us.

ACKNOWLEDGMENTS

This work was supported in part by Grant No. 0166 from the Smokeless Tobacco Research Council. The author thanks Ms. Mary Ross for her excellent assistance in preparing this manuscript.

REFERENCES

1. Cave DR, Mitchell DN, Kane SP, Brooke BN: Further animal evidence of a transmissible agent in Crohn's disease. Lancet 2:1120, 1973
2. Cave DR, Mitchell DN, Brooke BN: Evidence of an agent transmissible from ulcerative colitis tissue. Lancet 1:1311, 1976
3. Cave DR, Mitchell JDN, Brooke BN: Induction of granulomas in mice by Crohn's disease tissues. Gastroenterology 75:632, 1978
4. Cohen Z, Jersch D, Archibald S, et al: The production of granulomas in rabbit bowel. Gastroenterology 783:1152 (abstr), 1980
5. Mitchell DN, Rees RJW: Agent transmissible from Crohn's disease tissue. Lancet 2:168, 1970
6. Taub RN, Sachar D, Janowitz H, Slitzbach LE: Induction of granulomas in mice by inoculation of tissue homogenates from patients with inflammatory bowel disease and sarcoidosis. Ann NY Acad Sci 278:560, 1976
7. Bolton PM, Owen E, Heatley RV, et al: Negative findings in laboratory animals for a transmissible agent in Crohn's disease. Lancet 2:1122, 1973
8. Heatley RV, Bolton PM, Owen E, et al: A search for a transmissible agent in Crohn's disease. Gut 16:528, 1975
9. Simonowitz D, Block GE, Riddell RH, et al: The production of an unusual tissue reaction in rabbit bowel injected with Crohn's disease homogenates. Surgery 82:211, 1977
10. Cave DR, Mitchell DN, Brooke BN: Correspondence: induction of granuloms in mice by Crohn's disease tissues. Gastroenterology 77:202, 1979
11. Thayer WR, Jr: Executive summary of the AGA-NFIC sponsored workshop on infectious agents in inflammatory bowel disease. Dig Dis Sci 24:781, 1979
12. Burke DA, Axon ATR: Adhesive Escherchia coli in inflammatory bowel disease and infective diarrhoea. Br Med J 297:102, 1988
13. Blazer MJ, Hoverson D, Eli IG, et al: Studies of Campylobacter jejuni in patients with inflammatory bowel disease. Gastroenterology 86:33, 1984
14. Becken WL: Transmissible agents in inflammatory bowel disease. Med Clin North Am 64:1021, 1980
15. Halstensen TS, Mollnes TE, Fausa O, Brandtzaeg P: Deposis of terminal complement components in muscularis mucosae and submucosal vessels in ulcerative colitis and Crohn's disease of the colon. Gut 30:361, 1989
16. Thomas DW, Sinatra FR, Merritte RJ: Fecal alpha-1-antitrypsin excretion in young people with Crohn's disease. J Pediatr Gastroenterol Nutr 2:491, 1983

17. Allan A, Wyke J, Allan RN, et al: Plasma fibronectin in Crohn's disease. Gut 30:627, 1989

18. Sharon P, Stenson WF: Enhances synthesis of leukotriene B_4 by colonic mucosa in inflammatory bowel disease. Gastroenterology 86:453, 1984

19. Lauritsen K, Laursen LS, Bukhave K, Rask-Masden J: Effects of topical 5-aminosalicylic acid and prednisolone on prostaglandin E_2 leukotriene B_4 levels determined by equilibrium in vivo dialysis of rectum in relapsing ulcerative colitis. Gastroenterology 91:837, 1986

20. Wallace JL, MacNaughton WK, Morris GP, Beck PL: Inhibition of leukotriene synthesis markedly excellerates healing in a rat model of inflammatory bowel disease. Gastroenterology 96:29, 1989

21. Anton PA, Targon SR, Shananahan F: Increased neutrophil receptors for and response to the proinflammatory bacterial peptide formyl-methionyl-leucylphenylalanine in Crohn's disease. Gastroenterology 97:20, 1989

22. Kozarek RA, Patterson DJ, Gilfand MD, et al: Methotrexate induces clinical and histologic remission in patients with refactory inflammatory bowel disease. Ann Intern Med 110:353, 1989

23. Smith CW, Hollers JC, Patrick RA, Hassett C: Motility and adhesiveness in human neutrophils: effect of chemotactic factors. J Clin Invest 63:221, 1979

24. Chadwick VS: Enzyme in neutorphiles by intestinal bacteria in vitro and in vivo. Scand J Gastroenterol 23:121, 1988

25. Chester JF, Ross JS, Malt RA, Weitzman SA: Acute colitis produced by chemotactic peptides in rats and mice. Am J Pathol 125:284, 1985

26. Hodgson HJF, Potter BJ, Jewell DP: Immune complexes in ulcerative colitis and Crohn's disease. Clin Exp Immunol 29:187, 1977

27. Jewell DP, MacLennan ICM: Circulating immune complexes in inflammatory bowel disease. Clin Exp Immunol 14:219, 1977

28. Otto HF: Immunpathogenetische and ultrastrukturelle Aspekte der Colitis ulcerosa. Schwiz Med Wschr 111:768, 1981

29. Hodgson HJF, Potter BJ, Skinner J, Jewell DP: Immune complex-mediated colitis in rabbits. an experimental model. Gut 19:225, 1978

30. Mee AS, McLaughlin JE, Hodgson HJF, Jewell DP: Chronic immune colitis in rabbits. Gut 20:1, 1979

31. Rhodes JM, McLaughlin JE, Brown DJC, et al: Inhibition of leucocyte motility and prevention of immune-complex experimental colitis by hydroxychloroquine. Gut 23:181, 1982

32. Kemler BJ, Alpert E: Inflammatory bowel disease associated circulating immune complexes. Gut 21:195, 1980

33. Soltis RD, Hasz D, Morris MJ, Wilson ID: Evidence against the presence of circulating immune complexes in chronic inflammatory bowel disease. Gastroenterology 76:1380, 1976

34. Leroux-Roels GG, Wieme RJ, DeBroe ME: Occurrence of enzyme-immunoglobulin complexes in chronic inflammatory bowel disease. J Lab Clin Med 97:316, 1981

35. Winship DH: Immune complexes in inflammatory bowel disease: cause or coincidence? J Lab Clin Med 97:313, 1981

36. Hodgson HJF, Potter FJ, Jewell DP: C3 metabolism in ulcerative colitis and Crohn's disease. Clin Exp Immunol 29:490, 1977

37. Lake AJ, Stitzel AE, Urmson JR, Walker WA, Spitzer RE: Complement alterations in inflammatory bowel disease. Gastroenterology 76:1374, 1979

38. Lake AJ, Stitzel AE, Urmson JR, Walker WA, Spitzer RE: Complement alterations in inflammatory bowel disease. Gastroenterology 76:1374, 1979

39. Potter BJ, Hodgson HJF, Mee AS, Jewell DP: C1q metabolism in ulcerative colitis and Crohn's disease. Gut 20:1012, 1979

40. Lake AJ, Stitzel AE, Urmson JR, et al: Complement alterations in inflammatory bowel disease. Gastroenterology 76:1374, 1979

41. Ward M, Eastwood AS: Serum complement components C2 and C4 in inflammatory bowel disease. Digestion 13:100, 1979

42. Potter FJ, Brown DJC, Watson A, Jewell DP: Complement inhibitors and immunoconglutinins in ulcerative colitis and Crohn's disease. Gut 21:1030, 1980

43. Gould SR, Brash AR, Conolly ME: Increased prostaglandin production in ulcerative colitis. Lancet 2:98, 1977

44. Sharon P, Ligumsky M, Rachmilewitz D, Zor U: role of prostaglandins in ulcerative colitis. Enhanced production during active disease and

inhibition by sulfasalazine. Gastroenterology 75:638, 1978

45. Rampton DS, Sladen GE, Youlten LJF: Rectal mucosal prostaglandin E_2 release and its relation to disease activity, electrical potential difference, and treatment in ulcerative colitis. Gut 21:591, 1980

46. Hawkey CJ, Truelove SC: Effect of prednisolone on prostaglandin synthesis by rectal radioimmunoassay. Gut 22:190, 1981

47. Rachmilewitz D, Ligumsky M, Haimovitz A, Treves AJ: Prostanoid synthesis by cultured peripheral blood mononuclear cells in inflammatory diseases of the bowel. Gastroenterology 82:673, 1982

48. Sharon P, Ligumsky M, Rachmilewitz D, Zor U: Role of prostaglandins in ulcerative colitis. Enhances production during active disease and inhibition by sulfasalazine. Gastroenterology 75:638, 1978

49. Rampton DS, Sladen GE: Prostaglandin synthesis inhibitors in ulcerative colitis: flurbiprofen compared with conventional treatment. Prostaglandins 21:417, 1981

50. Modigliani R: Prostanoids in ulcerative colitis. Gastroenterology 82:819, 1982

51. Segal AW, Loewi G: Neutrophil dysfunction in Crohn's disease. Lancet 2:219, 221, 1976

52. Morain CO, Segal AA, Walker D, Levi AJ: Abnormalities of neutrophil function do not cause the migration defect in Crohn's disease. Gut 22:817, 1981

53. Wandall JH, Binder V: Leukocyte function in Crohn's disease. Gut 23:173, 1982

54. Rhodes JM, Potter BJ, Brown DJC, Jewell DP: Serum inhibitors of leukocyte chemotacis in Crohn's disease and ulcerative colitis. Gastroenterology 82:1327, 1982

55. Rhodes JM, Potter BJ, Brown DJC, Jewell DP: Serum inhibitors of leukocyte chemotacis in Crohn's disease and ulcerative colitis. Gastroenterology 82:1327, 1982

56. Rhodes JM, Jewell DP: Motility of neutrophils and monocytes in Crohn's disease and ulcerative colitis. Gut 24:73, 1983

57. Elmgreen J, Berkowicz A, Sorensen H: Defective release of C5a related chemo-attractant activity from complement in Crohn's disease. Gut 24:525, 1983

58. Mahida YR, Patel S, Gionchetti P, et al: Macrophage subpopulations in lamina propria of normal and inflamed colon and terminal ileum. Gut 30:826, 1989

59. Verspaget HW, Mieremet-Ooms MAC, Weterman IT, Pena AS: Partial defect of neutrophil oxidative metabolism in Crohn's disease. Gut 25:349, 1984

60. Verspaget HW, Pena AS, Weterman IT, Lamers CBHW: Diminished neutrophil function in Crohn's disease and ulcerative colitis identifies by decreased oxidative metabolism and low superoxide dismutase content. Gut 29:223, 1988

61. Broberger O, Perlmann P: Autoantibodies in human ulcerative colitis. J Exp Med 110:657, 1959

62. Carlsson HE, Lagercrantz R, Perlmann P: Immunological studies in ulcerative colitis VIII. Antibodies to colon antigen in patients with ulcerative colitis, Crohn's disease, and other diseases. Scand J Gastroenterol 12:707, 1977

63. Auer IO, Grosch L, Hardorfer C, Roder A: Ulcerative colitis specific cytotoxic IgG-autoantibodies against colonic epithelial cancer cells. Gut 29:1639, 1988

64. Haviland AE, Borowitz MJ, Lan MS, et al: Aberrant expression of monoclonal antibody-defined colonic mucosal antigens in inflammatory bowel disease. Gastroenterology 95:1302, 1988

65. Roche JK, Fiocchi C, Youngman K: Sensitization of human intestinal mucosa-derived mononuclear cells reactive with purified epithelial cell-associated components in vitro. J Clin Invest 75:522, 1985

66. Fiocchi C, Roche JK, Michener WM: High prevalence of antibodies to intestinal epithelial antigens in patients with inflammatory bowel disease and their relatives. Ann Intern Med 110:786, 1989

67. Bull DM, Ignaczak TF: Enterobacterial common antigen-induced lymphocyte reactivity in inflammatory bowel disease. Gastroenterology 64:43, 1973

68. Fanger MW, Shen L, Pugh J, Bernier GM: Subpopulations of human peripheral granulocytes and monocytes express receptors for IgA. Proc Natl Acad Sci USA 77:3640, 1980

69. Lowell GH, Smith LF, Griffiss JM, Grandt BL: Antibody-dependent monocyte-mediated antibacterial activity. J Exp Med 150:127, 1979

70. Keren DF, Nair M, Rosillo M, Schwartz SA:

Antigen-specific secretory IgA can mediate antibody-dependent cell-mediated cytotoxicity against eukaryotic target cells. Gastroenterology 78:1194 (abstr), 1980

71. Lowell GH, Smith LF, Griffiss JM, et al: Antibody-dependent mono-nuclear cell-mediated anti-meningococcal activity. J Clin Invest 66:260, 1980

72. Smith LF, Collins HH, Wilson SR, et al: Secretory IgA-dependent mononuclear cell-mediated antibacterial activity. Fed Proc 40:1974 (abst), 1981

73. Arnaud-Battandier F, Bundy BM, O'Neill M, et al: Cytotoxic activities of gut mucosal lymphoid cells in guinea pigs. J Immunol 121:1059, 1978

74. Capron M, Raousseaux J, Mazingue C, et al: Rat mast cell-eosinophil cytotoxicity to *Schistosoma mansoni* shistosomula. J Immunol 2518, 1978

75. Shorter RG, Cardoza M, Spencer RJ, Huizenga KA: Further studies of *in vitro* cytotoxicity of lymphocytes from patients with ulcerative and granulomatous colitis for allogeneic colonic epithelial cells including the effects of colectomy. Gastroenterology 56:304, 1969

76. Shorter RG, McGill DB, Bahn RC: Cytotoxicity of mononuclear cells for autologous colonic epithelial cells in colonic disease. Gastroenterology 86:13, 1984

77. Wijesinha SS, Steer HW: Studies of the immunoglobulin-producing cells of the human intestine: the defunctioned bowel. Gut 23:211, 1982

78. Soltoft J, Binder V, Gudmand-Hoyer E: Intestinal immunoglobulins in ulcerative colitis. Scand J Gastroenterol 8:293, 1973

79. Brandtzaeg P, Baklein K, Fausa O, Hoel PS: Immunohistochemical characterization of local immunoglobulin formation in ulcerative colitis. Gastroenterology 66:1123, 1974

80. Skinner JM, Whitehead R: The plasma cells in inflammatory disease of the colon: a quantitative study. J Clin Pathol 27:643, 1974

81. Green FHY, Fox H: The distribution of mucosal antibodies in the bowel of patients with Crohn's disease. Gut 16:125, 1975

82. O'Donoghue DP, Kumar P: Rectal IgE cells in inflammatory bowel disease. Gut 20:149, 1979

83. Rosekrans PCM, Meijer CJ, Van der Val AM, et al: Immunoglobulin containing cells in inflammatory bowel disease of the colon: a morphometric and immunohistochemical study. Gut 21:941, 1980

84. Schneider HM, Loos M, Storkel S, Gross M: Immunohistological differential diagnosis of inflammatory colonic diseases. Histopathology 8:583, 1984

85. Uchima H, Eishi Y, Takemura T, Hirokawa K: Immunohistochemical studies of ulcerative colitis with special reference to localization of immunoglobulins, secretory, component, and lysozyme in view of suffering periods. Acta Pathol Jpn 33:1183, 1983

86. MacDermott RP, Nash GS, Auer IO, et al: Alterations in serum immunoglobulin G subclasses in patients with ulcerative colitis and Crohn's disease. Gastroenterology 96:764, 1989

87. Scott MG, Nahm MH, Macke K, et al: Spontaneous secretion of IgG subclasses by intestinal mononuclear cells: differences between ulcerative colitis, Crohn's disease, and controls. Clin Exp Immunol 66:209, 1986

88. Kett K, Rognum TO, Brandtzaeg P: Mucosal subclass distribution of immunoglobulin-producing cells is different in ulcerative colitis and Crohn's disease of the colon. Gastroenterology 93:919, 1987

89. Keren DF, Appleman HD, Geisinger DR, Foley JL: Immunoglobulin-containing cells in inflammatory bowel disease: correlation of immunofluorescence findings with histopathology. Lab Invest 46:45A, 1982

90. Surawicz CM, Belic L: Rectal biopsy helps to distinguish ASLC from idiopathic inflammatory bowel disease. Gastroenterology 86:104, 1984

91. Nostrant TT, Kumar NB, Appelman HD: Histopathology differentiates ASLC from ulcerative colitis. Gastroenterology 92:318, 1987

92. van Spreeuwel JP, Lindeman J, Meijer CJLM: A quantitative study of immunoglobulin containing cells in the differential diagnosis of acute colitis. J Clin Pathol 38:774, 1985

93. Keren DF, Kumar NB, Appelman HD: Quantification of IgA-containing plasma cells as an adjunct to histiopathology in distinguishing acute self-limited colitis from active idiopathic inflammatory bowel disease. Pathol Immunopathol Res 6:435, 1987

94. Lloyd G, Green FHY, Fox H, et al: Mast cells

and immunoglobulin E in inflammatory bowel disease. Gut 16:861, 1975

95. O'Donoghue DP, Kumar P: Rectal IgE cells in inflammatory bowel disease. Gut 20:149, 1979

96. Heatley RV, Calcraft BJ, Rhodes J, et al: Disodium cromoglycate in the treatment of chronic proctitis. Gut 16:559, 1975

97. Rosekrans PCM, Meyer CJLM, Vander Wal AM, Lindeman J: Allergic proctitis, a clinical and immunopathological entity. Gut 21:1017, 1980

98. Murdoch DL, Piris J: Immunoglobulin E in non-specific proctitis and ulcerative colitis studies with a monoclonal antibody. Digestion 25:201, 1982

99. Wright R, Truelove SC: Circulating antibodies to dietary proteins in ulcerative colitis. Br Med J 2:142, 1965

100. Mee AS, Brown D, Jewell DP: Atopy in inflammatory bowel disease. Scand J Gastroenterol 14:743, 1979

101. Kett K, Brandtzaeg P, Fausa O: J-chain expression is more prominent in immunoglobulin A2 than in immunoglobulin A1 colonic immunocytes and is decreased in both subclasses associated with inflammatory bowel disease. Gastroenterology 94:1419, 1988

102. Verspaget HW, Pena AS, Weterman IT, Lamers CBHW: Disordered regulation of the in vitro immunoglobulin synthesis by intestinal mononuclear cells in Crohn's disease. Gut 29:503, 1988

103. Unanue ER, Beller DI, Lu CY, Allen PM: Antigen presentation: comments on its regulation and mechanism. J Immunol 132:1, 1984

104. Seldenrijk CA, Drexhage HLA, Meuwissen SGM, et al: Dendritic cells and scavenger macrophages in chronic inflammatory bowel disease. Gut 30:484, 1989

105. Kelleher D, Murphy A, Whelan CA, et al: Defective suppression in the autologous mixed lymphocyte reaction in patients with Crohn's disease. Gut 30:839, 1989

106. Elson CO, James SP, Graeff AS, et al: Hypogammaglobulinemia due to abnormal suppressor T-cell activity in Crohn's disease. Gastroenterology 86:569, 1984

107. Meyers S, Sachar DB, Taub RN, Janowitz HD: Anergy to dinitrochlorobenzene and depression of T-lymphocytes in Crohn's disease and ulcerative colitis. Gut 17:911, 1976

108. Fiske SC, Falchuk ZM: Impaired mixed-lymphocyte culture reactions in patients with inflammatory bowel disease. Gastroenterology 79:682, 1980

109. MacDermott RPM, Bragdon MJ, Thurmond RD: Peripheral blood mononuclear cells from patients with inflammatory bowel disease exhibit normal function in the allogeneic and autologous mixed leukocyte reaction and cell-mediated lympholysis. Gastroenterology 86:476, 1984

110. Selby WS, Jewell DP: The T lymphocyte subsets in inflammatory bowel disease: peripheral blood. Gut 24:99, 1983

111. Shanahan F, Leman B, Deem R, et al: Enhanced peripheral blood T-cell cytotoxicity in inflammatory bowel disease. J Clin Immunol 9:55, 1989

112. Herberman RB, Holden HT: Natural cell-mediated immunity. Adv Cancer Res 27:305, 1978

113. Ginsburg CH, Dambrauskas JT, Ault KA, Falchuk ZM: Impaired natural killer cell activity in patients with inflammatory bowel disease: evidence for a qualitative defect. Gastroenterology 85:846, 1983

114. Brown TE, Bankhurst AD, Strickland RG: Natural killer cell function and lymphocyte subpopulation profiles in inflammatory bowel disease. J Clin Lab Immunol 11:113, 1983

115. Sakane T, Steinberg AD, Reeves JP, Creen I: Studies of immune functions of patients with systemic lupus erythematosus. Complement-dependent immunoglobulin M anti-thymus derived cell antibodies preferentially inactivate suppressor cells. J Clin Invest 63:954, 1979

116. Ginsburg CH, Falchuk ZM: Defective autologous jixed-lymphocyte reaction and suppressor cell generation in patients with inflammatory bowel disease. Gastroenterology 83:1, 1982

117. Elson CO, Graeff AS, James SP, Strober W: Covert suppressor T cells in Crohn's disease. Gastroenterology 80:1513, 1981

118. Fiocchi C, Youngman KR, Farmer RG: Immunoregulatory function of human intestinal mucosa lymphoid cells: evidence for enhanced suppressor cell activity in inflammatory bowel disease. Gut 23:692, 1983

119. Holdstock G, Chastenay BF, Krawitt EL: Increased suppressor cell activity in inflammatory bowel disease. Gut 22:1025, 1981

120. Victorino RMM, Hodgson HJF: Spontaneous

suppressor cell function in inflammatory bowel disease. Dig Dis Sci 26:801, 1981

121. Ginsburg CA, Falchuk SM: Defective autologous mixed lymphocyte reaction and suppressor cell generation in patients with inflammatory bowel disease. Gastroenterology 83:1, 1982 ·

122. Hirata I, Berrebi G, Austin LL, et al: Immunohistological characterization of intraepithelial and lamina propria lymphocytes in control ileum and colon and in inflammatory bowel disease. Dig Dis Sci 31:593, 1986

123. Selby WS, Janossy G, Bofill M, Jewell DP: Intestinal lymphocyte subpopulations in inflammatory bowel disease: an analysis by immunohistological and cell isolation techniques. Gut 25:32, 1984

124. Roche JK, Fiocchi C, Youngman K: Sensitization to epithelial antigens in chronic mucosal inflammatory disease. Characterization of human intestinal mucosa-derived mononuclear cells reactive with purified epithelial cell associated components *in vitro* J Clin Invest 75:522, 1985

125. Dinarello CA: Biology of interleukin 1. FASEB J 2:108, 1989

126. Mahida YR, Wu K, Jewell DP: Enhanced production of interleukin 1-B by mononuclear cells isolated from mucosa with active ulcerative colitis or Crohn's disease. Gut 30:835, 1989

127. Fiocchi C, Hilfiker ML, Youngman KR, et al: Interleukin 2 activity of human intestinal mucosa mononuclear cells. Decreased levels in inflammatory bowel disease. Gastroenterology 86:734, 1984

128. Rosenberg SA: Immunotherapy of cancer using interleukin 2: current status and future prospects. Immunol Today 9:58, 1988

129. Kanof ME, Strober W: Lymphokine-activated killer-cell cytotoxicity in the intestinal immune system (editorial) Gastroenterology 98:222, 1989

130. Kusugami K, Youngman KR, West GA, Fiocchi C. Intestinal immune reactivity to interleukin 2 differs among Crohn's disease, ulcerative colitis and controls. Gastroenterology 97:1, 1989

131. Brynskov J, Freund L, Rasmussen SN, et al: A placebo-controlled, double-blind, randomized trial of cyclosporine therapy in active chronic Crohn's disease. New Engl J Med 321:845, 1989

132. James SA: Remission of Crohn's disease after human immunodeficiency virus infection. Gastroenterology 95:1687, 1988

133. Rabin BS, Rogers SJ: A cell-mediated immune model of inflammatory bowel disease in the rabbit. Gastroenterology 75:29, 1978

134. Glick ME, Falchuk ZM: Dinitrochlorobenzene-induced colitis in the guinea pig: studies of colonic lamina propria lymphocytes. Gut 22:120, 1981

135. Morris GP, Beck PL, Herridge MS, et al: Hapten-induced model of inflammation and ulceration in the rat colon. Gastroenterology 96:795, 1989

136. Selby WS, Janossy G, Mason DW, Jewell DP: Expression of HLA-DR antigens by colonic epithelium in inflammatory bowel disease. Clin Exp Immunol 53:614, 1983

137. Mayer L, Shlien R: Evidence for function of Ia molecules on gut epithelial cells in man. J Exp Med 166:1471, 1987

138. Elson CO, Kagnoff MF, Fiocchi C, et al: Intestinal immunity and inflammation: recent progress. Gastroenterology 91:746, 1986

139. Gill TJ, Cramer DV, Kunz HW: The major histocompatability complex—comparison in the mouse, man and the rat. Am J Pathol 90:737, 1978

140. Vachon A, Gebuhrer L, Betuel H: HL-A antigens in ulcerative colitis and Crohn's disease (abstract V-18). p. 170. In First International Symposium on HL-A and Diseases. Editions INSERM, Paris, 1976

141. Smolen JS, Gangl A, Polterauer P, et al: HLA antigens in inflammatory bowel disease. Gastroenterology 82:34, 1982

142. Delpre G, Kadish U, Gazet E, et al: HLA antigens in ulcerative colitis and Crohn's disease in Isracl. Gastroenterology 78:1452, 1980

143. Purrmann J, Zeidler H, Bertrams J, et al: HLA antigens in ankylosing spondylitis associated with Crohn's disease. Increased frequency of the HLA phenotype B27, B44. J Rheumatol 15:1658, 1988

144. Kagnoff MF, Brown FJ, Schanfield MS: Association between Crohn's disease and immunoglobulin heavy chain (Gm) allotypes. Gastroenterology 85:1044, 1983

4

Dysplasia in Inflammatory Bowel Disease

Robert H. Riddell

Carcinoma complicating inflammatory bowel disease (IBD) accounts for only a very small proportion of large bowel carcinomas, probably less than 1 percent. However carcinomas developing in this setting tend to be unlike those occurring in the noncolitic population. Large tumors tend to form strictures, whereas small tumors are often little more than slightly raised plaques or mucosal irregularities. Sometimes tumors are only found in histologic sections or on random biopsy in the absence of a macroscopic lesion. The median age of presentation for tumors is in the range of 40 to 45 years, and these tumors are often poorly differentiated and aggressive, with poor prognosis.

Although the reported crude prevalence rates of carcinoma complicating ulcerative colitis are 3 to 5 percent of all patients with the disease,[1,2] the risk increases as the duration of the disease increases, and is greater in individuals with extensive disease, which is somewhat arbitrarily defined as disease extending proximal to the mid-transverse colon.[3–5] Thus, the highest risk occurs in individuals with pancolitis of 10 or more years' duration, for which the risk exceeds that seen in a control population by 20- to 30-fold.[4,6–8] Statistical analysis of this high-risk group by actuarial methods reveals cancer rates in the range of 5 to 20 percent per decade (0.5 to 2 percent per year) after the first 10 years of ulcerative colitis.[1,3,8–11] Although the actual numbers of all of these studies are small, there remains a surprising degree of similarity between studies without an obvious and marked selection bias, and does not appear to have changed over several decades (Fig. 4-1). How-

ever, these data include some studies in which there is a referred patient population, including some with colorectal carcinoma at the time of referral; indeed, one of the major problems is that of obtaining accurate data for the cancer risk, as the method of expressing the risks varies considerably and is frequently not comparable between centers. For instance, Hendriksen et al. quote a 30 percent cumulative incidence of 1.4 percent after 30 years of disease, but include all patients with ulcerative colitis irrespective of the extent of disease.[12] Further, their colectomy rate is so high that numerically it could have included all of the patients with total colitis as well as a good proportion of those with extensive colitis (defined in this study as between ulcerative proctitis and total colitis). The number of patients at risk in this series is therefore likely very small indeed.

Cumulative totals are often not expressed over the same time frame. Thus Gilat has a 13.7 percent prevalence at 20 years,[13] Gyde et al. have 7.1 percent at 20 years but 24 percent at 30 years,[14] and Brostrom has 13 percent at 25 years.[15] Others provide a combined cumulative incidence of invasive carcinoma and high-grade dysplasia ("hazard rate").[16] If the risk is expressed as relative risk for that particular age group, one study of a total of 13 cancers suggested that this is increased 370-fold for those in the 20- to 39-year age group, 31-fold for those 40 to 59, and 9-fold for those 60 to 75.[11] This translates to about 0.5 percent per patient year in those having the disease for 10 to 20 years and 1.6 percent per patient year in those with more than 20 years of disease, with a cumu-

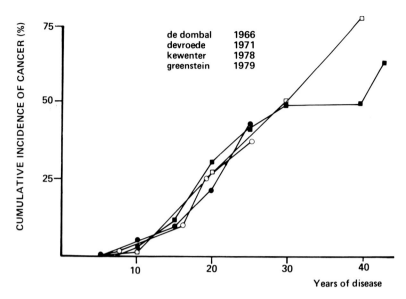

Fig. 4-1. Cumulative incidence of carcinoma in ulcerative colitis as shown in four separate studies. Although numbers after 25 years of disease are very small and not yet adequately confirmed prospectively, the 25-year figure of about 40 percent is impressively similar in all studies. (From Devroede,[62] with permission.)

lative cancer risk of 30 percent after 28 years.[8,11] However the data are expressed, in patients under surveillance there is a considerable lifetime risk of developing cancer. Data are accumulating to suggest that individuals with only intermittently active disease have a cancer risk similar to those with chronic continuous disease.[6,8,17]

WHICH PATIENTS ARE IN THE HIGH-RISK GROUP?

There is no argument that patients with total involvement of the large bowel diagnosed radiologically are at risk. What is much less clear is the nature of risk in patients with colitis that is other than total, is total microscopically but not by other criteria, or is extended to total colitis from distal disease, or even those having Crohn's colitis (unless colectomy has been carried out Crohn's ileitis may not be easily amenable to endoscopic examination and biopsy). Inevitably, case reports are published of carcinoma co-existing with left-sided or distal ulcerative colitis. However, it must be remembered that in countries at high risk of colorectal cancer about 4 to 6 percent of the population will develop this disease, and that in three-fourths of these (3 to 5 percent of the population) this will occur in the left colon, and in the rectosigmoid in particular. Well-controlled studies are therefore essential to demonstrate whether there really is an increased risk in patients with distal ulcerative colitis in whom the extent of disease has been accurately assessed by endoscopy and biopsy. This is probably best assessed following a relapse, preliminary evidence suggesting that the proximal extent of disease may regress endoscopically when the disease is in remission.[18]

All of these factors combine to produce a clinical problem for which there is no easy solution, the only alternatives available being either to carry out proctocolectomy fairly indiscriminately after about 10 years of disease, or to observe the patient closely and try to detect precarcinomatous (dysplastic) changes or carcinoma as early as possible. Although proctocolectomy might still be the best mode of therapy in some patients, such as those who appear unreliable, are easily lost to follow-up, or in whom total colonoscopy and biopsy is technically difficult, a surgical approach is often resisted by both patients and their physicians. The possibility that dysplasia might be used as a method of screening to detect patients within the group that might be at greatest clinical risk has contributed further to the demise of "routine" proctocolectomy as a method of cancer prevention when no other indications for the operation are present.

THE CONCEPT OF DYSPLASIA

Surveillance in ulcerative colitis has as its basic tenet the assumption that surveillance will reduce the mortality from colorectal cancer although the evidence that this is happening is very limited.[19] This would ideally have been proven in studies utilizing a control arm with patients not in a surveillance program, but this is obviously difficult to carry out ethically. In the absence of a controlled study, data are required showing that surveillance prevents the development of lethal cancers. One study used as a "control" patients that had been lost to follow-up, and indeed found 2 cancers in 1,168 patient-years of patients followed but with no mortality, compared with 5 cancers, 3 of which were lethal, in 315 patient-years of patients lost to follow-up.[20] Theoretically then, cancers which are resected but from which the patient survives are acceptable. Unfortunately, many surveillance studies include patients under surveillance who have both developed[3,15,21,22] and occasionally even died from carcinoma.[11,23,24] Many colitic cancers are flat or plaque-like, and readily escape endoscopic or radiologic detection[25]; and even if found there are few data showing that they really are less advanced pathologically.[11,20,26,27] Nevertheless, while several studies indicate that no lethal cancers developed, the number of patient-years of follow-up must be sufficiently high to allow determination of the number of cancers that might have been expected together with whether the

program actually showed a significantly different figure from this.

A second major tenet of surveillance is either that cancers can be detected before they have become lethal, or that a marker such as the presence of dysplasia precedes all carcinomas for a long-enough period of time to be detectable, analogous to the adenoma-carcinoma sequence in the noncolitic bowel.[28] Also, if dysplasia is present it must be both endoscopically detectable and morphologically identifiable. Considerable question has been raised regarding all of these issues.

The concept of dysplasia in ulcerative colitis is based on the principle that carcinoma also arises from a precarcinomatous lesion, and that the identification of dysplasia and excision of the large bowel in these patients prevents subsequent death from disseminated carcinoma. Conversely, patients with quiescent disease and no dysplasia could be followed and not subjected to unnecessary colectomy.

COMPARISON BETWEEN ADENOMAS AND DYSPLASIA

Although an analogy can be drawn between dysplasia in colitis and adenomas in noncolitics, it is also apparent that there are differences between the colitic and noncolitic precarcinomatous lesion at a morphologic level because of several factors.

Adenomas are usually discrete lesions, and are readily distinguishable macroscopically and microscopically from the surrounding mucosa, which is usually normal in noncolitics when assessed by both of these criteria. However, while true adenomas may occur in colitic patients (see the following discussion), the development of dysplasia is more frequently a gradual one in flat, otherwise unremarkable mucosa and part of a spectrum ranging from nondysplastic mucosa to neoplastic mucosa. The exact point at which the lesion becomes dysplastic, and therefore capable of giving rise directly to an invasive carcinoma, is therefore far more difficult to ascertain morphologically, since abrupt cut-off points often cannot be accurately defined. Adenomas in noncolitics tend to vary in their degree of dysplasia and accompanying mucous depletion, but appear to exhibit a reasonably consistent spectrum of dysplasia. In colitics, however, while the major spectrum is morphologically similar to that seen in adenomas, there are also numerous variations that are undoubtedly neoplastic and capable of giving rise directly to carcinomas yet are rarely seen in conventional adenomas.

The nuclear changes constituting dysplasia may be mimicked to a considerable extent when acute inflammation is present. However, it may pose problems of interpretation, primarily in crypts immediately adjacent to ulcers.

It should be stressed that dysplastic mucosa can by definition give rise directly to invasive carcinoma. Although invasive carcinoma might be thought to arise from a spectrum progressively involving low-grade, then high-grade dysplasia culminating in carcinoma in situ (the extreme of high-grade dysplasia) and finally in invasive carcinoma, carcinomas in colitics, noncolitics, and in a variety of different organs can be found arising from dysplastic epithelium that falls short of carcinoma in situ. Indeed, in the classic study of over 2,500 adenomas by Muto and colleagues,[28] the same conclusion was reached regarding adenomas in the noncolitic population. Further, carcinoma in situ is rare in ulcerative colitis in the absence of an invasive carcinoma.

Perhaps the major difference between adenomas in the noncolitic population and dysplasia in an ulcerative colitic population is the frequency with which the latter is associated with unsuspected invasive carcinoma.[29,30] While carcinomas are multiple in about 25 percent of patients presenting symptomatically, multiple carcinomas are rare in patients under surveillance. Simple excision of areas of dysplasia comparable to polypectomy is unlikely to provide adequate treatment; they can rarely be visualized and may also be a marker for other areas of dysplasia or carcinoma elsewhere in the large bowel.

The interpretation of biopsies from colitics is somewhat hazardous, particularly for pathologists seeing relatively few large bowel biopsies, in view of the potentially far-reaching clinical implications following a diagnosis of dysplasia (frequently leading to proctocolectomy). However, if both clinician and pathologist have an interest, and biopsies are taken at all stages of the disease, a pathologist may rapidly acquire an eye for the changes seen in all phases of colitis. Utilization of resected specimens, particularly those from long-standing disease or carcinoma, will add to the pathologist's skill in interpretation.

EVOLUTION OF DYSPLASIA IN INFLAMMATORY BOWEL DISEASE

The histologically identifiable precursor to carcinoma developing in ulcerative colitis was originally identified by Warren and Sommers in 1949.[31] However, confirmation has been lacking, with only occasional reports, such as that by Dawson and Pryse-Davies in 1959, to suggest a histologic relationship.[32] In 1967, Morson and Pang described "precancerous" changes in the mucosa of 23 colectomy specimens resected for carcinoma in ulcerative colitis that was extensive and involved the mucosa away from the site of carcinoma as well as in its immediate vicinity.[4] Similar changes were found retrospectively in 9 percent of large bowel resections for ulcerative colitis. A retrospective study of rectal biopsies revealed similar changes in biopsies from nine patients, and subsequent proctocolectomy revealed an unsuspected infiltrating carcinoma in five of these patients, implying that these changes were accompanied by a sufficiently high risk of invasive carcinoma to justify "prophylactic" proctocolectomy if such changes were found on rectal biopsy. This paper represented a milestone in both describing a series of histologic findings accurately and suggesting how they might be used clinically.

Since 1972 a series of papers emerged that were largely retrospective, although many now are prospective.[8,10,11,15,17,22–24,33–41] From these

studies several facts emerged, First, if proctocolectomy is carried out because of dysplasia found
on rectal biopsy, overall about 30 to 40 percent
of these patients will have an unsuspected carcinoma in the resected specimen.[42] Second, each
study has tended to define its own morphologic
criteria and grading system,[43] making it difficult
to compare these studies accurately, while morphologic problems have arisen because of difficulties in distinguishing postinflammatory from
neoplastic changes. Little information has therefore been forthcoming on the natural history
of dysplasia, there being only a retrospective
suggestion that, in the "average" patient, transition to early invasive carcinoma probably occurs
over a period of years.[5] Finally, there is no
method of follow-up that is known to be superior
to any other.

More recently an increase in the development
of intestinal carcinoma in patients with Crohn's
disease has also been recognized.[44-47] The tumors have much in common with carcinomas
occurring in ulcerative colitis, particularly their
tendency to occur in patients with long-standing
disease and at a younger age than is seen with
carcinoma in the general population. Dysplasia
has also been described in Crohn's disease[48,49]
and in the large bowel in chronic schistosomiasis
of the colon.[50] It is virtually identical to that
occurring in ulcerative colitis. The present classification of dysplasia formulated for ulcerative
colitis[51] should also be applicable to these other
forms of chronic colitis.

The large step from the pure concept of dysplasia to its applications in patient management
implies three major points. One is that prophylactic proctocolectomy in all patients in the high-
risk clinical group is unacceptable. The second
is that a laissez faire attitude is similarly not
condoned. Third, there is no good method of
easily anticipating which patients within the
clinical high-risk group will develop carcinoma.
Dysplasia is therefore best regarded as an aid
to predicting which patients are at greatest risk
of developing carcinoma, so that prophylactic
surgery would be offered only to this subgroup.

Many institutions have now attempted to use
dysplasia as part of the long-term follow-up

of colitics at greatest risk for developing carcinoma. It seems logical that those with these
changes should be at greater risk for having,
or for developing, invasive carcinoma compared
with their fellow colitics who do not have dysplasia. This appears to have been established
in view of the large proportion of patients undergoing proctocolectomy for rectal dysplasia that
are subsequently found to have an invasive adenocarcinoma (usually unsuspected) when the resected bowel is subjected to close pathologic
examination (see the previous discussion). Fortunately, most of these carcinomas are early
and have not infiltrated through the muscularis
propria or into the adjacent lymph nodes. The
cure rate for these early carcinomas is expected
to be over 90 percent. However, some unexpected carcinomas do extend through the wall
and into the lymphatics, and survival in this
group will be less favorable.

DYSPLASIA-ASSOCIATED LESIONS AND MASSES

The issue of dysplasia-associated lesions and
masses is critical in the management of colitis.
An endoscopic lesion may show only dysplasia,
either high or low grade, on biopsy, yet be
the superficial part of any invasive carcinoma.[29]
Indeed, that dysplasia has this potential is an
integral part of the definition of dysplasia. Both
the presence and utility of this concept have
been demonstrated.[40,52]

ABSENCE OF DYSPLASIA WITH INVASIVE CARCINOMA

Although studies examining adjacent and distant mucosa in patients presenting with clinical
carcinoma only find dysplasia in about 75 percent,[53] it is easy to argue that the invasive component outgrew and destroyed pre- or co-existing dysplasia, analogous to the lack of finding
an adenomatous edge to a carcinoma in noncolitic cancers. Nevertheless in the stomach the
preceding lesion for the diffuse variant of carci-

noma remains poorly defined and virtually impossible to diagnose on biopsies. As a proportion of colitic cancers are morphologically similar to this variant of gastric cancer, it may not be surprising if the same occasionally occurs in the large bowel. In addition, some carcinomas complicating ulcerative colitis have a very strong endocrine component and may be regarded as endocrine carcinomas, the preinvasive phase of which is again poorly defined irrespective of whether they occur in the setting of dysplasia or not. Finally, the precancerous phase may be very brief or dysplasia limited to the immediate vicinity of the carcinoma. Surveillance therefore now entails a deliberate search both for mucosal abnormalities that may prove on biopsy to be invasive carcinoma and areas of dysplasia with or without an underlying invasive element.

STANDARDIZED DEFINITION AND CLASSIFICATION OF DYSPLASIA

Dysplasia is defined as an unequivocal neoplastic alteration of the colonic epithelium that may be not only a marker or precursor of carcinoma, but may itself be malignant and associated with direct invasion into the underlying tissue.[51] Because dysplastic mucosa of any grade may give rise directly to an invasive carcinoma (carcinoma infiltrating into the submucosa or beyond), a positive diagnosis of dysplasia cannot be taken lightly. This definition of dysplasia is analogous to that used when speaking of adenomas in the colon, the rest of the gastrointestinal tract, and other sites in patients who do not have IBD. The classification (Table 4-1) consists of three major categories: *negative,* *indefinite,* and *positive* for dysplasia. It is essential that the pathologist be aware of the wide range of inflammatory and reparative changes that may affect the colonic mucosa in chronic IBD,[51,54] and that these be excluded before an unequivocal diagnosis of dysplasia is made. If the observer has any doubt at all regarding whether the changes are dysplastic/neoplastic,

Table 4-1. Classification of Large Bowel Mucosal Changes in IBD

Negative
  Normal large bowel epithelium
  Inactive (quiescent) colitis
  Active colitis ± regeneration

Indefinite
  Probably negative (probably inflammatory)
  Unknown
  Probably positive (probably dysplastic)

Positive
  Low-grade dysplasia
  High-grade dysplasia

the diagnosis is changed to that of *indefinite for dysplasia.*

MUCOSA NEGATIVE FOR DYSPLASIA

The classification of mucosa "negative for dysplasia" includes active and quiescent colitis, normal mucosa such as that seen proximal to areas of involvement in ulcerative colitis, and that seen in skip areas of the large bowel in patients with Crohn's disease (Fig. 4-2). Normal nuclei are small, indistinct, and either round or slightly ovoid when fixed in formalin. However, other fixatives—particularly those containing mercury or picric acid, which enhance nuclear detail—may allow small nuclei to be seen. The nuclear changes seen in both normal mucosa and quiescent colitis are essentially similar and negative for dysplasia (Fig. 4-3), but nuclei are larger adjacent to lymphoid follicles (Fig. 4-4).

ACTIVE COLITIS AND ITS RESOLVING PHASE

Active disease and its resolution causes most of the problems relating to interpretation of large bowel biopsies when the pathologist looks for dysplasia. Active colitis is usually not a problem, since the characteristic features of an intense mucosal inflammation—primarily involving crypts with crypt abscess formation,

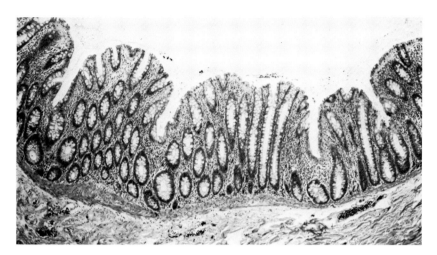

Fig. 4-2. Normal large bowel mucosa with regular surface undulations into which crypts may open (right and left). The latter should not be mistaken for crypt branching seen with formation of new crypts, which are invariably irregularly spaced and distorted. The small rim of nuclei and normal amount of mucus in each crypt is characteristic. (H&E, ×40.)

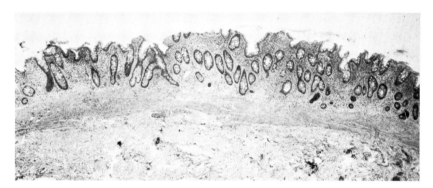

Fig. 4-3. Quiescent ulcerative colitis with a regenerated mucosa in which crypts are reduced in number (cf. Fig. 4-2), branched, and distorted. The muscularis mucosae is markedly thickened. (H&E, ×30.)

depletion of goblet cell mucin, and ulceration—are present (Fig. 4-5A). Mucosal vascular congestion with edema and focal hemorrhage is often present, and tends to be more prominent in severe cases of colitis.

The mucosal inflammatory infiltrate in active colitis includes an acute component associated with crypt abscess formation and a chronic component involving the lamina propria more diffusely, frequently with plasma cells or a band of lymphocytes immediately above the muscu-laris mucosae. Aggregates of neutrophils invade the crypt epithelium and form crypt abscesses that, when numerous, are characteristic and tend to correlate with clinical activity (Fig. 4-5B). Mucin depletion tends to be diffuse, affecting all crypts uniformly, and tends to be more pronounced in association with an intense inflammatory infiltrate. Restoration of mucin content, usually beginning in the most superficial portion of the crypts, occurs with resolution, and returns to normal levels in quiescent disease. Because

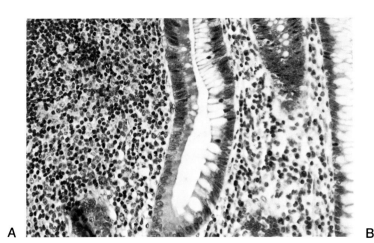
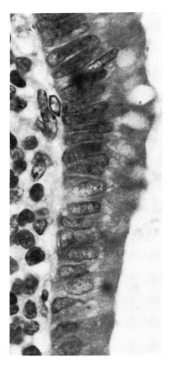

Fig. 4-4. Normal large bowel mucosa demonstrating increased nuclear size and decreased goblet cells that may be seen immediately adjacent to a lymphoid aggregate or follicle ("M-cells"). **(A)** Changes are most marked on the side of the crypt immediately adjacent to the follicle, but the other side of the crypt also contains nuclei that are increased in size when compared with the normal crypt on the right. **(B)** The part of the crypt immediately adjacent to the follicle shows increased nuclear size and lack of goblet cells. Nuclei are normochromatic. (H&E, Fig. A × 310, Fig. B ×1,250.)

mucin depletion may also be seen as the result of some bowel preparations and, most importantly, in dysplasia, the observation of mucus depletion should lead to an immediate search for its cause. A diagnosis of dysplasia should be made with extreme caution in the presence of acute inflammation, particularly if crypts are actively invaded by neutrophils.

Regeneration following relapse results from the proliferation of epithelium in the crypts adjacent to ulceration. Initially there is an outgrowth of cells over an ulcerated surface, or along a crypt in which the epithelium has been destroyed (Fig. 4-6A) by epithelium that is very attenuated, sometimes sufficiently so that the nucleus forms a bulge in its surface, analogous to the process of restitution in the stomach. These cells rarely have mitoses but gradually become cuboidal to low columnar, and are accompanied by nuclear changes that, while absolutely characteristic and typical of regenerating epithelium, may initially be mistaken for dysplasia. Nuclei are open, have large nucleoli, and may be situated anywhere within the cell. In contrast to what is seen in dysplasia, nuclear chromatin is sparse (Fig. 4-6B), and fewer nuclei are present, so that there is little tendency for nuclei to overlap or become stratified. The number of nuclei increases as the cells become columnar, but the nuclei at this phase have not yet returned to their normal location at the cell bases. At this point the distinction between resolving colitis and dysplasia may be most difficult; if the nuclear changes are very marked, some observers may be unconvinced that the changes are entirely the result of the repair process (unequivocally

Fig. 4-5. Active ulcerative colitis (negative for dysplasia). **(A)** There is superficial ulceration, marked mucin depletion, and polymorphs in the lamina propria, showing a distinct tendency to attack crypt epithelium. **(B)** Detail shows nuclei to be enlarged, but they are not hyperchromatic, there is no peripheral chromatin rim, and nucleoli are virtually indistinguishable. (H&E, Fig. A ×100, Fig. B × 400.)

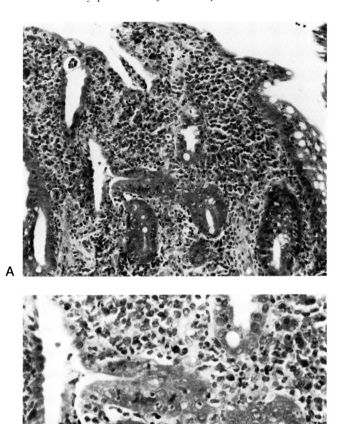

A

B

negative for dysplasia), and may feel obliged to employ the category "indefinite for dysplasia—probably negative" (see the following section).

CHANGES ASSOCIATED WITH ACTIVE REGENERATION

The majority of biopsies in this category were formerly classified as "indefinite for dysplasia—probably negative." One of the major changes in the last decade has been the increas-

ing comfort level of pathologists in recognizing the typical changes of restituting epithelium, which can be seen in any epithelial-lined tissue following ulceration, although the time frame in which they occur is still unclear (Figs. 4-6 to 4-8). Many pathologists now include these changes with "negative for dysplasia." This results in virtual elimination of the category of "indefinite for dysplasia—probably negative." If wildly exuberant changes are encountered that do not readily fit into this category, they are best included with "indefinite for dysplasia" (if a suffix is included, this is usually

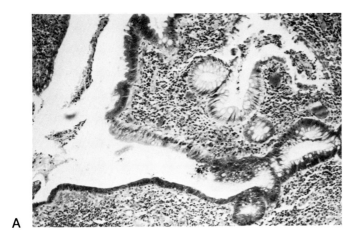

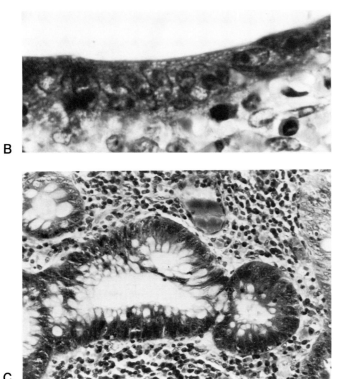

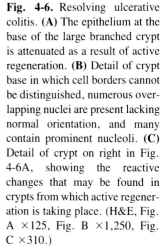

Fig. 4-6. Resolving ulcerative colitis. **(A)** The epithelium at the base of the large branched crypt is attenuated as a result of active regeneration. **(B)** Detail of crypt base in which cell borders cannot be distinguished, numerous overlapping nuclei are present lacking normal orientation, and many contain prominent nucleoli. **(C)** Detail of crypt on right in Fig. 4-6A, showing the reactive changes that may be found in crypts from which active regeneration is taking place. (H&E, Fig. A ×125, Fig. B ×1,250, Fig. C ×310.)

''unknown''), which includes the clinical implication of ensuring that they either regress with the inflammation or do not progress; this is usually achieved by recolonoscopy when the inflammation has at least partially resolved, and usually well before the next surveillance endoscopy. The differential diagnosis of this type of biopsy is inevitably with high-grade rather than low-grade dysplasia because the nuclei are usually scattered throughout the cells in a manner similar to that depicted in Figures 4-7 and 4-8, but rather more extreme.

Fig. 4-7. Mucosa ''indefinite for dysplasia—probably negative.'' **(A)** Columnar cells without production of mucus-containing enlarged stratified vesicular nuclei with prominent nucleoli but normal chromatin content. **(B)** In context these changes are found in a crypt that is actively regenerating and very close to the area depicted in Fig. 4-6A. (H&E, Fig. A ×1,250, Fig. B ×310.)

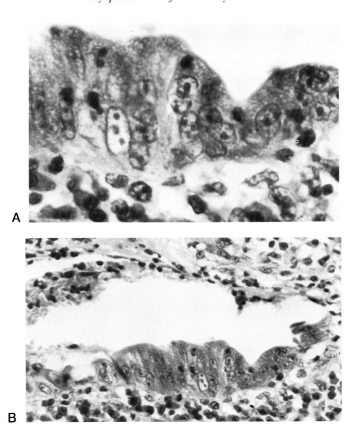

When the acutely inflamed and actively regenerating epithelium (described in the previous section) returns to its normal columnar appearance, there is a further opportunity for confusion with dysplasia. At this stage the nuclei tend to acquire a little more chromatin, particularly around the nuclear membrane, at a time when they are becoming more regular and are oriented in the same plane as the remainder of the cell, but are returning irregularly to their normal position at the base of the cell, sometimes while retaining a prominent nucleolus. The resulting nuclear stratification may be so similar to dysplastic epithelium that on isolated high-power micrograph it may appear indistinguishable from dysplasia (Fig. 4-7). There may be a little mucus production at the apices of some of the cells. Mitoses, including tripolar forms, can be found in both regenerating and dysplastic mucosa.

However, while dysplastic mucosa may contain numerous mitoses, they are surprisingly much less common in actively regenerating epithelium. The presence of numerous mitoses, particularly in mucin-depleted crypts and in the absence of acute inflammation, is a sinister feature, although one that still has to be interpreted in the light of the remaining nuclear characteristics.

The correct diagnosis of regenerative changes can usually be made because other features of inflammation and active regeneration can be found higher in the same crypt (Fig. 4-6), in adjacent crypts, or in biopsies from the same site. It is therefore sensible to interpret the whole biopsy or biopsies together with regard to the degree of activity, ulceration, and regeneration. Pronounced changes, although relatively uncommon, inevitably lead to some degree of doubt by the observer regarding whether the

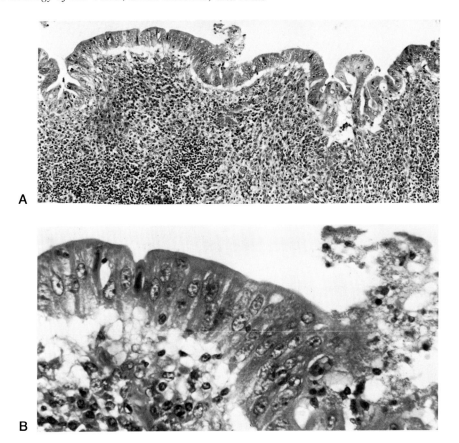

Fig. 4-8. Mucosa "indefinite for dysplasia—probably negative." **(A)** Active colitis in which new crypts are rudimentary (right). **(B)** High-power view shows tall columnar epithelium in which nuclei are stratified and vesicular and contain prominent nucleoli, although there is no increase in nuclear chromatin. Differentiation into goblet and absorptive cells has not yet occurred. Although the nuclear features are in many respects similar to those seen in Fig. 4-6B, they are much greater. They might be expected ultimately to return to normal, but as this cannot be stated unequivocally it is categorized in the "indefinite" category. In this instance the patient was adolescent and had a proctocolectomy after only 3 weeks of disease; nevertheless some might be sufficiently worried by these changes to request rebiopsy to ensure that the changes regress or might use the "indefinite for dysplasia—unknown" category, again with a request for rebiopsy. (H&E, Fig. A ×125, Fig. B ×500.)

changes can simply be ascribed to the inflammatory process (Fig. 4-8). Under these circumstances, whenever there really is doubt about the regenerative nature of the changes, it is best to employ the category of "indefinite for dysplasia." This may be followed by a comment noting that the changes are most likely reparative in nature (probably negative). This should not be necessary in any biopsy in which there is acute inflammation with a diffuse cryptitis, as diffuse acute inflammation virtually never involves dysplastic epithelium.[51] However, dysplastic epithelium can re-epithelialize ulcerated surfaces; resulting in highly atypical nuclei, and it is these changes that can cause problems (see below). Experience has shown that this is a rare phenomenon and that most of these lesions do in fact regress once the inflammation has resolved.

MUCOSA INDEFINITE
FOR DYSPLASIA

MODIFICATION TO THE ORIGINAL
CLASSIFICATION OF DYSPLASIA

The category of mucosa "indefinite for dysplasia" was originally subdivided into "probably negative," "unknown," and "probably positive" subgroups. Increasingly, the regenerative and reparative changes originally classified here are being recognized for what they really are, so that the number of biopsies in this category ("probably negative") has diminished over the last decade and its use is now relatively infrequent (see the preceding section). Functionally, the inclusion of active reparative changes with "negative for dysplasia" rather than with "indefinite for dysplasia—probably negative" leaves only the other two categories of "indefinite for dysplasia" ("unknown," and "probably positive") in the "indefinite for dysplasia" category. In practice, it is hardly worth vacillating between these two, as both have the same clinical implication of a need to gather more data by repeating the endoscopy and biopsies. This results in a simpler classification and suggested management of biopsies, as shown in Table 4-2.

The subcategorization of "probably positive" implies that the changes observed are most likely neoplastic but either fail to display sufficient nuclear changes to justify inclusions into that category or contain an overriding factor, usually active inflammation and regeneration, that results in caution on the grounds that they are

**Table 4-2. Modification of Biopsy Classification
of Dysplasia and Its Clinical Implications**

Biopsy Classification	Clinical Implications
Negative	Regular surveillance
Indefinite	Increased surveillance
Positive	
Low grade	Increased surveillance/
High grade	consider colectomy

unlikely to completely regress and may progress to unequivocal dysplasia. Also, as detection of aneuploidy becomes more frequent, there may be a trend to subdivide those patients in the "indefinite for dysplasia" group on this criterion rather than a subjective morphologic interpretation.

The category of mucosa "indefinite for dysplasia" specifically includes the following:

1. Exuberant regenerative features that cannot be accepted as unequivocally negative.
2. Chronic active disease with nuclear features beyond those usually associated with repair but which fail to reach criteria necessary for an unequivocal negative or positive diagnosis.
3. Quiescent disease with nuclei far larger than those usually associated with quiescent disease, and often with some degree of mucus depletion.
4. Other patterns that are unusual and that cause concern because, while they have not been observed to give rise directly to invasive carcinoma, their behavior is not known. Some may be confused with dysplasia.

The importance of this category is that it is not just a hedge for genuine ignorance but usually requires further biopsies within a relatively short period of time (usually months), so that the behavior of these lesions can be followed closely and their progress to dysplasia or regression documented.

This diagnosis of "indefinite for dysplasia" is one of exclusion and is made by asking two questions, namely, is the biopsy unequivocally negative for dysplasia, and is the biopsy unequivocally positive for dysplasia? If the answer to both of these is negative, then one is dealing with a biopsy that is indefinite for dysplasia. Because the "probably negative" label is increasingly uncommon, and because the "unknown" and "probably positive" categories have the same clinical implications for the patient, it is increasingly logical to use the generic term "indefinite for dysplasia" in an unqualified manner for all biopsies that are not unequivo-

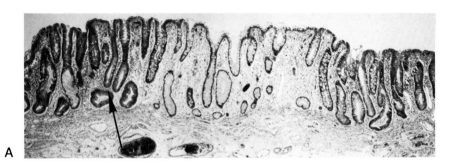

A

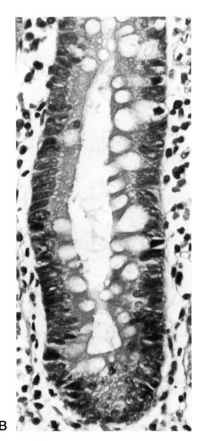

B

Fig. 4-9. Mucosa "indefinite for dysplasia—unknown." **(A)** Typical quiescent ulcerative colitis in which crypts appear full of mucin and the periphery of the crypt contains only a small rim of nuclei (center). These contrast with the areas on either side, where there is much less mucin and the nuclear rim at the periphery of the crypts is much more apparent. **(B)** Detail of crypt (arrow) shows the nuclei occupying up to half of the cell. They are also hyperchromatic but do not show the increase in number and stratification seen in dysplasia. Given the quiescent disease, the adjacent mucosa showing only typical features of quiescent colitis and the lack of any activity these changes cannot be ascribed in inflammation. Similarly lacking are features of dysplasia; they cannot be called "positive for dysplasia" or even "indefinite for dysplasia—probably positive." The only appropriate category is that of "indefinite for dysplasia—unknown." (H&E, Fig. A ×30, Fig. B ×500.)

cally positive or negative for dysplasia and in which short-term rebiopsy is required.

When subdivided, the "indefinite—unknown" category includes those biopsies that the observer cannot classify as belonging to either of the two subgroups "probably reactive" and "probably neoplastic," irrespective of the reason. Biopsies in this category may include the extremes of regeneration as described above: chronic active disease with nuclear features beyond those usually associated with repair, but not severe enough to justify a diagnosis of dysplasia (Fig. 4-9); or in quiescent disease, the

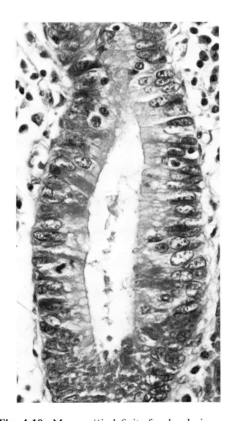

Fig. 4-10. Mucosa "indefinite for dysplasia—probably positive." Nuclei are increased in number and a little stratified but fall short of changes that might be seen in adenoma. In this example numerous Paneth cell granules can be seen in the supranuclear aspect of some cells along the sides of the crypt as well as most of the cells in the crypt base. (H&E, ×415.)

presence of nuclei far larger than those usually associated with quiescent disease (Fig. 4-10). These situations are often accompanied by some degree of mucus depletion that might represent early transition to dysplasia. It also includes other unusual patterns that may cause concern because, while they have not been observed to give rise directly to invasive carcinoma, their behavior is not known (see below).

The category of "indefinite for dysplasia—probably positive" is a rather difficult category, bridging that part of the histologic spectrum between "unknown," where the level of suspicion is increased, and that part which is "unequivocally dysplastic." It might best be regarded as "highly suspicious" yet not sufficient to contemplate colectomy. However, one or sometimes several features prevent an unequivocal diagnosis of dysplasia. Nuclei may be enlarged and hyperchromatic but fail to show the stratification typically seen in dysplasia in the presence of columnar epithelium that is reflecting its immaturity by the failure to produce goblet cells in the absence of any inflammation (Fig. 4-10). Alternatively, the epithelium may have features of dysplasia but an acute inflammation infiltrate may also be attacking the epithelium, raising the suspicion that some of the changes might regress when the inflammatory stimulus abates (Fig. 4-11). Interestingly, genuinely neoplastic epithelium often seems relatively uninvolved by acute inflammation. Although an unequivocal diagnosis of dysplasia in the presence of acute inflammation and ulceration can be made, extreme caution should be exercised when (1) acute inflammation affects virtually all of the crypts, and (2) when there is actively regenerating epithelium.

MUCOSA POSITIVE FOR DYSPLASIA

By definition, the category of mucosa "positive for dysplasia" includes only unequivocally neoplastic (dysplastic) mucosa. Any biopsy reported as positive for dysplasia must also, by

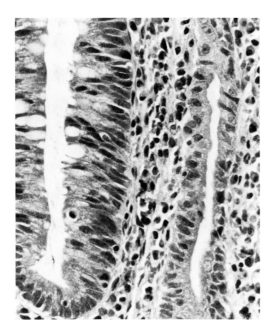

Fig. 4-11. Mucosa "indefinite for dysplasia—probably positive." The left crypt shows stratified hyperchromatic nuclei that while not severe enough to justify a diagnosis of dysplasia are nevertheless well beyond those usually seen following active disease. The adjacent crypt (right) shows typical regenerating features, raising the question of whether at least part of the changes may be the result of active disease. (H&E, ×500.)

definition, be capable of giving rise directly to an invasive adenocarcinoma. Thus, it is analogous to the adenoma in the noncolitic population.

Dysplastic mucosa is arbitrarily divided into two grades, namely "low-" and "high-grade." This division has been thought necessary in view of the potentially different implications for patient management. High-grade dysplasia corresponds to examples of severe, and sometimes moderate, dysplasia in the literature, and also includes carcinoma in situ. The latter is not included under a separate category because implications for therapy are the same as those for high-grade dysplasia.

Some low-power microscopic features have been described as characteristic of dysplasia in colitis, but these are not pathognomonic. How-

ever, their presence should raise the examiner's index of suspicion that dysplasia may be present, although ultimate confirmation depends on meeting the criteria for dysplasia. These changes include the following:

1. A villous configuration. Although typical of dysplastic mucosa, villous mucosa may occasionally be seen in active colitis in the absence of dysplasia, when the mucin depletion and full spectrum of regenerative changes may be present.
2. Budding of crypts. This is classically found in colitic mucosa as a result of epithelial destruction and regeneration, but is also found in dysplastic mucosa as a result of active budding of neoplastic crypts. Budding, therefore, is not a useful criterion. However, in contrast to the budding occurring in regenerated mucosa, which is usually accompanied by a reduced number of crypts, the crypts in dysplasia may be much closer together. Occasionally, long crypts running transversely may be found in dysplastic mucosa but are not seen in regenerative mucosa. However, these are relatively uncommon.

LOW-GRADE DYSPLASIA

Most biopsies of low-grade dysplasia pose little diagnostic problem, because of their morphologic similarity to tubular adenomas. Crypts are increased in size and lined by tall columnar cells in which there is frequently preservation of mucus, but the nuclei are enlarged and usually hyperchromatic (although occasionally they are open and vesicular, but with a heavy peripheral chromatin rim and several small nucleoli), and there is nuclear crowding with overlapping and stratification. Arbitrarily, the nuclei should be confined largely to the basal half of the cells in low-grade dysplasia (Fig. 4-12). In most instances the dysplasia is maximal at the luminal surface, and may not be apparent in the crypt base; however, in some patients the dysplasia is most marked at the base of the crypts and matures as the surface is approached; this is particularly true when the mucosa is villous.

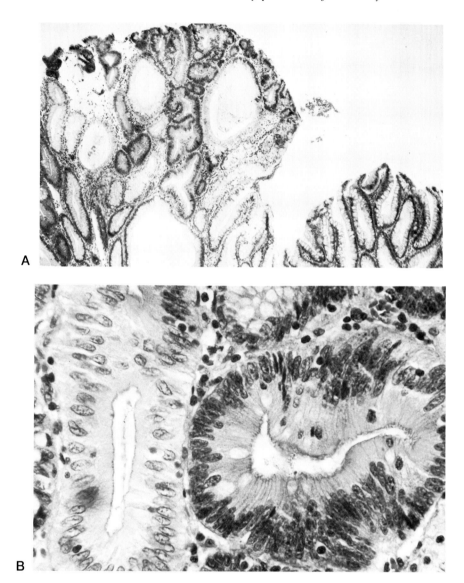

Fig. 4-12. Mucosa ''positive for dysplasia—low-grade.'' **(A)** Junction between colitic mucosa (right) and thicker dysplastic mucosa (left) in which the contrast between adenomatous crypts can be seen. **(B)** Detail contrasting dysplastic glands (right) and nondysplastic crypt. Typical hyperchromatic stratified nuclei are present. The designation of low-grade dysplasia is made because nuclei are largely confined to the basal portions of the cells. (H&E, Fig. A ×40, Fig. B ×680.)

The cells at the surface may be virtually indistinguishable from normal, except for their size. In such cases *the grade of dysplasia is determined using most dysplastic portion of the affected crypt,* in this case the base. The similarity to villous adenomas occurring in the rectum in noncolitic patients is apparent, while this pattern of maturation in both the colitic and noncolitic have in common the potential for an occult invasive carcinoma arising from the crypt bases.

While adenomatous mucosa typically accounts for most examples of low-grade dyspla-

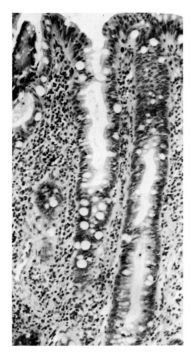

Fig. 4-13. Mucosa "positive for low-grade dysplasia" in which crypts also contain numerous goblet cells that have become rounded, producing an appearance similar to signet ring cells. (H&E, ×430.)

sia, other variants do occur. These may also be found in adenomas, although they are distinctly uncommon, and may involve all of the usual cell types found in the colitic bowel.

One variant form of low-grade dysplasia takes the form of epithelium that has the usual features of low-grade dysplasia, but the goblet cells are no longer goblet shaped; having become instead rounded, and bear a distinct resemblance to signet ring cells (Fig. 4-13). In addition there is usually some loss of polarity in the affected goblet cells, so that the nuclei may be on any side of the mucus droplet. These altered goblet cells have been called "dystrophic goblet cells" or, more euphemistically, "upside-down goblet cells." In some instances there appears to be a double layer of mucus-producing cells; those in the basal layer tend to be more normal, although both layers may contain rounded goblet cells. While the double layer of goblet cells tends only to occur in dysplastic mucosa, dystrophic goblet cells may occasionally be seen in otherwise unremarkable regenerated mucosa. However, most examples are found in patients with dysplasia or carcinoma elsewhere in their large bowel, so that if found in biopsies it should lead to a further search for other areas of dysplasia.

Some examples of low-grade dysplasia are accompanied by abundant mucin secretion (Fig. 4-14) or by excessive numbers of dysplastic endocrine and Paneth cells (Fig. 4-10). In both latter instances the granules may be entirely perinuclear, instead of having the usual subnuclear and supranuclear locations, respectively. Sometimes the granules appear to be dispersed randomly throughout the cell. Interestingly, al-

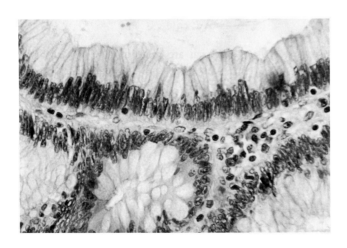

Fig. 4-14. Mucosa "positive for low-grade dysplasia" with abundant mucin production. The features are reminiscent of some villous adenomas, with virtually all cells containing a supranuclear mucin vacuole, a feature more characteristic of gastric than large-bowel mucosa. (H&E, ×430.)

though these two cell types may occur by themselves, they are often seen together, sometimes accompanied by dystrophic goblet cells. The presence of these relatively mature, specialized cell types is probably good reason to grade the dysplasia in the low-grade category, for the ability to form them seems to disappear rapidly when high-grade dysplasia is present. Although illustrated here, these cells may be found in virtually all phases of colitis. Their presence alone should therefore have no bearing on the classification of a biopsy. Other features as described above and below are key in making the diagnosis.

A form of dysplasia that is rather more problematic is characterized by the loss of specialized cells, so that the crypts are lined entirely by cells with eosinophilic cytoplasm, in contrast to the usual columns of goblet cells. Nuclei present are not crowded or stratified but are enlarged and hyperchromatic (Fig. 4-15). It is uncertain whether these crypts contain relatively undifferentiated cells or dysplastic absorptive cells. The term *incomplete maturation* may be used for this type of change. Most important is its tendency to give rise to carcinomas that, unlike most large bowel carcinomas, invade the lamina propria either as single cells or as small groups of cells—features that are distinctly reminiscent of the diffuse form of gastric carcinoma both in the manner by which they arise as well as in their pattern of infiltration.

HIGH-GRADE DYSPLASIA

"High-grade dysplasia" embraces all dysplastic biopsies not included in the low-grade category, and includes most biopsies that would formerly have been classified as moderate to severe change, including carcinoma in situ. It is not considered worthwhile to separate carcinoma in situ (Fig. 4-16) from the remainder of the high-grade category, since the implications for therapy are the same. In most instances, the appearances of the epithelium in this group so closely resemble those seen in adenomas in the noncolitic that the diagnosis is relatively

straightforward. Examples of the spectrum of high-grade dysplasia are illustrated in Figures 4-16 to 4-18. In contrast to low-grade dysplasia, in which the nuclei should be largely confined to the basal halves of the cells, high-grade dysplasia exhibits nuclear stratification that should cause the nuclei to extend frequently into the superficial (lumenal) parts of the cells. Nuclei may also exhibit loss of polarity, in addition to the usual stratification, or exhibit extremes of cytologic change. It should also be remembered that, as in the low-grade group, there will be frequent instances when the dysplasia is most marked at the surface, and occasional instances when high-grade dysplasia is found in the bases of the crypts, with progressive maturation as the surface is approached. The grade is judged wherever it is the most severe within the crypt.

Only two problems have been found when dealing with this category. One involves the problem of dysplastic biopsies that straddle the low-grade–high-grade interface (see Low-Grade Dysplasia above). The second involves the diagnosis of high-grade dysplasia in the presence of a heavy inflammatory infiltrate. This and other problems causing difficulty in diagnosis are discussed in the following section.

SITUATIONS CAUSING DIFFICULTY IN DIAGNOSIS

Situations that cause difficulty in diagnosis include biopsies in which serrated crypts are present that are more usually associated with hyperplastic (metaplastic) polyps, follicular inflammation, dysplasia involving one part of a crypt or one part of the biopsy, and the diagnosis of dysplasia in the presence of inflammation.

SERRATED CRYPTS

Occasional biopsies are encountered in which confusion arises because the superficial parts of the crypts contain the typical serrated or saw-

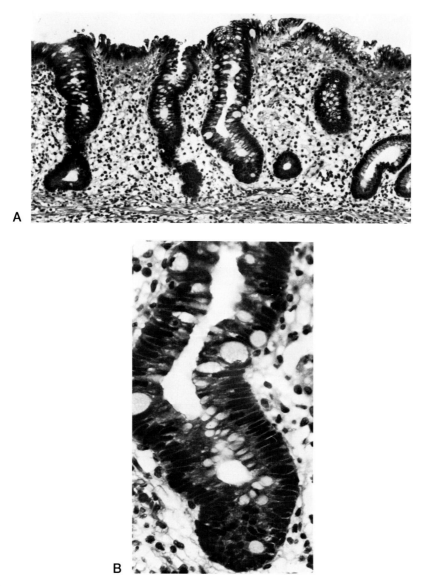

Fig. 4-15. Mucosa "positive for low-grade dysplasia" with incomplete maturation. **(A)** Mucosa is of normal thickness (not a prerequisite) and contains crypts that contain virtually no goblet cells. **(B)** Detail shows large, deeply hyperchromatic nuclei that do not show the stratification usually seen in dysplasia. However, such crypts tend to give rise to poorly differentiated adenocarcinomas. (H&E, Fig. A ×125, Fig. B ×500.)

tooth appearance associated with hyperplastic (metaplastic) polyps. While not a problem in the absence of dysplasia, sometimes the epithelium at the bases of the crypts may be frankly dysplastic (Fig. 4-19). Confusion also occurs because the dysplasia is usually limited to the bases of the crypts when the serrated pattern is present. The problem may be resolved using the criterion of grading crypts on the basis of their most dysplastic part, together with recognition that this pattern can be associated with dysplasia.

Fig. 4-16. Mucosa "positive for high-grade dysplasia" with carcinoma in situ. More conventional high-grade dysplasia is present in remaining crypts not showing the gland-within-gland pattern. (H&E, ×210.)

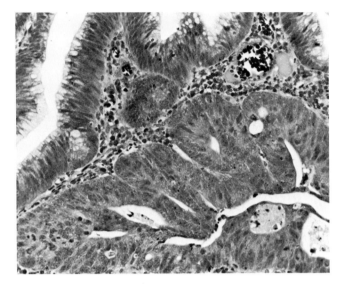

Fig. 4-17. Mucosa "positive for high-grade dysplasia" with numerous hyperchromatic stratified nuclei reaching the crypt lumen. (H&E, ×500.)

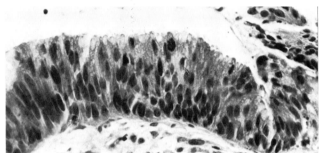

Interestingly, the serrated pattern tends to disappear as the epithelium becomes more dysplastic and the dysplasia extends toward the surface. However, examples of high-grade dysplasia are encountered in which remnants of a serrated pattern are still discernible. At this stage, the pattern is largely academic, being completely overshadowed by the obvious high-grade dysplasia.

FOLLICULAR INFLAMMATION

The presence of numerous lymphoid follicles, usually in rectal biopsies, is a poorly recognized phase of ulcerative colitis but can be found in other inflammatory diseases. It may be accompanied by any of the other stages of ulcerative colitis. Thus, a typical regenerated mucosa with

decreased numbers of crypts that are invariably branched or distorted can be accompanied by follicular inflammation. Dysplasia may be accompanied by similar changes, In practice, the phase associated with active regeneration causes the greatest difficulty (Fig. 4-20). As with hyperplastic polyp-like changes, it is important to remember that any phase of ulcerative colitis can be accompanied by follicular inflammation, and that the epithelium should be graded entirely on its own merit.

DYSPLASIA INVOLVING ONE PART OF THE CRYPT

As discussed and illustrated in the preceding sections on low-grade and high-grade dysplasia, that part of the crypt is graded where the displa-

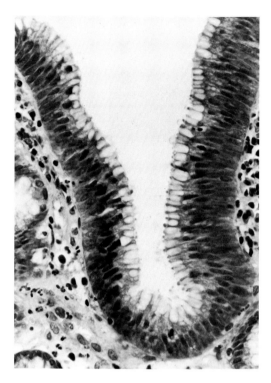

Fig. 4-18. Mucosa "positive for high-grade dysplasia." The appearances are similar to those seen in adenomas, and most of the nuclei are more than halfway to the surface of the crypt. Note that mucin is present not as goblet cells but as supranuclear mucin vacuoles. (H&E, ×400.)

sia is greatest. Usually the lumenal portion of the crypt is the part affected, as is seen in tubular adenomas.

DYSPLASIA INVOLVING ONE PART OF THE BIOPSY

Abnormal and sometimes dysplastic features are confined occasionally to one part of a biopsy. This causes two problems. First, it becomes difficult to determine how many crypts need to be involved to make a confident diagnosis of dysplasia. There is obviously no easy answer to this, but if crypts at the edge of an ulcer undergoing active regeneration are examined, exuberant features that might be confused with

dysplasia can be seen as far as three crypts from the ulcer's edge; thus, it might be tentatively suggested unless the disease is quiescent that at least four dysplastic crypts should be present to make a positive diagnosis. If quiescent, even one or two crypts indefinite for dysplasia may stand out sufficiently that the diagnosis is simple.

Second, the residual mucosa is often so typical of quiescent colitis (with crypts that are full of goblet cells containing nuclei that are small and regular) that an adjacent area containing cells depleted of mucus but having enlarged nuclei contrasts more strongly with it. This may lead the pathologist to use an inappropriately high grade. Nevertheless, the contrast is also useful, since ulceration in ulcerative colitis invariably occurs on a background of a heavy acute and chronic inflammatory infiltrate, except in some patients with fulminant disease. The presence of quiescent colitis with an adjacent area that is morphologically different is likely to represent either the focal changes seen in Crohn's disease or epithelium that is becoming dysplastic. Surprisingly, the latter is frequently accompanied by an increase in chronic, but not acute, inflammatory cells limited entirely to the vicinity of the abnormal epithelium. Whether this represents a host response as seen in dysplasia elsewhere in the body is speculative, but it is present often enough to be expected, and should not lead to its misinterpretation as being the result of recent inflammation.

DYSPLASIA IN INFLAMMATORY POLYPS

Dysplasia in inflammatory polyps is well documented but relatively uncommon. As with dysplasia occurring in nonpolypoid mucosa, an entire spectrum of changes ranging from postinflammatory to high-grade dysplasia may be found. These changes should be graded using the system proposed, but with the suffix that the lesion is from an inflammatory polyp. The major problem with these polyps is that they frequently show nuclear changes that are greater

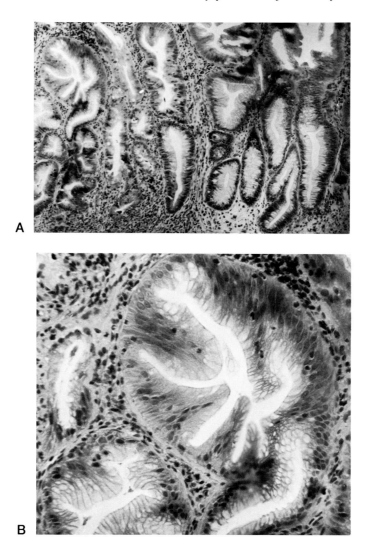

Fig. 4-19. Mucosa ''indefinite for dysplasia'' with serrated crypts. (**A**) The superficial part of the mucosa contains crypts having an infolded, sawtooth, or serrated appearance similar to that seen in hyperplastic polyps. The crypt bases contain enlarged hyperchromatic nuclei that fall just short of changes seen in adenomas and are therefore ''indefinite for dysplasia—probably positive.'' (**B**) Detail of crypt in the upper left of part A shows better the serrated pattern. (H&E, Fig. A ×125, Fig. B ×500.)

than those in the adjacent mucosa, although such changes usually fall short of unequivocal neoplasia (dysplasia) (Fig. 4-21). Nevertheless, examples of dysplasia occurring in inflammatory polyps are encountered, and ultimately the distinction between an inflammatory polyp and an adenoma may become blurred (Fig. 4-22). In dysplastic polyps, the possibility that the lesion began as an inflammatory polyp may only be considered because of the abnormal architecture of the polyp; which contains crypts that are markedly enlarged and contain cystic spaces in an abundant lamina propria, as seen in other inflammatory polyps.

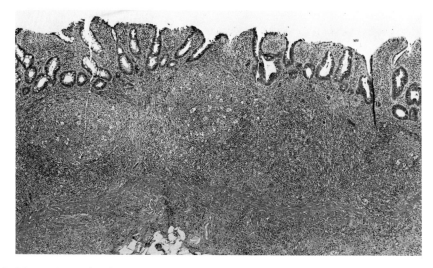

Fig. 4-20. Mucosa "negative for dysplasia" with follicular inflammation. Numerous germinal centers can be seen, primarily in the submucosa. However, the epithelium is graded as other epithelium, although regenerative changes may be very marked in this type of mucosa. (H&E, ×25.)

THE INFLUENCE OF ACUTE INFLAMMATION

The problems associated with an inflammatory infiltrate have long been a major stumbling block in the diagnosis of dysplasia in colitis. There are good reasons for this. First, the lack of definition of dysplasia as encompassing only unequivocally neoplastic changes meant that a variety of changes that fell short of this were reported as a mild or moderate type or dysplasia. Second, changes that in the current terminology would have been considered sequela of an acute inflammatory process or "indefinite for dysplasia" may also have been included under the general terms of *atypia* or *dysplasia*. The significance of such changes is very confusing to the clinician who cannot incorporate such information into a definitive plan of management for the patient. Familiarity with the spectrum of changes that are the result of an acute inflammatory process removes a potentially large source of error. If this situation is to be avoided in the future it is imperative that terms such as *inflammatory dysplasia* no longer be used and that *dysplasia* be used only in the context of neoplasia. Finally, the identification of the prob-lems discussed in the preceding sections removes additional sources of confusion. Nevertheless, this does leave a small number of biopsies that contain acute inflammatory cells and nuclear changes so exuberant that serious consideration has to be given to the possibility that the epithelium is dysplastic, as discussed in the section Mucosa Idenfinite for Dysplasia.

At one end of the spectrum there is no real doubt that neoplastic crypts are readily recognized in the presence of acute inflammation or ulceration. In the noncolitic, adenomas are often ulcerated or inflamed or contain crypt abscesses, but this never causes a diagnostic problem and represents little more than a pathologic curiosity (Fig. 4-23). This is true because if crypt abscesses are present they do not involve all the adenomatous crypts, and usually involve only one or two. The focality of the acute inflammation in the areas of dysplasia, together with the lack of a diffuse acute inflammatory reaction throughout the lamina propria that attacks the crypts (as seen typically in active ulcerative colitis), causes the inflammation to be ignored.

Unfortunately, there is currently no infallible method of making a definitive diagnosis in this

Fig. 4-21. Mucosa "indefinite for dysplastia—unknown," in an inflammatory polyp. (**A**) Typical low-power appearance of an inflammatory polyp. (**B**) Detail from the region of the arrow, showing marked mucin depletion and nuclear enlargement. (**C**) High-power view of part of the crypt in the upper right quadrant of part B shows that although nuclei are large and mitotic activity is prominent the nuclei are not hyperchromatic; indeed, it is difficult to make out any nuclear detail. In addition, there is not the increased number of nuclei usually seen in dysplastic epithelium. Because the criteria for dysplasia are not present unequivocally the epithelium is graded as "indefinite for dysplasia." The "unknown" suffix is because neither "probably negative" nor "probably positive" is applicable. Similar changes in active colitis have been known to resolve entirely within a month or two, but sometimes nuclei remain enlarged and similar to those seen in the crypts in Fig. 4-19A. Only time will show whether such mucosa has increased neoplastic potential. (H&E, Fig. A ×9, Fig. B ×100, Fig. C ×1,000.)

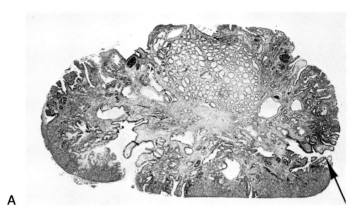

A

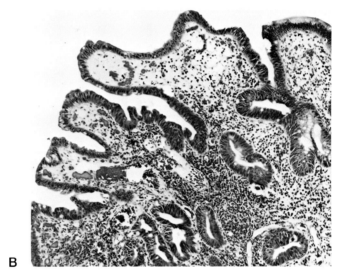

B

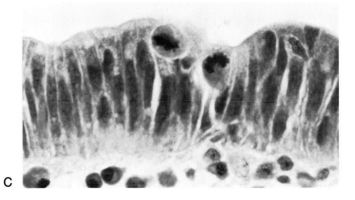

C

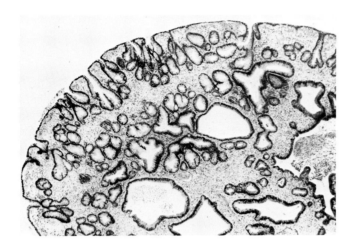

Fig. 4-22. Inflammatory polyp with mucosa "positive for low-grade dysplasia." The architecture of the polyp with an excess of lamina propria and dilated glands is frequently seen in inflammatory polyps, and it is likely that this polyp was originally inflammatory. When such polyps are excised, the adjacent mucosa should always be biopsied to ensure that the polyp is not part of a larger area of dysplasia when local excision of the polyp alone would be inadequate treatment. (H&E, ×20.)

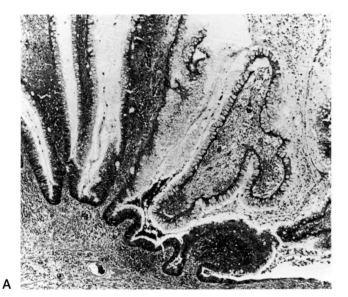

A

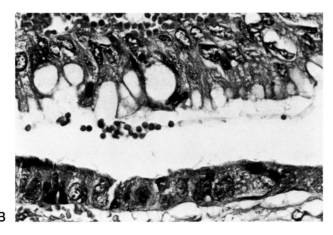

B

Fig. 4-23. (A) Mucosa "positive for dysplasia" with ulceration (bottom left). **(B)** Detail from the regenerating epithelium shows much greater pleomorphism and a greater chromatin content than seen in regenerating epithelium unassociated with dysplastic mucosa. (H&E, Fig. A ×100, Fig. B ×400.)

situation, although it should be noted that in the colitic bowel neoplastic epithelium seems to be relatively immune to a brisk inflammatory reaction in the adjacent mucosa.

Fortunately, this classification makes such biopsies relatively easy to deal with. Because there is at least a shadow of doubt concerning whether the lesion really is dysplastic, in view of the heavy acute inflammatory infiltrate present, such biopsies cannot be regarded as unequivocally neoplastic (dysplastic) and cannot therefore be called "positive for dysplasia." The category "indefinite for dysplasia" (but "probably dysplastic" if this suffix is deemed necessary) is best for such biopsies. Further, this category requires repeated biopsies within a short period of time (see the following discussion). These often help to resolve the question, since the changes may regress, particularly if treated with vigorous medical therapy. In this situation, it is not unreasonable for the pathologist to ask his clinical colleagues if medication can be increased in an attempt to resolve the inflammation and concomitant nuclear changes. Most clinicians conversant with this dilemma are willing to do this, particularly if the pathologist has involved them in the problem by reviewing the slides with them.

IMPLICATIONS OF BIOPSY RESULTS FOR PATIENT MANAGEMENT

This section is included because there is no "best" way of managing patients with colitis who are at risk for developing dysplasia, and because the pathologist's advice is invariably critical, particularly when the question of possible colectomy is raised. Routine follow-up of patients relies heavily on colonsocopy with multiple biopsies, and this is usually carried out at roughly annual intervals. Preliminary data indicated that double-contrast barium enemas may have a place in the localization of suspicious lesions to be biopsied but are not generally used.[55] Single-contrast barium enemas are fre-

quently worthless, because only gross lesions are detected; if these prove to be neoplastic the prognosis is usually extremely poor. Given our current lack of objective data, colonoscopy with multiple biopsies appears to be the best method of following patients and detecting early neoplastic changes. Recommendations following colonoscopy are very limited, and consist only of follow-up colonoscopy about 1 year later, follow-up at a shorter interval (increased surveillance), or a recommendation for colectomy (usually proctocolectomy).

REPRODUCIBILITY

The test system of classification rests on whether biopsy interpretations prove reasonably reproducible by the same pathologist and by other pathologists familiar with the system. As with all subjective assessments of a spectrum of changes that is somewhat arbitrarily divided and that depends to a certain extent on personal experience, reproducibility is not absolute. Nevertheless, given the relatively limited number of options available, false-negative and false-positive results will be relatively uncommon.[51] However, as these will occasionally occur, some form of confirmation should be sought when biopsy changes are a major indication for considering surgical intervention, preferably by the aid of a second pathologist familiar with the system or by repeated biopsies.[51] The latter is fraught with hazard, primarily because the endoscopic appearances of dysplasia remain very poorly documented so that it may be virtually impossible to return to what may have been a very small patch of dysplasia.

MANAGEMENT OF NEGATIVE BIOPSIES

A series of biopsies reflecting changes that may be seen in quiescent, active, or resolving colitis, or in biopsies that seem most likely to be the result of these processes, do not justify any increase in surveillance.

MANAGEMENT OF BIOPSIES INDEFINITE FOR DYSPLASIA

Biopsies showing changes that are "indefinite for dysplasia" cannot simply be dismissed, nor do such biopsies justify colectomy. In those instances when the changes are most likely due to an exuberant response to acute inflammation ("negative for dysplasia" or "indefinite for dysplasia—probably negative"), the time interval between colonoscopies may not need to be reduced, although the observer is always at liberty to suggest this. Where there is greater likelihood that a dysplastic lesion might be present (the categories "indefinite for dysplasia—unknown," or "probably positive"), a shorter-interval follow-up (within a few months) is indicated until the nature of the lesion becomes clear. An alternative mode of follow-up may then be recommended. Medical treatment of active disease may lead to resolution of a morphologic abnormality, but if the lesion in question is focal, it is imperative to try to return to and biopsy the same lesion or area; otherwise, apparent resolution may in fact be due to failure to rebiopsy the appropriate site. There is no way to know if an abnormal biopsy obtained from an otherwise unremarkable area of large bowel really resolved or whether it was focal and was not resampled. If the lesion persists, it can be carefully followed at whatever intervals appear most appropriate to ensure that it does not ultimately become neoplastic.

Increased surveillance is therefore appropriate, which implies repeating the colonoscopy and biopsies within a few months. If active disease was present this time frame is often adequate to allow inflammation to subside, particularly if treated. However, it should be recalled that the objective of therapy is to control the patient's symptoms and not the endoscopic or biopsy appearances, and in some patients it may be inappropriate to do this; particularly if it means adding systemic steroids, which may not be easily withdrawn. This may result in biopsies that are repeatedly indefinite for dysplasia. Provided that the morphologic features remain stable and do not progress to unequivocally dysplastic it is reasonable to lengthen the intervals between endoscopy until the usual intervals are again reached. Increasingly, the presence of aneuploidy may be one method of determining whether patients require increased surveillance,[56] but there are currently no good studies utilizing this parameter in this situation.

MANAGEMENT OF DYSPLASTIC BIOPSIES

Controversy continues regarding the management of dysplastic biopsies. The immediate problem is that there remains relatively little data regarding the likelihood of an underlying invasive carcinoma being present on which to base a rational decision. The notion that all patients must be managed on an individual basis continues to guarantee that data remain difficult to obtain. This is often the case because the decision for colectomy is rarely made on the basis of dysplasia alone, but on weighing both the risks and benefits of all courses of action. Numerous factors affect this, including the extent of disability from the disease, the attitude of both the patient and physician toward colectomy, age and life expectancy of the patient, the operative risk, and availability of and confidence in both the pathologist and surgeon, the latter particularly if a pouch procedure is contemplated.

However, there are circumstances in which there is relatively uniform agreement regarding a recommendation for colectomy. These include the presence of a dysplasia-associated lesion or mass on endoscopy; which probably stands a greater than 50 percent risk of being an invasive cancer on resection, particularly if found on the first (diagnostic) rather than subsequent (surveillance) colonoscopy.[29,40] The reason is that at the first endoscopy the length of time that a lesion has been present is unknown, while if seen at surveillance colonoscopy it is unlikely to have been present for extended periods of time. The same also holds true for the presence of dysplasia of any grade if seen at the first colonoscopy, thus its presence at first colonoscopy should lead to much more serious consideration of dysplasia than if it develops at surveillance colonscopy.

CONFIRMATION OF DYSPLASIA

The question of whether confirmation of dysplasia is required, and if so; how it is best confirmed, has become contentious. Confirmation by a second pathologist clearly depends on the competence of both pathologists and the degree of confidence that the gastroenterologist has in each pathologist. Most of the time the diagnosis of dysplasia is very straightforward, and therefore confirmation by a second pathologist is usually only necessary if either party is insecure. This assumes that there has been a distinct learning curve over the last decade, particularly in the distinction from reparative changes, which certainly appears to be the case. However, the likelihood of requesting a second opinion inevitably increases if colectomy is being considered primarily because of the biopsy diagnosis of dysplasia.

THE FOCALITY OF DYSPLASIA AND PROBLEMS OF SAMPLING

In contrast to patients presenting clinically with invasive carcinoma in whom dysplasia may be relatively widespread and cancers multiple,[4,53] in patients under surveillance both of these are uncommon. Dysplasia is frequently confined to small areas of the mucosa, and this causes major sampling problems for the endoscopist. Further, the endoscopic appearance of dysplasia is very poorly defined in the literature, and these largely reiterate gross pathologic descriptions. No prospective endoscopic study exists, and most accept that dysplasia (and sometimes invasive carcinoma) may occasionally be found on random biopsies in the absence of an endoscopic abnormality. Unless dysplasia is widespread or an area of dysplasia can be visualized endoscopically, confirmation of dysplasia by repeated endoscopy and biopsy is usually doomed to failure because it has repeatedly been shown that dysplasia is patchy.[22,33,35,53,57,58] Current sampling methods of taking 1 or 2 biopsies every 10 cm of bowel assume that perhaps 5 mm^2 of biopsy is representative of 100×100 mm^2 of mucosa, that is, at best 1/2000th of the mucosa is being sampled. Given this intense sampling problem, if one is fortunate enough to detect it on biopsy it makes little sense to ignore it if the criterion for colectomy is the development of dysplasia. To accentuate the sampling problem further, a 2×2 cm patch of dysplasia would require about 20 to 25 evenly spaced biopsies in a 10-cm length of bowel to reasonably guarantee its detection. In requesting an endoscopist to confirm the presence of dysplasia by repeating the endoscopy and the biopsies, we are clearly being incredibly optimistic and unrealistic, and should not be surprised if such missions fail.

OPTIONS FOR MANAGEMENT

Options for patient management are regular surveillance, increased surveillance, or resection. If resection is not recommended then the option is to repeat the endoscopy and biopsies; the only issue is when and how will the results affect the management algorithm. Some have criteria for consideration of colectomy, which variously include the repeated demonstration of dysplasia on endoscopic biopsy, the development of high-grade dysplasia, the repeated demonstration of low-grade dysplasia, or the development of a dysplasia-associated lesion or mass. All of these options are geared toward delaying colectomy, the assumption being that the risk of a potentially lethal cancer at this time is extremely low, a position for which there is little support, and which deliberately chooses to disregard that part of the definition of dysplasia stating that it may give rise directly to invasive carcinoma irrespective of the grade, and may also be the superficial part of an invasive carcinoma. It also ignores the fact that carcinomas may escape endoscopic detection, that it is impossible to time colectomy to the point of minimal invasion, or that strategies along these lines do not appear to have reduced the mortality from colorectal cancer in surveillance programs.

HIGH-GRADE DYSPLASIA

A biopsy or biopsies yielding high-grade dysplasia justify recommendation for colectomy, in view of the high risk of the patient having a synchronous occult carcinoma, as described previously. Clearly, if nothing is to be advocated in the face of the biopsy yielding high-grade dysplasia, then there is no point in having placed the patient in a cancer-prevention protocol. Nevertheless, this is only a recommendation, and it must always be remembered that the ultimate objective is the longevity of the patient. The recommendation must therefore be weighed against the immediate and long-term morbidity and mortality of the operation and its sequela, balanced against those doing nothing, with the understanding that the final decision regarding operation is the patient's.

LOW-GRADE DYSPLASIA

The most controversial and difficult issues regarding the management of biopsies are encountered with biopsies showing low-grade dysplasia and the presence of true adenomas in a patient with colitis. Patients that have biopsies showing low-grade dysplasia (that is, unequivocal neoplastic change but with relatively little dysplasia) pose a problem, because arguments can be made for a variety of different courses of management. The most serious is the recommendation that the patient undergo proctocolectomy, justifiable because the biopsy has demonstrated that the large bowel has the ability to form mucosa that can give rise directly to an invasive carcinoma (dysplasia). This is particularly true if the biopsy was taken from an endoscopically visible lesion, since this could prove to be an invasive carcinoma on resection.[29]

At the other extreme, it can be argued that there is no information regarding the behavior of these biopsies, and therefore the patient should be followed to gain information about the true significance of the biopsies. The obvious counterargument is that the development of an unequivocally neoplastic lesion could itself be regarded as an endpoint. A further difficulty is that if such patients are merely followed, what is to be the endpoint for these patients, particularly when it is known that even invasive carcinomas may not be detected even when biopsied?[29,40] (see the following discussion). The situation is perhaps analogous to following an adenoma in the noncolitic just to see if it will ultimately become invasive.

In summary, if low-grade dysplasia is found in the presence of an endoscopic lesion other than an adenoma (see below), this is a clear indication for colectomy and local lymphadenectomy, this being a typical dysplasia-associated lesion or mass. In the absence of an endoscopic lesion the options remain to recommend colectomy as a preventative measure or to repeat the endoscopy and biopsies. The advantages and disadvantages of the latter have been discussed above.

CHOICES OF OPERATION

The operation of choice is one that removes all large bowel mucosa, namely proctocolectomy with or without a pouch as appropriate; anything less than this leaves diseased large bowel in which further neoplasms may develop if not already present. Nevertheless, some patients, for a variety of understandable reasons, refuse the proctectomy part of the operation. If a decision is taken to comply with the patient's wishes, the necessity for continued close follow-up of all residual large bowel must be stressed. There is virtually no place for partial colectomy in the management of dysplasia. Finally, if a dysplastic biopsy comes from an endoscopic lesion that ultimately might prove to be a carcinoma, a radical lymphadenectomy should be carried out in that area, despite the lack of biopsy proof. This helps prevent the necessity to return and complete the lymphadenectomy should the lesion prove to be invasive following resection.

MANAGEMENT OF ADENOMAS IN ULCERATIVE COLITIS

The major concern of adenomas is that they may represent part of a larger area of dysplasia. If the latter is the case, then it will be impossible to excise the lesion completely colonoscopically, for the dysplastic mucosa will continue into the stalk and the adjacent mucosa. When the possibility of this situation is encountered endoscopically, the polyps should be snared if possible and multiple biopsies taken of the adjacent mucosa, particularly in patients who are in the adenoma-bearing age range. If the adjacent mucosa as well as the polyp proves to be dysplastic, polypectomy will not remove the entire lesion, and colectomy is recommended. However, there is theoretically no reason why colitic patients in the adenoma-bearing age group (for the sake of argument, over 50 years old) should not be just as susceptible to adenoma formation than the noncolitic population, and its removal protect them from the development of cancer, as seen in the noncolitic population.[59] The management of such lesions is currently controversial. At one extreme is such a lesion occurring in a 30-year-old patient with a 16-year history of colitis. It can be argued that he has demonstrated the potential of his large bowel to form neoplastic lesions and is therefore in a very high-risk category for the subsequent development of carcinoma. Logically, one could argue that the wisest course of action would be excision of the large bowel to ensure, as far as one can, the patient's longevity, irrespective of the presence or absence or dysplasia in the mucosa adjacent to the polyp.

At the other extreme might be a 68-year-old patient with a 10-year history of colitis who has two typical adenomas excised from his sigmoid colon, but no other evidence of dysplasia. The possibility that these may have been potentiated by the colitic process cannot be denied, but it currently seems most reasonable to treat such patients conservatively and to simply follow them carefully. The lack of dysplasia in the mucosa adjacent to the polyp would support this interpretation.

The most difficult patients to manage are those intermediate between these two examples, for example, a 42-year-old patient with an adenoma but no other evidence of dysplasia and a 12-year history of colitis. Arguably he could be treated conservatively. However, if he has two or three such lesions, the possibility that these are not simple adenomas but part of the colitic process is increased, and the chance that other undiscovered lesions are present also has to be borne in mind. Under these circumstances it is difficult to avoid suggesting colectomy. In such patients a variety of other clinical and personal factors tend to affect this decision. It is apparent from these examples that clinical judgment still has a large role to play in determining when a patient should undergo colectomy.

NEGATIVE RESECTION SPECIMENS FOLLOWING A DIAGNOSIS OF DYSPLASIA

A concern of some is that even if colectomy is carried out for the presence of dysplasia, at least half of the patients will *not* have an unsuspected carcinoma in the resected specimen, raising the possibility that the patient may never have developed a carcinoma and has therefore been subjected to an unnecessary operation. There is clearly no way of knowing whether a cancer would or would not have developed, and if it had developed whether it would have also been detected before dissemination had occurred; it is only known that a patient at high risk of developing colorectal cancer will now never develop it. Nevertheless some clinicians are disappointed if an invasive carcinoma is not present in the resected specimen, despite the good fortune of the patient. Often the presence of a "small" carcinoma that has usually been cured by the resection justified the resection for both clinician and patient. The patient with biopsy-proven dysplasia but without invasive carcinoma at resection is surely in the best clinical situation.

Many centers now have patients with dysplasia who have refused an operation, while some are following carefully selected patients with dysplasia. This is obviously not without hazard. However, we have no further follow-up information on such patients either undergoing subsequent operation or coming to autopsy. One study using patients lost to follow-up as controls found a definite mortality from cancer in that group, unlike those undergoing surveillance in whom this did not occur.[20]

Although uncommon, an embarrassing situation sometimes arises when numerous blocks of tissue fail to reveal any dysplasia at all after colectomy has been carried out for dysplasia. Further, this situation also arises, albeit rarely, when a biopsy has revealed an invasive adenocarcinoma. The only possible explanations are that (1) the lesion was completely removed by the biopsy, (2) the remainder of the lesion was present in the resected specimen but not observed or sampled, (3) the biopsy was somehow confused with that from another patient, or (4) the biopsy was misinterpreted. Although the most likely interpretations are the first two, particularly with a small lesion, the possibility of the last is the most disquieting. It only requires one encounter with a situation such as this for a clinician to lose confidence in the pathologist, to say nothing of the fall in the pathologist's own self-confidence. There is currently no objective knowledge on the frequency with which this occurs. Operative intervention (i.e., ''prophylactic'' proctocolectomy) also has its own small but definite risks.

A possible fifth reason for the failure of the blocks to reveal dysplasia is that there has been regression of dysplasia. Although not entirely impossible, there is little evidence to support this contention. However, there has been a suggestion that folate supplements may prevent the onset of dysplasia.[60]

EXAMINATION OF A BIOPSY FOR DYSPLASIA

This section is aimed at helping the practicing pathologist in interpreting biopsies that are taken for dysplasia. However, it should be remembered that good examples of dysplasia may often be found in the mucosa adjacent to carcinomas found in patients with colitis, therefore review of surgical pathology files may provide material with dysplasia for review. In addition, it cannot be stressed too greatly that in attempting to recognize dysplasia it is imperative that the pathologist be familiar with the range of changes that may be seen in all other phases of the disease.

ORIENTATION

The diagnosis of any phase of IBD is greatly facilitated by the examination of well-oriented biopsies. This can be accomplished by a technician, who can orient small biopsies when embedding them in paraffin, or by the endoscopist, who can orient biopsies for the pathologist by manually removing them from the forceps and orientating them on a mounting medium. When the biopsy is taken, the lumenal surface abuts the concave surface of the jaws of the forceps. When the jaws are opened following biopsy, the spike is placed directly onto a piece of millipore filter and the biopsy gently scraped from the spike using a fine needle; the submucosal surface is then in direct contact with the millipore filter and the lumenal surface is uppermost. The filter and biopsy are then placed directly into fixative, and both can be embedded and cut together. A variety of substances can be used for mounting biopsies, including pieces of filter paper, millipore filter, and even thinly sliced alcohol-fixed cucumber, all of which can be processed and cut without removing the biopsy from the material on which it has been oriented. Ideally, each biopsy should be placed in a separately labelled container together with the site. If the patient is charged directly according to the number of blocks utilized for the pathology, some include all biopsies from the same part of the large bowel in one block, or even color-code biopsies from each part of the colon with a different color dye to allow numerous biopsies to be included in one block.

EFFECTS OF PREPARATION FOR ENDOSCOPY

Some of the features associated with IBD may be mimicked to some extent by the purgation used prior to colonoscopy. Microscopically, at low power this is most commonly reflected by mucin depletion, which results in the crypts staining in an eosinophilic manner rather than showing the clear cytoplasmic staining that results from the presence of mucin. Eosinophilically-staining crypts are important to detect at low power because they may be seen in both active disease and dysplasia (see below). Most patients with colitis receive relatively little preparation prior to colonoscopy. In addition to mucin depletion there may be damage to the lumenal surface, reflected by an attenuated, actively regenerating epithelium, including occasional mitotic figures high in the crypts or on the surface and sometimes the presence of polymorphs in the same location.[61] Electrolytically and osmotically balanced preparatives seem not to affect morphology.

EFFECT OF FIXATIVES IN BIOPSY INTERPRETATION

The choice of fixative for biopsies has to be taken into account when interpreting biopsies in which the underlying question is whether dysplasia is present. When compared with formalin fixation, which causes nuclear chromatin to appear relatively condensed, other mercury- or picric- acid-based fixatives such as Bouin's, Hollande's, or B5 produce much more vesicular nuclei. These nuclear changes can lead to over-interpretation of dysplasia in active or resolving colitis, particularly when the effects of mucin depletion resulting from bowel preparation are also present.

BIOPSY EXAMINATION

Assuming the biopsy is adequate, the presence of dysplasia can frequently be suspected at low power, and microscopy at this power should seek to answer the following questions.

1. What is the surface configuration (flat, villous, ulcerated, hyperplastic polyp-like)? Flat or slightly convex surfaces are obtained with most mucosal biopsies. A villous appearance should immediately lead to a search for other features of acute inflammation and regeneration or dysplasia. An ulcerated surface is usually a feature of active disease, but may occur in all polyps and tumors. A hyerplastic polyp-like appearance should lead to careful examination of the crypt bases to ensure that these are not dysplastic. This type of mucosa is virtually unknown in active disease.

2. Is there mucus depletion in the crypts? (Are they pink or white?) Mucus depletion in crypts is due to preparative enemas, active disease, or dysplasia, and at low power constitutes one of the most important keys to the possibility that dysplasia is present. In a typically regenerated mucosa the presence of abundant mucus and only a small nuclear rim in the crypts virtually excludes dysplasia. Only a brief confirmatory glance at high power is usually required to confirm the low-power impression.

3. In the presence of such a signal, the next question is the following: Does the rim of crypt nuclei appear normal in size or more prominent?

4. Attention is then focused on the lamina propria to answer the following questions: What is the nature of the inflammatory infiltrate (normal plasma cells and lymphoid tissue, follicular inflammation)? Is it normal or increased, and is it diffuse or focal in the lamina propria? If

there is little or no increase in inflammatory cells, dysplasia and possibly preparation artifact will be the most likely diagnoses, and the changes should be evaluated at higher power. If follicular inflammation is present, evidence of active disease and regeneration should be sought. Great care should be taken before a diagnosis of dysplasia is made. If the inflammatory infiltrate is quantitatively normal, is there any focal abnormality in the epithelium that might reflect focal dysplasia? If the inflammatory infiltrate is focal (other than for the normal lymphoid aggregates that straddle the muscularis mucosae), is this a reflection of resolving disease, Crohn's disease (which may be reflected by focal disease within and between biopsies excluding inflammatory polyps), or focal nuclear changes that might be chronic inflammation in the vicinity of the changes only?

All of these features may be confirmed at higher power, but some become particularly important. If there is an increase in inflammatory cells, is there a polymorphonuclear component, and if so are they attacking the crypts? If yes, is this limited to a few crypts or is it diffuse? If the latter, are the nuclear changes consistent with those that may be found in the acute or regenerating phase of ulcerative colitis? Even a partially positive answer excludes a positive diagnosis of dysplasia.

ACKNOWLEDGMENTS

The author thanks Janice Butera and Barb Lahie for their word processing assistance.

REFERENCES

1. Devroede GJ, Taylor WF, Sauer WG, et al: Cancer risk and life expectancy in children with ulcerative colitis. N Engl J Med 285:17, 1971
2. Mottet NK: Histopathologic Spectrum of Regional Enteritis and Ulcerative Colitis. p. 220. WB Saunders, Philadelphia, 1971
3. Kewenter J, Ahlman H, Hulten L: Cancer risk in extensive ulcerative colitis. Ann Surg 88:824, 1978
4. Morson BC, Pang LSC: Rectal biopsy as an aid to cancer control in ulcerative colitis. Gut 8:423, 1967
5. Riddell RH: The precarcinomatous phase of ulcerative colitis. Cur Top Pathol 63:179, 1976
6. Devroede GJ, Dockerty MB, Sauer WG, et al: Cancer of the colon in patients with ulcerative colitis since childhood. Can J Surg 15:369, 1972
7. Fuson JA, Farmer RG, Hawk WA, et al: Endoscopic surveillance for cancer in chronic ulcerative colitis. Am J Gastroenterol 73:120, 1980
8. Lennard-Jones JE, Morson BC, Ritchie JK, et al: Cancer in colitis; assessment of the individual risk by clinical and histological criteria. Gastroenterology 73:1280, 1977
9. de Dombal FT, Watts JMcK, Watkinson G, Goligher JC: Local complications of ulcerative colitis; stricture, pseudopolyposis and carcinoma of colon and rectum. Br Med J 1:1442, 1966
10. Greenstein AJ, Sachar DB, Smith H, et al: Cancer in universal and left-sided ulcerative colitis: factors determining risk. Gastroenterology 77:290, 1979
11. Lennard-Jones JE, Morson BC, Ritchie JK, Williams CB: Cancer surveillance in ulcerative colitis. Lancet 2:149, 1983
12. Hendriksen C, Kreiner S, Binder V: Longterm prognosis in ulcerative colitis based on results from a regional group from the county of Copenhagen. Gut 26:158, 1985
13. Gilat T, Fireman Z, Grossman A, et al: Colorectal cancer in patients with ulcerative colitis. A population study in central Israel. Gastroenterology 94:870, 1988
14. Gyde SN, Prior P, Allan RN, et al: Colorectal cancer in ulcerative colitis: a cohort study of primary referrals from three centres. Gut 29:206, 1988
15. Brostrom O, Lofgberg R, Ost A, Reichard H: Cancer surveillance of patients with longstanding ulcerative colitis: a clinical, endoscopical, and histological study. Gut 27:1408, 1986
16. Lashner BA, Hanauer SB, Silverstein MD: Optimal timing of colonoscopy to screen for cancer in ulcerative colitis. Ann Int Med 108:274, 1988
17. Lennard-Jones JE, Misiewitz JJ, Parrish JA, et al: Prospective study of outpatients with extensive colitis. Lancet i:1065, 1974

18. Niv Y, Bat L, Theodor E: Changes in the extent of inflammatory extent in ulcerative colitis. Am J Gastroenterol 82:1046, 1987

19. Collins RH, Feldman M, Fordtran JS: Colon cancer, dysplasia, and surveillance in patients with ulcerative colitis. N Engl J Med 316:1654, 1987

20. Jones HW, Grogono J, Hoare AM: Surveillance in ulcerative colitis: burdens and benefits. Gut 29:325, 1988

21. Manning AP, Bulgim OR, Dixon MF, Axon ATR: Screening by colonoscopy for colonic epithelial dysplasia in inflammatory bowel disease. Gut 28:1489, 1987

22. Nugent FW, Haggitt RC, Colcher H, Kutteruf GC: Malignant potential of chronic ulcerative colitis: preliminary report. Gastroenterology 76:1, 1979

23. Biasco G, Miglioli M, DiFebo G, et al: Cancer and dysplasia in ulcerative colitis: preliminary report of a prospective study. Ital J Gastroenterol 6:212, 1984

24. Hulten L, Kewenter J, Ahren C: Precancer and carcinoma in chronic ulcerative colitis. Scand J Gastroenterol 7:663, 1972

25. Allen DC, Biggart JD, Pyper PC: Large bowel mucosal dysplasia and carcinoma in ulcerative colitis. J Clin Pathol 38:30, 1985

26. Rutegard JN, Ahsgren LR, Janunger KJ: Ulcerative colitis: colorectal cancer risk in an unselected population. Ann Surg 208:721, 1988

27. Turunen MJ, Jarvinen HJ: Cancer in ulcerative colitis: What failed in following up? Acta Chir Scand 151:669, 1985

28. Muto T, Bussey HJR, Morson BC: The evolution of cancer of the colon and rectum. Cancer 36:2251, 1975

29. Blackstone MO, Riddell RH, Rogers GBH, Levin B: Dysplasia-associated lesion or mass (DALM) detected by colonoscopy in longstanding ulcerative colitis: An indication for colectomy. Gastroenterology 80:355, 1981

30. Crowson T, Ferrante WF, Gathright JB: Colonoscopy: Inefficacy for early carcinoma detection in patients with ulcerative colitis. JAMA 236:2351, 1976

31. Warren S, Sommers SC: Pathogenesis of ulcerative colitis. Am J Pathol 25:657, 1949

32. Dawson IMP, Pryse-Davies J: The development of carcinoma of the large intestine in ulcerative colitis. Br J Surg 47:113, 1959

33. Cook MG, Goligher JC: Carcinoma and epithelial dysplasia complicating ulcerative colitis. Gastroenterology 68:1127, 1975

34. Dickerson RJ, Dixon MF, Axon ATR: Colonoscopy and the detection of dysplasia in patients with longstanding ulcerative colitis. Lancet 2:620, 1980

35. Evans DJ, Pollock DJ: In-situ and invasive carcinoma of the colon in patients with ulcerative colitis. Gut 13:566, 1972

36. Fenoglio CM, Pascal RR: Adenomatous epithelium, intraepithelial anaplasia and invasive carcinoma in ulcerative colitis. Am J Dig Dis 18:556, 1973

37. Gewertz BL, Dent TL, Appelman HD: Implications of precancerous rectal biopsy in patients with inflammatory bowel disease. Arch Surg 111:326, 1976

38. Kewenter J, Hulten L, Ahren C: The occurrence of severe epithelial dysplasia and its bearing on treatment of longstanding ulcerative colitis. Ann Surg 195:209, 1982

39. Myrvold HE, Kock NG, Ahren CHR: Rectal biopsy and precancer in ulcerative colitis. Gut 15:301, 1974

40. Rosenstock E, Farmer RG, Petras R, et al: Surveillance for colon carcinoma in ulcerative colitis. Gastroenterology 89:1342, 1985

41. Yardley JH, Keren DF: "Precancer" lesions in ulcerative colitis. A retrospective study of rectal biopsy and colectomy specimens. Cancer 34:835, 1974

42. Dobbins WO III: Current status of the precancer lesion in ulcerative colitis. Gastroenterology 73:1413, 1977

43. Yardley JH, Bayless TM, Diamond MP: Cancer and ulcerative colitis (editorial). Gastroenterology 76:221, 1979

44. Darke SG, Parks AG, Grogono JL, Pollock DJ: Adenocarcinoma and Crohn's disease—a report of 2 cases and an analysis of the literature. Br J Surg 60:169, 1973

45. Greenstein AJ, Sachar DB, Smith H, et al: Patterns of neoplasia in Crohn's disease and ulcerative colitis. Cancer 46:403, 1980

46. Gyde SN, Prior P, Macartney JCC, et al: Malignancy in Crohn's disease. Gut 21:1024, 1980

47. Weeden DD, Shorter RG, Ilstrup DM, et al: Crohn's disease and cancer. N Engl J Med 289:1099, 1973

48. Craft CF, Mendelsohn G, Cooper HS, Yardley

JH: Colonic "precancer" in Crohn's disease. Gastroenterology 80:578, 1981

49. Simpson S, Traube J, Riddell RH: The histological appearance of dysplasia (precarcinomatous change) in Crohn's disease of the small and large intestine. Gastroenterology 81:492, 1981

50. Ming-Chai C, Chi-Yaun C, Pei-Yu C, Jen-Chun H: Evolution of colorectal cancer in schistosomiasis: transitional mucosal changes adjacent to large intestinal carcinoma in colectomy specimens. Cancer 46:1661, 1980

51. Riddell RH, Goldman H, Ransohoff DF, et al: Dysplasia in inflammatory bowel disease: standardized classification with provisional clinical implications. Hum Pathol 14:931, 1983

52. Butt JH, Konoshi F, Morson BC, et al: Macroscopic lesions in dysplasia and carcinoma complicating ulcerative colitis. Dig Dis Sci 28:18, 1983

53. Ransohoff DF, Riddell RH, Levin B: Ulcerative colitis and colonic cancer. Problems in assessing the diagnostic usefulness of mucosal dysplasia. Dis Colon Rectum 28:383, 1985

54. Yardley JH, Donowitz M: Colo-rectal biopsy in inflammatory bowel disease. p. 50. In Yardley JH, Morson BC, Abell MR (eds): The Gastrointestinal Tract. Williams & Wilkins, Baltimore, 1977

55. Frank PH, Riddell RH, Feczko PJ, Levin B: Radiological detection of colonic dysplasia (precarcinoma) in chronic ulcerative colitis. Gastrointest Radiol 3:209, 1978

56. Lofberg R, Caspersson T, Tribukait B, Ost A: Comparative DNA analyses in longstanding ulcerative colitis with aneuploidy. Gut 30:1731, 1989

57. Riddell RH, Morson BC: Value of sigmoidoscopy and biopsy in the detection of carcinoma and premalignant change in ulcerative colitis. Gut 20:575, 1979

58. Vatn MH, Elgjo K, Bergan A: Distribution of dysplasia in colitis. Scand J Gastroenterol 19:893, 1984

59. Gilbertson VA, Nelms JM: The prevention of invasive carcinoma of the rectum. Cancer 41:1137, 1978

60. Lashner BA, Heindenreich PA, Su GL, et al: Effect of folate supplementation on the incidence of dysplasia and cancer in chronic ulcerative colitis. Gastroenterology 97:255, 1989

61. Meisel JL, Bergman D, Graney D, et al: Human rectal mucosa: proctoscopic and morphological changes caused by laxatives. Gastroenterology 72:1274, 1977

62. Devrode G: Cancer risk in IBD. p. 325. In Winnawer SJ, Schottenfeld D, Sherlock D, Sherlock P (eds): Colorectal Cancer. Raven Press, New York, 1980

5

Re-examination of the Spectrum of Ischemic Bowel Disease

H. Thomas Norris

Less than a quarter of a century has passed since the concept of ischemic bowel disease was originally proposed.[1] Recent advances have refined this concept and clarified the spectrum of diseases of the gastrointestinal tract involved in this process.[2-8]

Ischemic bowel disease refers to a sequential series of changes that occur following anoxia to the bowel wall. The etiology is multifactorial, involving (1) the state of the vessels supplying the segment of the bowel, (2) the virulence of bacteria located in the lumen of the affected segment of the gastrointestinal tract, and (3) the duration of the anoxic or hypoxic episode. Profound changes occur in the hemodynamics of the bowel wall. Complete occlusion of the vessels supplying the affected segment is usually absent and thromboemboli are rarely observed.[9] Ischemic bowel disease affects any age group,[10, 11] involves any area of the gastrointestinal tract, and can occur in healthy or severely ill patients.[12]

The pathogenesis of ischemic bowel disease is dependent on enough blood being supplied to prevent complete death of the involved segment, but insufficient blood flow to meet the metabolic needs of an injured bowel. A combination of necrosis and subsequent bacterial invasion develops as the mucosal barrier becomes ineffective.

The basic pathologic response is coagulative necrosis, which is initially observed in the mucosal layer—the layer most susceptible to anoxia. Ischemic changes in the small bowel occur initially at the tip of the villus. A series of sequential events then may occur involving subjacent layers of the affected bowel wall. The muscular and serosal layers are usually spared during the early phases of the process. The histologic picture is also influenced by the size of the area of involvement and whether blood flow to the affected segment of bowel can be re-established. Complete and permanent cessation of blood flow causes extensive coagulative necrosis. If blood flow is re-established (reflow), an acute inflammatory response will also develop. The duration of the ischemic event also plays a significant part in the outcome of the process.

The eventual outcome is manifested by one of three basic responses. Total restitution of structure can occur, partial restitution of structure with fibrosis can develop, or the process can progress until transmural infarction occurs.

It is now possible to measure under experimental conditions both the volume of blood flow through a segment of bowel and the distribution of blood flow to the various layers of gastrointestinal tract during normotensive conditions as well as hypoxic periods.

When in an animal, hypovolemic shock is induced to the degree that the mean arterial pressure is decreased to 50 percent of normal levels, profound hemodynamic events occur—even though this degree of shock is reversible with restitution of blood volume (Fig. 5-1). During hypovolemic shock, over 50 percent of the blood vessels of the microcirculation that are

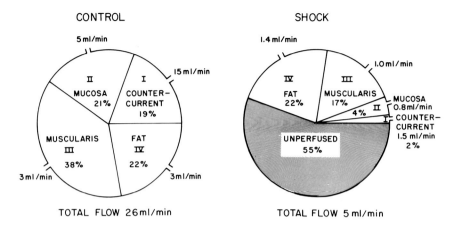

Fig. 5-1. Diagram of distribution of nutritional blood flow to the canine ileum during normotensive periods (control) and hypovolemic shock. Profound changes in hemodynamics occur with hypovolemic shock. The area of each circle represents the amount of microcirculation that is perfused. Numbers at the periphery of the circle represent the volume of blood flow to each layer. During shock, over 50 percent of the microcirculation is not perfused. The volume of total blood flow is decreased 81 percent. Only 19 percent of the mucosa and submucosa is perfused during shock. The volume of blood flow to the mucosa and submucosa is decreased to 16 percent of control levels. (From Norris,[5] with permission.)

perfused during normotensive conditions are without perfusion.[13, 14] The areas of perfused microcirculation of the mucosa/submucosa and the muscle layer are decreased to 19 percent and 45 percent of normotensive values. The volume of blood perfused in the mucosa and submucosa is decreased to 16 percent of normotensive values (from 5.0 ml/min to 0.8 ml/min). The volume of blood flow to the muscular layer is decreased to 33 percent of normotensive levels. These changes in hemodynamics are similar to the diving reflex encountered in aquatic animals, which enables them to dive to great depths. The diving reflex is thought to be a protective mechanism to provide blood to the heart and brain, while shunting blood away from the visceral and peripheral vascular beds. The lesions of ischemic bowel disease result from episodes of hypoxia or anoxia of a more prolonged nature. While redistribution of blood flow is a specific response to hypoxia, changes in blood flow distribution in ischemic bowel disease have not been studied in detail.

THE SPECTRUM OF ISCHEMIC BOWEL DISEASE

A variety of descriptive and pathogenetic terms have been applied to the spectrum of ischemic bowel disease that relate to the location of involvement within the gastrointestinal tract or on when the findings were initially described (Table 5-1). These include ischemic colitis, necrotizing entercolitis of premature infants, hemorrhagic necrosis of the gastrointestinal tract,

Table 5-1. The Spectrum of Ischemic Bowel Disease

Ischemic colitis
Necrotizing enterocolitis of the premature infant
Hemorrhagic necrosis of the gastrointestinal tract
Pseudomembranous enterocolitis
Staphylococcal enterocolitis
Hemorrhagic colitis attributable to *E. coli* 0157:H7
Radiation enterocolitis, delayed form
Uremic colitis
Potassium-induced stenotic ulcer
Stress ulceration

nonocclusive intestinal ischemia, nonocclusive mesenteric ischemia, hemorrhagic gastroenteropathy, certain presentations of pseudomembranous enterocolitis, staphylococcal enterocolitis, hemorrhagic colitis due to *Escherichia coli* O157:H7, radiation enterocolitis, ischemic enterocolitis, uremic colitis, potassium-induced stenotic ulcer, and stress ulceration of the gastrointestinal tract.

The purpose of this chapter is to re-examine the pathology of the various lesions currently classified as members of the spectrum of ischemic bowel disease, to examine their common pathogenesis, to explore experimental studies that led to a better understanding of these disease processes, and to comment on current diagnostic and therapeutic implications.

ISCHEMIC COLITIS

Ischemic colitis, first described in the 1960s, is probably the best understood of the lesions.[1, 15–21] Three clinical forms are recognized and have been studied extensively (Fig. 5-2). The least severe form is characterized by episodes of bloody diarrhea and healing without sequelae. The next most severe form is clinically manifested by healing of a focally ischemic segment of bowel by fibrosis with stricture formation. In the most severe form, transmural gangrene develops—the result of sequential involvement of the entire wall by the ischemic process. Any area of the large bowel may be involved. The splenic flexure is most frequently affected, as it is the anastomotic area between the colonic branches of the superior and inferior mesenteric arteries.

The gross pathology of the least severe form of ischemic colitis is usually only appreciated by the colonoscopist. A focally hemorrhagic, bluish-purple mucosa may be the only gross finding. More extensive disease is characterized by the appearance of mucosal ulceration. Healing of the more extensively involved colon may cause fibrosis of the submucosa, resulting in a fusiform stricture that may reach 15 cm in length. Gross examination of severely affected bowel wall reveals patchy to confluent areas of bluish mucosal discoloration. Often several areas of the bowel wall are involved at the same time (Fig. 5-3). If mucosal ischemia is extensive and blood flow has been re-established, pseudomembrane formation may be present.

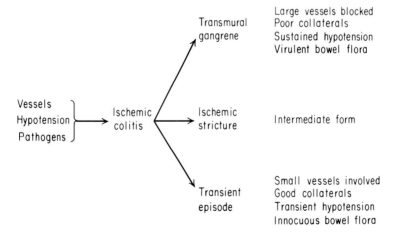

Fig. 5-2. Schema depicting the pathogenesis of ischemic colitis, indicating that multiple factors are involved in the pathogenesis of the lesion, with outcome dependent on the severity of involvement. (Modified from Marston et al.,[1] with permission.)

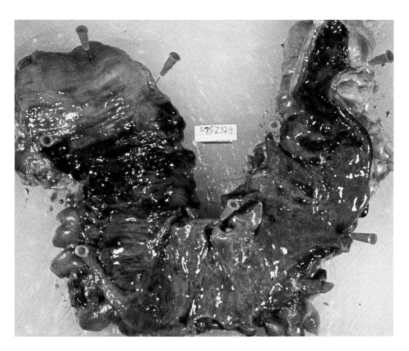

Fig. 5-3. Gross photograph of the mucosal surface of a segment of colon removed for ischemic colitis. Multiple areas of involvement are present.

Examination of a cross section of the severely affected bowel reveals hyperemia of the mucosal surface and significant edema of the submucosa. The edema may be so extensive that focal areas of the mucosa and submucosa protrude into the lumen of the bowel as polypoid masses. These polypoid masses are transient but are readily demonstrated by radiographic examination of the colon, producing the "thumbprint" sign. It is only in the most severe form that the serosa of the bowel is involved. This involvement is the sequela of progressive ischemia that starts in the mucosa and extends through the submucosa and muscular layers. The most extensive form of ischemic colitis leads to transmural infarction.

Histologic examination of the least severe form of ischemic colitis shows changes limited to the mucosal layer. The changes are prominent in the epithelium and lamina propria of the most superficial aspect of the mucosa. The capillaries in this area are severely congested, and extravasation of erythrocytes is frequent. Focal coagula-

tive necrosis of the epithelium and adjacent lamina propria may also be seen. An acute inflammatory response is usually not present. As the lesion becomes more extensive, edema formation develops initially in the mucosa and then in the subjacent submucosa. Focal loss of the entire thickness of the mucosa, with resulting ulceration, may occur.

Cases presenting with stricture formation usually demonstrate extensive fibrosis of the submucosa and muscular layer. At the time of resection, the histologic architecture of the mucosa and submucosa may be completely restored, or patchy superficial ulcerations and granulation tissue response may be present.

In the more severe forms of ischemic colitis, diffuse coagulative necrosis of the mucosa, muscularis mucosae, and submucosa is encountered, while the muscular layer and serosa initially remain intact (Fig. 5-4). The microcirculation demonstrates severe congestion and extravasation of erythrocytes into the lamina propria (Fig. 5-5). Hemosiderin deposition may be present.

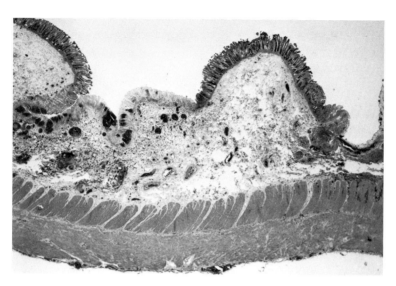

Fig. 5-4. Cross section of the entire width of a segment of ischemic colitis showing multiple areas of coagulative necrosis of the mucosa with severe congestion of the vessels of the submucosa and marked edema formation in the submucosa. The muscular layer is uninvolved by the process. The area of coagulative necrosis of the mucosa are evidenced by the lack of cellular detail in those areas. (H&E, × 15.)

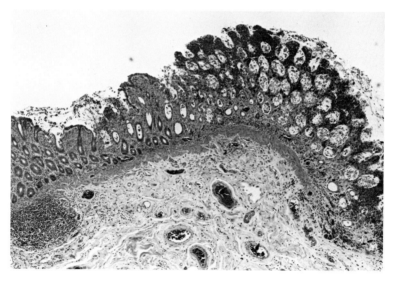

Fig. 5-5. Histologic section of the mucosa and submucosa of ischemic colitis. The mucosa on the left side of the figure is intact. Progressive changes occur, starting with the development of hemorrhage within the lamina propria, loss in staining characteristics of the epithelial cells, and finally, on the right edge of the figure, the early stages of coagulative necrosis of the mucosa and subjacent muscularis mucosae. (H&E, × 60.)

Extensive edema formation is present, with polypoid masses of edematous mucosa and submucosa protruding into the lumen (Fig. 5-6). An acute inflammatory process may be seen, with cryptitis and crypt abscess formation present where the architectural scaffold of the mucosal layer can be recognized. Pseudomembranes arise from the area of mucosal damage. The membranes are composed of necrotic mucosa, acute inflammatory cells, fibrin, and bacteria. The pseudomembrane may cover the more severely affected mucosa and extend over the less severely affected mucosa. The process becomes self-perpetuating, with involvement of the more superficial muscle layers by coagulative necrosis. Finally, with the development of coagulative necrosis of the deeper portions of the muscular layer and serosa, transmural gangrene is established.

Experimental studies of ischemic colitis are based on the historical observation that led to the recognition of the disease process. The discovery that ischemic colitis occurred most frequently at the splenic flexure was the result of complications encountered after ligation of the inferior mesenteric artery during abdominal aortic aneurysm surgery. Experimental studies of ischemic colitis rely on complete occlusion of the vasculature for varying periods of time.[22–34] The results obtained closely resemble the clinical findings of the disease. At least 1 hour of complete cessation of blood flow is necessary to produce the experimental lesion. While little morphologic damage can be appreciated after 1 hour of ischemia, derangement in sodium transport does occur. Usually 3 hours of ischemia are necessary for extravasation of erythrocytes and coagulative necrosis to develop as the microcirculation loses its structural integrity. If blood flow is re-established, marked submucosal edema develops and hemorrhage occurs in the necrotic mucosa. These changes are followed by an acute inflammatory cell infiltrate into the devitalized mucosa and submucosa. Increased intraluminal pressure has also been shown to contribute to the pathogenesis of this lesion.[32] The microcirculation of the muscular layer remains intact, with only minimal changes occurring in this layer.

Additional insight into an understanding of the pathogenesis of ischemic bowel disease has been provided by the pivotal studies of Granger,

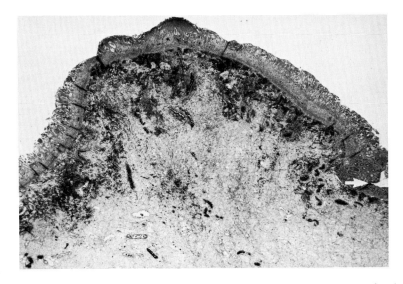

Fig. 5-6. Histologic section of the mucosa and submucosa of ischemic colitis. Except for the right edge of the photograph, the entire mucosa is infarcted. There is marked congestion in the submucosa beneath the infarcted mucosa and severe edema formation within the submucosa, causing a polypoid projection into the lumen of the bowel. The usual height of the mucosa is indicated by an arrow. (H&E, × 15.)

Parks, and their colleagues.[35-43] These biochemical studies have convincingly demonstrated that it is not hypoxia per se that causes the ischemic damage in the bowel but the generation of reactive oxygen metabolites (ROMs), including superoxide, hydrogen peroxide, hydroxyl radical, and hypohalous acids, during *reperfusion* that is responsible for the tissue damage. The hydroxyl radical, whose formation requires the presence of iron, is the most damaging of the ROMs. The ROMs are thought to alter vascular permeability of endothelial cells and cause necrosis of epithelial cells by a variety of mechanisms, including peroxidation of the cell membrane. The ROMs are also strongly chemotactic for neutrophils and may help to explain the acute inflammatory response that is occasionally seen.

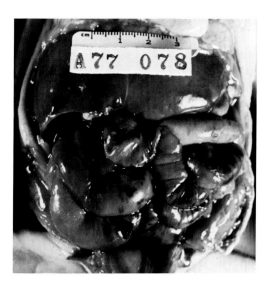

Fig. 5-7. Gross photograph of necrotizing enterocolitis. Multiple areas of infarction are present in loops of the small and large intestine.

NECROTIZING ENTEROCOLITIS OF PREMATURE INFANTS

It is now well established that necrotizing enterocolitis of premature infants belongs within the spectrum of ischemic bowel disease.[44-49] The onset of necrotizing enterocolitis usually occurs within the first week of life of some premature and low-birthweight infants. It is thought that three preconditions must occur before the premature infant can develop necrotizing enterocolitis. These include (1) the establishment of feeding, (2) an episode of ischemic injury to the intestinal mucosa, and (3) the presence of bacteria in the lumen of the affected portion of the gastrointestinal tract. The terminal ileum and right colon are involved with the greatest frequency, although any area of the gastrointestinal tract, including the stomach, may occasionally be involved. While the pathologic findings are definitive, they may mimic autolytic changes. For this reason, examination of tissue soon after resection and prompt fixation is imperative.

The findings at surgery or at autopsy may be very dramatic (Fig. 5-7). The affected segments of bowel are dilated, necrotic, hemorrhagic, and very friable. Bubbles of gas (pneumatosis intestinalis) may be present in the bowel wall (Fig. 5-8), mesenteric veins, and portal vein. The histopathologic consequences of pneumatosis may be difficult to preserve, especially if fixation has been delayed. Stricture formation may occur as early as 5 weeks after the initial episode in those infants who survive. Strictures occur most frequently in the ascending colon and ileum.

Microscopically, the earliest changes occur in the most superficial mucosa (Fig. 5-9). The capillaries are congested; extravasation of erythrocytes occurs into the injured lamina propria. Coagulative necrosis without an accompanying acute inflammatory response is present in the lamina propria. Edema formation occurs, followed by focal mucosal ulceration. The ischemic process then extends to the subjacent layers. A pseudomembrane composed of necrotic epithelium, fibrin, and inflammatory cells may develop. Overt perforation also occurs as the ischemic process involves the entire thickness of the bowel wall. When stricture formation develops, it is due to the deposition of fibrous connective tissue in the submucosa and muscular layers.

The experimental models of neonatal entero-

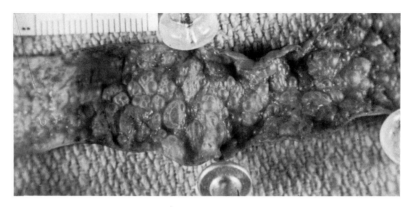

Fig. 5-8. Gross photograph of the mucosal aspects of a segment of small intestine demonstrating pneumatosis intestinalis. The mucosal surface is distorted by numerous bubbles of gas.

colitis rely on simulation of the perinatal period.[50, 51] The hypoxic episode is postulated to occur during delivery or shortly thereafter. Decreased mucosal resistance develops, allowing bacteria to invade the bowel wall. No specific causal organism has been identified.[52] The normal indigenous flora of the gastrointestinal tract has been found sufficient to aid in the development of necrotic bowel. Passive enteric immunity supplied by macrophages of breast milk can be protective in controlling the gut flora, while feeding artificial hyperosmolar formulas tends to encourage development of the lesions. As a result formulas for premature infants are now less hyperosmolar. Experimental studies using neonatal piglets indicate that there are no changes in total blood volume or total cardiac output following induced hypoxia. Redistribu-

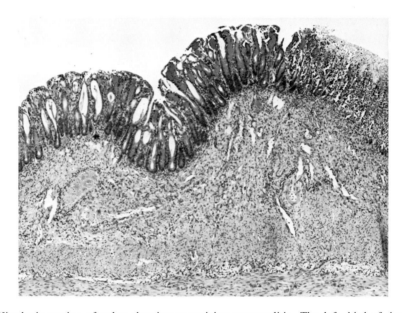

Fig. 5-9. Histologic section of colon showing necrotizing enterocolitis. The left third of the mucosa is relatively intact; the middle third shows severe congestion in the lamina propria, while the right third shows coagulative necrosis. There is slight edema in the submucosal layer. The muscular layer is intact. (H&E, × 40.)

tion of blood flow to the gastrointestinal tract occurs with reduction in blood flow to the mucosa. The decreased perfusion is most severe in the stomach, distal ileum, and colon. Perhaps this is the reason perforation occurs most frequently in these sites. Multiple episodes of stress may be necessary to cause the lesion. An experimental model developed by Gonzalez-Crussi and his co-workers to simulate necrotizing enterocolitis has provided significant advancement in our understanding of this disease.[52–56] Their model utilizes the intra-aortic injection of synthetic platelet activating factor or a combination of platelet activating factor and bacterial endotoxin in the rat. These investigators suggested that secondary mediators, especially leukotrienes, participate in the pathogenesis of bowel necrosis. Very recently, it has been shown that a more fundamental role may be played by the superoxide radical formed during reperfusion in the pathogenesis in this or other experimental models of necrotizing enterocolitis.[57, 58]

Normal birthweight infants can also develop necrotizing enterocolitis. These infants have associated hyperviscosity syndrome, polycythemia vera, or have been exposed to cocaine while in utero.[59, 60] Necrotizing enterocolitis in older infants, a complication of severe gastroenteritis, may also be on an ischemic basis.[61, 62]

OTHER PATHOLOGIC LESIONS INCLUDED IN ISCHEMIC BOWEL DISEASE

In 1965, Ming[63] summarized cases of hemorrhagic necrosis of the gastrointestinal tract occurring as secondary phenomenona in patients with severe infections, shock, or poor cardiovascular status. Clinically, these patients have shock, gastrointestinal hemorrhage, and abdominal complaints. Pathologic changes are similar in all cases. On gross examination the mucosa was dark red with patchy areas or confluent areas of hemorrhage (Fig. 5-10). Shallow ulcerations were present. The serosa appeared purple or dark red owing to the large amount of blood in the lumen. Thrombosis of major mesenteric vessels was noted infrequently. Microscopically, changes similar to those just described were seen. There was diffuse hemorrhage in the mucosa and submucosa, with coagulative necrosis starting at the surface of the mucosa and extending to involve the entire mucosa. Extension of the necrotic process into the sub-

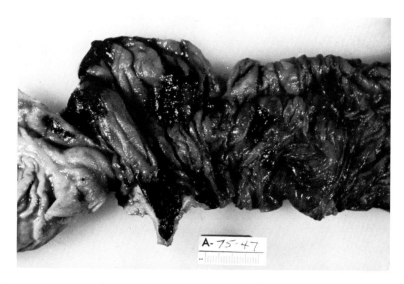

Fig. 5-10. Gross photograph of another form of ischemic colitis showing hemorrhagic necrosis of the small intestine. Numerous areas of infarction are present within this segment of small intestine.

mucosa occurred (Fig. 5-11). Varying degrees of edema in the submucosa were present, and an occasional focus of mild acute inflammatory infiltrate was also noted. Pseudomembrane formation was infrequent in these cases. The muscular layers and serosal layers were usually not involved.

While pseudomembranous colitis is associated with a variety of specific infectious agents and their products, including *Clostridium difficile* toxin, well-documented cases of pseudomembranous colitis have occurred in which no infectious agent could be demonstrated.[64] Even Penner and Bernheim in their original description of staphyloccal enterocolitis alluded to its possible ischemic etiology.[65] The histopathologic findings are similar to those seen in other forms of ischemic disease, namely, congestion, edema, and coagulative necrosis beginning in the mucosal layer. In these cases, however, the appearance of an acute inflammatory response results in pseudomembrane formation. Recent studies indicate that yet another bacterium with its toxins should be included in the spectrum of ischemic bowel disease. *E. coli* 0157:H7 and its associated verotoxin cause hemorrhagic colitis, which is also associated with the development of hemolytic uremic syndrome in children and thrombotic thrombocytopenic purpura in adults.[66-70]

It is also now well accepted that uremic colitis, the delayed changes occurring in the large and small bowel following irradiation, potassium-induced stenotic ulcers[71, 72] (Fig. 5-12), and the multiple shallow stress ulcers occurring in the upper gastrointestinal tract (Fig. 5-13) all have an ischemic etiology. In fact, ischemic colitis is now considered the most frequent colonic complication of renal transplantation.[73, 74] Histopathologic changes present in these lesions mirror the pathologic sequences described in previous paragraphs (Fig. 5-14). Experimental models of stress ulceration confirm that the basic process is nonocclusive focal ischemia.[75-78] Focal reduction in mucosal blood flow has been demonstrated. For focal coagulative necrosis of the gastric mucosa to develop requires 15 minutes of nonlethal shock, whereas 45 minutes of hypoxia are necessary for focal gastric erosions to develop. Recent experimental studies of stress ulceration have focused on changes in intracellular calcium homeostasis. With

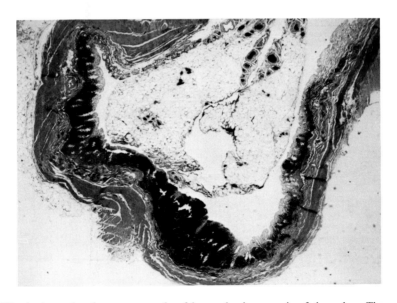

Fig. 5-11. Histologic section from an example of hemorrhagic necrosis of the colon. The entire colonic mucosa is infarcted with varying degrees of congestion beneath it. In the center of the section there is marked extravasation of erythrocytes into the submucosa. (H&E, × 15.)

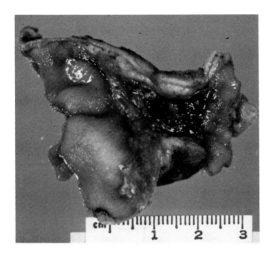

Fig. 5-12. Gross photograph of potassium-induced stenotic ulcer of the small bowel. Stricture formation is present. The overlying mucosa is focally ulcerated.

UNIQUE PRESENTATIONS AND COMPARISON OF ISCHEMIC BOWEL DISEASE WITH OTHER HISTOPATHOLOGIC RESPONSES OF THE GASTROINTESTINAL TRACT

While a number of responses to injury of the gastrointestinal tract may superficially mimic ischemic bowel disease, the degree of coagulative necrosis is usually either quite minimal or absent (see Ch. 2). Extensive coagulative necrosis that appears to begin in the mucosa and then progress to involve the other layers of the gastrointestinal tract is the hallmark of ischemic bowel disease. The muscular layer and serosal layer are not involved until the process has become quite extensive. While occlusion of the intramural vessels or acute vasculitis is usually absent in ischemic bowel disease, cholesterol emboli in vessels to areas of the bowel demonstrating ischemic change are being reported with greater frequency.[82] The vasospastic effects of cocaine also occur in the gastrointestinal tract, and cases of intestinal ischemia are being reported following its use or ingestion.[83, 84] The presence of primary vasculitis in the vessels of the bowel wall is associated with rheumatoid

ischemia, there is a significant increase in intracellular calcium.[79] It has been speculated that the increased amount of intracellular calcium may have a significant role in mediating irreversible ischemic injury. Slow calcium channel blockers such as Verapamil prevent or significantly reduce the occurrence of experimentally produced stress ulcers in the stomach.[80, 81]

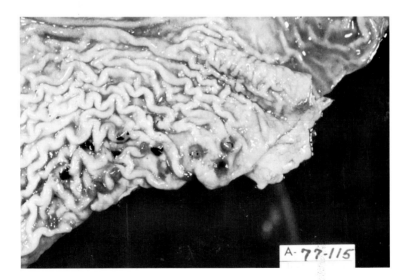

Fig. 5-13. Gross photograph showing multiple stress ulcers of the stomach.

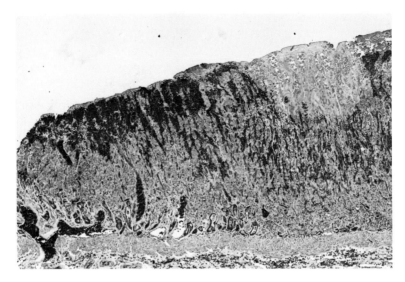

Fig. 5-14. Histologic section of one of the stress ulcers in Fig. 5-13. There is severe congestion of the mucosa, especially in the most superficial aspect. A focal area of coagulative necrosis of the superficial portion of the mucosa is present on the right side of the photograph. (H&E, × 80.)

disease, systemic lupus erythematosus, allergic phenomenon, or dermatomyositis. The pathologic findings of ischemic colitis may rarely be encountered in polyarteritis[85] and systemic lupus erythematosus.[86] The location and type of vessels involved by vasculitis as well as associated clinical laboratory data provide a means of differentiating these processes. Intramural fibrinoid necrosis of small arteries occurs more frequently in systemic lupus erythematosus, whereas involvement of serosal and mesenteric vessels is the hallmark of polyarteritis. Metastatic carcinoid tumors may present initially as an episode of massive intestinal ischemia[87, 88] owing to the development of elastic vascular sclerosis in intestinal vessels with resultant decreased blood flow to the bowel.

IMPACT ON CURRENT DIAGNOSTIC PRACTICES AND SPECULATION ON FUTURE DEVELOPMENTS IN DIAGNOSIS AND THERAPY

As the various manifestations and types of responses of the gastrointestinal tract to ischemic bowel disease were appreciated, improvements in diagnosis, therapy, and eventual outcome resulted. This is particularly true of necrotizing enterocolitis of premature infants,[89–91] but also has been seen in other forms of the disease process. Neither angiographic imaging nor scanning techniques using radionuclides have been as useful as initially anticipated.[92–96]

Currently, many attempts are being made to arrive at an earlier diagnosis of ischemic bowel disease and related lesions. In necrotizing enterocolitis of the infant, studies are directed at analyzing increases in breath hydrogen or other metabolites as a reflection of gas production from necrotic bowel.[47] Doppler ultrasound, laser Doppler, perfusion fluorometry, transserosal oxygen determinations, intramural pH determinations, and the use of fluorescein dye during endoscopy may more precisely indicate the extent of involvement of the bowel by ischemic processes.[97–103]

Now that the biochemical events occurring during ischemia and reperfusion are better understood, significant advances in therapy should be forthcoming. The therapeutic modalities will be directed at preventing formation of injurious compounds or blocking the action of these compounds once produced.

The spectrum of ischemic bowel disease has been re-examined. Recent studies have reaffirmed that many of the lesions previously proposed as members of this spectrum indeed belong in this grouping, because they share a common pathogenesis and similar pathologic changes. Our greater understanding of the pathogenesis may significantly influence therapy in this disease.

REFERENCES

1. Marston A, Pheils MT, Thomas ML, Morson BC: Ischaemic colitis. Gut 7:1, 1966
2. Allen AC: A unified concept of the vascular pathogenesis of enterocolitis of varied etiology: a pathophysiologic analysis. Am J Gastroenterol 55:347, 1971
3. Fagin RR, Kirsner JB: Ischemic diseases of the colon. Adv Intern Med 17:343, 1971
4. Sullivan JF: Vascular disease of the intestines. Symposium on gastrointestinal physiology. Med Clin North Am 58:1473, 1974
5. Norris HT: Ischemic bowel disease: its spectrum. p. 15. In Yardley JH, Morson BC, Abell MR (eds): The Gastrointestinal Tract. International Academy of Pathology Monograph No. 18. Williams & Wilkins, Baltimore, 1977
6. Saegesser F, Roenspies U, Robinson JWL: Ischemic diseases of the large intestine. p. 303. In Ioachim HL (ed): Pathobiology Annual. Vol. 9. Raven Press, New York, 1979
7. Norris HT: Re-examination of the spectrum of ischemic bowel disease. p. 109. In Norris HT (ed): Contemporary Issues in Surgical Pathology. Vol. 2. Pathology of the Colon, Small Intestine and Anus. Churchill Livingstone, New York, 1983
8. Norris HT: Recent advances in ischemic bowel disease. p. 69. In Fenoglio-Preiser CM (ed): Progress in Surgical Pathology XI. WW Norton New York/London, 1990
9. Qizilbash AH: The nonspecific nature of fibrin thrombi in ischemic bowel disease. Can Med Assoc J 8:807, 1978
10. Clark AW, Loyd-Mostyn RH, Sadler MR, De C: "Ischaemic" colitis in young adults. Br Med J 4:70, 1972
11. Duffy TJ: Reversible ischaemic colitis in young adults. Br J Surg 68:34, 1981
12. Heer M, Repond F, Hany A, et al: Acute ischaemic colitis in a female long distance runner. Gut 28:896, 1987
13. Wolfe EA Jr, Sumner DS: Redistribution of intestinal blood flow during hypotension. Surg Forum 24:20, 1973
14. Norris HT, Sumner DS: Distribution of blood flow to the layers of the small bowel in experimental cholera. Gastroenterology 66:973, 1974
15. Morson BC: Pathology of ischaemic colitis. Bibl Gastroenterol 9:134, 1970
16. Byrne JJ, Wittenberg J, Grimes ET, Williams LF Jr: Ischemic diseases of the bowel. Pt. II. Ischemic colitis. Dis Colon Rectum 13:283, 1970
17. Marcuson RW: Ischemic colitis. Clin Gastroenterol 1:745, 1972
18. Morson BC: The pathology of colitis and other inflammatory diseases of colon. Deutsche Roentgengesellschaft, Refrante uber die Tagung 54:308, 1973
19. Whitehead R: Reversible ischaemic colitis. Practitioner 213:54, 1974
20. Alschibaja T, Morson BC: Ischaemic bowel disease. J Clin Pathol 30 (suppl, R Coll Pathol): 11:68, 1977
21. Sakai L, Keltner R, Kaminski D: Spontaneous and shock-associated ischemic colitis. Am J Surg 140:755, 1980
22. Boley SJ, Schwartz S, Lash J, Sternhill V: Reversible vascular occlusion of the colon. Surg Gynecol Obstet 116:53, 1963
23. Brown RA, Chiu CJ, Scott HJ, Gurd FN: Ultrastructural changes in the canine ileal mucosal cell after mesenteric arterial occlusion: a sequential study. Arch Surg 101:290, 1970
24. Robinson JWL, Rausis C, Basset P, Mirkovitch V: Functional and morphological response of the dog colon to ischaemia. Gut 13:755, 1972
25. Aho AJ, Arstila AU, Ahonen J, et al: Ultrastructural alterations in ischacmic lesions of small intestinal mucosa in experimental superior mesenteric artery occlusion: effect of oxygen breathing. Scand J Gastroenterol 8:439, 1973
26. Manohar M, Tyagi RPS: Experimental intestinal ischemia shock in dogs. Am J Physiol 225:887. 1973
27. Robinson JWL, Haroud M, Winistorfer B, Mirkovitch V: Recovery of function and structure of dog ileum and colon following two hours acute ischemia. Eur J Clin Invest 4:443, 1974
28. Katz S, Wahab A, Murray W, Williams LF:

New parameters of viability in ischemic bowel disease. Am J Surg 127:136, 1974

29. Bounous G: Ischemic bowel disease: mucosal injury in low flow states. Can J Surg 17:434, 1974

30. Ming SC, McNiff J: Acute ischemic changes in intestinal muscularis. Am J Pathol 82:315, 1976

31. Mishima Y, Horie Y: Experimental studies of ischemic enterocolitis. World J Surg 4:601, 1980

32. Saegesser F, Sandblom P: Ischemic lesions of the distended colon: a complication of obstructive colorectal cancer. Am J Surg 129:309, 1975

33. Bailey RW, Bulkley GB, Hamilton SR, et al: Pathogenesis of nonocclusive ischemic colitis. Ann Surg 203:590, 1986

34. Bailey RW, Bulkley GB, Hamilton SR, et al: Protection of the small intestine from non-occlusive mesenteric ischemic injury due to cardiogenic shock. Am J Surg 153:108, 1987

35. Granger DN, Parks DA: Role of oxygen radicals in the pathogenesis of intestinal ischemia. Physiologist 26:159, 1983

36. Parks DA, Granger DN, Bulkley GB, et al: Soybean trypsin inhibitor attenuates ischemic injury to the feline small intestine. Gastroenterology 89:6, 1985

37. Bulkley GB, Kvietys PR, Parks DA, et al: Relationship of blood flow and oxygen consumption to ischemic injury in the canine small intestine. Gastroenterology 89:852, 1985

38. McCord JM: Oxygen-derived free radicals in postischemic tissue injury. N Engl J Med 312:159, 1985

39. Parks DA, Granger DN: Contributions of ischemia and reperfusion to mucosal lesion formation. Am J Physiol 250:G749, 1986

40. Bulkley GB: Free radical-mediated reperfusion injury: a selective review. Br J Cancer 55 (Suppl):66, 1987

41. Hernandez LA, Grisham MB, Granger DN: A role for iron in oxidant-mediated ischemic injury to intestinal microvasculature. Am J Physiol 253:G49, 1987

42. Granger DN: Role of xanthine oxidase and granulocytes in ischemia-reperfusion injury. Am J Physiol 255:H1269, 1988

43. Grisham MB, Granger DN: Neutrophil-mediated mucosal injury. Role of reactive oxygen metabolites. Dig Dis Sci 33:6S, 1988

44. Hopkins GB, Gould VE, Stevenson JK, Oliver TK Jr: Necrotizing enterocolitis in premature infants: a clinical and pathologic evaluation of autopsy material Am J Dis Child 120:229, 1970

45. Stevenson JK, Stevenson DK: Necrotizing enterocolitis in the neonate. In Nyhus LM (ed): Surgery Annual. Vol. 9. Appleton-Century-Crofts, New York, 1976

46. deSa DJ: The spectrum of ischemic bowel disease in the newborn. Perspect Pediatr Pathol 3:273, 1976

47. Kliegman RM, Fanaroff AA: Necrotizing enterocolitis. N Engl J Med 310:1093, 1984

48. Milner ME, de la Monte SM, Moore GW, et al: Risk factors for developing and dying from necrotizing enterocolitis. J Pediatr Gastroenterol Nutr 5:359, 1986

49. Cheromcha DP, Hyman PE: Neonatal necrotizing enterocolitis. Inflammatory bowel disease of the newborn. Dig Dis Sci 33:78S, 1988

50. Touloukian RJ, Posch JN, Spencer R: The pathogenesis of ischemic gastroenterocolitis of the neonate: selective gut mucosal ischemia in asphyxiated neonatal piglets. J Pediatr Surg 7:194, 1972

51. Barlow B, Santulli TV: Importance of multiple episodes of hypoxia or cold stress on the development of enterocolitis in an animal model. Surgery 77:687, 1975

52. Musemeche CA, Kosloske AM, Bartow SA, Umland ET: Comparative effects of ischemia, bacteria, and substrate on the pathogenesis of intestinal necrosis. J Pediatr Surg 21:536, 1986

53. Gonzalez-Crussi F, Hsueh W: Experimental model of ischemic bowel necrosis: the role of platelet-activating factor and endotoxin. Am J Pathol 112:127, 1983

54. Hsueh W, Gonzalez-Crussi F, Arroyave JL: Platelet-activating factor-induced ischemic bowel necrosis: an investigation of secondary mediators in its pathogenesis. Am J Pathol 122:231, 1986

55. Lefer AM: Leukotrienes as mediators of ischemia and shock. Biochem Pharmacol 35:123, 1986

56. Hsueh W, Gonzalez-Crussi F, Arroyave JL: Sequential release of leukotrienes and norepinephrine in rat bowel after platelet-activating factor. A mechanistic study of platelet-activating factor-induced bowel necrosis. Gastroenterology 94:1412, 1988

57. Cueva JP, Hsueh W: Role of oxygen derived

free radicals in platelet activating factor induced bowel necrosis. Gut 29:1207, 1988

58. Crissinger KD, Granger DN: Mucosal injury induced by ischemia and reperfusion in the piglet intestine: influences of age and feeding. Gastroenterology 97:920, 1989

59. Dunn SP, Gross KR, Scherer, LR, et al: The effect of polycythemia and hyperviscosity on bowel ischemia. J Pediatr Surg 20:324, 1985

60. Telsey AM, Merrit TA, Dixon SD: Cocaine exposure in a term neonate. Necrotizing enterocolitis as a complication. Clin Pediatr 27:547, 1988

61. Rodin AE, Nichols MM, Hsu FL: Necrotizing enterocolitis occurring in full-term neonates at birth. Arch Pathol 96:335, 1973

62. Takayanagi K, Kapila L: Necrotising enterocolitis in older infants. Arch Dis Child 56:468, 1981

63. Ming S-C: Hemorrhagic necrosis of the gastrointestinal tract and its relation to cardiovascular status. Circulation 32:332, 1965

64. Goulston SJM, McGovern VJ: Pseudo-membranous colitis. Gut 6:207, 1965

65. Penner A, Bernheim AI: Acute postoperative enterocolitis: a study on the pathologic nature of shock. Arch Pathol 27:966, 1939

66. Riley LW, Remis RS, Helgerson SD, et al: Hemorrhagic colitis associated with a rare *Escherichia coli* serotype. N Engl J Med 308:681, 1983

67. Kelly JK, Pai CH, Jadusingh IH, et al: The histopathology of rectosigmoid biopsies from adults with bloody diarrhea due to verotoxin-producing *Escherichia coli*. Am J Clin Pathol 88:78, 1987

68. Dalal BI, Krishnan C, Laschuk B, Duff JH: Sporadic hemorrhagic colitis associated with Escherichia coli, type O157:H7: unusual presentation mimicking ischemic colitis. Can J Surg 30:207, 1987

69. Richardson SE, Karmali MA, Becker LE, et al: The histopathology of the hemolytic uremic syndrome associated with verocytotoxin-producing *Escherichia coli* infections. Hum Pathol 19:1102, 1988

70. Griffin PM, Ostroff SM, Tauxe RV, et al: Illnesses associated with Escherichia coli O157:H7 infections. A broad clinical spectrum. Ann Intern Med 109:705, 1988

71. Windsor CWO: Ischaemic strictures of the small bowel. Clin Gastroenterol 1:707, 1972

72. Grosdidier J, Boissel P, Bresler L, Vidrequin A: Stenosing and perforated ulcers of the small intestine related to potassium chloride in enteric-coated tablets. Apropos of 11 cases. Chirurgie 115:163, 1989

73. Gomella LG, Flanigan RC, Hagihara PF, et al: The influence of uremia and immunosuppression on an animal model for ischemic colitis. Dis Colon Rectum 29:724, 1986

74. Stylianos S, Forde KA, Benvenisty AI, Hardy MA: Lower gastrointestinal hemorrhage in renal transplant recipients. Arch Surg 123:739, 1988

75. Schellerer W: The role of mucosal blood flow in the pathogenesis of stress ulcers. Acta Hepatogastroenterol (Stuttg) 21:138, 1974

76. Menguy R, Desbaillets L, Masters YF: Mechanism of stress ulcer. Pt. IV: Influence of hypovolemic shock on energy metabolism in the gastric mucosa. Gastroenterology 66:46, 1974

77. Menguy R, Masters YF: Mechanism of stress ulcer. Pt. IV: Influence of fasting on the tolerance of gastric mucosal energy metabolism to ischemia and on the incidence of stress ulceration. Gastroenterology 66:1177, 1974

78. Cheung LY, Ashley SW: Gastric blood flow and mucosal defense mechanisms. Clin Invest Med 10:201, 1987

79. Cheung JY, Bonventre JV, Malis CD, et al: Calcium and ischemic injury. N Engl J Med 314:1670, 1986

80. Ogle CW, Cho CH, Tong MC, et al: The influence of verapamil on the gastric effects of stress in rats. Eur J Pharmacol 112:399, 1985

81. Wait RB, Leahy AL, Nee MJ, et al: Verapamil attenuates stress-induced gastric ulceration. J Surg Res 38:424, 1985

82. Moolenaar W, Kreuning J, Eulderink F, Lamers CB: Ischemic colitis and acalculous necrotizing cholecystitis as rare manifestations of cholesterol emboli in the same patient. Am J Gastroenterol 84:1421, 1989

83. Nalbandian H, Sheth N, Dietrich R, Georgiou J: Intestinal ischemia caused by cocaine ingestion: report of two cases. Surgery 97:374, 1985

84. Fishel R, Hamamoto G, Barbul A, et al: Cocaine colitis. Is this a new syndrome? Dis Colon Rectum 28:264, 1985

85. Wood MK, Read DR, Kraft AR, Barreta TM: A rare cause of ischemic colitis: polyarteritis nodosa. Dis Colon Rectum 22:428, 1979

86. Kistin MG, Kaplan MM, Harrington JT: Diffuse ischemic colitis associated with systemic

lupus erythematosus—response to subtotal colectomy. Gastroenterology 75:1147, 1978

87. Qizilbash AH: Carcinoid tumors, vascular elastosis, and ischemic disease of the small intestine. Dis Colon Rectum 20:554, 1977

88. Payne-James JJ, Lovell D, Gow NM, et al: Metastatic carcinoid tumour in association with small bowel ischaemia and infarction. J R Soc Med 83:54, 1990

89. Stevenson JK, Oliver TK, Jr, Graham CB, et al: Aggressive treatment of neonatal necrotizing enterocolitis: 38 patients with 25 survivors. J Pediatr Surg 6:28, 1971

90. Santulli TV: Acute necrotizing enterocolitis: recognition and management. Hosp Pract 9:129, 1974

91. Schullinger JN, Mollitt DL, Vinocur CD, et al: Neonatal necrotizing enterocolitis: survival, management, and complications: a 25-year study. Am J Dis Child 135:612, 1981

92. Westcott JL: Angiographic demonstration of arterial occlusion in ischemic colitis. Gastroenterology 63:486, 1972

93. Bookstein JJ: Nonocclusive ischemic colitis: angiographic aspects in a canine model. Invest Radiol 13:506, 1978

94. Zarins CK, Skinner DB, Rhodes BA, James AE Jr: Prediction of the viability of revascularized intestine with radioactive microspheres. Surg Gynecol Obstet 138:576, 1974

95. Moossa AR, Skinner DB, Stark V, Hoffer P: Assessment of bowel viability using 99^m technetium-tagged albumin microspheres. J Surg Res 16:466, 1972

96. Haase GM, Sfakianakis GN, Lobe TE, Boles ET: Prospective evaluation of radionuclide scanning in detection of intestinal necrosis in neonatal necrotizing enterocolitis. J Pediatr Surg 16 (No. 3): 241, 1981

97. Lynch TG, Hobson RW, Kerr JC, et al: Doppler ultrasound, laser doppler, and perfusion fluorometry in bowel ischemia. Arch Surg 123: 483, 1988

98. Johansson K, Ahn H, Lindhagen J: Assessment of small-bowel ischemia by laser doppler flowmetry. Some case reports. Scand J Gastroenterol 21:1147, 1986

99. Krohg-Srensen K, Kvernebo K: Laser Doppler flowmetry in evaluation of colonic blood flow during aortic reconstruction. Eur J Vasc Surg 3:37, 1989

100. Lim KH, Catinella F, Anselmo M, et al: Transserosal pO_2 as a predictor of intestinal viability after acute arterial occlusion. Curr Surg 43:214, 1986

101. Fiddian-Green RG, Amelin PM, Herrmann JB, et al: Prediction of the development of sigmoid ischemia on the day of aortic operations. Indirect measurements of intramural pH in the colon. Arch Surg 121:654, 1986

102. Schiedler MG, Cutler BS, Fiddian-Green RG: Sigmoid intramural pH for prediction of ischemic colitis during aortic surgery. A comparison with risk factors and inferior mesenteric artery stump pressures. Arch Surg 122:881, 1987

103. Galandiuk S, Fazio VW, Petras RE: Fluorescein endoscopy. A technique for noninvasive assessment of intestinal ischemia. Dis Colon Rectum 31:848, 1988

6

Small Bowel Biopsy in Malabsorptive States

William O. Dobbins III

The method of processing and interpreting intestinal biopsies outlined in this chapter is the sometimes controversial, always exceedingly demanding, even rigid system recommended by C. E. Rubin. Because the technique of processing and interpreting gastrointestinal mucosal biopsy requires considerable skill, it merits the same specialization within pathology that has been so useful in the interpretation of needle biopsy specimens of the liver, the lung, and the kidney. It is desirable to have the same technician process all biopsy specimens of the gastrointestinal mucosa and to have a select group of pathologists with a major interest in gastrointestinal histopathology interpret the biopsies.

Rubin points out that there are five main sources of misinterpretation of small bowel biopsy specimens: (1) failure of the clinician to orient and handle the biopsy optimally, (2) failure of the technician to process and section the biopsy adequately, (3) failure of the clinician to provide adequate information to the pathologist, (4) inadequate appreciation by the pathologist of the spectrum of normal intestinal histology, and (5) failure of the pathologist to

appreciate the clinical significance of his interpretation.

BIOPSY PROCESSING

Only a brief discussion of the method of obtaining biopsy specimens, the complications of biopsy, and the appropriate method of handling and processing the biopsies is given in this chapter. Readers with more than a passing interest in the intestinal mucosa should review the detailed discussion relating to suction biopsy technique in the paper by Rubin and colleagues.[1] Because proximal small intestine lesions may be patchy, it is advisable to use the multipurpose tube (as recommended by Rubin), which obtains four separate biopsies each time. This will permit processing of three of the biopsies for routine light microscopy, and special processing of the fourth biopsy for electron microscopy or biochemical analysis. When using suction biopsy techniques, the intestinal biopsy specimens should be taken routinely at the easily identified fluoroscopic landmark, the region of the ligament of Treitz, which is located at the duodenojejunal junction. This standardizes biopsy location and facilitates comparison among patients and assessment of a therapeutic response in the same patient.

I no longer recommend suction biopsy (which requires fluoroscopy) but recommend instead that the specimens be obtained endoscopically. This permits sampling areas that show the greatest changes grossly and permits more accurate sampling of patchy lesions. I prefer the

This chapter is based heavily on the magnificent review of the subject of small intestinal biopsy published by Cyrus E. Rubin, M.D., and two of his colleagues in 1975,[1] on my review of the diagnostic value of intestinal biopsy published in the first edition of this volume,[2] and on my atlas of diagnostic pathology of the intestinal mucosa.[3] Many of the illustrations in this chapter were supplied by C. E. Rubin, and I am very grateful to him and to his former fellows for making these illustrations available.

"jumbo" biopsy forceps (Olympus FB 13K), but the standard forceps obtains specimens that are quite adequate in size for intreptation.[4] The specimens should be obtained as far distally as possible unless proximal lesions are noted, keeping in mind that confusing artifacts are more likely present in the proximal than the distal duodenum. Nevertheless, the proximal duodenum accurately reflects the distal duodenum.[4]

Prior to taking the biopsy specimen from a patient with malabsorption, the prothrombin time should be shown to be normal and a careful history obtained to discern evidence of bleeding. If a history suggestive of a bleeding problem is obtained, a complete clotting workup is probably indicated. Further, it is advisable for patients to avoid aspirin for 72 hours before the biopsy procedure.

The specimens obtained should be carefully handled and oriented before fixation, and then embedded and serially or step sectioned. It is important that the physician who performs the biopsy be familiar with the method of orienting the tissue without traumatizing it. The carefully flattened intestinal biopsy specimen should be mounted on a monofilament plastic mesh so that there will be no doubt about the proper orientation of the specimen at the time of sectioning by the laboratory technician. The value of the monofilament mesh is that it leaves no material adherent when the mesh is removed prior to sectioning. This protects the cutting edge of the microtome knife from needless injury. After the specimen is oriented on mesh, it is immediately placed in Bouin's fixative or in Hollande's fixative for at least 2 hours. I prefer Bouin's fixative, whereas Rubin prefers Hollande's fixative. Hollande's-fixed tissue is easier to section than formalin-fixed tissue. More importantly, there is less shrinkage in tissue fixed in Bouin's fixative or in Hollande's fixative and thus there are few artifactual gaps in the tissue sections. Because it is important to section the biopsy specimen serially, it is preferable to embed the tissue in Peel-a-way paraffin (56 to 58°C temperature range). The biopsy specimen is gently removed from the monofilament plastic mesh just prior to embed-

ding. The use of Tissue Tek stainless steel base molds (#4121) for embedding facilitates the ease with which the tissue can be oriented for appropriate sectioning. The paraffin block is then attached to the microtome chuck and trimmed closely so that two to three ribbons per slide containing approximately 30 serial sections per ribbon can be obtained (Fig. 6-1A). The biopsy specimens are sectioned at 4-μm intervals through the limits of the central core (Fig. 6-1B). Serial sectioning of small intestine biopsies is not essential, although it is very helpful in ascertaining the presence or absence of four normal villi in a row in normal biopsy specimens. Step sectioning of small bowel biopsies is a reasonable alternative. However, serial sectioning of rectal biopsies is helpful to detect focal lesions and granulomas in inflammatory bowel disease. Three to four slides should be stained and examined carefully. Rubin recommends hematoxylin and eosin (H&E) with Alcian blue and saffron staining. The saffron stains collagen and differentiates edema from collagenous scar. I prefer to use routinely both H&E staining and periodic acid-Schiff (PAS)-hematoxylin staining of separate slides. It is reasonable to retain several unstained slides for those occasions when special stains may also be required.

BIOPSY INTERPRETATION

NORMAL VILLOUS ARCHITECTURE

Villous architecture should be assessed initially. There is considerable variation in villous shape and length, and this must be appreciated in order to avoid interpretive errors. A variety of methods are available for the quantitative assessment of villous architecture, but these are rarely required for routine diagnostic assessment of small bowel biopsies. There is no substitute for extensive experience in biopsy interpretation, a major reason why intestinal biopsy interpretation should receive the same attention from specialized pathologists as does kidney biopsy interpretation.

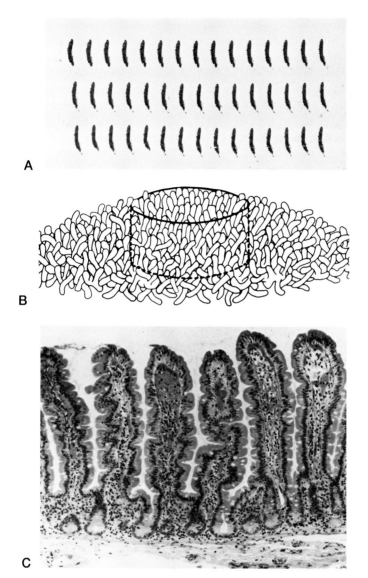

Fig. 6-1. Serial sectioning. **(A)** Photograph of a typical slide containing three ribbons totaling 45 serial sections. Rubin prefers two carefully centered ribbons per slide in order to reduce the problem of fading of the stain in sections placed too close to the edge of the slide. **(B)** Diagram of an oriented biopsy to illustrate the central core, which is most likely to contain sections with the best oriented villi. **(C)** Normal section of proximal jejunum from the central core demonstrating four normal villi in a row. The differences in length of adjacent villi are explained by the fact that some villi are bent and others are not. (H&E, × 132.) (Fig. B from Perea et al,[1] with permission.)

In addition to assessment of villous architecture, the other key features include assessment of the surface epithelium, the cellular content of the lamina propria, and the structures of the submucosa. Villi are not necessarily all perfectly tall, finger-like structures standing in a row perpendicular to the muscularis mucosae. Rather, many villi may bend in various directions, and may vary in their structure from slender, finger-like structures to leaf-shaped structures. It is reasonable to follow Rubin's dictum that if there are four normal finger-like villi in a row in *any* serial section of a biopsy specimen, then the biopsy can be considered to be normal (Fig. 6-1C). There are times when one may modify this dictum, especially when given small biopsy specimens.

Tangentially sectioned villi are the most common source of misinterpretation of normal biopsy specimens. This artifact can be avoided completely by attention to appropriate orientation of the specimen prior to fixation, during embedding, and during attachment of the block to the microtome chuck. It is also avoided by ascertaining that the sections obtained are within the central core of the biopsy specimen (Figs. 6-1B and 6-2). Tangential sectioning is easily recognized by the presence of multilayered cross sections of crypts, or when villi appear to be broad and short and contain a surface epithelium that appears to be multilayered. Intestinal biopsy specimens obtained from the proximal duode-

num rather than from the distal duodenum are more likely to have Brunner gland artifact.[1] Brunner glands found in the first and second portions of the duodenum may distort the overlying villi so that they are broadened and shortened (Fig. 6-3A to C). Distorted villi may be present even when Brunner glands are not included within the biopsy specimen. Although Brunner glands may be found in the distal duodenum, the most common reason for their presence is that the biopsy tube moved inadvertently into the proximal duodenum just prior to obtaining the biopsy specimen. Occasional small bowel biopsy specimens appear to consist of gastric antral mucosa. In this case, it is likely that the suction biopsy tube was inadvertently placed in the stomach rather than in the small bowel. Such a problem should not occur during endoscopic biopsy.

Shallow biopsy specimens that do not include the muscularis mucosae often have villi that appear to be shortened and broadened because

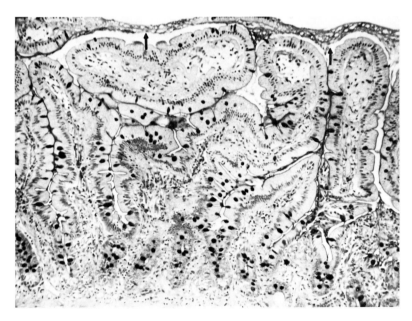

Fig. 6-2. Normal section of duodenojejunal biopsy obtained in a patient with giardiasis. The section illustrated here was not obtained within the central core of the biopsy specimen and shows apparent irregularity in the shape of the villi and differences in length of the villi, both of which are artifacts. The homogeneous material (arrows) seen above the villi consists of a massive number of giardial trophozoites. (PAS-hematoxylin, × 132.)

they lack the underlying muscle bundle to hold them together. Biopsy trauma may be very subtle. Generally, separation of the epithelium from the underlying lamina propria and gaps in epithelial continuity without inflammatory changes in the underlying lamina propria are due to trauma. Lymphoid follicles are occasionally found within the normal mucosa and may distort adjacent villi so that they appear abnormal (Fig. 6-3D).

Most of the artifacts described above are easily recognized and should be no source of interpretive error. Such artifacts, even unrecognized, should not be confused with severe mucosal lesions such as those seen in celiac sprue. However, if patchy mucosal changes are clinically likely, additional specimens may be necessary in order to distinguish artifacts from patchy pathologic changes.

NORMAL EPITHELIUM

Tall columnar absorptive cells predominate in the epthelium of villi of biopsy specimens obtained at the duodenojejunal junction (Fig. 6-1C). Occasional goblet cells are seen between the absorptive cells, and approximately one intraepithelial lymphocyte for every five epithelial cells is usually present.[5] Mitoses are found only in the crypt region, and Paneth cells are located at the bases of crypts. Enteroendocrine cells can occasionally be discerned in H&E-stained sections, and the presence of undifferentiated crypt cells (best defined by electron microscopy) rounds out the epithelial cell population.

NORMAL LAMINA PROPRIA

Suction used in obtaining the biopsy specimen often results in mild hemorrhage and edema within the lamina propria. The presence of these changes must be interpreted with great caution. Plasma cells tend to be the most common cells found within the lamina propria, whereas lymphocytes and macrophages are less common. Fibroblasts align themselves parallel to the basal lamina. Occasional lymphoid nodules are present in normal individuals (Fig. 6-3D). Macrophages, often containing prominent inclusions, are occasionally found at the tips of villi. Eosinophilic leukocytes, when looked for, are frequently observed within the lamina propria, but only rarely are polymorphonuclear (PMN) leukocytes seen outside of blood vessels in normals. Leukocytes within areas of artifactual hemorrhage obviously have no pathologic significance.

It is important to note that lymphoid cells are normally found within the lamina propria, and their numbers vary widely depending on the patient's country of origin. The intestinal mucosa of individuals who live in tropical areas of the world tends to contain increased numbers of round cells. When this alone is observed, it is better to indicate that the round cell content of the lamina propria appears to be increased, rather than that there is presence of chronic inflammation.

NORMAL MUSCULARIS MUCOSAE

The intestinal mucosa, consisting of epithelium and lamina propria, is separated from the submucosa by a thin layer of smooth muscle called the *muscularis mucosae*, the third component of the intestinal mucosa. This muscle layer is generally poorly developed, but may on occasion be prominent, and consists of an inner layer of circular fibers and an outer layer of longitudinally arranged fibers. This thin layer of muscle lies just beneath the intestinal glands that open into the crypts of Lieberkuhn. Occasional muscle cells extend from this thin muscle layer into the villus core.

THE ABNORMAL BIOPSY

Villous architecture is altered in most mucosal disorders of the intestine. Thus, the severity of a mucosal abnormality should be graded first according to changes in villous architecture. Abnormal specimens should be graded as showing

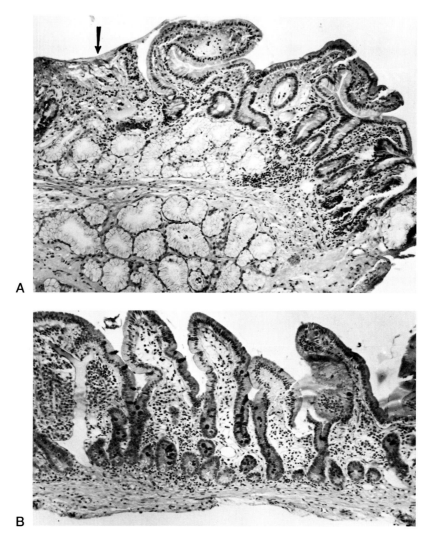

Fig. 6-3. (A) Section of biopsy obtained from the duodenal bulb showing severe Brunner gland artifact. The presence of Brunner glands both below and above the muscularis mucosae is noted. The villi are shortened and distorted and contain an increased cellular content within the lamina propria. Further, there is severe traumatic artifact (arrow) and some hemorrhagic artifact in the lamina propria. Traumatic artifact is more likely to occur in the presence of Brunner gland hypertrophy. **(B)** Normal section of biopsy of the duodenal bulb obtained only a few millimeters away from the biopsy illustrated in Fig. A. There are four normal villi in a row, but these are shortened and broadened and contain an increased cellular content in the lamina propria. Note the very broad leaf-shaped villus on the left, which contains a prominent central lacteal. The pallisading of nuclei of the epithelium at the apex of this villus is an artifact of tangential sectioning. (*Figure continues.*)

a mild, moderate, or severe abnormality in villous architecture. There is excellent agreement among experienced observers regarding the interpretation of moderate and severe abnormalities when biopsy specimens are read in a coded fashion. It may be more difficult to distinguish consistently a mild abnormality from the normal.[6]

In the *mild* villous abnormality, many villi are branched, broadened, or fused above the

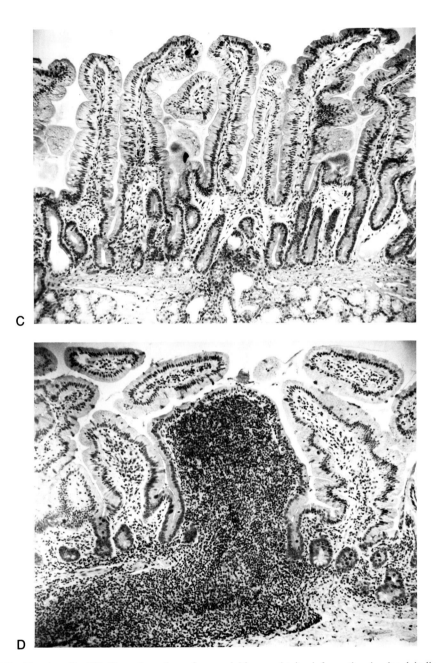

C

D

Fig. 6-3. (*Continued*). (**C**) Normal section of peroral biopsy obtained from the duodenal bulb showing that villous architecture may be perfectly normal even in the presence of Brunner glands. Generally, proximal duodenal biopsies accurately reflect jejunal biopsies in both normal individuals and individuals with diffuse diseases of the intestine.[4,83] (**D**) Section of proximal duodenal biopsy in which a small lymphoid nodule distorts a single villus in an otherwise normal biopsy specimen. (H&E, Figs. A–D × 132.)

crypt region. Other villi may be normal in appearance. The surface epithelium is often abnormal, with a loss of nuclear polarity and an increase in intraepithelial lymphocytes (Fig. 6-4). Sometimes the epithelial changes will be more striking than changes in villous structure. Mitotic figures may be more prominent and may be found just above the crypt level. The number of round cells and of acute inflammatory cells may be increased in the lamina propria. However, a slight increase in number of cells within the lamina propria in the absence of villous changes or changes in the surface epithelium is more likely a normal variant.

The *moderate* lesion is characterized by broadened and shortened villi (Fig. 6-5). The surface epithelium over the tips of villi may be cuboidal, and the round cell content of the lamina propria will be unequivocally increased. Intraepithelial lymphocytes appear to be greatly increased in number.

The *severe* lesion is easily recognized because villi are almost completely absent (Fig. 6-6). The cellular content of the lamina propria is obviously markedly increased, and intraepithelial lymphocytes are generally quite numerous.

The above classification is based on assessment of villous architecture alone.[1] Other changes may be found in the epithelium regardless of the degree of villous change. For example, the surface epithelium may be severely vacuolated, the vacuoles generally representing cell injury or collections of fat. Frank macrocytosis is sometimes a feature of the surface epithelium. The presence of more than occasional PMN leukocytes within the lamina propria generally represents an abnormality if hemorrhagic artifact has been excluded. Clearly excessive numbers of PMN leukocytes may justify the pathologic diagnosis of *acute inflammation.* Other isolated inflammatory changes that are occasionally observed include crypt abscesses, microulcerations, and the presence of granulomas. These changes are more likely to be detected if many sections are examined. Changes that may be observed in the submucosa include changes in blood vessels and nerves, presence of granulomas, dilated lymphatics, and lymphomatous infiltration.

Some prefer to examine the biopsy specimen using a hand lens or a dissecting microscope prior to processing of the specimen. This may be worthwhile because the observation of a grossly flat mucosa leaves little doubt that the

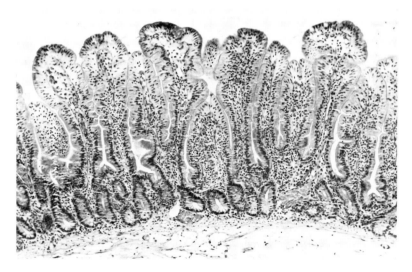

Fig. 6-4. Mild villous abnormality of proximal jejunal mucosa showing broadened villi, loss of nuclear polarity of the surface epithelium, increased numbers of intraepithelial lymphocytes, and a slight increase in the cellular content of the lamina propria. Two of the villi are branched. (H&E, × 100.)

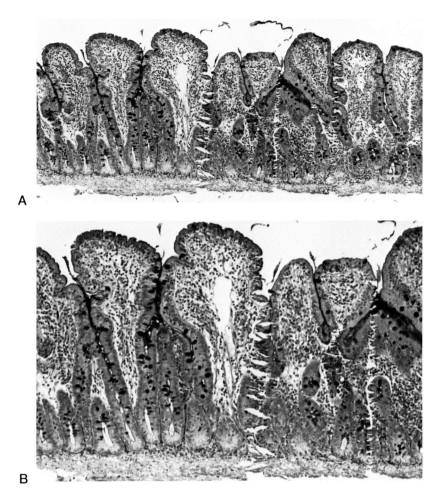

Fig. 6-5. **(A)** Moderate villous abnormality of the proximal jejunal mucosa in a North American patient with tropical sprue acquired during a trip to the Philippines. The villi are clearly broadened, there is a marked increase of cellular content within the lamina propria, and the epithelium is somewhat flattened with a marked increase in number of intraepithelial lymphocytes. The crypts are slightly lengthened, this change being best determined by the upward displacement of mitoses from the bases of the crypts toward the lumen. **(B)** Higher-power magnification of the protion of section in Fig. A that illustrates more clearly the epithelial changes and increased numbers of intraepithelial leukocytes. (PAS-hematoxylin, Fig. A × 80, Fig. B × 132.)

specimen will be abnormal when processed histologically. Although a grossly flat mucosa usually means celiac sprue in North America, a wide variety of specific histopathologic abnormalities can only be revealed after careful sectioning. The hand lens (the ''poor man's dissecting microscope'') is best used as an aid in orienting the specimen.

CLASSIFICATION AND INTERPRETATION OF ABNORMAL SPECIMENS

Rubin (personal communication) classifies the abnormal small bowel biopsy as (1) flat biopsy, either nonspecific (nondiagnostic) or diagnostic); (2) variably abnormal villi, either nonspecific or diagnostic; and (3) normal villi

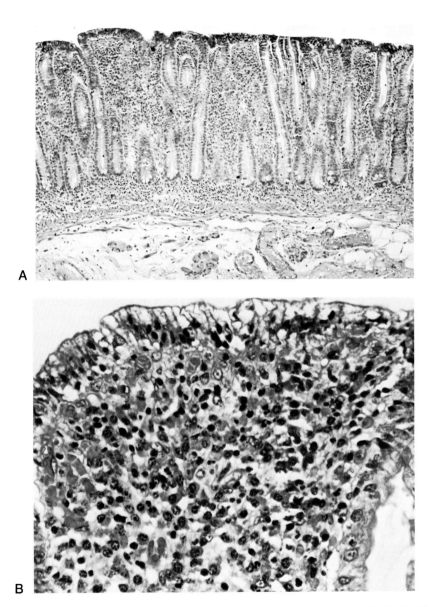

A

B

Fig. 6-6. **(A)** Characteristic severe abnormality of the proximal jejunum in an individual with untreated celiac sprue. Note absence of villi, flattened surface epithelium, lengthened crypts, and increased cellular content of the lamina propria. **(B)** Severe epithelial cell injury in an intestinal biopsy specimen of another patient with untreated celiac sprue. Marked vacuolization of the surface epithelial cells and the marked plasma cell infiltrate in the lamina propria may be seen. The crypt epithelial cells on the right have a more normal appearance but are still flattened and cuboidal in shape. (H&E, Fig. A × 132, Fig. B × 500.)

but diagnostic abnormality present (Table 6-1). The definitive diagnosis often requires not only an abnormal biopsy but a second diagnostic criterion, usually one relating to specific therapy.

In the discussion that follows, lesions are described as either diffuse or patchy in distribution. In diffuse lesions, every biopsy specimen taken at the duodenojejunal junction is abnormal. In patchy lesions, some specimens show histologic changes, whereas others do not. When a lesion is described as *severe*, this means that the abnormal tissues always lack villi. On the other hand, use of the term *variable* implies that biopsy specimens exhibit a spectrum of changes ranging from normal to severe in the same patient or in different patients with the same disease.

DISEASES ASSOCIATED WITH A FLAT SMALL BOWEL BIOPSY

Table 6-2 lists the diseases associated with a flat small bowel biopsy (severe lesion) but in which the histologic changes are nonspecific and the diagnosis hinges on a therapeutic response. Table 6-3 lists the diseases associated with a flat small bowel biopsy in which the histologic changes are diagnostic.

CELIAC SPRUE

Patients with untreated celiac sprue, who present with overt malabsorption or with various deficiencies secondary to malabsorption, show a severe abnormality of the villous architecture

Table 6-1. Rubin Classification of Small Bowel Biopsy

Flat biopsy
  Nonspecific
  Diagnostic
Variably abnormal villi
  Nonspecific
  Diagnostic
Normal villi
  Diagnostic

(Courtesy of C. E. Rubin.)

Table 6-2. Flat Small Bowel Biopsy—Nonspecific (Nondiagnostic)

Disease	Treatment Response With:
Symptomatic celiac sprue	Gluten-free diet
Other protein injury	Soy-, chicken-, milk-free diet
Refractory sprue	Unknown
IgA deficiency (rare)	Unknown
Some tropical sprue	Antibiotic + folic acid
Childhood kwashiorkor	Adequate-protein diet
Familial enteropathy	Unknown
Drug-induced injury (rare)	Withdrawal of drug
Infectious gastroenteritis (rare)	Self-limited illness
Some stasis syndromes	Antibiotics; surgical procedure

in the proximal jejunal mucosa (Fig. 6-6).[6] Almost all North Americans with this intestinal lesion turn out to have celiac sprue. The intestinal lesion is characteristic but is not diagnostic because it is seen in several other diseases that are rare in North America. Celiac sprue appears to be the result of a genetically determined defect in intestinal absorption whose pathogenesis is related to intestinal mucosal injury by gluten.[7] Gluten is a component of proteins found in wheat, rye, barley, and possibly oats. Malabsorption disappears in these patients when gluten is removed from the diet. Thus, the diagnosis requires demonstration of the characteristic severe intestinal mucosal lesion, as well as a clinical response to a gluten-free diet.

Table 6-3. Flat Small Bowel Biopsy—Diagnostic

Disease	Diagnostic Histology
Collagenous sprue	Broad band of collagen below surface epithelium
Late-onset immunodeficiency (common variable hypogammaglobulinemia)	Virtually absent lamina propria plasma cells; nodular lymphoid hyperplasia
Whipple's disease (some)	Typical macrophages in lamina propria
Eosinophilic gastroenteritis (some)	Eosinophilic infiltrate
Primary intestinal lymphoma (some) (immunoproliferative small intestinal disease)	Malignant lymphoid cells in lamina propria

The severe mucosal lesion of the untreated patient generally shows the absence of villi. The surface epithelium may be cuboidal, vacuolated, and basophilic, and contains many intraepithelial lymphocytes. The infiltration of the lamina propria and of the epithelium with lymphocytes suggests that the lesion is immune mediated.[8] Occasional PMN leukocytes may be seen in the epithelium. In some patients the surface epithelium may be almost normal despite the presence of the flat lesion. Crypts are elongated, as evidenced by the presence of scattered mitoses extending from the base of the crypts almost to the surface of the specimen. Crypt epithelial cells tend to be normal in appearance.

The cell content of the lamina propria is obviously increased. Plasma cells predominate, while lymphocytes, eosinophils, and PMN leukocytes are also increased in number but to a lesser extent. Crypt abscesses may occasionlly be seen. The number of crypts is not decreased, and the mucosal thickness is generally normal. In one patient, metaplasia of the mucosa to gastric fundal glands was reported.[2]

The mucosal lesion is more severe in the proximal intestine than in the distal intestine. This may relate to the fact that the proximal intestine is exposed to higher concentrations of gluten than is the distal intestine. In fact, in patients with little or no steatorrhea, only the most proximal jejunum is abnormal. However, in those patients with severe steatorrhea, the whole small bowel, including the ileum, tends to be severely involved.[9] As the patient improves in response to a gluten-free diet, the ileal lesion repairs itself much more rapidly than does the jejunal lesion. Several years or more may be required for the lesion at the duodenojejunal junction to return to normal in patients on strict gluten-free diets (Fig. 6-7). Most frequently, the proximal jejunum only shows evidence of partial improvement, even though the distal jejunum and the ileum may show return to complete normality. Further, many patients fail to adhere completely to an absolutely gluten-free diet, and this may account for the continued evidence of injury in the proximal jejunum. The pathologist must remind the clinician that a persistent

proximal mucosal abnormality does not necessarily reflect the state of the rest of the jejunum, and is not a cause for concern if the patient is doing well clinically. If the patient can adhere to an absolutely gluten-free diet, the intestinal mucosa will eventually return to normal in virtually all of these patients. Few individuals are capable of such a strict diet, particularly when they find that they suffer few clinical consequences by occasional gluten ingestion.

The rare individual who fails to respond to a gluten-free diet may have *refractory sprue* or *unclassified sprue*.[10] Some of these patients with refractory sprue will recover with corticosteroid therapy, or with cyclophosphamide[11] or cyclosporine[12] (Fig. 6-7). Rarely these patients are refractory to all therapy, and the disease pursues a relentless and generally fatal course. One individual was shown to require not only a gluten-free diet but a diet free of egg, chicken, and tuna.[10] Occasionally other lesions may be confused with the lesion of celiac sprue. In those patients with apparent celiac sprue who fail to respond to a gluten-free diet, the original biopsy specimen should be re-examined to look for such lesions as collagenous sprue, hypogammaglobulinemic (late-onset immunodeficiency) sprue, intestinal lymphoma, and treatable infections, such as giardiasis or coccidiosis, which may have been missed on the original biopsy specimen. The unusual causes, at least in North America, of the severe nonspecific jejunal abnormality must be ruled out by the therapeutic response to appropriate treatment (Table 6-2). Additional biopsies may be indicated to look for diseases with a patchy distribution, such as collagenous sprue and intestinal lymphoma. There is an increased incidence of abdominal lymphoma in patients with celiac sprue. Thus, lymphoma should be considered in patients who respond suboptimally to the initial gluten-free diet, or who relapse while on the diet.

The diagnosis of celiac sprue in children is often complicated by the fact that these children have often been placed on gluten-free diets without obtaining a prior intestinal biopsy. Response to a gluten-free diet without prior determination of the characteristic intestinal lesion does *not*

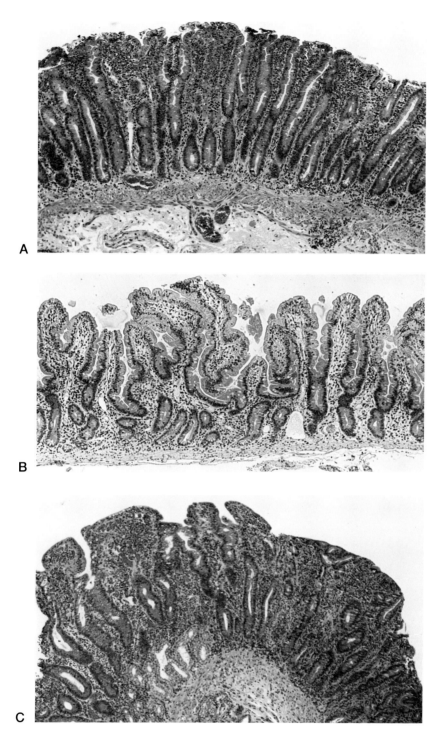

Fig. 6-7. Reversible abnormality in celiac sprue and in unclassified sprue. **(A)** Severe abnormality in the proximal jejunum of a patient with untreated celiac sprue. **(B)** Mild abnormality indicating improvement in the mucosa in the same patient after 5 months of a gluten-free diet. Contrast in the epithelium before and after treatment may be seen. **(C)** Severe abnormality in duodenum of a patient with unclassified sprue unresponsive to a gluten-free diet. (*Figure continues.*)

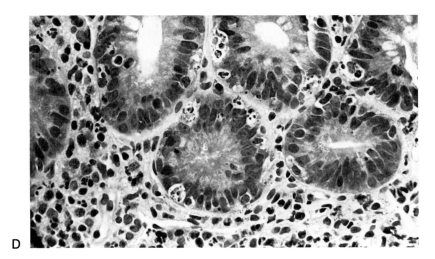

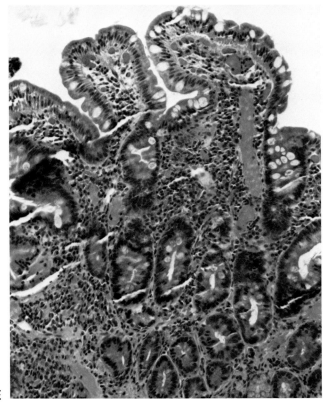

Fig. 6-7 (*Continued*). **(D)** High magnification of the specimen illustrated in Fig. C showing a striking degree of single cell necrosis (apoptosis) in the crypt epithelium, indicating immume-mediated injury. PMN leukocyte infiltrate is seen in the lamina propria and in some areas of the epithelium. **(E)** Mild abnormality in the duodenum of the same patient following treatment with corticosteroids. There was also a dramatic clinical response in this patient, who had failed to respond to a gluten-free diet. (H&E, Figs. A,B,C × 100, Fig. D × 500, Fig. E × 250.)

make the diagnosis of celiac sprue. Such patients should undergo biopsy examination because an established diagnosis of celiac sprue requires a life-long gluten-free diet. Rubin found that most children diagnosed as having celiac sprue by a therapeutic trial of the gluten-free diet early in life proved not to have the disease when intestinal biopsy specimens were taken after institution of a high-gluten diet. Some of these children who were thought to have celiac sprue probably had infectious gastroenteritis, which may induce a transient but severe intestinal mucosal abnormality in children (Fig. 6-8).[2] Some children with established celiac sprue may abandon the gluten-free diet after responding to it and yet continue to do well. However, a repeat

small bowel biopsy will still show the presence of the characteristic jejunal lesions.

It may be that celiac sprue is more often a subclinical disorder than a disorder that presents with overt malabsorption. For example, family studies have revealed asymptomatic members with severe intestinal mucosal lesions.[2, 7] Some patients may present with an isolated deficiency of absorption, such as iron-deficiency anemia secondary to iron malabsorption, or osteomalacia secondary to calcium and vitamin D malabsorption. Biopsy specimens in these patients reveal the characteristic severe lesion of celiac sprue. Two thirds of patients with *dermatitis herpetiformis* have the characteristic severe lesion of celiac sprue (Fig. 6-6).[9] Even though

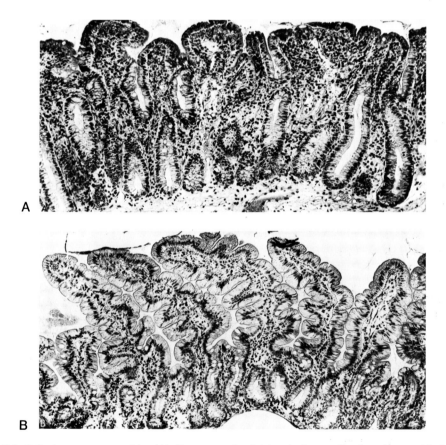

Fig. 6-8. Infectious gastroenteritis. **(A)** Severe proximal jejunal abnormality in a 7-year-old child with acute gastroenteritis. No pathogens were cultured. **(B)** Normal proximal jejunal biopsy specimen in the same child taken 6 weeks after biopsy (Fig. A) and 12 weeks after onset of illness. The patient was completely well at the time of the biopsy. (H&E, × 184). (From Perea et al,[1] with permission.)

these patients do not have apparent malabsorption, both the intestinal lesion and the skin lesions respond to treatment with a gluten-free diet if it is strict and of long duration. A small number of patients with dermatitis herpetiformis have a normal small intestine mucosa. However, when two such patients were placed on a high-gluten diet, their intestinal mucosa became abnormal.[2] Thus, it appears that most (if not all) patients with dermatitis herpetiformis have a latent form of celiac sprue, usually clinically latent but sometimes both morphologically and clinically latent. The vast majority of patients with dermatitis herpetiformis can be shown, using direct immunofluorescence, to have IgA deposits in the skin lesions.[13] Similar deposits of IgA have not been detected in intestinal mucosal biopsies of these patients.[13]

OTHER PROTEIN INJURY

Severe gastrointestinal reactions to the introduction of a new protein into the diet of an infant are rarely observed.[14] The normal proximal jejunal mucosa became acutely inflamed and lost its villi within 12 hours after soy protein ingestion by one susceptible infant.[15] This infant concomitantly developed shock, fever, and mild gastrointestinal bleeding. The severe lesion produced was indistinguishable from that seen in untreated celiac sprue. Similar reactions to various dietary proteins, especially those in milk, have been detected. It should be noted that one adult has been shown to require not only a gluten-free diet but a diet free of egg, chicken, and tuna in order to correct the severe intestinal mucosal lesion.[10]

REFRACTORY (UNCLASSIFIED) SPRUE AND ULCERATIVE JEJUNOILEITIS

Patients with refractory unclassified sprue have the characteristic severe lesion of untreated celiac sprue, and they do not respond to a strict gluten-free diet.[15] This is a diagnosis of exclusion and may well represent more than one as

yet unidentified disease process. There appear to be two clinical categories of this syndrome, one in which malabsorption is not life threatening and one in which malabsorption runs a fulminant course. The latter group has often been reported as having *ulcerative jejunoileitis*.[16] Occasionally the benign syndrome will evolve into a "malignant" syndrome, but long survival with variable disability is often the case. Patients in both categories may respond initially to a gluten-free diet, only later becoming unresponsive. Some of these patients eventually turn out to have abdominal lymphoma. Whether the lymphoma has been a primary event or has developed as a complication of pre-existing celiac sprue generally cannot be determined.[15] Paneth cells may be absent in a few patients with unclassified sprue, but the significance of this observation is not at all clear.[1] The presence of single crypt cell necrosis (apoptosis) suggests an immune-mediated (presumably not gluten-related) mechanism (Fig. 6–7C to E). (See Graft-versus-Host Disease, below.)

COLLAGENOUS SPRUE

Villi are completely absent and all other characteristic features of the severe lesion of untreated celiac sprue are found in intestinal biopsy specimens from patients with collagenous sprue.[17] In addition, the unique and diagnostic feature is a strikingly broad band of collagen found just below the epithelial basal lamina (Fig. 6-9). Most patients with this rare lesion have a fulminant and generally fatal course. There is no known treatment for this syndrome. Some of the patients do respond transiently to a gluten-free diet, and it is reasonable to recommend a prolonged gluten-free diet in all of the patients. Immunosuppressive agents such as corticosteroids and cyclophosphamide may be tried.[11, 12] Collagen deposition is not uniformly present early in the disease. Biopsy specimens may be required at repeated intervals in order to establish the diagnosis.

Collagenous sprue may be an end stage of unclassified sprue, or even of celiac sprue that

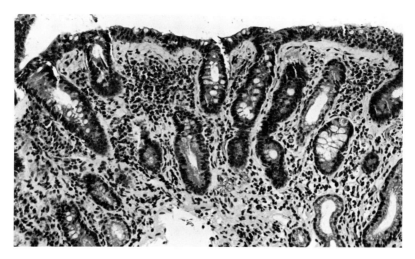

Fig. 6-9. Collagenous sprue. Severe proximal jejunal abnormality in a patient with fatal malabsorption. A broad hyaline band of collagen separating the surface epithelium from the underlying lamina propria is seen. (H&E, × 184.)

has become refractory to treatment. Because its course is different from that of celiac sprue, and because the long-term prognosis is grim, it is reasonable to classify this as a separate diagnostic entity until it can be more clearly defined. Bossart and colleagues[18] suggest that collagenous sprue is nothing more than a varient of celiac sprue, and that it does not deserve a separate classification. Rubin (personal communication) points out that Bossart did not demonstrate the presence of a broad band of collagen below the epithelium, but only the expanded basement membrane complex seen in any flat lesion.

IMMUNODEFICIENCY

The two major adult immunodeficiency syndromes are (1) late-onset immunodeficiency, or common variable hypogammaglobulinemia (CVH), and (2) selective IgA deficiency.[19] CVH is represented by two major subgroups, one in which there is variable deficiency of immunoglobulins, especially IgA and IgM, and one in which there may or may not be clinically significant T-cell deficiency. The other subgroups of CVH is manifested by predominant T-cell defi-

ciency, with antibody deficiency being less prominent. CVH is characterized by two major presentations, one in which there is recurrent respiratory tract infection, and the other in which the predominant clinical manifestation is chronic diarrhea and malabsorption (hypogammaglobulinemic sprue) with recurrent gastrointestinal giardiasis. These two clinical syndromes tend to be mutually exclusive. Chronic diarrhea, malabsorption, and protein-losing enteropathy are common features of CVH. The key pathologic finding is a marked reduction or even absence of plasma cells in the intestinal mucosa (Fig. 6-10). Plasma cells are also absent or markedly diminished at other sites such as the bone marrow and spleen. Mucosal structure varies from normal in appearance to a flat lesion comparable to that seen in individuals with celiac sprue (Fig. 6-10). There is no clinical or histologic response to a gluten-free diet. *Giardia lamblia* is often found on careful search of serial sections, and may be more easily seen in Giemsa-stained smears of mucus adherent to the specimen.[20] Generally, the flat mucosa will return to a more normal appearance following successful treatment of giardiasis.[19, 20] Alternatively, it has been shown that a relatively normal-appearing mucosa in patients with CVH

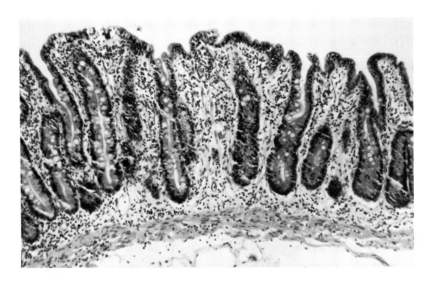

Fig. 6-10. Severe jejunal mucosal lesion in a patient with late-onset immunodeficiency (CVH), the lesion seeminly indistinguishable from that seen in untreated celiac sprue. However, plasma cells were absent in the lamina propria, and the patient had severe deficiency of serum IgG, IgA, and IgM. (H&E, × 132.)

will progress over a period of years, in association with recurrent diarrheal illnesses, to a flat mucosal appearance. This progression is usually, but not always, related to recurrent giardiasis. Nodular lymphoid hyperplasia (NLH), consisting of hyperplastic lymphoid follicles containing immature B cells, may be found throughout the gastrointestinal tract. These follicles create a characteristic and often diagnostic nodular appearance of the small bowel when examined using barium contrast media. Suction biopsy specimens may include whole benign lymphoid follicles within the lamina propria. The villi overlying the follicles may be distorted, and the intervening mucosa may be normal or may show a variable abnormality in villous architecture. At one time it was thought that NLH was a separate entity from CVH. Today it is generally thought that NLH is one of the manifestations of CVH, and it tends to develop in these patients as they become older. NLH may represent "compensatory" hyperplasia of immatue B cells that are genetically defective and unable to mature as plama cells. The histologic and radiologic changes of NLH may rarely be found in otherwise normal individuals.[21]

The most common adult immunodeficiency syndrome is that of *selective IgA deficiency*.[19] The incidence of this syndrome is approximately one in 700 individuals. Many individuals with selective IgA deficiency have no apparent clinical abnormalities, possibly because they have a "compensatory" increase in serum IgM and presumably of secretory IgM. Other individuals with selective IgA deficiency, especially if deficient in the IgG subclasses, IgG2 and IgG4, present with three types of illness: sinopulmonary disease, malabsorption syndrome, or autoimmune disease. There is *no* predisposition to the intestinal parasite, *Giardia*. Pathologically, the intestinal mucosa is generally normal, although there is a decrease or absence of IgA-bearing cells in the gut. IgM- and IgG-staining plasma cells are present in normal numbers. A single intriguing patient has been reported with a severe villous abnormality of the small intestine, associated with selective IgA deficiency.[22] The patient did not respond to a strict gluten-free diet. Indirect immunofluorescent studies revealed in his serum an IgG antibody that bound to epithelial cells in control intestine, but not to cells in the patient's diseased mucosa. Following treatment with cyclophosphamide, the serum antibody titer slowly declined, and the appearance of the patient's intestinal mucosa returned to normal. These unique findings suggested an autoimmune etiology for the intestinal mucosal damage in this single individual.[22] There may be an increased incidence of celiac sprue in patients with selective IgA deficiency. These patients have a severe intestinal mucosal lesion and respond to a gluten-free diet.

Structural alterations of the intestinal mucosa may sometimes be found in the large variety of immunodeficiency syndromes found in the pediatric age group.[23–25] Certainly the increased incidence of gastrointestinal symptoms in children with severe combined immunodeficiency and in some children with isolated T-cell deficiency suggests that an intact cellular immune system is essential for the normal function of the intestinal tract.[23] There is usually no histologic abnormality other than absence of plasma cells in the lamina propria in the majority of these patients.[24] Plasma cells are not present in biopsies of patients with infantile X-linked agammaglobulinemia and in most children with CVH. Plasma cells are easily recognized in biopsies of patients with ataxia-telangiectasia, selective IgA deficiency, immunodeficiency syndrome with normal serum gamma globulins, and X-linked immunodeficiency with hyper-IgM. Multiple small bowel biopsies are necessary to assess the morphology in all symptomatic children with immunodeficiency, because the villous architecture may often vary from normal to severely abnormal in different biopsies obtained at the same time from the same individual.[25]

CHRONIC GRAUNLOMATOUS DISEASE

Chronic granulomatous disease of childhood is an inherited illness manifested by repeated bacterial infections.[23] The phagocytic cells of these patients can ingest but not kill certain microorganisms. Two of nine children with CGD had steatorrhea, and six of the patients had mild to moderate vitamin B_{12} malabsorption. In seven of eight of the patients biopsied, there were clumps of characteristic vacuolated pigmented macrophages within the lamina propria adjacent to the crypts and occasionally within the villous core (Fig. 6-11). Small bowel morphology was otherwise completely normal. The macrophages were PAS positive and contained a yellowish-brown pigment. Unlike untreated Whipple's disease, the villous architecture was completely normal, and there were far fewer macrophages in the lamina propria.[23] Large foamy macrophages may be seen in the lamina propria of intestinal biopsies of patients with macroglobulinemia. These macrophages are not pigmented but may be faintly PAS positive, and should be easily distinguished from the macrophages seen in CGD and in Whipple's disease.

TROPICAL SPRUE SYNDROME

Many asymptomatic people living in certain areas of the world such as Ceylon, Puerto Rico, Haiti, India, and Hong Kong show mild or moderate nonspecific abnormalities in the proximal jejunum. Some of these apparently clinically well people may even have a severe nonspecific abnormality that is indistinguishable from that seen in untreated celiac sprue.[26] Nonspecific mucosal abnormalities may be found in individuals who have lived in those parts of the world for short periods of time, generally after a few years but sometimes after only a few months (Fig. 6-12). The pathogenesis of this syndrome is not clear, but most evidence favors enterotoxin production by an infectious agent, in addition to intestinal injury caused by unknown influences in the environment. When severe, the characteristic features of this syndrome include chronic diarrhea, steatorrhea, macrocytic anemia, glossitis, and emaciation, all attributable to intestinal malabsorption of fat, carbohydrate, vitamin B_{12}, and folic acid.

Jejunal biopsy in symptomatic patients, as well as in asymptomatic individuals residing in tropical areas, will show abnormalities of villous structure ranging from mild to severe (Fig. 6-13).[1] A North American returning from

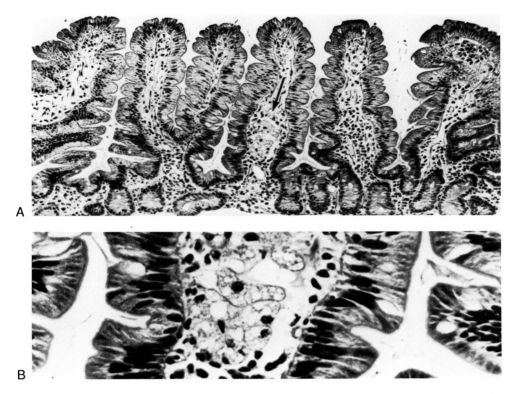

Fig. 6-11. Section of small bowel biopsy obtained from a patient with chronic granulomatous disease. The villous architecture is normal. **(A)** A cluster of macrophages is present in the lamina propria of the middle villus (arrow). **(B)** The macrophages show a typical vacuolated appearance. (H&E, Fig. A × 184, Fig. B × 736.) (From Perea et al.,[1] with permission. Courtesy of Dr. Marvin Ament, Los Angeles.)

a tropical area of the world with malabsorption and who is found to have a severe nonspecific lesion may have either tropical sprue or celiac sprue. If the patient has tropical sprue, treatment with folic acid and a broad-spectrum antibiotic such as tetracycline generally results in a prompt remission of symptoms, often with improvement in intestinal structure. If the patient fails to respond to such treatment, a gluten-free diet should be tried in order to exclude celiac sprue.

It is essential to remember that biopsy specimens obtained from patients residing in the tropical areas of the world cannot be interpreted by the same criteria as those from patients residing in North America.[1, 26] The range of normal in small bowel morphology of asymptomatic individuals residing in tropical areas must be established for each country. Intestinal biopsy in normal asymptomatic individuals residing in

tropical countries often show mild villous abnormalities when compared with biopsy specimens of North Americans. Further, mucosal changes in both asymptomatic people and clinically ill individuals with malabsorption may look worse in Haiti or Vietnam than they do in Puerto Rico.[26]

Childhood Kwashiorkor

Kwashiorkor is one of the most common illnesses of children in "undeveloped" areas of the world.[27] In growing children, protein deficiency per se has been shown to cause severe nonspecific proximal jejunal abnormalities indistinguishable from those of untreated celiac sprue.[27] The same lesion can be produced experimentally in growing animals by depriving them

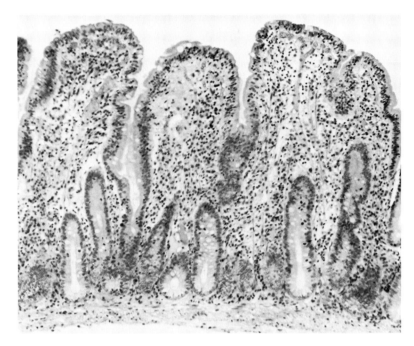

Fig. 6-12. Proximal jejunal biopsy specimen showing a severe villous abnormality in a Puerto Rican patient with tropical sprue. There is a marked increase in number of lymphocytes and a modest increase in plasma cells in the lamina propria. There is the striking increase in number of intraepithelial lymphocytes, possibly the most characteristic histologic feature in tropical sprue. (Formalin fixation, H&E, × 540.)

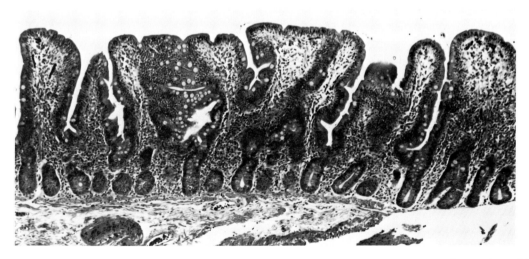

Fig. 6-13. Proximal jejunal biopsy specimen showing a mild abnormality in a Puerto Rican patient with tropical sprue. The villous architecture is only slightly altered, but again there is an increase in number of lymphocytes and plasma cells in the lamina propria, and in the number of intraepithelial lymphocytes. (Formalin fixation, H&E, × 80.)

of proteins. These patients will respond to a normal diet containing adequate amounts of high-quality protein, and with concomitant improvement in the appearance of the intestinal mucosa. The intestinal lesion in kwashiorkor may be patchy, mild to moderate in degree, and impossible to differentiate from abnormalities characteristically seen in tropical sprue. The diagnosis is established on the basis of response to protein feeding.

Familial Enteropathy (Microvillus Inclusion Disease)

Familial enteropathy is a new syndrome described in nine infants residing near Toronto, Canada.[28] It is a syndrome of protracted diarrhea from birth and failure to thrive, with intestinal mucosal changes comparable in severity to those seen in celiac sprue. No consistent hematologic or immunologic defects were found in the infants. Duodenal biopsies showed a severe mucosal lesion, crypt hypoplasia without an increase in mitoses, the absence of an inflammatory cell infiltrate in the lamina propria, and, most remarkably, absence of the brush border. Electron microscopy confirmed the absence of the brush border, the microvilli being

found within intracytoplasmic inclusions. Similar changes were also present in the rectum. Celiac sprue was easily excluded, because the infants either had not ingested gluten or had failed to respond to total parenteral nutrition. There were some similarities to kwashiorkor. However, in kwashiorkor there is a marked increase in inflammatory cells in the lamina propria, and those patients respond to adequate nutritional intake, features lacking in familial enteropathy. Because other types of small intestine cells (goblet cells, Paneth cells, and enteroendocrine cells) were normal, the abnormality may be restricted to one of absorptive cells. The abnormality may be one of failure of normal maturation and differentiation of crypt cells.[28]

DISEASES ASSOCIATED WITH VARIABLY ABNORMAL VILLI— NONSPECIFIC

Table 6-4 lists the diseases associated with variably abnormal villi (mild to moderate lesions) in which the histologic changes are nonspecific, and again require a treatment response in order to establish a diagnosis.

CELIAC SPRUE AND DERMATITIS HERPETIFORMIS

Subclinical celiac sprue and dermatitis herpetiformis are discussed above under Celiac Sprue, above.

INFECTIOUS GASTROENTERITIS

Infectious gastroenteritis is probably caused by a variety of viral and bacterial pathogens, most of which have not been clearly identified.[29, 30] Jejunal lesions are generally mild to moderate in severity and are nonspecific, but may be severe with a flat biopsy (Fig. 6-8). The clinical picture of acute gastroenteritis at the onset of symptoms and the usually temporary

Table 6-4. Variably Abnormal Villi—Nonspecific

Disease	Treatment Response With:
Subclinical celiac sprue (dermatitis herpetiformis)	Gluten-free diet
Infectious gastroenteritis	Spontaneous cure
Stasis syndromes	Antibiotics
Some tropical sprue	Antibiotics + folic acid
Geographic variation	Environmental improvement
Zollinger-Ellison syndrome (gastrinoma)	Omeprazole
Graft-versus-host disease (Immune-mediated injury)	Steroids; antithymocyte globulin
Ischemia, hyalinosis, vasculitis	Unknown
Sarcoidosis	Unknown
Drug-induced injury	Withdrawal of drug

nature of symptoms suggest the diagnosis. Moderate to severe changes were documented in the intestinal mucosa of 31 infants and children with "nonbacterial" gastroenteritis.[2] Repeat biopsy specimens in some of those children, when they became asymptomatic, showed improvement or return to normality.[2] Histologically, there may be an acute inflammatory process with formation of early crypt abscesses. Rubin has noted rare patients with infectious enteritis in whom malabsorption with acute inflammatory changes in the biopsy specimens continued for months before the lesions and symptoms finally disappeared.[1] Pathogenic *Escherichia coli* may produce diarrhea, with a flat intestinal lesion and even death in infants.[29] Fluorescent antibody staining for the presence of *E. coli* may be required to establish the invasive nature of the organism.[1, 29]

STASIS SYNDROMES

Steatorrhea and/or macrocytic anemia may arise in patients with bacterial overgrowth in the proximal small intestine.[31] This bacterial overgrowth is secondary to a variety of causes of impaired intestinal transit, including the presence of surgical blind loops, intestinal strictures, jejunal diverticulosis, chronic idiopathic pseudo-obstruction, scleroderma, and diabetes mellitus. The etiology of malabsorption is probably multifactorial. In many of these patients, bacterial conversion of conjugated bile salts to unconjugated bile salts is of importance. Patchy intestinal abnormalities (Fig. 6-14), whether attributable to toxicity of unconjugated bile salts or the presence of the bacteria themselves, are often present in varying severity and may contribute to the malabsorption.

The diagnosis of stasis syndromes is based on three criteria: the presence of increased volumes of proximal jejunal contents, demonstration of increased concentrations of bacteria in the proximal jejunum, and clinical and laboratory responses to an appropriate antibiotic. Most normal individuals will have bacterial counts within the proximal jejunum of 10^3/ml or less, whereas most individuals with stasis syndromes will have counts greater than 10^7/ml. It is important to make a firm diagnosis of stasis syndrome because some patients may have surgically correctable lesions, whereas others may require periodic administration of antibiotics.

ZOLLINGER-ELLISON SYNDROME

One-third of patients with Zollinger-Ellison syndrome (ZES) have diarrhea, and 7 percent present with diarrhea as their major manifestation.[32] Steatorrhea is sometimes present in these patients. Patchy nonspecific abnormalities may be seen in the proximal segment of the jejunum in these patients.[32, 33] The diagnosis is based on finding elevated serum gastrin levels in individuals with hypersecretion of gastric acid. Because these patients may have evidence of severe mucosal abnormalties in the proximal small bowel on barium studies of the upper gastrointestinal tract, small intestinal biopsies may be obtained when the diagnosis of ZES has not been suspected clinically. The patchy lesions identified in the biopsy are generally mild in degree, and very uncommonly severe in degree (Fig. 6-15). Three structural responses of the intestinal mucosa to excessive gastric acid production have been described. The most common response is an inflammatory response with surface microulcerations, PMN leukocyte infiltration of the lamina propria, and edema of the lamina propria and submucosa.[33] Plasma cells may be increased in the lamina propria, but not to the degree seen in celiac sprue. The second response is that of gastric surface mucous cell metaplasia of intestinal absorptive cells.[32] The third structural response is that of electron microscopic evidence of injury to intestinal absorptive cells that appear to be normal when examined by light microscopy.[32] The steatorrhea seen in these patients is largely related to acid inactivation of intraluminal enzymes, whereas the structural abnormalities in

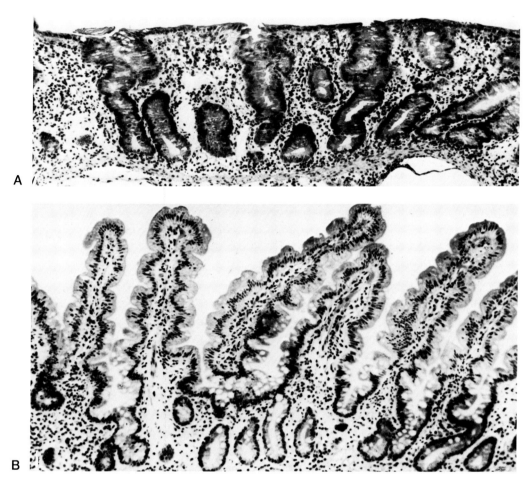

Fig. 6-14. (A) Severe proximal jejunal lesion in a patient with intestinal stasis, steatorrhea, bacterial overgrowth, and intestinal pseudo-obstruction. **(B)** Adjacent normal biopsy specimen obtained with the four-hole multipurpose tube at the same time, illustrating the patchiness of the lesion. (H&E, × 184.) (From Perea et al.,[1] with permission.)

the intestinal mucosa probably play only a small part in this regard.

GRAFT-VERSUS-HOST DISEASE (IMMUNE-MEDIATED INJURY)

Graft-versus-host disease (GVHD) is an immunologic illness that results in skin, liver, and gastrointestinal mucosal damage. It is usually seen in humans as an iatrogenic process following bone marrow transplantation.[34] Prior to transplantation, the patients must be given immunosuppressive therapy so that the marrow graft will not be rejected by the host. This therapy generally consists of a combination of total-body irradiation and chemotherapeutic drugs such as cyclophosphamide. This conditioning often results in damage to the liver and the intestinal mucosa. The changes are discussed later in this chapter (See Macrocytosis below.) These changes are only present for up to 20 days after conditioning therapy.

Acute GVHD starts 3 to 7 weeks after transplantation and may be accompanied by crampy abdominal pain, profuse watery diarrhea, and

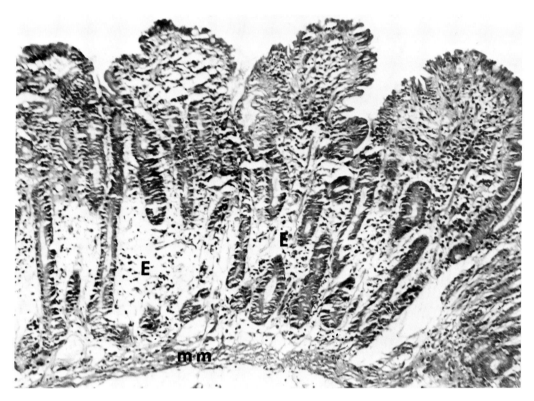

Fig. 6-15. Moderate villous abnormality in a biopsy specimen taken at the duodenojejunal junction of a patient with Zollinger-Ellison syndrome and severe diarrhea. The villi are broadened and there is a mild increase in number of plasma cells in the lamina propria. The surface epithelium is slightly flattened and irregular in appearance. There is moderate edema (*E*) of the lamina propria just above the muscularis mucosae (*mm*). (H&E, × 132.)

jaundice.[34] The lesions of acute GVHD range from necrosis of individual crypt cells to a total loss of mucosa, with the most severe involvement occurring in the ileum and right colon. When severe, there may be sheets of bacteria, fungi, and debris lining the few epithelial cells remaining. The earliest and mildest change seen in GVHD is that of necrosis of individual crypt cells, a change also seen following chemotherapy and irradiation injury. The necrosis of individual crypt cells has an unusual appearance sometimes called *apoptosis* or *exploding crypt cells* (ECC), (Fig. 6-7D). ECC is not specific, may occasionally be seen in any form of crypt injury, and is commonly found in the presence of concomitant cytomegalovirus (CMV) involvement of the gut and in AIDS enteropathy in the absence of CMV involvement.[35] AIDS enteropathy is characterized by a mild mucosal lesion and by crypt cell necrosis (ECC) in the absence of identifiable pathogens.[35] The presence of ECC in the severe mucosal lesion of refractory sprue suggests an immune (non-gluten) mediated injury. Changes of grade II severity include crypt abscess and crypt cell flattening, with or without crypt cell necrosis. In grade III severity, there is, in addition to the above changes, dropout of one or more whole crypts in a biopsy specimen, and in grade IV severity there is total denudation of the epithelium. The lamina propria does not appear to be histologically altered, but with appropriate immunofluorescent staining a marked depletion of IgA- and IgM-bearing plasma cells can be demonstrated.

Intestinal infections owing to bacteria, viruses, fungi, and parasites are the most troublesome complication in these patients, and evidence for their presence may be obtained from appropriate examination of mucosal biopsies. Clinically, rectal biopsy is more useful, and safer, then proximal small intestine biopsy for detecting mucosal changes in GVHD.[34]

Involvement of the small intestine is uncommon in patients with chronic GVHD. Chronic GVHD develops insidiously 3 to 12 months after transplantation in up to 40 percent of long-term survivors of allogeneic marrow transplants. Intestinal involvement in chronic GVHD is manifested by intractable diarrhea, malabsorption, abdominal pain, and severe malnutrition. Understandably, few peroral intestinal biopsies have been obtained in such patients, but those obtained have been normal. Rubin (personal communication) has observed abnormal intestinal biopsy changes in one patient with chronic GVHD. Autopsy specimens may show the presence of focal fibrosis in the lamina propria and segmental fibrosis of the submucosal and serosal layers, extending from stomach to colon.[34]

DISEASES ASSOCIATED WITH VARIABLY ABNORMAL VILLI— DIAGNOSTIC

Table 6-5 lists the causes of variably abnormal villi in which the histologic changes are diagnostic.

WHIPPLE'S DISEASE

Whipple's disease is an uncommon, systemic bacterial illness, affecting primarily middle-aged white men. It is characterized morphologically by the presence, in virtually all organ systems, of macrophages that are intensely stained by the PAS stain. However, there is a unique predisposition for involvement of the lamina propria of the small intestine, mesenteric lymph nodes, the mitral and aortic valves of the heart, and of the central nervous system.[36] Bacilli,

Table 6-5. Variably Abnormal Villi—Diagnostic

Disease	Diagnostic Histology
Whipple's disease	Typical macrophages filling lamina propria
Mycobacterium intracellulare	Macrophages containing acid-fast bacilli
Eosinophilic gastroenteritis	Clumps of eosinophils
Primary intestinal lymphoma	Malignant lymphoid cells in lamina propria
Parasitic diseases	Infection with *Strongyloides, Giardia,* Coccidia, Microsporidia, *Capillaria, Schistosoma,* or *Leishmania*
Fungal diseases	Infection with *Histoplasma, Candida,* or *Torula*
Viral diseases	Infection with cytomegalovirus, herpes, Rotavirus, or Norwalk virus
Macroglobulinemia	Hyaline masses in lamina propria
Lymphangiectasia (primary or secondary)	Dilated lymphatics in lamina propria
Irradiation, chemotherapy	Deficiency of mitoses
Late-onset immunodeficiency (common variable hypogammaglobulinemia)	Virtually absent plasma cells; nodular lymphoid hyperplasia
Severe B$_{12}$ or folate deficiency	Epithelial macrocytosis
Polyposis; Cronkhite Canada	Inflammatory polyp

most appropriately called *Whipple bacilli*, with all of the structural characteristics of bacteria have been observed within the intestinal mucosa, Kupfer cells of the liver, the mesenteric and peripheral lymph nodes, the heart, the central nervous system, the eye, and the lung.[36, 37] These patients may have impaired immunologic defenses, but this has not been clearly established.[38]

Because the lamina propria of the proximal intestine almost always contains characteristic macrophages, biopsy examination of tissue from the intestine usually provides the definitive diagnosis. The typical Whipple macrophages are easily recognizable on routine H&E staining (Fig. 6-16A & B), and thus it is not necessary to routinely perform a PAS stain, although it is generally helpful to do so. It should be noted

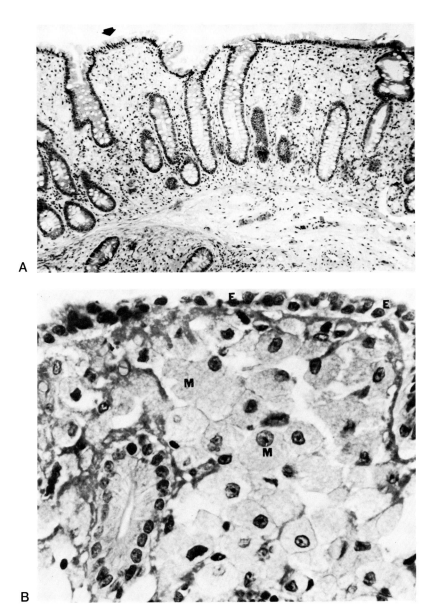

Fig. 6-16. **(A)** Severe proximal jejunal lesion in a patient with untreated Whipple's disease, showing marked infiltration of the lamina propria by macrophages that, with this stain and at this magnification, appear to be rather indistinct. A rather normal-appearing surface epithelium (arrow) is noted. **(B)** Section of biopsy obtained adjacent to the biopsy illustrated in Fig A showing at this magnification the foamy appearance of the macrophages (*M*) in the lamina propria, and illustrating a markedly flattened surface epithelium (*E*). (H&E, Fig. A × 132, Fig. B × 500.) (*Figure continues.*)

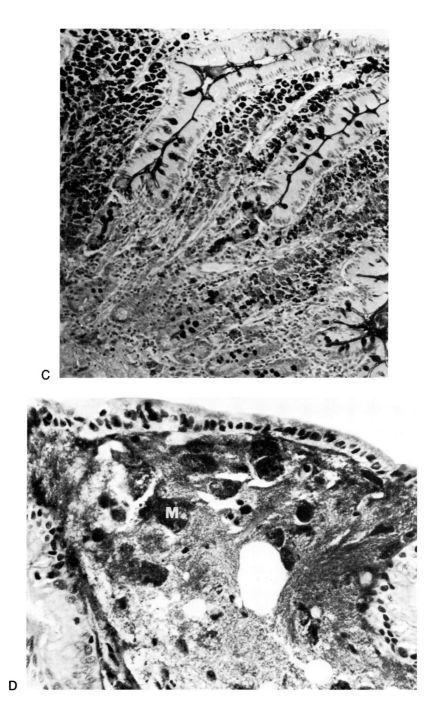

Fig. 6-16 *(Continued).* **(C)** Section of jejunal biopsy obtained in a patient with Whipple's disease after 6 weeks of antibiotic treatment. Note that the lamina propria still contains numerous macrophages that react intensely with the PAS stain. **(D)** Section of biopsy of proximal jejunum of a patient with untreated Whipple's disease illustrating a severe abnormality. Marked flattening of the surface epithelium, the indistinct, but clearly PAS-positive macrophages *(M)*, and diffuse amorphous material scattered throughout the lamina propria and shown to be a great mass of rod-shaped bacilli by electron microscopy can be seen. Using the Brown and Brenn stain and oil-immersion microscopy, this amorphous material can be seen to consist of numerous rod-shaped organisms. (PAS-hematoxylin, Fig. C × 132, Fig. D × 500.)

that macrophages in general are PAS positive, and therefore this feature alone does not distinguish the Whipple macrophage from macrophages seen in other conditions. There are three occasions when numerous PAS-positive macrophages in the intestinal lamina propria may be misleading: (1) acquired immunodeficiency syndrome (AIDS) with *Mycobacterium intracellulare* (MI) infection, (2) in systemic histoplasmosis, and (3) in macroglobulinemia. The pathologist should easily distinguish the faintly staining homogeneously PAS-positive macrophages of macroglobulinemia and the large, PAS-positive, rounded, encapsulated histoplasma organisms in macrophages from those of Whipple's disease.[39] More care must be taken to distinguish Whipple's disease from the intestinal mucosa in patients with AIDS and with a lamina propria packed with macrophages containing MI. In the latter caes, the bacilli are acid fast and easily cultured, and have a characteristic electron-microscopic appearance different from that of Whipple bacilli.[36] In Whipple's disease the villous architecture is distorted to varying degrees by the expanded and infiltrated lamina propria; the changes are generally mild to moderate in degree, but are sometimes severe. Absorptive cells at the apex of villi are often flattened and can be shown by electron microscopy to be infiltrated by bacilli. There are several recent reports of Whipple's disease with minimal or with *no* intestinal involvement.[36] The diagnosis has been established in these patients by appropriate light- and electron-microscopic examinations of lymph nodes or of brain biopsy.

Intestinal biopsies obtained during antibiotic treatment show improvement in the appearance of the surface epithelium within 1 week (Fig. 6-16C). Free bacilli have been reported to persist within the lamina propria for up to 9 weeks. These bacilli can be observed at light microscopy using Brown and Brenn stains of paraffin-embedded sections, and in PAS-stained sections (Fig. 6-16D). However, the bacilli are more easily detected when biopsy samples are prepared for electron microscopy, and sectioned at 1 μm intervals for light microscopic examination.[1, 37] The macrophages, which at electron microscopy are filled with bacilli in various stages of degeneration, clear at a much slower rate, so that even at 6 months and 1 year, the lamina propria often contains prominent macrophages, although free bacilli are no longer identifiable. The macrophages remaining after treatment tend to predominate in the lamina propria around crypt bases and in the submucosa. These macrophages may persist within the lamina propria for as long as 11 years after successful treatment.[36]

Antibiotics are the treatment of choice. Patients have been reported to respond to a great variety of antibiotics, but I currently recommend treatment with parenteral penicillin G and streptomycin for 10 to 14 days followed by twice daily oral ingestion of a double-strength tablet of trimethoprim-sulfamethoxazole for 1 year.[36] The latter drug provides effective activity within the central nervous system. Some patients have relapsed during treatment with one antibiotic and have required a new antibiotic to complete successful treatment.

EOSINOPHILIC GASTROENTERITIS

Patients with eosinophilic gastroenteritis generally have substantial eosinophilic leukocytosis in the peripheral blood and gastrointestinal symptoms characterized by nausea, vomiting, diarrhea, abdominal pain, and sometimes by steatorrhea and protein-losing enteropathy.[2] Eosinophilic infiltration of the intestine may be extramucosal (in the muscularis externa or subserosa), or the infiltration may be found in more distal portions of the small bowel, where peroral biopsy is difficult. When the eosinophilic infiltration involves the mucosa of the proximal jejunum, it can be established by peroral biopsy. The mucosal lesion tends to be very patchy, and multiple biopsies may be necessary in order to detect the eosinophilic infiltration. Rubin recommends that a minimum of eight specimens be examined before concluding that there is no involvement of the proximal jejunum.[2] Note that eosinophilic leukocytes are normally present in the lamina propria, but in this disease eosinophils are abnormally numerous and may occur in clumps within the lamina propria, submucosa, and/or epithelium (Fig. 6-17). There may be massive infiltration by eosinophilic leukocytes and complete loss of villi.[2, 40]

The pathogenesis of eosinophilic gastroenteritis, often attributed to allergy, is unclear. Only about half of the cases occur in atopic patients, a group in whom food allergy is uncommon. Those patients with the allergic form of eosinophilic gastroenteritis have an atopic history or food sensitivity, and may have very high circulating levels of serum IgE. Fluorescent staining of biopsy specimens from these patients may show a marked increase in IgE-staining plasma cells.[2] This suggests that this form of eosinophilic gastroenteritis is associated with IgE-mediated reactions arising in the gut. This does not establish a role for food allergy, however. Some patients appear to respond to removal of certain foods from their diet, particularly milk and meat products, whereas many require long-term treatment with low doses of corticosteroids.[2] The gastric mucosa may be more consistently involved than the intestinal mucosa

and hence gastric mucosal biopsy may establish the diagnosis when intestinal mucosal biopsy specimens are equivocal or negative for eosinophilic infiltration.[41] Rarely, there may be esophageal involvement.[42]

PRIMARY INTESTINAL LYMPHOMA
(MEDITERRANEAN LYMPHOMA)

Primary intestinal lymphoma usually presents with malabsorption and abdominal pain in patients in their second or third decade.[1, 43] It is not generalized lymphoma, in which small intestine involvement may or may not be found. It is confined to the bowel and abdominal lymph nodes, and is more likely to be found in "undeveloped" areas of the world. It is often associated with an abnormal production of α-heavy chain. Hence, it is sometimes called *heavy-chain disease.*[44] The Mediterranean form of primary intestinal lymphoma may present initially as a diffuse and intense lymphoplasmacytic infiltration of the intestinal mucosa and hence is frequently termed *immunoproliferative small intes-*

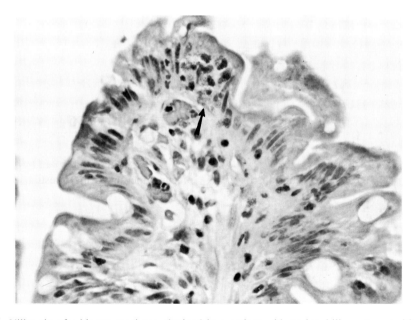

Fig. 6-17. Villus tip of a biopsy specimen obtained in a patient with eosinophilic gastroenteritis. There is marked eosinophilic infiltration in the lamina propria, and of the epithelium (arrow). (H&E, × 500.)

tinal disease (IPSID).[44] This proliferation may be secondary to intense bacterial antigenic stimulation and antibiotic treatment may inhibit evolution of an apparently benign disorder into a malignant stage.[44] The most constant histologic finding in IPSID is a dense infiltrate of the lamina propria by mature-appearing (polyclonal) plasma cells. If malignant lymphoma develops, the superficial lamina propria often retains its dense plasma cell infiltrate, whereas the cytologically malignant cell (often containing α heavy chain without light chain) is seen in the deeper portions of the mucosa, with invasion of the crypts and involvement of submucosa and muscularis. The malignant lymphoma seen in IPSID is variously designated as lymphoplasmacytoid, follicular, diffuse follicular-center-cell, or B-immunoblastic lymphoma. In the majority of these neoplasms, the malignant cells do *not* contain light or heavy chains. Lesser degrees of lymphoplasmacytic infiltration of the intestinal mucosa are common in individuals with tropical sprue from Southeast Asia, India, and Africa and should not be confused with IPSID.

If there is extensive disease with involvement of the proximal jejunum and/or duodenum, per-oral biopsy often makes the diagnosis (Fig. 6-18). The malignant lymphoid infiltrate is found throughout the lamina propria, crypts are sparse, and the villi may no longer be present. Patchy involvement of the proximal intestine by the lymphoma can be detected, but it often requires scanning of many biopsy specimens to find the few malignant cells that make the diagnosis. The changes may be indistinguishable from those seen in celiac sprue, with no malignant cells being found in some sections, while sparse malignant lymphoid cells are found in other sections.[43] Rubin notes that scattered malignant lymphoid cells were seen only in a few serial sections of eight biopsy specimens from the proximal jejunum of a patient with primary intestinal lymphoma.[1, 43] Pseudolymphoma (focal lymphoid hyperplasia) involving the small intestine alone is distinctively uncommon.[45] There are two reports of jejunal pseudolymphoma and approximately 20 reports of ileal pseudolymphoma.[45] The key histologic feature is a polymorphous cell population of infiltrating lymphocytes usually with a pronounced, reactive-appearing, follicular component throughout the lesion. Local resection, when required for obstructive symptoms, appears to be curative.

PARASITIC DISEASES

The four parasitic diseases that may cause proximal intestinal mucosal abnormalities in North Americans include giardiasis, coccidiosis, microsporidiosis and strongyloidiasis. Outside North America, schistosomiasis, leishmaniasis, and capillariasis must be considered. Infection with the flagellated protozoan *G. lamblia* is now recognized as a common cause of diarrhea in both adults and children. Many patients, particularly adults, with this infestation are asymptomatic, but others have watery diarrhea, frank steatorrhea, and chronic abdominal pain. The symptoms may easily be confused with those of irritable bowel syndrome. Giardial cysts may be found in the stool of these patients, and stool examination is the first diagnostic procedure that should be performed. However, if giardiasis is strongly suspected and cysts are not found in the stool, the diagnostic procedure is duodenal biopsy with examination of duodenal contents and mucus adherent to the biopsy for the presence of the protozoan by Giemsa stain of a dried smear. The parasite may be found in H&E-stained sections, but this may be difficult. The use of PAS-hematoxylin staining brings out the parasite very nicely (Fig. 6-19). Sometimes, the parasite can only be found in mucus adhering to the intestinal specimen, and it is advisable to prepare smears of intestinal juice when giardiasis is suspected.[20] The smears can then either be stained routinely with the Giemsa method or be stained at a later date if the parasite has not been found on the routine sections. Mucus and intestinal juice obtained at the time of biopsy should be spread thinly on a glass slide and air dried for at least 2 hours. The smears can then be fixed in absolute methanol for 20 minutes and stained for 20 min-

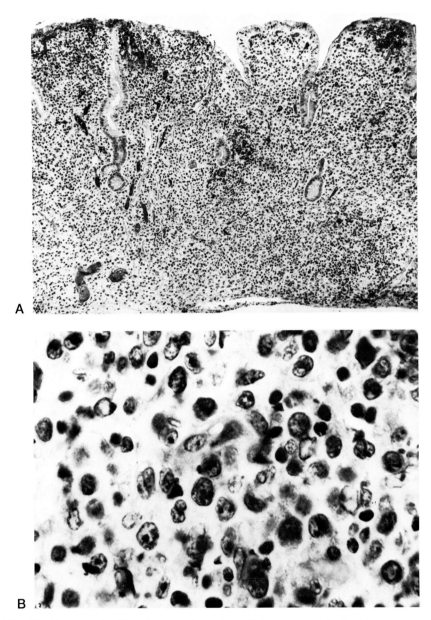

Fig. 6-18. **(A)** Absence of villi and destruction of crypts in primary intestinal lymphoma. Round cell infiltration replaces the lamina propria. **(B)** High-power magnification of the infiltrate reveals it to be made up of malignant lymphoid cells. (H&E, Fig. A × 184, Fig. B × 1,840.) (From Perea et al., [1] with permission.)

utes in dilute Giemsa solution. This technique should be performed in all patients in whom small intestine biopsy is being performed because of a suspected diagnosis of giardiasis.[20]

Villous architecture in patients with giardial infestation is usually normal. Sometimes patchy lesions of mild to moderate severity may be seen, and, exceedingly rarely, a severe mucosal lesion may be detected.[46, 47] The organism may rarely invade the intestinal mucosa, an observa-

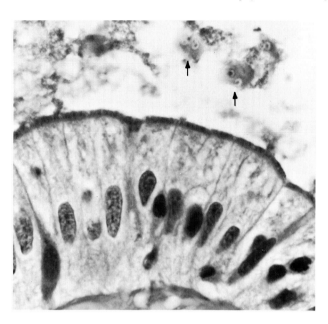

Fig. 6-19. High-power magnification view of a villous tip from the biopsy section illustrated in Figure 6-2 of a patient with giardiasis. The giardial organisms (arrows) appear to be free in the lumen and unattached to adjacent epithelial cells. (H&E, × 1250.)

tion first noted by Brandborg[2] and confirmed by other investigators.[2] Giardiasis is the most common cause of diarrhea and steatorrhea in patients with late-onset immunodeficiency (CVH).[19] It also accounts for most of the morphologic abnormalities of the intestinal mucosa in CVH. Giardiasis is not increased in frequency in patients with selective IgA deficiency.[19]

All patients with giardiasis should be treated with quinacrine hydrochloride (Atabrine), or with metronidazole if quinacrine fails to eradicate the infestation.

Within the subphylum Sporozoe and the subclass Coccidia, are two protozoan parasites (*Cryptosporidium* and *Isospora belli*) that may produce mucosal abnormalities of the small intestine.[48–50] Patients with coccidial infestations present as an obscure problem of unrelenting chronic malabsorption, or present with watery diarrhea. Intestinal biopsy is probably the best method for diagnosing this disease, even though it is sometimes difficult to find the causative organisms microscopically. *Cryptosporidium* is located intracellularly, just below the

plasma membrane, and appears to be intimately attached to the microvillous plasma membrane of intestinal epithelial cells when examined by electron microscopy.[3] Jejunal biopsies show mild to severe injury and attachment of numerous tiny 2- to 4-μm organisms on the epithelial surface (Fig. 6-20). Treatment is generally ineffective although the cryptosporidiosis cleared after discontinuation of an immunosuppressive agent in one individual.[2]

In contrast, *I belli,* another member of the Coccidia family, invades the intestinal epithelial cell and is found in an intracytoplasmic position. The villous architecture of intestinal biopsy varies from normal to severely abnormal, and the lesion is patchy. Various developmental forms of the coccidia may be seen within the epithelium or immediately beneath it (Fig. 6-21).[49] The various stages of schizogony are easiest to see, and a Colophonium-Giemsa stain may highlight the schizonts. Multiple sections must be examined by oil-immersion microscopy in order to detect these organisms. Diagnosis is important, because improvement may follow

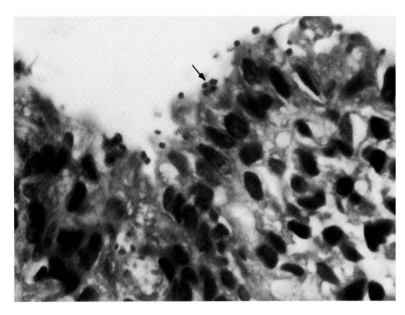

Fig. 6-20. High-power magnification view of attachment of cryptosporidial organisms (arrow) to the brush border of epithelial cells of a duodenojejunal biopsy of a patient with profuse watery diarrhea and cryptosporidiosis. Electron microscopy shows a junctional-like attachment of these organisms to the brush border. This same biopsy specimen showed a mild to moderately severe villous abnormality with a moderate increase in round cells in the lamina propria. (H&E, × 1,250.)

treatment with a combination of pyrimethamine and sulfadiazine, or treatment with cotrimoxazole.

Microsporidia have been shown to be an occasional cause of diarrhea and of malabsorption in patients with AIDS.[48] Microsporidia, like coccidia, are intracellular parasites that frequently infect invertebrates and have been reported to infect all classes of vertebrates, but until the advent of AIDS were an exceedingly rare cause of disease in man.[51] The organisms invade intestinal epithelial cells, are too small and too poorly stained to be seen easily at light microscopy, and must generally be identified at electron microscopy.[3, 48, 51] The spores are too small to be identified in feces.

Strongyloidiasis, resulting from infestation by the nematode *Strongyloides stercoralis,* most commonly causes mild gastrointestinal symptoms with little change in the villous architecture. The infestation may result in severe injury to the intestinal mucosa, with a flat lesion and complete loss of villi, thereby producing severe malabsorption. On occasion the illness can be quite serious. The diagnosis is made by confirming the presence of adult worms and larvae within intestinal crypts.[1, 52]

Schistosome ova may be seen in small bowel biopsy specimens of patients with shistosomiasis, although villous structure is not altered from that seen in normal individuals living in endemic areas of schistosomiasis.[53]

The nematode *Capillaria philippinensis* inhabits the intestinal lumen and can be seen adhering to the tissue in biopsy sections.[2] There are no changes in the villous architecture that are not seen in uninfected control subjects living in the Philippines.

Visceral leishmaniasis (kala azar) is generally characterized by fever, anemia, and splenomegaly. A minority of patients have diarrhea and even steatorrhea. Weight loss and hypoalbuminemia may be extreme. The causative agent is a genus of parasitic protozoa of the family

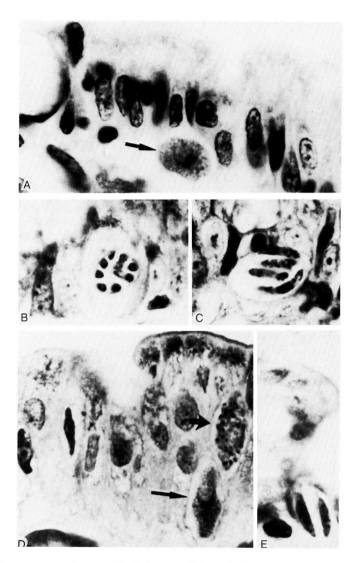

Fig. 6-21. Various stages of *Isospora belli* in a small bowel biopsy specimen. **(A)** Immature schizont below the villous epithelium (arrow). (H&E, × 1,500.) **(B&C)** Developing merozoites within schizonts. **(D)** Two merozoites on the left within the absorptive cell layer. The upper organism on the right is a macrogametocyte (thick arrow), whereas the one below is an immature schizont (thin arrow). **(E)** Two meroxoites within a schizont. (Colophonium Giemsa, Figs. B–E × 1,500.) (From Perea et al.,[1] with permission. Courtesy of Dr. Lloyld L. Brandborg, San Francisco.)

Trypanosomatidae that is found predominantly in macrophages of the skin and viscera. *Leishmania* parasites were found in 5 of 10 pretreatment duodenal biopsy specimens and in none of post-treatment specimens in a report from Kenya.[54] Parasites were found in macrophages mainly in villous tips, rarely in the submucosa, and were free in the lamina propria only on one occasion. The epithelium was normal and there was a mild to moderate lymphocytic infiltrate. Plasma cells were sparse. The mucosal lesion ranged from mild to moderate in degree and was patchy in distribution.

FUNGAL DISEASES

Gastrointestinal involvement occurs in up to 75 percent of patients with disseminated histoplasmosis, but is clinically obvious in only about 25 percent of patients.[55] The definitive diagnosis depends on culture of the organism from involved tissues, but presumptive diagnosis may be made by biopsy evidence of yeast in the diseased tissues. The fungus was reported to involve the small bowel and to cause malabsorption in one patient.[39] The lamina propria was greatly distended, with macrophages that contained encapsulated fungi. Treatment of that patient with amphotericin was successful, and the repeat intestinal biopsy showed reversion to normal appearance.

The most frequently encountered fungal infection in immunosuppressed patients (including AIDS patients) is due to *Candida* species. Mucosal lesions in the gastrointestinal tract generally involve the esophagus. Gastric and duodenal candidiasis are most unusual.[56] There is one report of an immunosuppressed patient with thickened duodenal and jejunal mucosal folds that led to the endoscopic diagnosis of duodenal candidiasis, based on the presence of multiple, small white patches in the entire duodenum. Biopsy specimens showed no alteration in villous structure other than for acute inflammatory changes in the lamina propria.[56] Direct smear of brushings from the duodenal plaques demonstrated yeast and pseudohyphae of *Candida* species. The patient responded to treatment with amphotericin B and with a return to a normal mucosal appearance.

There may rarely be involvement of the gastrointestinal tract in torulosis (cryptococcosis).

VIRAL DISEASES

Two viral diseases, cytomegalovirus (CMV) and herpes simplex virus, may produce characteristic and diagnostic alterations in the intestinal mucosa. Patients who are debilitated or immunosuppressed are susceptible to gastrointestinal involvement by CMV.[57] Its characteristic appearance is difficult to miss if it is sought, but may be easily overlooked if not sought. Cells invaded by CMV are enlarged, with a large oval intranuclear inclusion having a prominent surrounding halo.[57, 58] CMV infection occurs in up to 90 percent of patients who have had renal transplantation and who are maintained on immunosuppressive therapy.[58] Duodenal Brunner's glands seem to be the elective site for gut involvement. There is no correlation between the presence of CMV with symptoms or with morphologic changes. The CMV is probably not a pathogen in this setting. CMV does appear to be pathogenic in AIDS patients, in whom there may be diffuse gastroenterocolitis with extensive presence of CMV in the stomach, duodenum, and colon.[3]

Infection with Norwalk virus often results in clinical gastroenteritis and mildly abnormal intestinal histology characterized by mucosal inflammation, absorptive-cell abnormalities, shortening of villi, crypt hypertrophy, and increased numbers of epithelial-cell mitoses.[30, 59] The virus has not been detected within involved mucosal cells by electron microscopy, possibly because of the small size of the virus and its patchy distribution. The mucosal lesion disappears within 2 weeks.[30]

Duodenal biopsy specimens obtained from infants and young children with rotaviral diarrhea also reveal mucosal abnormalities similar to those described with Norwalk virus. Unlike Norwalk virus, rotaviral particles can be visualized by electron microscopy in the intestinal epithelial cells of biopsy specimens.[3]

MACROGLOBULINEMIA

Macroglobulinemia is considered to be a malignant neoplasm of the lymphoreticular system, similar to lymphoma and multiple myeloma. It is distinguished from multiple myeloma by its longer, more benign course, and by its lack of bone lesions, renal complications, and amyloidosis. Two cases have been reported in which involvement appeared to be limited to the small bowel and bone marrow.[1] The patients presented with malabsorption. There is also a report of a patient presenting with diarrhea who was found to have macroglobulinemia with intestinal involvement.[60] The diagnostic feature in intestinal biopsy specimens is the presence of hyaline, amorphous masses in an extracellular location within the lamina propria (Fig. 6-22). This same hyaline material is often found between the epithelial cells as well. The accumulation of this material may give the villi a clubbed shape. The hyaline material is moderately to intensely eosinophilic and is PAS positive. This material has been shown by specific immunofluorescent stains to be composed of a monoclonal IgM macroglobulin.[1] Lymphangiectasia secondary to macroglobulinemia with increased viscosity of lymph has been reported.[3]

LYMPHANGIECTASIA

Primary lymphangiectasia is a rare congenital obstructive defect of the lymphatics that was first described by Waldmann in 1961.[61] Waldmann reported a group of patients with "idiopathic hypoproteinemia" who had protein-losing enteropathy in whom he demonstrated the presence of marked lymphatic dilatation in intestinal biopsies. These patients also have steatorrhea. The lymphatic abnormality may be a generalized one, therefore the patients may also have chylothorax, chyluria, chylous ascites, or a lymphedematous limb, either singly or in combination. When there is intestinal involvement, numerous dilated lymphatics may be seen throughout the mucosa and submucosa. Some give the appearance of rupturing into the lumen. In the area of lymphangiectasia, overlying villi may be distorted, whereas in areas devoid of dilated lymphatics, the villous architecture is usually completely normal (Fig. 6-23). These patients may respond to a low-fat diet, particularly when supplemented with medium-chain triglycerides. Occasional patients have responded to surgical lymphovenous anastomoses.[1]

Secondary lymphangiectasia may be seen in a variety of diseases, including constrictive pericarditis, primary myocardial disease, Behcet's disease, intestinal lymphoma and carcinoma, retractile mesenteritis, and sarcoidosis.[62] Patients with constrictive pericarditis may mimic primary intestinal lymphangiectasia in every respect, and thus it is important to show presence of normal central venous pressure in all patients thought to have primary intestinal lymphangiectasia. Localized lymphangiectatic cysts of the small bowel may be found in random locations at postmortem examination. Most are submucosal and would be missed by suction biopsy.[1]

DRUG AND IRRADIATION INJURY (MACROCYTOSIS)

Severe vitamin B_{12} and folic acid deficiency, acute radiation reaction, and chemotherapeutic drugs used for treatment of malignancy all inhibit DNA synthesis, with resulting impairment of epithelial cell replacement.[2, 3, 63–66] Crypt mitotic activity is reduced, epithelial cells are enlarged, and villous abnormalities vary from mild changes to complete loss of villi. Macrocytosis may be readily apparent or may be quite inapparent. When present, it is often irregularly distributed from villus to villus or crypt to crypt.

Even when a severe lesion is present, it is generally easy to differentiate it from a lesion of celiac sprue because of the presence of macrocytosis, decreased number of mitoses, and a less-dense cellular content of the lamina propria. In celiac sprue, macrocytosis is not seen, mitoses are increased in number, and there is a dense cellular infiltrate in the lamina propria. Following treatment with folic acid or vitamin B_{12}, or following cessation of drug therapy, the changes in the intestinal mucosa revert to normal. Radiation-induced changes also revert to normal, unless the radiation has been excessive.[2, 65]

A variety of drugs have been implicated in production of intestinal malabsorption.[63] Administration of these drugs may result in malabsorption of specific substances such as vitamin B_{12} or folic acid by inhibiting their specific transport mechanisms in the intestine. These drugs do not ordinarily result in light-microscopic evidence of morphologic injury to the intestinal mucosa, but injury may be identifiable by elec-

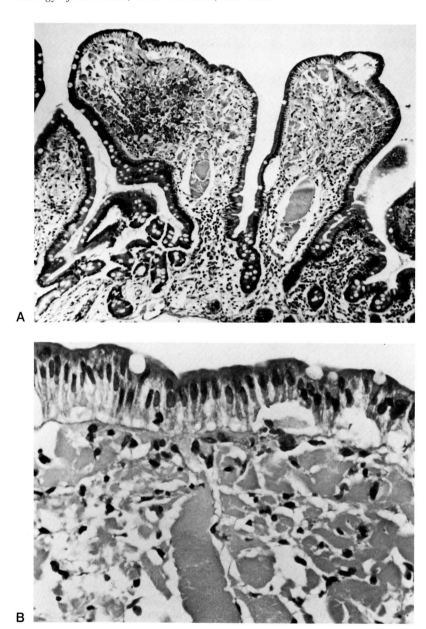

Fig. 6-22. (**A**) Intestinal biopsy specimen of a patient with macroglobulinemia showing the lamina propria to be filled with amorphous hyalin emasses. (**B**) Higher-power magnification of the biopsy specimen showing the amorphous extracellular masses of macroglobulin. (H&E, Fig. A × 150, Fig. B × 540.)

tron microscopy. The most severe gut injury reported has been that produced by MER-29 (triparanol), a drug once used in the treatment of hypercholesterolemia. This drug resulted in ectodermal changes, including cataracts, icthyo-sis, and alopecia. An intestinal lesion, indistinguishable from that of severe celiac sprue, with resulting malabsorption, was found in two subjects. The intestinal lesion was reversed by withdrawing the drug while the patients were main-

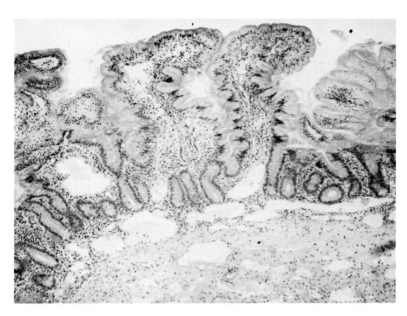

Fig. 6-23. Proximal jejunal biopsy specimen from a patient with congenital lymphangiectasia manifested by protein-losing enteropathy and chylous ascites. Dilated lacteals distort villous structure and can be seen throughout the submucosa. In other uninvolved areas of the biopsy specimen, the villi were normal. (H&E, × 132.)

tained on a normal diet. A lesion of similar severity, reversible on withdrawal of the drug, has been induced by the NSAID sulindac (Clinoril).[64] Sulindac also may induce marrow aplasia, Stevens-Johnson toxic epidermal necrolysis syndrome, pneumonitis, pancreatitis, hepatitis, and life-threatening hypersensitivity.

Antimetabolites, colchicine, and antibiotics, especially neomycin, have produced morphologic injury to the intestinal mucosa easily identifiable at light microscopy. Neomycin's effect on the intestine has been thoroughly studied.[3] Light-microscopic changes induced by neomycin include shortening of villi and infiltration of the lamina propria with inflammatory cells and pigment-containing macrophages.

ISCHEMIA (AND HYALINOSIS)

Ischemic injury to the duodenum, though unusual, may be detected in biopsy specimens of individuals with vasculitis or following hypotensive episodes.[67] Features of acute damage include desquamation of the upper third of villi or retention of irregular cubic epithelium over shortened villi, and flattening of crypt cells. When injury is severe, there may be denudation of villi and hemorrhage into the lamina propria.[67] Atheromatous emboli may be found in small vessels of the lamina propria. Mucosal injury in patients with severe vasculitis is presumably due to vasculitis (Fig. 6-24A&B). Acute duodenitis with mucosal ulcerations was reported to be secondary to submucosal vasculitis (with deposits of IgA and C3) of Henoch-Schönlein purpura.[68]

Hyalinosis is a new familial syndrome found to affect three of seven siblings in which ischemic injury may have accounted for the intestinal manifestations.[69] Pathologically there was marked and progressive hyalinosis (thickened hyalin walls like those seen in diabetic patients) of capillaries, and often of arterioles and small veins of the gut, kidneys, and calcified areas of the brain. Diarrhea, malabsorption, rectal bleeding, and protein-losing enteropathy were lethal in the proband. Electron microscopy

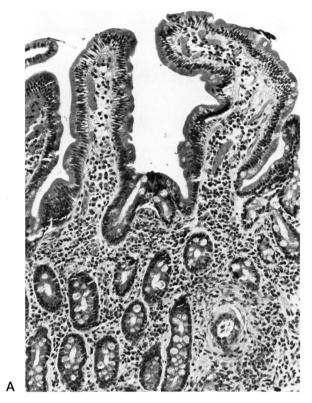

Fig. 6-24. (A) Intestinal biopsy specimen of 31-year-old woman with severe lupus erythematosus, diarrhea, and malabsorption. There is fairly normal villous architecture and focal crypt injury. *(Figure continues.)*

showed that the hyaline substance about the capillaries consisted of concentric layers of basal lamina-like deposits within a fine granular fluffy material.

POLYPOSIS SYNDROMES

Although there may be focal involvement of the duodenum in the various polyposis syndromes, only in the Cronkhite-Canada syndrome is there a diffuse mucosal lesion.[70] This is a nonfamilial syndrome of diffuse gastrointestinal (inflammatory) polyposis associated with cutaneous hyperpigmentation, alopecia, and nail dystrophy. The mucosa of the entire gastrointestinal tract may be flattened and replaced by distorted and often cystic glands separated by a loose stroma (Fig. 6-24C). Paneth and endocrine

cells may be greatly diminished.[70] These changes may result from loss of normal proliferation in the crypts and are potentially reversible.

DISEASES ASSOCIATED WITH NORMAL VILLI—DIAGNOSTIC

Table 6-6 lists the diseases in which normal villi are present but in which there is a diagnostic histologic change.

A-β-LIPOPROTEINEMIA

A-β-lipoproteinemia was first described by Bassen and Kornzweig in 1950, and is characterized by steatorrhea, retinitis pigmentosa, spine-shaped red cells in the peripheral blood (acantho-

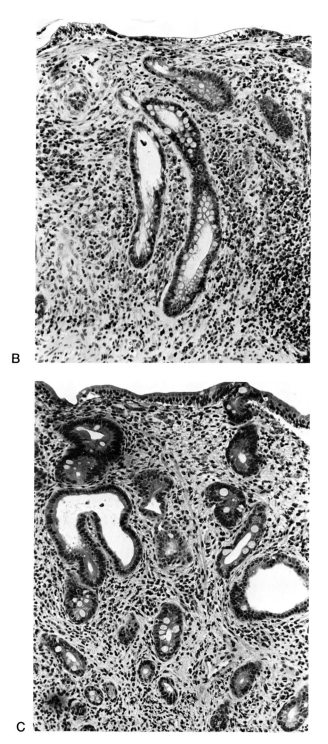

B

C

Fig. 6-24. (*Continued*). **(B)** Intestinal biopsy specimen obtained 2 weeks later while the patient was acutely ill. There is a severe lesion, the surface epithelium is flattened and vacuolated, and there is extensive dropout of crypts. The patient had a dramatic clinical response following high dose corticosteroid treatment. **(C)** Intestinal biopsy specimen of a 83-year-old woman with Cronkhite-Canada syndrome manifested by diarrhea, malabsorption, alopecia, and nail dystrophy. Multiple biopsy specimens showed a flat mucosa with cystic dilatation of many glands and a mild inflammatory infiltrate in the lamina propria. (H&E, × 200.)

Table 6-6. Normal Villi—Diagnostic

Disease	Diagnostic Histology
A-β-lipoproteinemia	Fasting absorptive cells loaded with fat
Crohn's disease	Noncaseating granulomas
X-linked immunodeficiency	Virtually absent lamina propria plasma cells
Lipid storage diseases	Vacuolated ganglion cells, capillaries, and macrophages
Amyloidosis	Congo red-positive material in capillaries/lamina propria
Chronic granulomatous disease	Pigmented, vacuolated macrophages in lamina propria
Melanosis intestini	Densely pigmented macrophages in lamina propria
Mastocytosis	Mast cell infiltrate

cytosis), and neurologic changes similar to those seen in Friedreich's ataxia.[2] These patients are unable to synthesize apoprotein B, which is required for the synthesis and transport of very low-density lipoproteins (β-lipoproteins) and chylomicrons. There is normal uptake of fatty acids by absorptive cells, but they cannot be synthesized into chylomicrons. Absorptive cells thus are stuffed with large intracytoplasmic fat particles that are unable to exit into the lamina propria to reach lacteals. Failure to absorb essential fatty acids may explain the defective lipid membrane of the red cell, accounting for their acanthocytic or thorny appearance. The progressive neurologic disease may also be related to a deficiency of essential fatty acids.

Intestinal biopsies obtained from these patients show normal villous architecture, but the intestinal absorptive cells are found to be packed with large droplets of triglyceride (Fig. 6-25).[1 2] The diagnostic feature in biopsy specimens processed for routine histologic examination is the extremely vacuolated cytoplasm of the absorptive cells covering the upper third of villi (Fig. 6-25A). These vacuoles can be shown to contain fat in frozen sections stained with oil red O. Light-microscopic sections of osmium-fixed epoxy-embedded specimens stained with toluidine blue show the presence also of the striking accumulation of lipid in varying-sized droplets

in intestinal absorptive cells (Fig. 6-25C). The intestinal lamina propria appears to be normal except for the presence of an unusual number of macrophages containing bizarre inclusions.[2]

CROHN'S DISEASE

The distal ileum and/or colon are the usual sites of involvement in Crohn's disease. The proximal intestine and duodenum may rarely be involved, and the diagnosis can be established by small bowel biopsy.[71, 72] The proximal involvement may not be detected by radiographic examination or by endoscopy, but noncaseating epithelioid granulomas with giant cells may be found on biopsy (Fig. 6-26). The presence of such epitheloid granulomas is very supportive of the diagnosis of Crohn's disease, especially if the clinical and radiologic findings are appropriate. The presence of granulomas is not specific for Crohn's disease because they may be found rarely in other conditions, such as sarcoidosis.[73] Rubin has observed a solitary granuloma in a biopsy specimen from a patient with unclassified sprue and from one patient with celiac sprue and dermatitis herpetiformis. Numerous epithelioid and giant cell granulomas were observed in jejunal biopsy specimens of a patient with malabsorption and a moderate intestinal lesion. Because the patient had a complete clinical and histologic remission on a gluten-free diet, the granulomatous lesion was considered to be a manifestation of celiac sprue.[74] Five patients were reported who had simultaneously celiac sprue and sarcoidosis, with the gastro-intestinal lesion of celiac sprue and pulmonary manifestations of sarcoidosis.[75]

Schuffler and Chaffee have shown that a spectrum of abnormalities ranging from mild to severe may be found, in the absence of granulomas, by peroral mucosal biopsy in patients with Crohn's disease involving the duodenum. The abnormalities are patchy, and include flattened mucosa and abnormal surface epithelium that is infiltrated by large numbers of PMN leukocytes, increased plasma cells and PMN leuko-

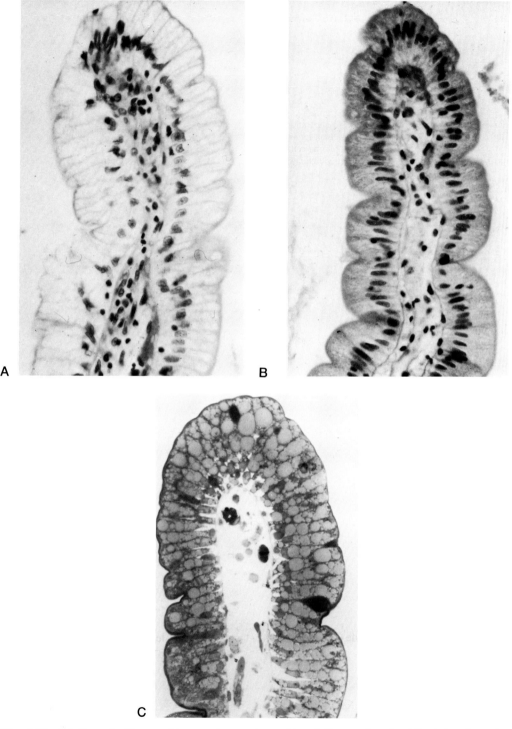

Fig. 6-25. **(A)** Normal villous architecture in a patient with a-β-lipoproteinemia. All of the absorptive cells covering the upper third of the villus are severely vacuolated, an appearance resulting from extraction of the excess lipid from these cells during processing. **(B)** Appearance of a villus from a normal individual for comparison with that seen in Fig. A. (H&E, Figs. A & B × 500) **(C)** Thick section of osmium-fixed plastic-embedded specimen showing striking accumulation of lipid droplets in epithelial cells. (Toluidine blue, × 750.)

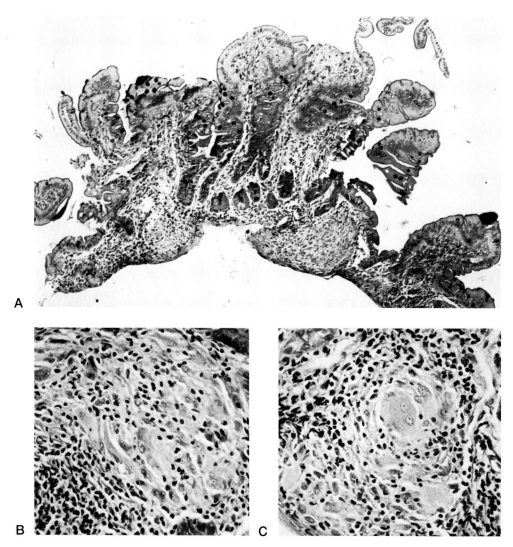

Fig. 6-26. **(A)** Endoscopically obtained duodenal biopsy specimen illustrating normal villous architecture in a patient with Crohn's disease involving the terminal ileum, but without apparent disease of the upper intestine. The presence of granulomas below the crypts may be seen. **(B&C)** High-power magnification showing that the granulomas consist of multiple epitheloid cells surrounded by a thin rim of round cells. (H&E, Fig. A × 132, Fig. B × 270.)

cytes in the lamina propria, crypt abscesses, erosions, and pyloric gland metaplasia.[72]

LIPID STORAGE DISEASES

Lipid storage diseases may be suspected when the ganglion cells of Meissner's plexus are vacuolated. Vacuolated ganglion cells have been reported in Fabry's disease,[2] and Rubin has observed them in Niemann-Pick disease.[1] Electron microscopic, histochemical, and biochemical studies of biopsy specimens may help make the diagnosis in lipid storage diseases.[2] In cholesterol ester storage disease, the lamina propria may be greatly distended by numerous foamy-appearing macrophages, all filled with cholesterol esters and carotenes.[2] In Tangier disease,

numerous foamy macrophages filled with cholesterol esters are found at the muscularis mucosae and in the submucosa.[2] In contrast to cholesterol ester storage disease, the small intestine
mucosa in Tangier disease does not contain
foamy macrophages. The myenteric plexus also
shows vacuolization owing to cholesterol ester
deposits.[2]

AMYLOIDOSIS

Rectal biopsy is preferable for the diagnosis
of systemic amyloidosis because it is easy to
perform and is generally safe.[1] Both primary
and secondary amyloidosis may involve the
small intestine. Amyloid is demonstrated using
special stains, or by electron microscopy.[1] The
use of Congo red staining and demonstration
of dichroism by polarized light microscopy is
favored. Small bowel biopsy may provide the
diagnosis when rectal biopsy examination is
negative and amyloidosis is still suspected
clinically.[76] Serious consideration should be
given to obtaining small bowel biopsies with
this diagnosis in mind in patients with obscure
causes of malabsorption, and in whom rectal
biopsy is negative for the presence of amyloid.[76]

MELANOSIS

Melanosis of the gastrointestinal tract consists
of a black pigmentation in the mucosa that commonly occurs only in the colon and generally
stops abruptly at the ileocecal valve. Extracolonic melanosis is a rare finding, although it
has been noted in the ileum as an isolated manifestation. Several cases of duodenal melanosis
are documented.[77] The villous architecture in
duodenal biopsies was normal but the lamina
propria was filled with macrophages containing
an intense brown-black pigment. The pigment
was similar to that observed in melanosis coli
and histochemically did not stain like melanin
or lipofuscin.[77] The pigment is largely composed of iron and sulfur.

MASTOCYTOSIS

There may be a mucosal or submucosal infiltrate of mast cells in the intestine of individuals
with systemic mast cell disease, but the villous
architecture remains normal. Several patients
with systemic mast cell disease have also had
celiac sprue (i.e., they had a severe intestinal
mucosal lesion that responded to a gluten-free
diet). The severe mucosal lesion in this setting
has been both free of mast cell infiltration, or
infiltrated with up to 30 mast cells per high-
power field on toluidine blue staining. Mast
cells, like eosinophils, are easily found when
looked for in the intestinal mucosa and thus
their presence must be quantitated before drawing conclusions about their significance.[78]

NORMAL PROXIMAL JEJUNAL BIOPSY

There are conflicting reports that a variety
of other disease may result in abnormalities of
the proximal jejunum. Most investigators have
been unable to confirm that these diseases indeed
result in abnormalities, and it is likely that many
of the reported abnormalities are related to artifacts. Table 6-7 lists the disease entities that
reportedly result in abnormalities of the jejunum, a finding not confirmed by Rubin and
the many individuals who have worked with
him in his laboratory.[1]

Table 6-7. Normal Proximal Jejunal Biopsy

Dermatoses other than dermatitis herpetiformis
Pancreatitis
Alcoholism
Cirrhosis
Hepatitis
Iron deficiency anemia
Ulcerative colitis
Postgastrectomy without bacterial overgrowth
Malignant disease outside the small intestine
Cholera[a]
Hookworm disease[a]

[a] Normal by local geographic standards (i.e., same as
in uninfected controls in the same environment).
(From Perea et al.,[1] with permission.)

ENDOSCOPIC BIOPSY OF THE DUODENAL BULB

With the ready availability of fiberoptic duodenoscopes, it is difficult for the endoscopist to refrain from obtaining numerous tiny mucosal biopsy specimens of any abnormality that he might perceive in the duodenum. Biopsy specimens obtained with both the "jumbo" and standard forceps are interpretable.[4]

It is important for the endoscopist to communicate clearly to the pathologist just why the biopsy specimen was taken. Generally biopsy specimens are taken from the duodenal bulb to determine whether nonulcerative changes represent significant mucosal disease. If the endoscopist uses appropriate terms such as *erythema, swelling,* and *deformity* and avoids pathologic terms such as *inflammation, edema,* and *scar,* the pathologist is more likely to be of help in interpreting the specimens. Quite frequently, the biopsy specimens are clearly normal even though there was an "apparent" abnormality seen by the endoscopist. Often, histologic abnormalities will be found in biopsy specimens obtained from apparently normal duodenal bulbs. Whether these histologic abnormalities can account for the patient's symptoms has not yet been determined. Hopefully, prospective studies of duodenal bulb biopsy specimens and their comparison with endoscopic finding will clarify many of the unknowns of interpretation of duodenal bulb biopsy specimens.[4, 73, 79–82] A helpful discussion of the problem of duodenitis and its histologic grading, from the pathologist's viewpoint, may be found in the text by Whitehead[81] and from the gastroenterologist's viewpoint in the paper by Weinstein.[82]

NORMAL HISTOLOGY OF THE DUODENAL BULB

The histology of proximal duodenal biopsies generally reflects the appearance of distal duodenal biopsies.[4, 83] Slight to moderate increases in lamina propria cell content and slight to moderate shortening of villi in proximal duodenal biopsies are usually not confused with specific pathologic states. Mucosa overlying Brunner's glands may occasionally be flattened, while biopsy specimens from the ligament of Treitz are normal. Villi in the proximal duodenum tend to vary somewhat more in their height than do villi in the distal duodenum, and the cellular content of the lamina propria tends to be slightly greater in the proximal duodenum. Histologic findings in the proximal duodenum that are of questionable significance include the presence of hemorrhage, gastric surface epithelium, heteroptic fundic gland mucosa, and mild inflammatory changes. Hemorrhage is commonly observed in endoscopic biopsy specimens, and one can never be sure that it is not due to trauma of obtaining the biopsy. Villi in the proximal duodenum are often lined with cells similar to surface mucus cells of the stomach, and this finding appears to be more frequent in individuals with high gastric acid output than in those with lose acid output. Nevertheless, it may be observed in specimens that are otherwise normal, and little significance can be attached to its finding (Fig. 6-27). On one occasion, I was able to correctly suggest the diagnosis of Zollinger-Ellison syndrome when I observed extensive surface mucus cell metaplasia of the intestinal epithelium in a jejunal biopsy specimen of a patient with chronic diarrhea. Heterotopic fundic gland mucosa in the duodenum has been observed for many years, and has no diagnostic significance.[1, 79] The presence of mild increases in the round cell content of the lamina propria, and of occasional PMN leukocytes in the lamina propria of the proximal duodenum are of doubtful significance. Only if other pathologic changes are present can any significance be placed on this observation.

The term *nonspecific duodenitis* should apply to changes seen in the mucosa obtained adjacent to duodenal ulcers, as well as to the changes seen in celiac sprue and Crohn's disease. In full-blown nonspecific duodenitis not attributable to specific inflammatory diseases such as celiac sprue, the villi are blunted and the surface epithelium has an abnormal appearance.[1, 82] The changes in the surface epithelium are often simi-

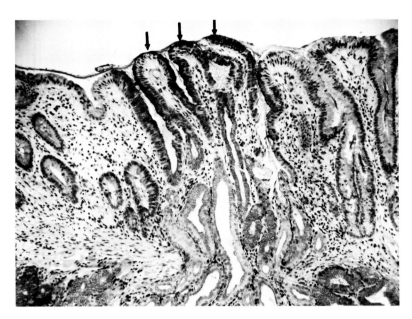

Fig. 6-27. Biopsy specimen obtained from duodenal bulb showing characteristic appearance of gastric surface mucous cell metaplasia in which three of the villi in the middle are covered by gastric-type epithelium (arrows) rather than by an absorptive type epithelium. A portion of the villus to the right and a portion of the villus to the left of the three central villi is also lined in part by gastric surface mucus cells, with a sharp demarcation between the gastric type and absorptive type epithelium. There is also the presence of a Brunner gland artifact. (PAS-hematoxylin, × 150.)

lar to those seen in reactive atypia. The surface epithelium in acute duodenitis resembles the surface epithelium seen in gastritis rather than the epithelial changes seen in celiac sprue.[82] The lamina propria contains a marked increase in the number of round cells and PMN leukocytes. PMN leukocytes tend to invade the surface epithelium, and mitotic figures are increased within the crypt epithelium. The histologic spectrum ranges from mild changes that affect the surface epithelium only to severe changes that on occasion may be difficult to distinguish from celiac sprue. The pathologic significance of so-called nonspecific duodenitis has not been adequately defined and requires long-term prospective clinicopathologic studies to determine their significance, if any.[82] Thus, there is usually no need to biopsy duodenal erosions unless a specific cause (such as Crohn's disease, celiac sprue, or Whipple's disease) is suspected.

ILEAL BIOPSY

With the ability to enter the ileum almost routinely during colonoscopy, the endoscopist faces the same temptations in the ileum as he does in the proximal duodenum and tends to obtain biopsy specimens from all "abnormalities," whether apparent or real. Many of the precautions in interpreting proximal duodenal biopsy specimens also apply to interpretation of ileal biopsy specimens.[84] The normal structure of the distal ileum is similar to that of the rest of the intestine, with a villus: crypt ratio of 3:1 to 4:1. Both villi and crypts are shorter than they are in the jejunum. There are more goblet cells and increased cellularity of the lamina propria when compared to the jejunum. Lymphoid follicles (Peyer's patches) may be prominent in the ileum and may distort the overlying mucosa, just as lymphoid follicles distort the duodenal mucosa.

Our knowledge of pathology of the ileum is necessarily less extensive than our knowledge of duodenojejunal pathology. Villus shortening with inflammation in the lamina propria alone, especially when chronic, is nonspecific and must be interpreted with great caution. This finding is frequently observed and often overinterpreted. In celiac sprue, the ileal mucosa ranges from normal in appearance to that of a severe lesion similar to that of the jejunum.[1] When there is acute ischemic injury to the ileum, the lesion seen is a characteristic bland hemorrhagic necrosis with minimal inflammation. A flat ileal lesion was noted in a patient with chronic ischemic injury.[85] The patient had Raynaud's phenomenon, purpura, eosinophilia, chronic diarrhea, and steatorrhea with bile acid malabsorption. The proximal intestine was normal, whereas ileal biopsy showed a flat mucosa with tufts of thrombosed convoluted capillaries.[85] Histologic features that support the diagnosis of Crohn's ileitis include a minimum of spotty necrosis and injury of surface epithelium and a

PMN leucocyte infiltrate (Fig. 6-28). The presence of shortened villi, crypt abscesses, and frank ulcerations provide further evidence for the diagnosis. Granulomas along with the other inflammatory changes described are strongly suggestive of Crohn's disease, but granulomas in the ileum in the absence of other inflammatory changes may be nonspecific. "Backwash" ileitis seen in ulcerative colitis may mimic Crohn's ileitis.

An ileal pouch-anal anastamosis (IPAA) is constructed following subtotal colectomy and mucosal proctectomy, and utilized in the treatment of ulcerative colitis and of familial polyposis coli.[86] A syndrome called "pouchitis" develop in up to 20 percent of patients having this procedure for treatment of ulcerative colitis, but very rarely follows this procedure in patients with polyposis. Pouchitis is characterized by high stool frequency, watery stools, cramps, fat malabsorption, and occasionally by nocturnal leakage, incontinence, and rectal bleeding.[86] There is a poor correlation between the endo-

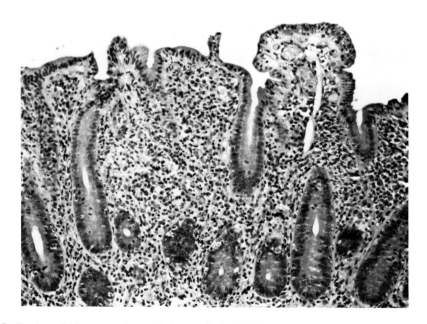

Fig. 6-28. Section of biopsy specimen of ileum obtained during colonoscopy in a patient with Crohn's disease. There is a moderate to severe lesion and the lamina propria is infiltrated with lymphocytes, plasma cells, and PMN leukocytes. PMN leukocyte infiltrate of the crypt epithelium may be noted. (H&E, × 200.)

scopic appearance and biopsy findings. Biopsy specimens may show changes similar to those seen in the colon and include mild to moderate villous abnormalities and PMN leukocyte infiltrate of the mucosa, including crypt abscesses. The rapid clinical response to treatment with metronidazole suggests that anaerobic bacterial toxins and bile salt deconjugation play a role in the pathogenesis of the pouchitis.

ACKNOWLEDGMENTS

Supported in part by Merit Review Funding from the Veterans Administration of the United States.

REFERENCES

1. Perea DR, Weinstein WM, Rubin CE: Small intestinal biopsy. Hum Pathol 6:157, 1975
2. Dobbins WO III: Small bowel biopsy in malabsorptive states. p. 121. In Norris HT (ed): Pathology of the Colon, Small Intestine, and Anus. Churchill Livingstone, New York, 1983
3. Dobbins WO III: Diagnostic Pathology of the Intestinal Mucosa. An Atlas and Review of Biopsy Interpretation. Springer-Verlag, New York, 1990
4. Dandalides SM, Carey WD, Petras R, Achkar E: Endoscopic small bowel biopsy: A controlled trial evaluating forceps size and biopsy location in the diagnosis of normal and abnormal mucosal architecture. Gastrointest Endosc 35:197, 1989
5. Austin LL, Dobbins WO III: Intraepithelial leukocytes of the intestinal mucosa in normal man and in Whipple's disease: a light and electron microscopic study. Digest Dis Sci 27:311, 1982
6. Rubin CE, Brandborg LL, Phelps PC, et al: Studies of celiac disease. Pt. I: The apparent identical and specific nature of the duodenal and proximal jejunal lesion in celiac disease and idiopathic sprue. Gastroenterology 38:28, 1960
7. Sollid L, Markussen G, Ek J, et al.: Evidence for a primary association of celiac disease to a particular HLA-DQ alpha/beta heterodimer. J Exp Med 169:345, 1989
8. Targan SR, Kagnoff MF, Brogan MD, Shanahan F: Immunologic mechanisms in intestinal disease. Ann Intern Med 106:853, 1987
9. Brow J, Parker F, Weinstein W, et al: The small intestinal mucosa in dermatitis herpetiformis. Pt. I: Severity and distribution of the small intestinal lesion and associated malabsorption. Gastroenterology 60:355, 1971
10. Baker AL, Rosenberg IH: Refractory sprue: recovery after removal of nongluten dietary proteins. Ann Intern Med 89:505, 1978
11. Walker-Smith JA, Unsworth DJ, Hutchins P, et al.: Autoantibodies against gut epithelium in a child with small-intestinal enteropathy. Lancet 1:566, 1982
12. Bernstein EF, Whitington PF: Successful treatment of atypical sprue in an infant with cyclosporine. Gastroenterology 95:199, 1988
13. Katz SI, Hall RP III, Lawley TJ, et al: Dermatitis herpetiformis: the skin and the gut. Ann Intern Med 93:857, 1980
14. Ament M, Rubin CE: Soy protein—another cause of the flat intestinal lesion. Gastroenterology 62:227, 1972
15. Trier JS, Falchuk ZM, Carney MC, et al: Celiac sprue and refractory sprue. Gastroenterology 75:307, 1978
16. Baer AN, Bayless TM, Yardley JH: Intestinal ulceration and malabsorption syndromes. Gastroenterology 79:754, 1980
17. Weinstein W, Saunders D, Tytgat G, et al: Collagenous sprue—an unrecognized type of malabsorption. N Engl J Med 283:1297, 1970
18. Bossart R, Henry K, Booth CC, et al: Subepithelial collagen in intestinal malabsorption. Gut 16:18, 1975
19. Dobbins WO III: Gut immunophysiology: a gastroenterologist's view with emphasis on pathophysiology. Am J Physiol 242:G1, 1982
20. Ament M, Rubin CE: Relation of giardiasis to abnormal intestinal structure and function in gastrointestinal immunodeficiency syndromes. Gastroenterology 62:216, 1972
21. Matuchansky C, Touchard G, Lemaire M, et al.: Malignant lymphoma of the small bowel associated with diffuse nodular lymphoid hyperplasia. N Engl J Med 313:166–171, 1985
22. McCarthy DM, Katz SI, Gazze L, et al.: Selective IgA deficiency associated with total villous atrophy of the small intestine and an organ-specific antiepithelial cell antibody. J Immunol 120:932, 1978
23. Ochs HD, Ament ME, Davis SD: Structure and function of the gastrointestinal tract in primary

immunodeficiency syndromes (IDS) and in gran-
ulocyte dysfunction. Birth Defects 11:199, 1975

24. Keren DF: Immunology and Immunopathology
of the Gastrointestinal Tract. p. 45. American
Society of Clinical Pathologists, Educational
Products Division, Chicago, 1980

25. Ament M, Ochs H, Davis S: Structure and function of the gastrointestinal tract in primary immunodeficiency syndromes: a study of 39 patients.
Medicine 52:227, 1973

26. Brunser O, Eidelman S, Klipstein FA: Intestinal
morphology of rural Haitians: a comparison between overt tropical sprue and asymptomatic subjects. Gastroenterology 58:655, 1970

27. Brunser O, Reid A, Monkeberg F, et al: Jejunal
biopsies in infant malnutrition: with special reference to mitotic index. Pediatrics 38:605, 1966

28. Cutz E, Rhodes JM, Drumm B, et al: Microvillus
inclusion disease: an inherited defect of brush-
border assembly and differentiation. N Engl J
Med 320:646, 1989

29. Drucker MM, Polliade A, Yeivin R, et al: Immunofluorescent demonstration of enteropathic *E.
coli* in tissues of infants dying with enteritis.
Pediatrics 46:855, 1970

30. Schreiber D, Blacklow N, Trier J: The intestinal
lesion in acute infectious nonbacterial gastroenteritis. N Engl J Med 288:1318, 1973

31. Ament M, Shimoda S, Saunders D, et al: Pathogenesis of steatorrhea in three cases of small
intestinal stasis syndrome, Gastroenterology
63:728, 1972

32. Fang M, Ginsberg AL, Glassman L, et al: Clinical conference: Zollinger-Ellison Syndrome with
diarrhea as the predominant clinical feature. Gastroenterology 76:378, 1979

33. Shimoda S, Saunders D, Rubin CE: The Zollinger-Ellison syndrome with steatorrhea. Pt. II.
The mechanism of fat and vitamin B_{12} malabsorption. Gastroenterology 55:705, 1968

34. McDonald GB, Shulman HM, Sullivan KM,
Spencer GD: Intestinal and hepatic complications
of human bone marrow trnsplantation. Gastroenterology 90:460, 770, 1986

35. Kotler DP, Gaetz HP, Lange M, et al: Enteropathy associated with AIDS. Ann Intern Med
101:421, 1984

36. Dobbins WO III: Whipple's Disease. Charles
C Thomas, Springfield, IL, 1987

37. Trier JS, Phelps PC, Eidelman E, et al: Whipple's disease: light and electron microscopic correlation of jejunal mucosal histology with antibi-

otic treatment and clinical status.
Gastroenterology 48:684, 1965

38. Dobbins WO III: Is there an immune deficit in
Whipple's disease? Dig Dis Sci 26:247, 1981

39. Bank S, Trey C, Gaus I, et al: Histoplasmosis
of the small bowel with "giant" intestinal villi
and secondary protein-losing enteropathy. Am
J Med 39:492, 1965

40. Keshavarzian A, Saverymuttu TP-C, Thompson
M, et al: Activated eosinophils in familial eosinophilic gastroenteritis. Gastroenterology 88:1041,
1985

41. Katz AJ, Goldman H, Grand RJ: Gastric mucosal
biopsy in eosinophilic (allergic) gastroenteritis.
Gastroenterology 73:705, 1977

42. Dobbins JW, Sheahan DG, Behar J: Eosinophiic
gastroenteritis with esophageal involvement.
Gastroenterology 72:1312, 1977

43. Eidelman S, Parkins RA, Rubin CE: Abdominal
lymphoma presenting as malabsorption: a clinicopathologic sutdy of nine cases in Israel, and
a review of the literature. Medicine 45:111, 1966

44. Matuchansky C, Touchard G, Babin P, et al:
Diffuse small intestinal lymphoid infiltration in
nonimmunodeficient adults from Western Europe. Gastroenterology 95:470, 1988

45. Gudjonsson H, Jones M, Krawitt EL, Kaye MD:
Pseudolymphoma of the jejunum. Digest Dis
Sci 32:1314, 1987

46. Levinson JD, Nastro LJ: Giardiasis with total
villous atrophy. Gastroenterology 74:271, 1978

47. Hartong WA, Gourlay WK, Aravantakis C: Giardiasis: clinical spectrum and functional-structural
abnormalities of the small intestinal mucosa.
Gastroenterology 77:61, 1979

48. Dobbins WO III, Weinstein WM: Electron microscopy of the intestine and rectum in AIDS.
Gastroenterology 88:738, 1985

49. Liebman WM, Thaler MM, DeLorimier A, et
al: Intractable diarrhea of infancy due to intestinal
coccidiosis. Gastroenterology 78:579, 1980

50. Current WL, Reese NC, Ernst JV, et al: Human
cryptosporidiosis in immunocompetent and immunodeficient persons. Studies of an outbrake
and experimental transmission. N Engl J Med
308:1252, 1983

51. Rijpstra AC, Canning EU, vanKetel RJ, et al:
Use of light microscopy to diagnose small-intes-
tinal microsporidiosis in patients with AIDS. J
Infect Dis 157:827, 1988

52. Weller PF: Case records of the Massachusetts

General Hospital Intestinal *Strongyloides stercoralis* infestation. N Engl J Med 314:903, 1986

53. Witham RR, Mosser RS: An unusual presentation of schistosomiasis duodenitis. Gastroenterology 77:1316, 1979
54. Muigai R, Shaunak S, Gatei DG, et al: Jejunal function and pathology in visceral leishmaniasis. Lancet 2:476, 1983
55. Miller DP, Everett ED: Gastrointestinal histoplasmosis. J Clin Gastroenterol 1:233, 1979
56. Joshi SN, Garvin PJ, Sunwoo YC: Candidiasis of the duodenum and jejunum. Gastroenterology 80:829, 1981
57. Freeman HJ, Shnitka TK, Piercey JRA, et al: Cytomegalovirus infection of the gastrointestinal tract in a patient with late onset immunodeficiency syndrome. Gastroenterology 73:1397, 1977
58. Franzin G, Muolo A, Griminelli T: Cytomegalovirus inclusions in the gastroduodenal mucosa of patients after renal transplantation. Gut 22:698, 1981
59. Blacklow NR, Cukor G: Viral gastroenteritis. N Engl J Med 304:397, 1981
60. Brandt LJ, Davidoff A, Bernstein LH, et al: Small-intestinal involvement in Waldenstrom's macroglobulinemia: case report and review of the literature. Digest Dis Sci 26:174, 1981
61. Waldmann TA, Steinfeld JL, Dutcher TF, et al: The role of the gastrointestinal system in "idiopathic hypoproteinemia." Gastroenterology 41:197, 1961
62. Popovic OS, Brkic S, Bojic P, et al: Sarcoidosis and protein losing enteropathy. Gastroenterology 78:119, 1980
63. Longstreth GF, Newcomer AD: Drug-induced malabsorption. Mayo Clin Proc 50:284, 1975
64. Freeman HJ: Sulindac-associated small bowel lesion. J Clin Gastroenterol 8:569, 1986
65. Wiernik G: Changes in the villous pattern of the human jejunum associated with heavy radiation damage. Gut 7:149, 1966
66. Smith FP, Kisner DL, Widerlite L, et al: Chemotherapeutic alteration of small intestinal morphology and function: a progress report. J Clin Gastroenterol 1:203, 1979
67. Haglund L, Hulten L, Ahren C, Lundgren O: Mucosal lesions in the human small intestine in shock. Gut 16:979, 1979
68. Morichau M, Touchard G, Marie P, et al: Jejunal IgA and C3 deposition in adult Henoch-Schön-

lein prupura with severe intestinal manifestations. Gastroenterology 82:1438, 1982
69. Rambaud J-C, Galian A, Touchard G, et al: Digestive tract and renal vessel hyalinosis, idiopathic nonarteriosclerotic intracerebral calcifications, retinal ischemic syndrome, and phenotypic abnormalities. A new familial syndrome. Gastroenterology 90:930, 1986
70. Freeman K, Anthony PP, Miller DS, Warin AP: Case report. Cronkhite Canada syndrome: a new hypothesis. Gut 26:531, 1985
71. Hermos J, Cooper H, Kramer P, et al: Histological diagnosis by peroral biopsy of Crohn's disease of the proximal intestine. Gastroenterology 59:868, 1970
72. Schuffler MD, Chaffee RG: Small intestinal biopsy in a patient with Crohn's disease of the duodenum: the spectrum of abnormal findings in the absence of granulomas. Gastroenterology 76:1009, 1979
73. Sprague R, Harper P, McClain S, et al: Disseminated gastrointestinal sarcoidosis. Case report and review of the literature. Gastroenterology 87:421, 1984
74. Bjornklett A, Fausa O, Refsum SB, et al: Jejunal villous atrophy and granulomatous inflammation responding to a gluten-free diet. Gut 18:814, 1977
75. Douglas JG, Logan RFA, Gillon J, et al: Sarcoidosis and celiac disease. An association ? Lancet 2:13, 1984
76. Mordechai R, Sohar E: Intestinal malabsorption: First manifestation of amyloidosis in familial Mediterranean fever. Gastroenterology 66:446, 1974
77. Rey DK, Jersild RA Jr: Further characterization of the pigment in pseudomelanosis duodeni in three patients. Gastroenterology 95:177, 1988
78. Fishman RS, Fleming CR, Li C-Y: Systemic mastocytosis with review of gastrointertinal manifestations. Mayo Clin Proc 54:51, 1979
79. Shousa S, Barrison IG, El-Sayeed W, et al: A study of incidence and relationship of intestinal metaplasia of gastric antrum and gastric metaplasia of duodenum in patients with nonulcer dyspepsia. Digest Dis Sci 29:311, 1984
80. Scott BB, Jenkins D: Endoscopic small intestinal biopsy. Gastrointest Endosc 27:162, 1981
81. Whitehead R: Major Problems in Pathology. Vol 3. Mucosal Biopsy of the Gastrointestinal Tract. 2nd Ed. WB Saunders, London, 1985
82. Weinstein WM: The diagnosis and classification

of gastritis and duodenitis. J Clin Gastroenterol 3(suppl 2):7, 1981

83. Scott BB, Losowsky MS: Patchiness and duodenal-jejunal variation of the mucosal abnormality in coeliac disease and dermatitis herpetiformis. Gut 17:984, 1976

84. Goldman H, Antonioli DA: Mucosal biopsy of the rectum, colon, and distal ileum. Hum Pathol 13:981, 1982

85. Halphen M, Galian A, Certin M, et al: Clinicopathological study of a patient with idiopathic villous atrophy and small vessel alterations of the ileum. Digest Dis Sci 34:111, 1989

86. Nasmyth DG, Godwin PGR, Dixon MF, et al: Ileal ecology after pouch-anal anastamosis or ileostomy. A study of mucosal morphology, fecal bacteriology, fecal volatile fatty acids, and their interrelationship. Gastroenterology 96:817, 1989

7

Polyps of the Colon and Small Intestine, Polyposis Syndromes, and the Polyp-Carcinoma Sequence

Thomas H. Kent and Frank A. Mitros

A *polyp* is defined as any growth or mass protruding from a mucous membrane. Although carcinomas and other large masses are technically polyps, they are generally excluded from this category. Polyps are much more common in the colon than in the small intestine, and are more common in the rectosigmoid colon than more proximally. Most colon polyps fit into one of a few well-defined types, whereas small intestinal polyps represent a wider variety of lesions, none of which is common.

This chapter begins by presenting the basic types of colon polyps, followed by briefer accounts of rarer types of colon polyps and small intestinal polyps. Discussions of intestinal polyposis syndromes utilize the morphology presented earlier in the discussions of colon polyps. Finally, the relationship of benign polyps to the development of cancer is summarized.

The challenge of intestinal polyps lies in their morphologic classification and how knowledge of their age distribution, genetics, and relationship to cancer is used to predict their behavior and select treatment. We stress definitions, classification, morphology, pathogenesis, and the most important clinical circumstances associated with the various types of polyps.

The literature on intestinal polyps is vast, but there are few comprehensive sources of information on intestinal polyps other than those by Morson.[1-3] References used in this chapter have been selected on the basis of their coverage of the topic, currentness, and their references to the remaining literature on the topic.

CLASSIFICATION AND FREQUENCY

The simple classifications of *hamartomatous, hyperplastic,* and *neoplastic* encompass most intestinal polyps. Hamartomas are characterized morphologically by cellular components that are normal for the area, but not normally organized. Hamartomas can occur in infancy and childhood, although some appear later in life.

Hyperplastic polyps are so named by default. Morphologically, they are a focal increase in relatively normal cells with a relatively normal arrangement, that is, they lack the cellular crowding and atypia of neoplasms and the disorganization of hamartomas. Hyperplastic polyps of the colon appear, however, to be an entity distinct from hyperplastic polyps of the stomach, and hyperplastic polyps are not recognized as an entity in the small intestine. Like adenomas, hyperplastic polyps of the colon are most common in the elderly but may be seen as early as the teen years.

Neoplastic polyps are mostly adenomas, that is, benign neoplasms of glandular epithelium, regardless of whether they form acini, tubules, or villi. They are distinguished morphologically from hamartomas and hyperplastic polyps by their cellular crowding and atypia, and from carcinoma by their lack of invasiveness. Adenomas occur predominantly in older adults, and are uncommon under 40 years and exceedingly rare under 30 years of age except when part of a familial syndrome. In familial syndromes they begin to appear at about age 15 years. Adenomas vary greatly in their behavior, so subclassification is useful even though uniform criteria for subclassification have not yet been established.

Hyperplastic polyps of the colon are undoubtedly the most common of gastrointestinal polyps, but they are not the most common lesions seen by surgical pathologists, since they are asymptomatic and often are not biopsied. Adenomas make up the majority of lesions biopsied and present the problems of subclassification, exclusion of cancer, and exclusion of polyposis to the pathologist.

Of the hamartomatous polyps, the solitary juvenile polyp in children, although uncommon, appears to have a very constant and predictable occurrence rate. The various polyposis syndromes occur in clusters associated with dominant inheritance and as rare sporadic cases. Other types of colon polyps and all types of

Table 7-1. Classification of Polyps of the Intestine

Basic types of colon polyps
  Hyperplastic
  Adenomatous polyp (tubular adenoma)
  Villous adenoma
  Tubulovillous adenoma
  Juvenile polyp
  Peutz-Jeghers polyp
Other colonic polyps
  Inflammatory polyps
  Lymphoid polyp
  Carcinoid
  Leiomyoma of the muscularis mucosae
  Lipoma
Small intestinal polyps
  Inflammatory fibroid polyp
  Brunner's gland "adenoma"
  Adenomatous polyp
  Villous adenoma
  Neurogenic polyps
  Lymphangiectatic cyst
Polyposis syndromes
  Familial polyposis coli
  Gardner's syndrome
  Turcot's syndrome
  Multiple adenomas
  Juvenile polyposis syndromes
  Peutz-Jeghers syndrome
  Cronkhite-Canada syndrome
  Cowden's (multiple hamartoma) syndrome
  Nodular lymphoid hyperplasia (lymphoid polyposis)
  Small intestinal lipomatosis

small intestinal polyps can be classified as rare. The classification used in this chapter is given in Table 7-1.

BASIC TYPES OF COLON POLYPS

Rectosigmoid polyps comprise the majority of intestinal polyps, and hyperplastic polyps, adenomas, and juvenile polyps comprise the majority of rectosigmoid polyps. Peutz-Jeghers polyp, although rare in the colon, is discussed here because it is one of the basic morphologic types of intestinal polyps that must be distinguished from the others.

HYPERPLASTIC POLYP OF THE COLON

The hyperplastic polyp of the colon[4-12] is a distinct morphologic entity of unknown cause characterized by focal enlargement of crypts owing to crowding of cells and mucus depletion at the base of the crypt (hyperplasia), and by excessive cytoplasm toward the mouth of the crypt, producing a serrated epithelium. This lesion has also been called *metaplastic polyp*.

Gross Pathology

Most hyperplastic polyps are sessile, smooth, pale gray polyps less than 5 mm in diameter (Fig. 7-1). A few reach 10 mm or greater. Lesions on mucosal folds may appear pedunculated. Larger lesions may appear similar to small adenomas.

Microscopic Pathology

When cut perpendicularly, the maintenance of normal crypt configuration can be appreciated in these small focal lesions (Fig. 7-2). The nuclei at the base of the crypt are crowded, and cytoplasmic mucus is depleted. When cut tangentially, the bases of crypts may be mistaken for

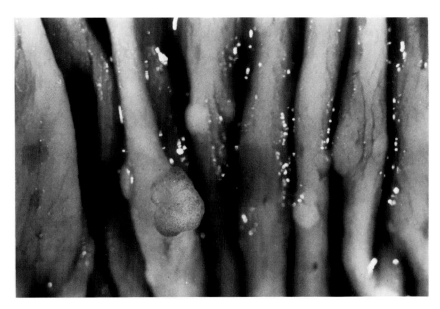

Fig. 7-1. Multiple hyperplastic polyps; the tendency to appear at the tip of a fold may be noted. The single adenoma is larger, darker, and has a bossellated surface.

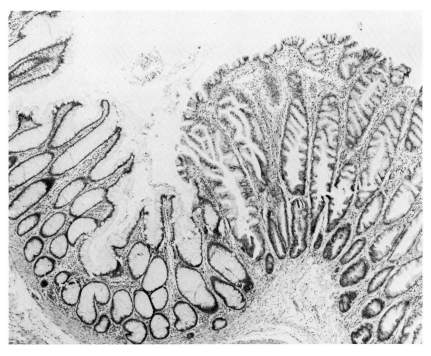

Fig. 7-2. Hyperplastic polyp.

an adenoma. Reconstruction of a tangentially cut lesion will, however, reveal the typical changes found in the upper portion of the crypts. Toward the mouth of a crypt the cytoplasm of absorptive-type cells becomes abundant and buckles to give the characteristic serrated appearance, whereas the nuclei are basally oriented and not crowded. Tangential sections of gland lumina have a characteristic stellate configuration, in contrast to the round or oval contours seen in adenomas. The subsurface collagen table is thickened focally, providing another clue to recognition.

Pathogenesis

No specific cause has been identified for these common focal hyperplasias. The cells of the upper crypt are retained longer than normal and hence are hypermature.[7, 9] Hyperplastic polyps increase in frequency with age.[4] The comparative histogenesis of hyperplastic polyps and adenomas has been extensively studied.[5–10] The proliferative zone, as measured by mitotic activity, is confined to the basal portion of the crypt, although this zone is expanded compared to normal epithelium. This is in contrast to adenomas, in which the proliferative activity is spread throughout the lesion.

Location

These lesions are confined to the colon, including the vermiform appendix.[11] They are often found in association with carcinoma, although this probably is because the resection provides the opportunity to discover them.

Multiplicity

Numbers may vary from one to many, with multiplicity as a typical feature. In a few cases the occurrence of multiple, large hyperplastic polyps in patients as young as 27 years of age has simulated familial polyposis.[12]

Age and Sex

Hyperplastic polyps are more often found in older people, but it is difficult to judge the age distribution because they are always discovered incidentally. They can be found as early as the teens. They occur frequently in both sexes, although there is a suggestion that they are more common in men.[12]

Behavior

It is not known whether these lesions can regress, but it is clear that they rarely become very large and do not produce symptoms. Although they have been generally considered as not being directly related to the development of colon cancer, new evidence suggests that this may not always be the case. A new subtype, the mixed hyperplastic adenomatous polyp, has recently been described. Another term proposed to describe these lesion, *serrated adenoma,* stresses the key morphologic features.[13] The architecture is that of a hyperplastic polyp (serrated), whereas the nuclear features more closely resemble those of an adenoma. Severe atypia (carcinoma in situ) and intramucosal carcinoma have been noted in these lesions, even in some less than 1 cm in diameter.

ADENOMATOUS POLYP (TUBULAR ADENOMA)

The adenomatous polyp of the colon[1–3,10,13–23] is a benign neoplasm of colonic epithelium characterized by a glandular proliferation composed chiefly of tubules, as seen in standard section. It is also called *tubular adenoma.*

Gross Pathology

A typical lesion at diagnosis is an ovoid to spherical mass slightly less than 1 cm in diameter with an irregular surface somewhat darker and redder than the surrounding mucosa attached

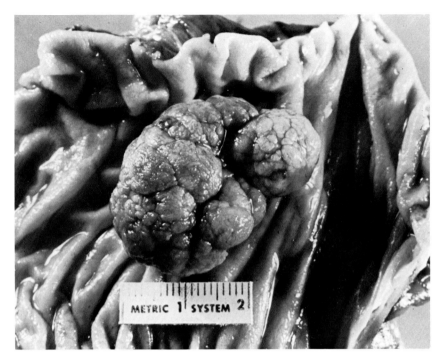

Fig. 7-3. Large pedunculated tubular adenoma. The characteristic surface may be noted.

to the colon by a stalk lined by normal mucosa (Fig. 7-3). Smaller lesions may be indistinguishable from hyperplastic polyps. The diameter can vary from less than 0.1 cm to greater than 3 cm. It is important to note that up to 32 percent of adenomatous polyps are sessile. Larger lesions are more likely to have recognizable stalks.[14] Exceptionally long (7 to 9 cm) stalks are sometimes found in those located in the sigmoid colon.

Microscopic Pathology

The usual appearance is that of closely packed epithelial tubules, usually appearing in cross section, suggesting a horizontal relationship to the muscularis mucosae. Near the center of the lesion, the tubules can appear more oblong, approaching a perpendicular relationship to the muscularis mucosae (Fig. 7-4). In many sections, presumably from the periphery of the polyps, neoplastic tubules can be seen overlying normal mucosa (Fig. 7-5); the inverse relationship is never seen. The basement membrane and lumenal surfaces of the tubules usually have a smooth contour with no papillary infolding, in spite of apparent crowding of the nuclei (Fig. 7-6). The nuclei tend to be large and hyperchromatic, often having a pencil-shaped contour; stratification is often prominent. Mitotic activity is increased. The amount of mucin is variable, but is most often decreased in amount as compared to normal mucosa. The cytoplasm is usually distinctly basophilic. Paneth and neuroendocrine cells are commonly present scattered throughout the tumor, but do not appear to be of any significance.[15] The subsurface collagen table is thinner than that of normal mucosa. Variable degrees of atypia have been recognized, although criteria for separating grades have been difficult to establish. Practically speaking, grading of atypia is not usually done except when it is severe; severe atypia is usually characterized by pronounced budding or a frank cribriform pattern.

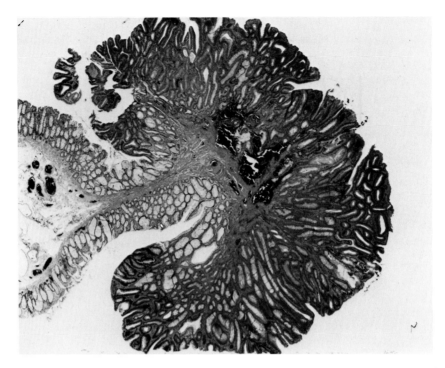

Fig. 7-4. Adenomatous polyp composed entirely of tubular structures embedded in lamina propria with a well-defined stalk.

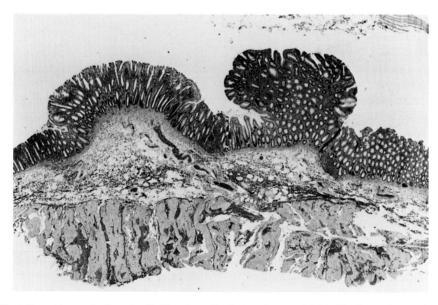

Fig. 7-5. Adjacent hyperplastic polyp (left) and small tubular adenoma (right). The hyperchromatic epithelial cells are at the base of the former, but at the surface of the latter.

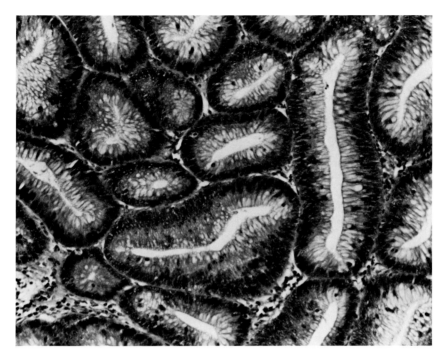

Fig. 7-6. Tubules: benign neoplastic colonic epithelium surround a central lumen and embedded in lamina propria. Many are seen in cross section.

Benign adenomatous epithelium in the stalk of an adenoma (most commonly tubular, but also villous and tubulovillous) is called *pseudocarcinomatous invasion* (misplaced epithelium). Originally described by Muto,[22] this finding is probably more common than formerly thought, appearing in up to 10 percent of excised polyps.[23] It usually occurs in larger polyps, and is thought to be due to trauma to the polyp with subsequent regeneration. The entrapped epithelium is similar to the surface of the adenoma, and does not elicit a desmoplastic response. Hemosiderin is almost always present in the stalk (Fig. 7-7). Dilated spaces filled with mucin or mucin lying free in the stalk is common. These spaces can be acellular or lined by a flattened layer of epithelial cells. If clusters of epithelial cells are present "floating" in the mucin, the diagnosis of mucinous (colloid) carcinoma is virtually certain.

Pathogenesis

Adenomas are usually found in increased frequency in those populations with an increased frequency of colon cancer; it is believed that similar mechanisms are operative in causing both.[1] Based on epidemiologic studies, it is believed that both genetic and environmental factors are involved. The latter appear to be of more importance, and are believed by most to be related to dietary factors, particularly the high fat and meat content of most Western diets. There is likely a complex interrelationship with bile acid metabolism. Whatever the initiating event, the sequence that has emerged from multiple studies[10, 16–18] involving serial sectioning and/or incorporating tritiated thymidine into adenomas is that of neoplastic transformation occurring first in the normal proliferative zone near the base of a crypt or several adjacent

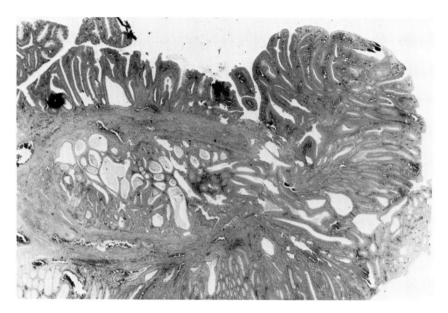

Fig. 7-7. Pseudocarcinomatous invasion with adenomatous epithelium beneath the muscularis mucosal. Focal mild cystic dilatation is present; there is dense deposition of hemosiderin.

crypts, then spreading to involve the full thickness. The surface epithelium consistently appears more mitotically active than that underneath, suggesting spread along the surface or recruitment of adjacent tubules.

Location

The distribution within the colon appears to depend somewhat on the age of the patient, the size of the polyp, and perhaps the geography of the population studied. In general, there is a distal predilection, although not so pronounced as for colon cancer. In one series[19] of 3,725 adenomatous polyps, the distribution was as follows: right colon, 11 percent; transverse colon, 12 percent; descending colon, 24 percent; sigmoid, 48 percent; and rectum, 5 percent. With polyps over 1 cm in diameter, the distribution more closely approaches that of colon cancer.

Age and Sex

The incidence of adenomas increases with age, but they can be found from the teens (very rarely) to senescence.[14] In younger patients, evidence for familial polyposis coli should be sought. The average age at which polyps are diagnosed will vary, depending on whether the patients are symptomatic (61.9 years) or otherwise healthy and asymptomatic (50.2 years).[14] It will also vary considerably according to the population studied (e.g., an age-adjusted prevalence of 63 percent in Hawaiian-Japanese males versus an 11 percent age adjusted prevalence in Colombians (Cali)).[20] There is usually a slight male predominance at any age in a given population.

Behavior

It is not known what percentage of tumors remain asymptomatic, nor for how long. The relatively high incidence in asymptomatic adults suggests that the majority are clinically silent. The most common symptom is rectal bleeding. Cancer risk in adenomas correlates with tumor size. Those under 1 cm, which constitute about 74 percent of all adenomatous polyps, contain invasive cancer 1.0 percent of the time; those over 2 cm, which constitute about 5 percent of all adenomatous polyps, contain invasive cancer 35 percent of the time.[21] With multiple adenomas, the cancer risk appears to increase with the number of adenomas.

VILLOUS ADENOMA

The villous adenoma of the colon[1-3, 16, 24, 25] is a benign neoplasm of colonic epithelium characterized by an epithelial proliferation composed chiefly of villi, as seen in standard sections. It has a well-established high cancer risk.

Gross Pathology

The characteristic appearance at the usual time of diagnosis is of a round to oval exophytic mass that is several centimeters in diameter and has a shaggy, often friable surface (Fig. 7-8). About 90 percent of villous adenomas are clearly sessile, but otherwise typical villous adenomas can have a definite stalk.[24] The junction between

tumor and surrounding mucosa tends to be less distinct than with adenomatous polyps. There can be areas of surface ulceration or induration; these should always occasion histologic examination, because they frequently mark areas of malignant change. Although the mean size has been reported as 3.4 cm,[24] sizes can range from 0.3 to 20 cm. Even completely benign lesions can be circumferential.

Microscopic Pathology

The appearance of individual cells within the lesion is indistinguishable from that of adenomatous polyps, although overall these lesions are more likely to contain a larger amount of mucus, at times even more than the surrounding mucosa. The characteristic histologic feature is the presence of many slender villi (Fig. 7-9), many of which appear to arise directly from the area of the muscularis mucosae (Fig. 7-10). Serial reconstructions and stereologic examination have shown that the villi are in reality platelike struc-

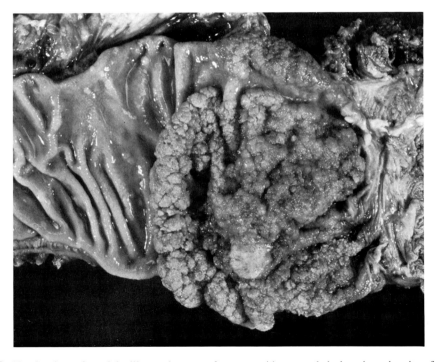

Fig. 7-8. Nearly circumferential villous adenoma of rectum with a rounded elevation, the site of a focus of invasive carcinoma. Several hyperplastic polyps are present.

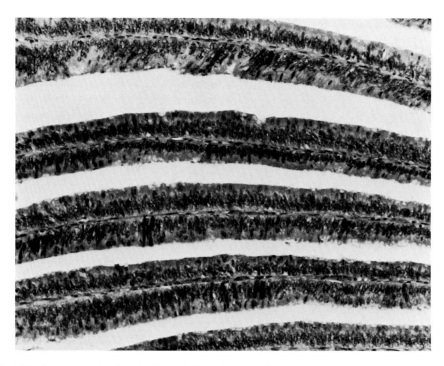

Fig. 7-9. Villi: benign neoplastic colonic epithelium lining delicate cores of lamina propria. The fact that these are apparently perfectly oriented longitudinal sections is evidence that these structures are plates and not fingerlike projections.

tures, or folia.[25] This would account for the fact that cross sections of fingerlike villi are not commonly seen in standard sections.

Pathogenesis

The pathogenesis of villous adenoma is believed to be similar to that described for adenomatous polyps. The tritiated thymidine studies again show the most prominent incorporation near the surface,[16] with perhaps even more intense mitotic activity here than in tubular adenomas.

Location

The distribution shows a distal predominance approaching that seen for colon cancer. There is a slightly increased occurrence in the cecum and ascending colon, and a very definite peak in the rectum, where over 74 percent of the lesions are located.[24]

Multiplicity

Villous adenomas are infrequently multiple. In one study, only 4 of 215 (1.9 percent) patients had more than one villous adenoma.[24] Although adequate quantitation is lacking, villous adenomas frequently co-exist with adenomatous polyps.

Age and Sex

The mean age at time of diagnosis is 58 years. The sex incidence is approximately equal.

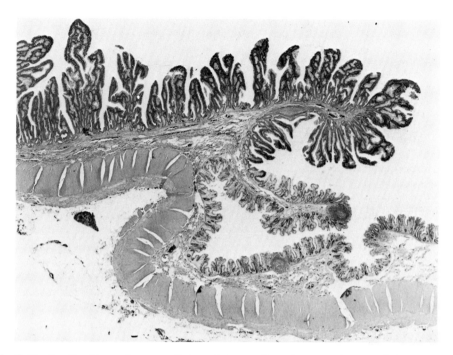

Fig. 7-10. Sessile villous adenoma with long flat area of attachment to the muscularis mucosae.

Behavior

Villous adenomas are more likely to be symptomatic than tubular adenomas. Bleeding (65 percent) and diarrhea or extrusion of mucus (43 percent) are the most important of these, but many patients (13 percent) are asymptomatic.[24] Unlike tubular adenomas, villous adenomas frequently (12 percent) recur after excision.[24] The propensity for malignancy is high and is related to tumor size. The presence of severe atypia or carcinoma in situ is even more frequent. In most series, about 30 percent of villous adenomas contain invasive carcinoma at the time of diagnosis.

TUBULOVILLOUS ADENOMAS

Many have recognized the existence of an intermediate form of benign neoplasm of colonic epithelium between adenomatous polyp (tubular adenoma) and villous adenoma. Synonyms for this type have included *mixed* or *intermediate form*, *villoglandular adenoma*, and *papillary adenoma*.[1–3, 19, 21, 26, 27] Several definitions

have been published; the most widely accepted is that of Morson as it appears in the World Health Organization monograph[3]: ''an adenoma that may have both tubular and villous patterns or a pattern that seems to be intermediate between tubular and villous.'' He also notes that polyps with the intermediate structure are more common than those containing mixtures of typical tubules and villi; these structures are described as broad and stunted villi deep to which are tubules similar to those in a tubular adenoma.[2] Note that any quantification of a tubular or villous components is scrupulously avoided. Others[19, 21, 26, 27] have insisted that a certain percentage of the area of a two-dimensional section be occupied by the villous component (e.g., 5 to 50 percent or 25 to 75 percent), although what constitutes a villus is not always clearly defined. A comparison of several series is given in Table 7-2. Occasional series have included tubulovillous adenomas but give no criteria for defining the category. It has frequently been noted that the percentage falling into the tubulovillous category increases with more extensive sampling.

Table 7-2. Relative Frequency and Occurrence of Carcinoma in Tubular, Tubulovillous, and Villous Adenomas

Source and Criteria	Tubular			Tubulovillous			Villous		
	Number of Polyps	% of All Polyps	% With Invasive Cancer	Number of Polyps	% of All Polyps	% With Invasive Cancer	Number of Polyps	% of All Polyps	% With Invasive Cancer
A	1,875	75	4.7	380	15	22.4	234	9	41.9
B	250	38	0	304	45	2.3	123	18	8.1
C	3,725	64	2.8	1,542	27	8.4	519	9	9.4
D	314	53	0.3	159	27	0.6	120	20	13.3

A. As defined by Morson.[20]
B. Adenoma: <5% villous, tubulovillous; 5.50% villous, villous; >50% villous.[26]
C. Adenoma: <25% tubulovillous; 25–75% villous, villous; >75% villous.[19]
D. Adenoma: purely tubules, tubulovillous; any villous component, villous; purely villi.[27]

Gross and Microscopic Pathology, Pathogenesis, Location, Multiplicity, Age, and Sex

These features are similar to those already described for adenomatous polyps and villous adenomas. The percentage that are pedunculated or sessile is uncertain, but in general there is a tendency toward a broad flat base. Typical tubules and villi are commonly present (Fig. 7-11). The broad stunted villus described by Morson is the only unique feature, although is not always present (Fig. 7-12).

Behavior

The practical reason for separating benign neoplasms of the colon into three categories rather than two has to do with a difference in biologic behavior. The cancer risk in tubulovillous adenomas appears to be significantly greater than in tubular adenomas, and more closely approximates that of villous adenoma in most series. This is true even after a correction is made for the size of the polyp.

JUVENILE POLYP

A juvenile polyp[28–30] is a non-neoplastic polyp composed of epithelium indigenous to the site of origin, which is often disorganized with cystic dilation of glandular structures and fibroblastic stroma containing inflammatory cells. Most consider it a hamartomatous lesion. The term *retention polyp* was used as a synonym in the past.

Gross Pathology

The well-developed juvenile polyp tends to be spherical, deep red, and smooth surfaced, and has a distinct narrow stalk. Cross sections demonstrate small cystic areas (Fig. 7-13). Early lesions are less pedunculated and resemble inflammatory polyps.

Microscopic Pathology

The classic appearance includes a narrow stalk of normal mucosa and submucosa, and a core composed of dilated glands filled with mucus and/or inflammatory cells, an abundant fibroblastic stroma containing many chronic inflammatory cells, and a smooth, partially ulcerated surface with the remainder covered by a single layer of columnar epithelium (Fig. 7-14). Hemosiderin is often present in the stroma. The earliest lesions appear as focal protrusions of granulation tissue, but with increasing size the cystic glands become more prominent. The early lesions are safely recognized as juvenile polyps when occurring in children

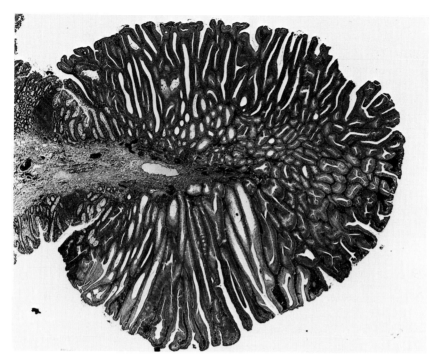

Fig. 7-11. Pedunculated tubulovillous adenoma; the central portion is clearly tubular, whereas well-defined villi are found at the periphery.

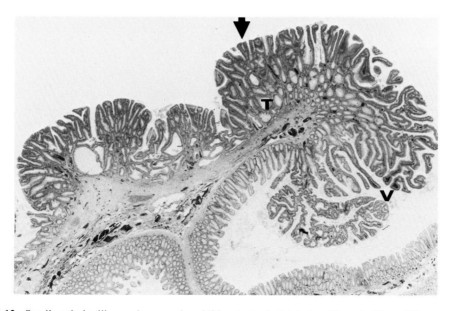

Fig. 7-12. Sessile tubulovillous adenoma. In addition to typical tubular (*T*) and villous (*V*) areas, short blunted villi (arrow) are present.

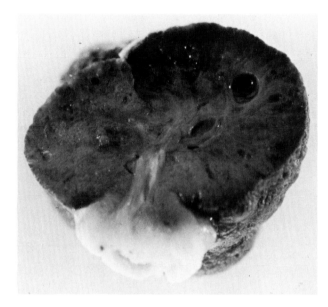

Fig. 7-13. Cut surface of juvenile polyp with cystically dilated glands. The outer surface is hemorrhagic and irregular.

under 10 years of age or when occurring in association with other well-developed juvenile polyps, but in adults the distinguishing criteria from inflammatory polyp or a site of injury are less definite.

Pathogenesis

The argument for the hamartomatous nature is based on morphology and circumstances of occurrence. Morphologically, juvenile polyps

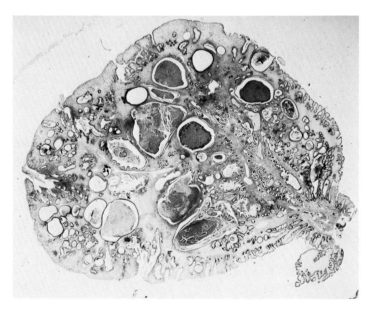

Fig. 7-14. Juvenile polyp with dilated glands, inflamed edematous stroma, and partially ulcerated surface.

are composed of elements indigenous to the site of origin that are neither histologically nor biologically neoplastic. Most are found in children under 10 years of age, suggesting that they either are congenital or develop at an early age. They also occur as multiple, familial lesions, a feature favoring hamartomatous origin over an acquired injury and repair reaction.

Location

The typical lesions of children are predominantly (85 percent) located in the rectosigmoid colon, but may occur anywhere in the colon. The location of the much rarer scattered lesions of adults is less clearly defined. Multiple juvenile polyposis syndromes are discussed later in this chapter.

Multiplicity

The typical childhood lesions are solitary (85 percent), but several may be present. If many are present, and especially if the patient is over 10 years of age, the possibility of multiple juvenile polyposis should be considered.

Age and Sex

The age distribution of childhood lesions is bell shaped, peaking at 4 to 5 years and ranging from 1 to 10 years, with a tail extending into the early teens. There is no age pattern associated with the few solitary lesions found in patients over 15. There is no sex preference.

Behavior

Most lesions become symptomatic at some stage and are removed. Bleeding is by far the most common symptom (90 percent), but some autoamputate or prolapse through the anus. The failure to find more of these lesions in adults,

either because of symptoms or incidentally, suggests that most eventually become symptomatic or, perhaps, autoamputate and are never discovered. Regression of such large lesions seems unlikely. There is no evidence that neoplasms develop in juvenile polyps, although some juvenile polyposis families also may have an increased frequency of neoplastic polyps and carcinoma, as is discussed later.

PEUTZ-JEGHERS POLYP

A Peutz-Jeghers polyp[31-33] is a non-neoplastic polyp composed of mature epithelium indigenous to the site of origin arranged on a treelike proliferation of muscularis mucosae. Most consider it a hamartomatous lesion. Although originally described as part of a hereditary syndrome that includes polyps of stomach, small intestine, and colon associated with mucocutaneous pigmentation, it can also occur as a solitary lesion in a patient without a family history.

Gross Pathology

Peutz-Jeghers polyps vary in size but may be quite large. They are usually pedunculated and have a smooth or lobulated surface similar to that of adenomatous polyps (Fig. 7-15).

Microscopic Pathology

The most characteristic feature is the treelike ramification of muscularis mucosae (Fig. 7-16). This is associated with a disorganized appearance of the relatively normal-appearing epithelial cells. In contrast to the juvenile polyp, the epithelial component makes up a larger portion of the polyp, and cystic change in glands is not prominent and stroma is scant. The disorganized muscularis mucosae intermingled with epithelium is easily misinterpreted as invasion (Fig. 7-17). Occasionally some degree of atypia in the epithelium has been noted.

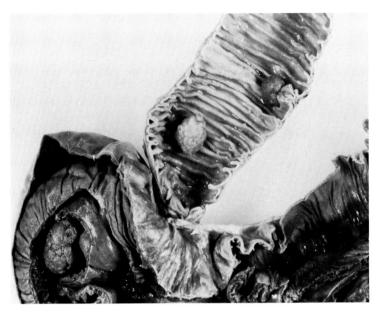

Fig. 7-15. Three Peutz-Jeghers polyps and resulting intussusception. (Photo by Elliott Foucar.)

Pathogenesis

Peutz-Jeghers polyps were first described as part of a dominant hereditary syndrome, but nonfamilial cases[31] and single polyps with similar histology occur without evidence of the syndrome.[32] The occurrence of the syndrome in a patient without a family history can be attributed to mutation or failure to detect the familial nature, owing to incomplete examination and/or incomplete forms of the syndrome. The occurrence of solitary lesions without fam-

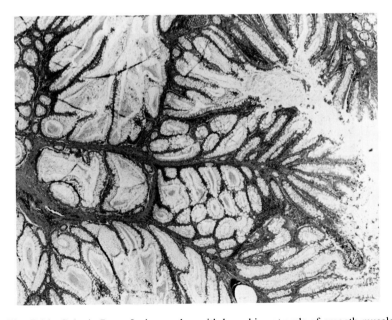

Fig. 7-16. Colonic Peutz-Jeghers polyp with branching strands of smooth muscle.

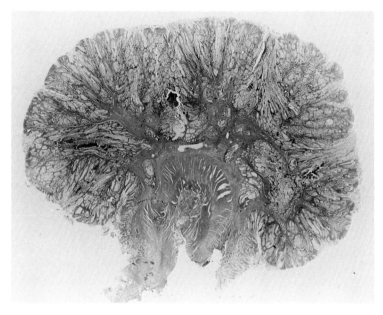

Fig. 7-17. Full-thickness section of Peutz-Jeghers polyp with pseudoinvasion. (Slide courtesy of Elliott Foucar.)

ily history or other manifestations of the syndrome is poorly documented and needs further study.

Location

Isolated polyps may occur in the stomach, small intestine, or colon.[32] (Their distribution in Peutz-Jeghers syndrome is discussed later in this chapter.)

Multiplicity

Emphasis in the literature has been on Peutz-Jeghers syndrome, in which multiple polyps occur. The number of polyps is highly variable, and new polyps may develop over time.

Age and Sex

The most common age of onset of the syndrome is adolescence and early adulthood, but onset may occur in childhood or in older adults.

Further, new lesions may develop with age. There is no sex preference.

Behavior

The behavior of solitary lesions is not clear at this time. Some may behave like solitary juvenile polyps (i.e., once removed there is no further problem), and others may be the first manifestation of the syndrome. Follow-up for many years is indicated to detect new polyps.

OTHER COLONIC POLYPS

Inflamed granulation tissue and redundant mucosa at sites of previous operations or biopsy sites are not infrequently encountered, and are biopsied to distinguish them from adenomas. The term *inflammatory polyp* tends to be restricted to inflamed redundant mucosal excrescences in patients with ulcerative colitis or, less commonly, other types of inflammatory bowel disease (IBD). Small lymphoid follicles are not unusual in a series of biopsies of rectal polyps.

Carcinoids and leiomyomas of the muscularis mucosa are less common but more distinctive, and will be encountered in any large series of rectal polyps. Lipomatous polyps are more likely to be encountered at autopsy or in surgical resection specimens. Inflammatory fibroid polyp and neurogenic polyps are rare in the colon, and are discussed with small intestinal polyps, below. Other neoplasms or conditions such as endometriosis are so rarely encountered as polyps that they do not merit specific discussion.

INFLAMMATORY POLYPS

Inflammatory polyps[1, 34] are non-neoplastic proliferations of mucosa and granulation tissue that appear to be a response to injury by the colonic mucosa. They are seen most frequently in ulcerative colitis. They have also been called *pseudopolyps*. These cylindrical to rounded outgrowths of mucosa are similar in appearance to the surrounding mucosa and vary from minute nodules to several centimeters in size. There is usually no sharp distinction between head and stalk (Fig. 7-18). The tip of the polyp may be bifid. Bridges from one portion of the mucosa to another can form. They occur throughout the colon, but the rectum is usually spared. Some polyps are merely raised bridges of mucosa with a small amount of muscularis mucosae and submucosa. However, there is usually a prominent inflammatory infiltrate, but the amount is quite variable. Granulation tissue can be identified frequently, and in those polyps occurring in conditions other than ulcerative colitis and Crohn's disease, the entire polyp may consist of a rounded mass of granulation tissue[1] (Fig. 7-19). Occasionally there may be such prominent cystic dilatation of the glands that confusion with juvenile polyps can occur if close attention is not paid to the state of the surrounding mucosa and to the clinical situation. Inflammatory polyps are usually multiple, although one report suggests that up to 25 percent of patients with ulcerative colitis have solitary lesions.[34]

LYMPHOID POLYPS

Lymphoid follicles are common in the rectum, particularly in children, in patients with

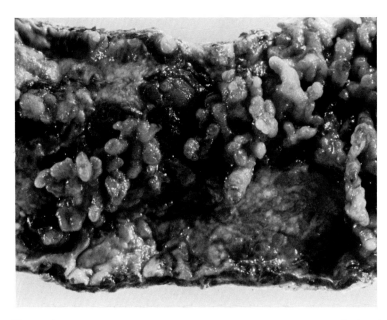

Fig. 7-18. Multiple irregularly shaped inflammatory polyps with no distinct head.

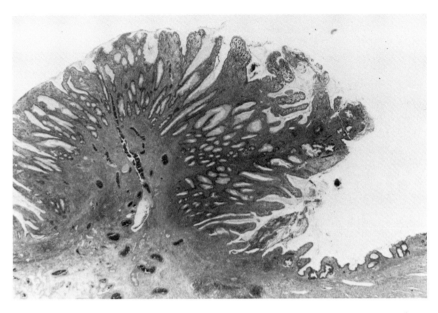

Fig. 7-19. Inflammatory polyp composed of chronically inflamed, slightly disorganized, protruberant mucosa.

IBD, and in older persons. Occasionally these tiny, gray, slightly elevated lesions are mistaken for hyperplastic polyps or early adenomas, and are biopsied.[35–37] The pathologist should be aware that a lymphoid follicle may be the explanation for biopsy in a specimen that appears otherwise normal. Larger lymphoid polyps do occur, and are almost always in the rectum and tend to be sessile.[35–37] They are appropriately termed *focal lymphoid hyperplasia* or *lymphoid polyps*, and in the past have been called *benign lymphoma of the rectum*. These lesions may occur at any age and may cause bleeding. Excisional biopsy is adequate for treatment and to exclude lymphoma.

CARCINOID

Small carcinoids[38, 39] of the rectosigmoid produce rounded polypoid elevations of the mucosa that appear as gray nodules. Microscopically, the typical carcinoid cells form a submucosal mass that partially involves and elevates the mucosa (Fig. 7-20).

The vast majority of lesions less than 1 cm in diameter are benign, and complete excision is adequate treatment,[38] although small lesions occasionally metastasize.[39] Lesions over 2 cm having a sheetlike pattern and nuclear atypia are more likely to metastasize than are small lesions having a ribbonlike histologic pattern.[39]

LEIOMYOMA OF THE MUSCULARIS MUCOSAE

Leiomyoma of the muscularis mucosae consists of a small spherical mass that produces a rounded polypoid elevation of the mucosa having an endoscopic appearance similar to that of a small carcinoid. The mucosa over the nodule is usually intact (Fig. 7-21). This rare lesion is encountered incidentally from time to time, and is cured by excisional biopsy.

LIPOMA

Lipoma of the colon[40, 41] is a localized tumor of mature adipose tissue in the submucosa.[40] Lipoma should be distinguished from lipomatous hypertrophy of the ileocecal valve, a common finding associated with excess adipose tissue in the submucosa of the colon at the junction with the ileum. Lipomas vary greatly in size

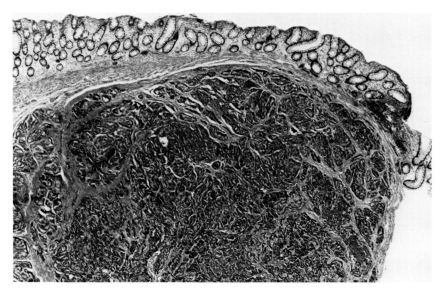

Fig. 7-20. Rectal carcinoid with mass of tumor cells in the submucosa.

and may be large. Radiologically, they produce a smooth filling defect whose shape can be altered by position and pressure.[41] They are most common in older adults in the right colon, with a female predominance.[40] Lipomas are about twice as common in the colon as they are in the small intestine.

SMALL INTESTINAL POLYPS

It is difficult to separate polyps appearing as pedunculated mucosal excrescences from tumors that protrude into the lumen of the small intestine in a nonspecific manner. Thus, the literature does not focus on ''polyps'' of the

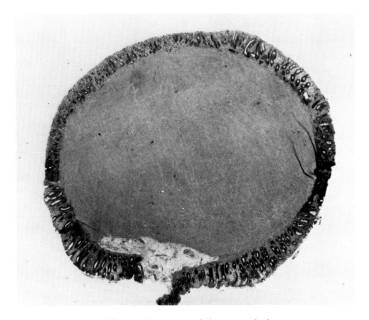

Fig. 7-21. Leiomyoma of the muscularis mucosae.

small intestine in the same manner as it does colon polyps. In this section we describe several polypoid lesions of the small intestine that may be of special interest to the surgical pathologist. We do not discuss malignant neoplasms, which are adequately covered in general textbooks, and, in particular, carcinoids, which are discussed in another chapter.

Polyps formed by inflammatory lesions in the small intestine are limited, with inflammatory fibroid polyp being the most definite entity. Hyperplastic polyps analagous to those in the colon and stomach are not described. Nodular lymphoid hyperplasia is discussed in the section on polyposis syndromes, below. Hamartomatous polyps, probably the most common type of epithelial polyp, are discussed in the section on colon polyps, above, and that on polyposis syndromes, below.

This leaves mainly benign neoplasms for consideration. In a comprehensive review in 1956, River, Silverstein, and Tope[42] analyzed 1,399 benign neoplasms of the small intestine and demonstrated their great diversity. At that time epithelial neoplasms were not well classified, but made up less than 25 percent of the benign neoplasms. The wide variety of nonepithelial lesions included, in order of frequency, lipoma, myoma, fibroma, angioma, neurogenic tumors, lymphangiomas, and other miscellaneous types.

INFLAMMATORY FIBROID POLYP

Inflammatory fibroid polyp[43, 44] is a benign lesion of unknown etiology that can form a polypoid mass anywhere in the gastrointestinal tract, although it is most frequent in stomach and small intestine. Most consider it to be inflammatory rather than neoplastic. Usually solitary, the majority of the small intestinal lesions occur in the ileum.[43, 44] These lesions can be sessile or, more commonly, pedunculated. Although the size varies greatly, they tend to be rather bulky in the small intestine (average diameter of 4 cm in a recent series of 10 cases).[44] They appear to arise in the submucosa and are covered by mucosa, which is frequently ulcerated. Encapsulation is not a feature, but the lesion is

usually well circumscribed. They can occasionally be dumbbell shaped, with a serosal component.

The polyps are composed primarily of loose connective tissue, often with a myxoid appearance (Fig. 7-22). They have a prominent vascular component, with many lesions containing a distinctive zone of loose connective tissue around some of the larger vessels (Fig. 7-23). There is considerable variability in the degree of cellularity. Eosinophils are a frequent and prominent component, and are spread evenly throughout the lesion. Mature plasma cells, lymphocytes, histiocytes, polymorphonuclear leukocytes, and mast cells are frequently observed. At times small lymphoid aggregates are present. Patients often present with signs of small intestinal obstruction, and intussusception is frequent. Peripheral eosinophilia is not a feature. There is no malignant potential.

BRUNNER'S GLAND "ADENOMA"

Localized overgrowth of mature-appearing Brunner's glands is a rare lesion occurring in the first portion of the duodenum or occasionally more distally.[45] The presence of Paneth cells, maturity of the glands, and ill-defined margins suggests that the lesion is a focal hyperplasia or a hamartoma rather than a true neoplasm. The lesion is quite rare, may occur at any age, and may produce nonspecific symptoms such as hemorrhage or obstruction. It is unassociated with other conditions, and is cured by simple removal.

ADENOMATOUS POLYP

Adenomatous polyp (tubular adenoma) morphologically similar to that in the colon is exceedingly rare in the small intestine. In the early literature, many epithelial lesions classified as adenomas were probably hamartomas, inflammatory lesions, villous adenomas, or Brunner's gland adenomas. Tubular adenomas very rarely occur in the ileum in patients with familial polyposis coli,[46] and they have been illustrated in

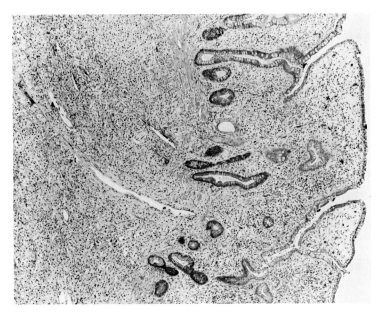

Fig. 7-22. Inflammatory fibroid polyp of small intestine with connective tissue and inflammatory infiltrate occupying submucosa and lamina propria. The glandular epithelium is unremarkable.

the duodenum[47] and stomach[47, 48] in Japanese. A tubulovillous lesion was found in the jejunum of a patient with juvenile polyposis.[49] From our own experience and review of the literature we are unsure whether solitary tubular adenomas occur as an entity in the small intestine. At best, they are very rare.

VILLOUS ADENOMA

In contrast to tubular adenoma, villous adenoma of the small intestine[50–52] appears to be a distinct but rare entity, with most lesions occurring proximally, mostly in the duodenum. One has been found in a Meckel's diverticulum.[50] The morphology and age distribution appear to be the same as for villous adenoma of the colon.[51, 52] Many occur in the region of the papilla of Vater and some obstruct it, causing jaundice. Villous architecture is found in the majority of small intestinal adenomas, probably reflecting the fact that villi are a normal architectural feature in this area. The predilection for carcinoma is higher than in the colon, with as many as 65 percent of such lesions having been reported to contain carcinoma.[53]

NEUROGENIC POLYPS

Neoplasms of nerve origin in the small intestine include neurofibroma, neurilemoma, ganglioneuroma, and paraganglioma. These lesions arise in the wall, probably most often in Auerbach's plexus, and may extend serosally or bulge into the lumen to produce a polyp or mass. Only a small portion of patients with Von Recklinghausen's disease have gastrointestinal lesions, and most of these are in the stomach.

Neurofibroma and neurilemoma are the most common nerve tumors in the small intestine but only a small portion are associated with neurofibromatosis.[54] Solitary lesions may be found at any level in the small intestine.

Ganglioneuromas are very rare in the gastrointestinal tract, may be found from stomach to rectum, with over half occurring in the stomach and appendix, and have been multiple in a few cases.[55–57]

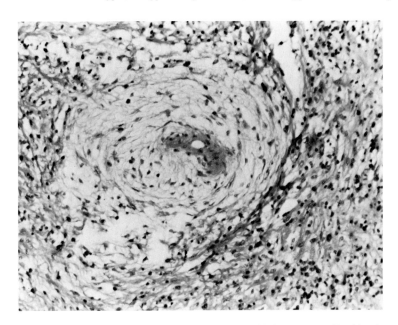

Fig. 7-23. Characteristic clear area around vessel of inflammatory fibroid polyp.

Gangliocytic paragangliomas are uncommon neoplasms that usually arise in the duodenal mucosa near the ampulla, although they may be found in the jejunum. They are most commonly seen in males in the fifth decade, and present as polypoid submucosal lesions about 2 cm in diameter. They may ulcerate and cause gastrointestinal bleeding. Histologically a mixture of elements may be found, including those resembling typical neurofibroma, ganglion cells associated with Schwann cells, and clusters of clear epithelioid cells with a neuroendocrine appearance. The tumor usually contains multiple polypeptide hormones, although these do not ordinarily produce clinical manifestations. The course is usually benign.[58-61]

LYMPHANGIECTATIC CYST

Lymphangiectatic cysts of the small intestine are thin-walled cystic spaces of the submucosa filled with yellow to milky fluid. They are often multiple, are more common proximally, and are usually only slightly elevated but occasionally polypoid. A large polypoid lesion is illustrated in Figure 7-24. They are usually unilocular but may be multilocular, and may extend into the mucosa. They are asymptomatic and are rarely encountered in surgical material, but are found in up to 20 percent of autopsies.[62]

POLYPOSIS SYNDROMES

The types of polyps found in polyposis syndromes resemble those found singly or in small numbers, and so the pathologist must be aware of the number of polyps present, the age of the patient, the family history, and other information that will serve to identify a patient with polyposis. In the past, families with polyposis have gone undiscovered because of a failure to consider isolated polyps as potential indicators of polyposis. Recent studies of polyposis have resulted in the discovery of more types, each with its own behavior pattern.

FAMILIAL POLYPOSIS COLI

Familial polyposis coli is a genetic disease in which the strong tendency to form multiple

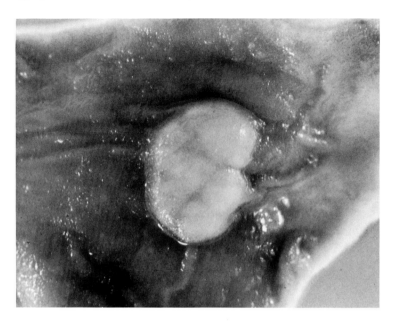

Fig. 7-24. Lymphangiectatic cyst of small intestine filled with creamy white fluid.

(greater than 100) adenomas in the colon is transmitted in an autosomal dominant fashion.[63]

Gross Pathology

The adenomas (and cancers derived from them) are identical in appearance to those of individually occurring tubular, tubulovillous, and villous adenomas. However, villous adenomas are relatively uncommon. Almost all the polyps are less than 1.0 cm in diameter at the time of diagnosis, and the majority of these are less than 0.5 cm[63] (Fig. 7-25).

Microscopic Pathology

Although the appearance of the individual polyps is identical to that described for singly occurring adenomas, a characteristic feature is the presence of multiple small adenomas involving only a few adjacent crypts, or even only a single crypt or portion thereof (Fig. 7-26). Ultrastructural differences have been reported.[64, 65]

Pathogenesis

The pathogenesis is uncertain, although clearly the genetic aspect is dominant. Penetrance is estimated at about 80 percent. It is not certain what contribution is made by environmental factors in susceptible individuals.

Location

The adenomas are found throughout the colon, including the appendix. In general, the numbers of polyps increases distally, although occasionally the area with the largest number of polyps will be the right colon or, rarely, the transverse colon.

Multiplicity

In 39 carefully counted cases, the number of polyps ranged from 104 to 5,000, with an average of 1,000.[63] No clearly familial cases with less than 100 polyps have been reported, and this number has been used as a somewhat arbitrary minimum number of lesions for a diagnosis of familial polyposis coli.

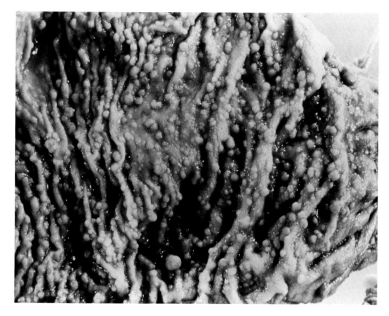

Fig. 7-25. Familial polyposis coli with colonic mucosa carpeted with small tubular adenomas.

Age and Sex

Approximately equal numbers of men and women are affected. The typical age sequence has been reported as follows: adenomas appear at 24.5 years; symptoms appear at 33.0 years; adenomas are diagnosed at 35.8 years; and cancer appears at 39.2 years.[63] The youngest patient diagnosed with adenomas was 4 years old, although diagnosis prior to 10 years of age is

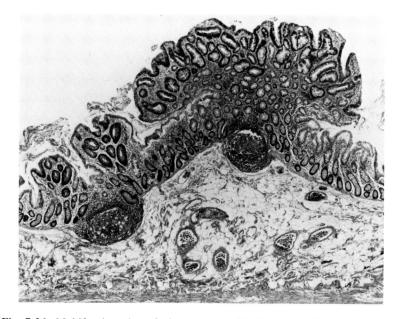

Fig. 7-26. Multifocal patches of adenomatous epithelium in familial polyposis coli.

distinctly uncommon; the adenomas in family members do not usually appear until the early teenage years. In the largest series (at St. Mark's Hospital)[63] the oldest patient at the time of diagnosis was 53 years old, although occasionally even older patients are discovered to have polyposis.

Behavior

Polyposis coli may be completely asymptomatic. Symptoms, when present, include rectal bleeding and, less commonly, a mucous discharge. Cancer develops in virtually all patients not treated with a colectomy. The incidence is about 10 percent in patients observed for 5 years, but about 50 percent in those observed for 20 years. Multiple cancers are frequent, with synchronous lesions occurring in 40.9 percent and metachronous lesions in 6.7 percent. The cancers appear to arise from adenomas in many instances; 36.2 percent of the cancers have identifiable contiguous adenomas, compared with 10.6 percent of the cancers in nonpolyposis patients. In many patients, a rectal stump is left behind. The adenomas have been observed to regress in the stump, but can reappear. Of 89 patients whose rectal stump was carefully observed, 2 patients developed carcinoma.

GARDNER'S SYNDROME

Gardner's syndrome is similar if not identical to familial polyposis coli with regard to inheritance and the colonic lesion. The difference is the presence of extracolonic lesions. At least one of a variety of lesions is present in affected patients.[66] These include osteomas, particularly of the mandible and maxilla. A variety of soft tissue tumors, including desmoids, often of the mesentery or abdominal wall, and subcutaneous lesions such as lipomas, fibromas, and epidermoid cysts, are common and appear at a young age. This often allows early diagnosis in affected family members. A variety of polypoid lesions involving the stomach and adenomas of the small intestine, particularly the duodenum, have been documented. Periampullary carcinoma also appears in some affected family members.

Controversy exists concerning whether this represents a distinct entity or one end of a spectrum continuous with familial polyposis coli. At least 50 of approximately 200 families with adenomatous polyps in the St. Mark's Hospital register of polyposis patients have at least one member with Gardner's syndrome.[63] The line between classic familial polyposis coli and Gardner's syndrome has been blurred by the frequent demonstration by means of sensitive radiologic techniques of bony jaw lesions in patients with polyposis but no other lesions of Gardner's syndrome.[67] Also, a similar group, when examined carefully endoscopically and histologically, showed a high incidence of a variety of gastric polyps.[50]

It has been reported that there appear to be fewer polyps in the colon and that these are more widely distributed in patients with Gardner's syndrome, compared with classic familial polyposis coli.[68] This has not been confirmed by the material in the St. Mark's Hospital registry.[63] In all other aspects, the appearance and behavior of the lesions in Gardner's syndrome and those in classic familial polyposis appear to be identical with regard to the colon.

TURCOT'S SYNDROME

The combination of malignant central nervous system neoplasms and familial polyposis coli has been called *Turcot's syndrome*.[69, 70] It has been noted in a very small number of individuals, with apparent autosomal recessive inheritance in the first two families described.[69, 70] No unique aspects of the morphology of the colonic polyposis are described.

MULTIPLE ADENOMAS

The presence of multiple (less than 100) adenomas in the colon defines a group of patients who do not have so clearly a genetic disorder as has been observed in familial polyposis coli, but who do have an increased risk for carcinoma of the colon.

In a survey of patients with intestinal neoplasms at St. Mark's Hospital,[1] 1,846 had one or more adenomas, either wholly benign or with a focus of malignant change. Of these, 27.9 percent had more than one adenoma. Only 83 patients (4.5 percent) had more than five adenomas, and 58 of these patients had evidence for familial polyposis coli. In this series the group with familial polyposis had a minimum of about 200 polyps, whereas the nonfamilial group had a maximum of 48 polyps. Occasional patients reported elsewhere with nonfamilial multiple adenomas have had up to 70 polyps. For this reason, the presence of 100 adenomas has been used as a convenient, somewhat arbitrary, boundary between multiple adenomas and familial polyposis coli.

The percentage of patients with associated carcinoma increases with increasing numbers of adenomas; in the material from the St. Mark's Hospital survey, this percentage was 80 percent in the group with 6 to 48 polyps.

JUVENILE POLYPOSIS SYNDROME

The term *juvenile polyposis*[49, 71, 72] is used here to include patients with multiple juvenile polyps of the colon (more than a few) and juvenile polyps involving stomach and small intestine, with or without colonic involvement. It is likely that this classification includes more than one disease or syndrome. Some patients may also have adenomatous polyps or even villous adenomas, but these are not present in the numbers characteristic of familial polyposis coli.

Juvenile polyposis of infancy is the most distinct subgroup, although it is quite rare.[71] Onset of symptoms occurs within the first year of life. Large numbers of polyps involve the colon, small intestine, and stomach, and have typical juvenile polyp histology. Severe clinical problems, including hemorrhage, malnutrition, and intussusception, usually lead to a fatal outcome

by age 2 years in spite of therapy. No family history of polyposis has been found in these patients.

Cases of juvenile polyposis in older children and adults vary in their age of onset, number of polyps, location of polyps, development of further polyps, and histology of the polyps. The clinical course is variable, depending on number and location of polyps. Family history may be negative or may show a dominant inheritance pattern. Some families have associated gastrointestinal malignancies, which occur in patients with polyps or their relatives, often at a young age and in an unusual location.[49] Some families appear to have only colonic polyps,[72] hence the term *juvenile polyposis coli*. Involvement of stomach, small intestine, and large intestine is termed *generalized juvenile polyposis*. More cases will be needed to determine if this classification is justified.

Gross Pathology

The typical appearance of juvenile polyposis of infancy is illustrated in Figure 7-27. Juvenile polyposis in older patients varies in number of polyps, size of polyps, and location of polyps. Several patients have developed massive gastric involvement, which tends to involve the gastric body with sparing of the antrum (Fig. 7-28).

Microscopic Pathology

In the infantile form of juvenile polyposis, the age, abundance of polyps to be removed, and typical histology present no problems in diagnosis. The polypoid form of Menetrier's disease may mimic gastric juvenile polyposis, because both involve the body mucosa and both are microcystic. In Menetrier's disease the cystic change should involve the base of the glands with preservation of overlying glands. Juvenile polyps are more disorganized, edematous, and inflamed, and tend to be more polypoid. Some patients have had both adenomatous and juvenile polyps and polyps with mixed features in the colon.

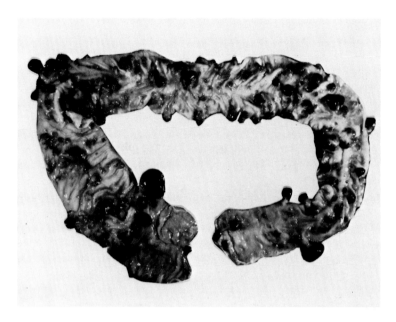

Fig. 7-27. Colon in infantile juvenile polyposis.

Age and Sex

Most children from 1 to 10 years of age with juvenile polyps have a solitary polyp or a few polyps; this should not be considered polyposis.

The diagnosis of juvenile polyposis is based on the age of the patient, the number of polyps, the location of the polyps (usually higher than the rectum), and family history. In patients over 10 years of age, the occurrence of juvenile pol-

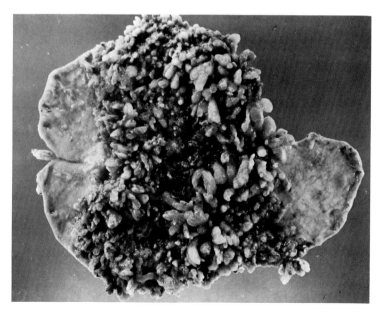

Fig. 7-28. Multiple gastric polypoid lesions with antral sparing in an adult with multiple juvenile polyposis.

yps takes on a greater chance of being part of the polyposis syndrome, and clinical investigation of family history and search for other polyps in the gastrointestinal tract should be considered.

Pathogenesis

Juvenile polyposis of infancy has not been associated with a positive family history; it could be due to a dominant mutation or a recessive trait. In older patients, juvenile polyposis of the colon and more generalized juvenile polyposis of the gastrointestinal tract sometimes show a dominant mode of inheritance and sometimes occur sporadically. Obtaining an accurate family history is much more difficult than with familial polyposis coli because the disease has onset at variable ages, cannot be excluded by a simple examination such as sigmoidoscopy, and may be manifest in variable ways. In a few families, gastrointestinal carcinomas, have developed in patients with juvenile polyposis or their relatives, often at a young age and at unusual locations. Since the carcinomas do not appear to arise in the polyps, and since they may occur at all levels of the gastrointestinal tract, prophylactic treatment is impractical and early diagnosis difficult.

PEUTZ-JEGHERS SYNDROME

A patient with the full syndrome[31–33, 73–75] will have (1) multiple polyps of Peutz-Jeghers type, which may involve small intestine, colon, and/or stomach; (2) mucocutaneous pigmentation; and (3) a family history suggestive of dominant inheritance pattern. The family history may be negative and the patient and/or family members may have polyps without pigmentation or pigmentation without polyps.

Gross Pathology

Data on the average number of polyps are lacking because total resection is not undertaken and polyps continue to develop over time. How-

ever, most patients have several to many polyps. Size varies from a few millimeters to a few centimeters. Although resected polyps tend to be large and pedunculated, they may be sessile. Intussusception, obstruction, and ulceration with hemorrhage are common.

Microscopic Pathology

Variations on the typical morphology previously described include superimposed inflammation, entrapped mucus, mild atypia, and pseudoinvasion. Care should be taken not to overdiagnose carcinoma. Carcinoma developing in a Peutz-Jeghers polyp is rare.[75]

Pathogenesis

The syndrome is caused by a dominant gene with variable expressivity. It may also arise by mutation, with up to 45 percent of cases lacking family history.[31]

Location

Most patients have jejunal or ileal polyps. Polyps of the colon, stomach, duodenum, and appendix occur less frequently, in that order.

Age and Sex

There is no sex preference. Age of onset is variable, ranging from early childhood to late adulthood, but most are first manifest in patients 10 to 30 years old.

Behavior

Asymptomatic patients may be discovered on the basis of family history or a finding of mucocutaneous pigmentation. It is not known whether the polyps can be present at birth, but it is clear that new ones can continue to develop at variable intervals throughout life. The usual sequence is for the polyps to become large enough to cause partial obstruction, intussusception, or hemorrhage and be removed surgically. Because of the liability of developing more polyps, preservation of bowel takes a high priority. The early literature suggested a higher cancer risk, but this was shown to be largely attributable to overdiagnosis of pseudoinvasion. For a number of years the cancer risk, based on gastrointestinal primary lesions with metastases, has been estimated at 2 to 3 percent.[73] Recent evidence suggests that this may be an underestimate with regard to the gastrointestinal lesions and especially to tumors arising outside the gastrointestinal tract.[74] These extraintestinal tumors include some highly characteristic for Peutz-Jeghers syndrome (sex cord tumors with annular tubules) as well as some more common neoplasms (primary tumors in the breast, pancreas, endometrium, cervix, and lung) appearing at an early age.

CRONKHITE-CANADA SYNDROME

Cronkhite-Canada syndrome,[76, 77] first described in 1955,[76] is an acquired, non-neoplastic polypoid change that usually involves stomach, small intestine, and colon, and is associated with pigmentation of the skin, loss of hair, and dystrophy of the nails. The diarrhea, protein-losing enteropathy, and weight loss, along with the associated skin changes and polypoid changes in gastrointestinal mucosa, distinguish this rate, distinct entity of unknown cause. The gross appearance varies from diffuse micronodularity of the mucosa to larger more pedunculated polyps that may appear gelatinous. Microscopically, there is usually diffuse mucosal change, with cystic dilation of glands and variable edema and chronic inflammatory changes in the mucosa. The nonuniformity of these changes and regenerative activity result in polypoid mucosa. The lesions differ from juvenile polyps in that they are diffuse rather than isolated hamartomatous masses, and they occur in older adults. The gastric lesions may resemble those of Menetrier's disease grossly because of the cystic change.

Cronkhite-Canada lesions are usually found in stomach, small intestine, and colon, and may involve esophagus. They are usually described as diffuse polyposis or pseudopolyposis. Patients with this condition are over 30 years of age, with mean age of 60 years, and there is a slight male predominance. Some patients have died from the effects of the disease but most die from other causes. Remissions have occurred, especially with steroid therapy, and polypoid lesions have regressed, supporting the concept of an inflammatory cause.

COWDEN'S SYNDROME (MULTIPLE HAMARTOMA)

Cowden's syndrome,[78, 79] described in 1963[78] and named after the family in which it occurred, is a very rare condition, probably autosomal dominant, with multiple orocutaneous hamartomas, proliferative lesions of breast and thyroid in women, and variable other hamartomatous/proliferative lesions, including polyps of the entire gastrointestinal tract. The polyps, which have been studied in only a few cases, appear to vary in size, shape, number, and location, and microscopically exhibit cystic dilation of glands, inflammation, and regenerative changes. Many of these polypoid lesions contain mature ganglion cells and neural fibers in the lamina propria and have been designated *ganglioneuromas*. Onset in the second decade and the morphology of the polyps mimic juvenile polyposis, but the occurrence of other hamartomatous features distinguishes the two syndromes.

NODULAR LYMPHOID HYPERPLASIA (LYMPHOID POLYPOSIS)

Multifocal lymphoid follicles[37, 80, 81] or aggregates that extrude into bowel lumen to form small, rounded polyps do not really represent a syndrome, but rather a manifestation of lymphoid hyperplasia. The term *nodular lymphoid hyperplasia* is preferred.

The small nodules of lymphoid tissue in the lamina propria and superficial submucosa containing follicles with germinal centers should be easily distinguished from the very rare nodular lymphomatous polyposis of the intestines. Nodular lymphoid hyperplasia can be divided into three etiologic categories: (1) idiopathic, (2) reactive, and (3) associated with hypogammaglobulinemia. The idiopathic group is most common, and may involve small intestine and/or colon. It may be found in children as an incidental finding, in persons suspected of having appendicitis, and in older persons. Reactive nodular lymphoid hyperplasia has been observed in the ileum of patients with ulcerative colitis and familial polyposis.[80] In the latter condition the polyps may appear grossly similar to early adenomas (Fig. 7-29). Nodular lymphoid hyperplasia associated with acquired late-onset hypogammaglobulinemia is usually confined to the small intestine and exhibits a paucity of plasma cells in the adjacent mucosa. Giardiasis is associated with this form, but not with the other types. Most patients with hypogammaglobulinemia do not have nodular lymphoid hyperplasia.

OTHER POLYPOSIS SYNDROMES

There are several other unusual polyposis syndromes. These include colon adenomas associated with multiple sebaceous cysts (Oldfield's syndrome), colon adenomas associated with cartilaginous exostoses (Zanca's syndrome), colon hamartomas associated with variable congenital anomalies (Ruvalcaba-Myhre-Smith syndrome), and inflammatory-type polyps of stomach and ileum (Devon family syndrome). An excellent overview of miscellaneous polyposis syndromes is to be found in a recent major gastrointestinal pathology text.[82]

POLYP-CARCINOMA SEQUENCE

The local effects produced by intestinal polyps are more easily dealt with than their potential for malignancy. The pathologist, however, is most often called on to evaluate the malignant potential of polyps at both a theoretical and practical level.

One can state that there is no evidence of

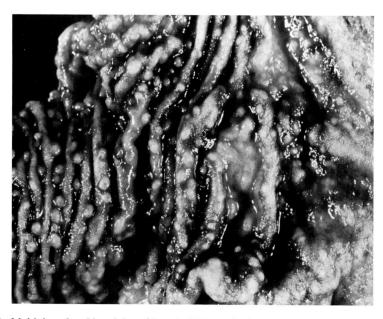

Fig. 7-29. Multiple polypoid nodules of lymphoid tissue in the terminal ileum mimicking adenomas.

malignant potential for hyperplastic polyps of the colon, nonfamilial solitary juvenile polyps of the colon in childhood, leiomyoma of the muscularis mucosae, lipoma, inflammatory fibroid polyp, Brunner's gland "adenoma," and lymphangiectatic cyst. Further, solitary Peutz-Jeghers polyps and neurogenic polyps do not appear to undergo malignant transformation, although patients with Peutz-Jeghers syndrome and Von Recklinghausen's disease have a slight tendency to develop carcinomas and neurogenic sarcomas, respectively. Cronkhite-Canada syndrome, Cowden's syndrome, nodular lymphoid hyperplasia, and small intestine lipomatosis are not clearly related to the development of malignancy.

The evidence for a relationship between colon adenomas and the subsequent development of colonic cancer is now incontestable. The majority of colon cancers appear to arise in pre-existing adenomas. The smaller the colon cancer, the more likely it is that one will find a residual component of benign adenoma. Size is the feature of paramount importance. In classic studies, it has been shown that the risk for invasive carcinoma is approximately 1.3 percent in those adenomas less than 1 cm in greatest diameter, 9.5 percent for those between 1 and 2 cm in greatest diameter, and 46 percent for those over 2 cm in greatest diameter.[1] When corrected for size, the degree of villous architecture then becomes the next most important feature. For example, in polyps under 1 cm in diameter 1 percent of tubular adenomas, 3.9 percent of tubulovillous adenomas, and 9.5 percent of villous adenomas will show foci of malignant transformation. In those lesions over 2 cm in greatest diameter, the corresponding percentage of adenomas showing malignant change is 34.7, 45.8, and 52.9 percent, respectively. One must be careful that malignant degeneration is carefully defined. In its earliest stage, epithelial changes will be present in a group of tubules within the adenoma and will be confined by their basement membranes. Although this can be properly referred to as *carcinoma in situ,* most laboratories report such change as *severe atypia*. The next step would be penetration of the basement membranes by the atypical glands into the surrounding lamina propria. This uncommon lesion

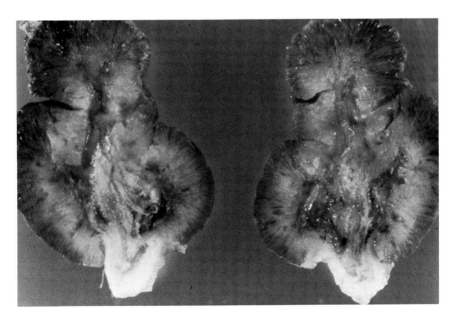

Fig. 7-30. Well-fixed adenoma bisected along its stalk; cautery has left an ashen white discoloration at the resection margin.

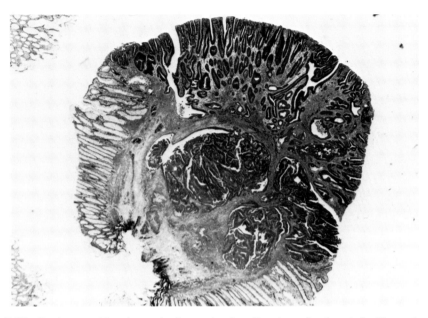

Fig. 7-31. Carcinoma with a desmoplastic reaction invading the stalk of a tubulovillous adenoma.

is referred as *intramucosal carcinoma*. Neither severe atypia (carcinoma in situ) nor intramucosal carcinoma has been clearly shown to be capable of distant metastases. The diagnosis of invasive carcinoma should not be made until the tumor has been shown to extend through the muscularis mucosae. This may be done if the biopsy specimen is sufficiently large that architecture is discernible; alternatively, the diagnosis can be made presumptively by the presence of a desmoplastic reaction to the atypical glands. Once a diagnosis of invasive carcinoma has been established, there still remain several tasks for both the pathologist and the clinician. There has been an ever-increasing number of polypectomy specimens appearing in surgical pathology laboratories. When invasive carcinoma is found in one of these specimens, the pathologist must provide information helpful in determining whether further therapy is needed. Currently, three parameters are evaluated in order to determine whether a polypectomy is sufficient therapy for a malignant polyp.[83–85] If the tumor is of high grade, is present in capillary-lymphatic spaces, or is present in the margin of resection, further surgical therapy is indicated. In order to report reliably on these parameters, meticulous handling of the polypectomy specimen from the time it arrives in the laboratory is of great importance; proper fixation and orientation are key elements to proper handling of polypectomy specimens (Figs. 7-30 and 7-31).

GENETIC ALTERATIONS IN COLORECTAL TUMORS

Much recent work has been done in this area. Several important genetic alterations have been noted in colorectal neoplasms.[86] One of the most important of these is *ras*-gene mutations, which may be a frequent early event in the genesis of colon tumors. Such mutations have been found in about half of both carcinomas and adenomas. Another important alteration in colorectal neoplasms is the allelic deletion of chromosome 5. A locus, referred to as the *fap* locus, has been mapped to the long arm of chromosome 5. It has been hypothesized that the *fap* locus may encode a tumor-suppressor gene. This locus has been reported to be lost in approximately one-third of colon adenomas and carcinomas. It has also been reported that there is loss of chromosome 17 and 18 sequences in colon carcinoma. There is also some evidence that, while alterations in chromosomes 5, 17, and 18 are particularly common in colon neoplasms, alterations may occur in other chromosomes. Current speculation suggests that there may be accumulated alterations affecting at least one dominantly acting oncogene and several tumor suppressor genes, which leads to the development of colorectal adenomas and, subsequently, carcinomas.

REFERENCES

1. Morson BC: The Pathogenesis of Colorectal Cancer. WB Saunders, Philadelphia, 1978
2. Morson BC, Dawson IMP: Gastrointestinal Pathology. Blackwell, Oxford, 1979
3. Morson BC, Sobin LH, et al: Histologic Typing of Intestinal Tumors. International Histologic Classification of Tumors. No. 15. World Health Organization, Geneva, 1976
4. Arthur JF: Structure and significance of metaplastic nodules in the rectal mucosa. J Clin Pathol 21:735, 1968
5. Goldman H, Ming S, Hickock DF: Nature and significance of hyperplastic polyps of the human colon. Arch Pathol 89:349, 1970
6. Lane N, Kaplan H, Pascal RR: Minute adenomatous and hyperplastic polyps of the colon: divergent patterns of epithelial growth with specific associated mesenchymal changes. Gastroenterology 60:537, 1971
7. Kaye GI, Pascal RR, Lane N: The colonic pericryptal fibroblast sheath: replication, migration and cytodifferentiation of a mesenchymal cell system in adult tissue. Gastroenterology 60:515, 1971
8. Kaye GI, Fenoglio CM, Pascal RR, Lane N: Comparative electron microscopic features of normal, hyperplastic, and adenomatous human colonic epithelium. Gastroenterology 64:926, 1973
9. Hayashi T, Yatani R, Apostol J, Stemmermann GN: Pathogenesis of hyperplastic polyps of the colon: a hypothesis based on ultrastructure and in vitro cell kinetics. Gastroenterology 66:347, 1974
10. Wiebeck B, Brandts A, Eder M: Epithelial proliferation and morphogenesis of hyperplastic adenomatous and villous polyps of the human colon. Virchows Arch [A] 364:35, 1974
11. Qizilbash AH: Mucoceles of the appendix. Their relationship to hyperplastic polyps, mucinous cystadenomas, and cytadenocarcinomas. Arch Pathol 99:548, 1975
12. Williams GT, Arthur JF, Bussey HJR, Morson BC: Metaplastic polyps and polyposis of the colorectum. Histopathology 4:155, 1980
13. Longacre TA, Ferroglio-Preiser CM: Mixed hyperplastic adenomatous polyps/serrated adenomas. Am J Surg Pathol 14:524, 1990
14. Grinnell RS, Lane N: Benign and malignant adenomatous polyps and papillary adenomas of the colon and rectum. An analysis of 1,856 tumors in 1,335 patients. Int Abstr Surg 106:519, 1958
15. Gibbs NM: Incidence and significance of argentaffin and Paneth cells in some tumors of the large intestine. J Clin Pathol 20:826, 1967
16. Deschner EE, Lipkin M: Proliferative patterns in colonic mucosa in familial polyposis. Cancer 35:413, 1975
17. Lane N, Lev R: Observations on the origin of adenomatous epithelium of the colon. Cancer 16:751, 1963
18. Maskens AP: Histogenesis of adenomatous polyps in the human large intestine. Gastroenterology 77:1245, 1979
19. Shinya H, Wolff WI: Morphology, anatomic distribution and cancer potential of colonic polyps. Ann Surg 190:679, 1979
20. Correa P, Strong JP, Reif A, Johnson WD: The epidemiology of colorectal polyps. Cancer 39:2258, 1977
21. Muto T, Bussey HJR, Morson BC: The evolution of cancer of the colon and rectum. Cancer 36:2251, 1975
22. Muto T, Bussey JR, Morson BC: Pseudo-carcinomatous invasion in adenomatous polyps of the colon and rectum. J Clin Pathol 26:25, 1973
23. Qizilbash AH, Meghji M, Castelli M: Pseudocarcinomatous invasion in adenomas of the colon and rectum. Dis Colon Rectum 23:529, 1980
24. Quan SH, Castro EB: Papillary adenomas (villous tumors): a review of 215 cases. Dis Colon Rectum 14:267, 1971
25. Elias H, Hyde DM, Mullens RS, Lambert FC: Colonic adenomas: Sterology and growth mechanisms. Dis Colon Rectum 24:331, 1981
26. Appel MF, Spjut HJ, Estrada RG: The signifi-

cance of villous component in colonic polyps. Am J Surg 134:770, 1977

27. Kurzon RM, Ortega R, Rywlin AM: The significance of papillary features in polyps of the large intestine. Am J Clin Pathol 62:447, 1974

28. Horrilleno EG, Eckert C, Ackerman LV: Polyps of the rectum and colon in children. Cancer 10:1210, 1957

29. Roth SI, Helwig EB: Juvenile polyps of the colon and rectum, Cancer 16:468, 1963

30. Silverberg SG: "Juvenile" retention polyps of the colon and rectum. Am J Dig Dis 15:617, 1970

31. Bartholomew LG, Dahlin DC, Waugh JM: Intestinal polyposis associated with mucocutaneous melanin pigmentation (Peutz-Jeghers syndrome). Gastroenterology 32:434, 1957

32. Gannon PG, Dahlin DC, Bartholomew LG, Beahrs OH: Polypoid glandular tumors of the small intestine. Surg Gynecol Obstet 114:666, 1962

33. Bartholomew LG, Moore CE, Dahlin DC, Waugh JM: Intestinal polyposis associated with mucocutaneous pigmentation. Surg Gynecol Obstet 115:1, 1962

34. Dawson IMP, Pryse-Davies A: The development of carcinoma of the large intestine in ulcerative colitis. Br J Surg 47:113, 1959

35. Helwig EB, Hansen J: Lymphoid polyps (benign lymphoma) and malignant lymphoma of the rectum and anus. Surg Gynecol Obstet 92:233, 1951

36. Cornes JS, Wallace MH, Morson BC: Benign lymphomas of the rectum and anal canal: a study of 100 cases. J Pathol Bacteriol 82:371, 1961

37. Ranchod M, Lewin KJ, Dorfman RF: Lymphoid hyperplasia of the gastrointestinal tract. Am J Surg Pathol 2:383, 1978

38. Tiedemann RN, McDivitt RM, Thorbjarnarson B: Carcinoid tumor of rectum. NY State J Med 72:559, 1972

39. Genre CF, Roth LM, Reed RJ: "Benign" rectal carcinoids: a report of two patients with metastases to regional lymph nodes. Am J Clin Pathol 56:750, 1971

40. Castro EB, Sterns MW: Lipoma of the large intestine. Dis Colon Rectum 15:441, 1972

41. Wolf BS: Lipoma of the colon. JAMA, 235:2225, 1976

42. River L, Silverstein J, Tope JW: Benign neoplasms of the small intestine. Int Abstr Surg 102:1, 1956

43. LiVolsi VA, Perzom LJ: Inflammatory pseudo-tumors (inflammatory fibrous polyps) of the small intestine: a clinicopathologic study. Dig Dis Sci 20:325, 1975

44. Johnstone, JM, Morson BC: Inflammatory fibroid polyp of the gastrointestinal tract. Histopathology 2:349, 1978

45. ReMine W, Brown P, Gomes M, Harrison R: Polypoid hamartomas of Brunner's glands. Arch Surg 100:313, 1970

46. Hamilton SR, Bussey HJR, Mendelsohn G, et al: Ileal adenomas after colectomy in nine patients with adenomatous polyposis coli/Gardner's Syndrome. Gastroenterology 77:1252, 1979

47. Ranzi T, Castagnone D, Valio P, et al: Gastric and duodenal polyps in familial polyposis coli. Gut 22:363, 1981

48. Watanabe H, Enjoji E, Yao T, et al: Accompanying gastroenteric lesions in familial adenomatous coli. Acta Pathol Jpn 27:823, 1977

49. Stemper TJ, Kent TH, Summers R: Juvenile polyposis and gastrointestinal carcinoma. Ann Intern Med 83:639, 1975

50. Adbel-Bari W: Villous adenomas with focal adenocarcinoma in a Meckel's diverticulum. Am J Clin Pathol 48:183, 1967

51. Mir-Madjlessi SH, Farmer RG, Hawk WA: Villous tumors of the duodenum and jejunum. Am J Dig Dis 18:467, 1973

52. Komorowski RA, Cohen EB: Villous tumors of the duodenum: a clinicopathologic study. Cancer 47:1377, 1981

53. Perzin KH, Bridge MF: Adenomas of the small intestine: a clinopathological review of 51 cases and a study of their relationship to carcinoma. Cancer 48:799, 1981

54. Sivak MV, Sullivan BH, Farmer RG: Neurogenic tumors of the small intestine. Gastroenterology 68:374, 1975

55. Gemer M, Feuchtwanger MM: Gangiloneuroma of the duodenum. Gastroenterology 51:689, 1966

56. Donnelly WB, Sieber WK, Yunis EJ: Polypoid ganglioneurofibromatosis of the large bowel. Arch Pathol 87:537, 1969

57. Shuster M, Causing WC, Zito PF: Ganglioneurofibromatous polyposis of the gastrointestinal tract. Am J Gastroenterol 55:58, 1971

58. Taylor HB, Helwig EB: Benign nonchromaffin paragangliomas of the duodenum. Virchows Arch [A] 335:356, 1962

59. Kepes JJ, Zacharias DL: Gangliocytic paragangliomas of the duodenum. Cancer 27:61, 1971

60. Perrone T, Sibley RK, Roasi J: Duodenal gangli-

ocytic paraganglioma: an Immunohistochemical and ultrastructural study and a hypothesis concerning its origin. Am J Surg Pathol 9:31, 1985

61. Hamid QA, Dhillon AP, Sibley RK: Duodenal gangliocytic paragangliomas: a study of 10 cases with immunocytochemical neuroendocrine markers. Hum Pathol 17:403, 1986

62. Shilkin KB, Zerman BJ, Blackwell JB: Lymphangiectatic cysts of the small bowel. J Pathol Bacteriol 96:353, 1969

63. Bussey HJR: Familial Polyposis Coli. Johns Hopkins University Press, Baltimore, 1975

64. Dawson PA, Filipe MI, Bussey HJR: Ultrastructural features of the colonic epithelium in familial polyposis coli. Histopathology 1:105, 1977

65. Birbeck MSC, Dukes CG: Electron microscopy of rectal neoplasms. Proc R Soc Med 56:793, 1963

66. Naylor EW, Lebenthal E: Gardner's syndrome: recent developments in research and management. Dig Dis Sci 25:945, 1980

67. Ooya K, Yamamoto H, Lay KM: Sclerotic masses in the mandible of a patient with familial polyposis of the colon. J Oral Pathol 5:305, 1976

68. McKusick VA: Genetic factors in intestinal polyposis. JAMA 182:271, 1962

69. Turcot J, Despres JP, St. Pierre F: Malignant tumors of the central nervous system associated with familial polyposis of the colon. Dis Colon Rectum 2:465, 1959

70. Baughman FA, List CF, Williams JR, et al: The glioma-polyposis syndrome. N Engl J Med 281:1345, 1969

71. Sachatello CR, Carrington CG: Juvenile gastrointestinal polyposis in a female infant: report of a case and review of the literature of a recently recognized syndrome. Surgery 75:107, 1974

72. Grotsky HW, Rickert RR, Smith WD, Newsome JF: Familial juvenile polyposis coli. Gastroenterology 82:494, 1982

73. Reid JD: Intestinal carcinoma in the Peutz-Jeghers syndrome. JAMA 229:833, 1974

74. Giardiello FM, Welsh SB, Hamilton SR, et al: Increased risk of cancer in Peutz-Jegher's syndrome. N Engl J Med 316:1511, 1987

75. Matuchansky C, Babin P, Coutrot S, et al: Peutz-Jeghers syndrome with metastasizing carcinoma arising from a jejunal hamartoma. Gastroenterology 77:1311, 1979

76. Cronkhite LW Jr, Cancada WF: Generalized gastrointestinal polyposis. N Engl J Med 252:1011, 1955

77. Nonomura A, Ohta G, Ibata T, et al: Cronkhite-Canada syndrome associated with sigmoid cancer. Acta Pathol Jpn 30:825, 1980

78. Lloyd KM II, Dennis M: Cowden's disease. Ann Intern Med 58:136, 1963

79. Weinstock JV, Kawanishi H: Gastrointestinal polyposis with orocutaneous hamartomas (Cowden's disease). Gastroenterology 74:890, 1978

80. Fieber SS, Schaefer HJ: Lymphoid hyperplasia of the terminal ileum—a clinical entity? Gastroenterology 50:83, 1966

81. Shaw EB Jr, Hennigar GR: Intestinal lymphoid polyposis. Am J Clin Pathol 61:417, 1974

82. Fenoglio-Preiser CM, Lantz PE, Listrom MB, et al: Gastrointestinal Pathology: An Atlas and Text. Raven Press, New York, 1989

83. Cooper HS: Surgical pathology of endoscopically removed malignant polyps of the colon and rectum. Am J Surg Pathol 7:613, 1983

84. Haggitt RC, Glotybach RE, Soffer EE, et al: Prognostic factors in colorectal carcinomas arising in adenomas. Gastroenterology 89:328, 1985

85. Cranley JP, Petras RE, Carey WD, et al: When is endoscopic polypectomy adequate therapy for colonic polyps containing invasive carcinoma? Gastroenterology 91:419, 1986

86. Vogelstein B, Fearon ER, Hamilton SR, et al: Genetic alterations during colorectal-tumor development. N Engl J Med 319:525, 1988

8

Carcinoma of the Colon and Rectum

J. Ross Slemmer and Harry S. Cooper

Carcinoma of the colon and rectum is the second most common neoplasm (excluding non-melanoma skin cancer and carcinoma in situ) seen in the United States, with an estimated 155,000 new cases reported in 1989. By the end of 1990, this neoplasm will have been responsible for 11 percent and 13 percent of cancer deaths in males and females, respectively.[1] As pathologists our role is not only to diagnose this malignancy, but also to provide meaningful clinicopathologic correlation in order to afford the patient the best care possible. The literature regarding colorectal cancer is voluminous. Although this chapter is not intended to be a complete review, it focuses on the more recent literature in order to provide updated information on such topics as incidence, staging, survival, early colorectal cancer, oncogenes, cytogenetics, flow cytometry, and tumor antigens. It is hoped that the subjects presented encompass major points and will be helpful to the surgical pathologist.

EPIDEMIOLOGY

The incidence of large bowel carcinoma shows wide variation throughout the world. Colon cancer occurs much more frequently in North America and Northern Europe than in South America and is quite rare in Africa and Asia.[1] It is thought to be a disease of affluence, associated with a lifestyle in which large amounts of beef and fatty foods are consumed. Consumption of these foods may be responsible for the production of great amounts of cholesterol and its metabolites, which may be carcinogenic.[2]

The highest rates are recorded in Scotland, but these rates represent the rural beef-consuming areas.[3] The Seventh-Day Adventists in the United States, who consume less meat than others, have a relatively low rate of colon cancer.[2] One must recognize, however, that rates of carcinoma of the lower rectum and possibly of the cecum do not depend on socioeconomic factors. Studies have shown that the incidence of rectal cancer (at the 10-cm level or lower) and cecal cancer does not vary between the population in Hawaii and Cali, Columbia, although carcinomas of other areas of the large bowel show a marked increase in frequency among the more affluent Hawaiian population.[4] In Japan, colon cancer is much less common than in the United States, although the incidence of rectal cancer is similar. In Japan, those patients with colon cancer have a higher socioeconomic status and eat a more Westernized diet than patients with rectal cancer.[5] Studies of migrant communities have produced interesting data. Migrants from countries where the risk of colon cancer is low will acquire the increased risk of the new host country. An excellent example of this is the Hawaiian Japanese, in whom the incidence of colon cancer is the same as that of whites.[6]

SITE, SEX, AND AGE DISTRIBUTION

Traditional teaching has emphasized that two-thirds of all colorectal cancers are within the reach of the sigmoidoscope, and that 50 percent can be felt digitally.[7] In the United States, many

225

investigators have noted a changing site distribution of colorectal cancer, and this may have profound effects on screening procedures. Welch[8] found that the average incidence of rectal cancer fell from 42.7 to 33.2 percent over a 40-year period, whereas the incidence of sigmoid and ascending colon cancers rose during this period. Rhodes and colleagues[9] found a statistically significant decrease in rectal cancers and a significant rise in proximal lesions over a 30-year period (1946 to 1975). In 1946, 82 percent of lesions were found in the rectum, rectosigmoid, and sigmoid region, whereas in 1975, 60 percent of cancers were located in this region. Similarly, Cady and co-workers[10] have shown that over 40 years (1928 to 1967), right-sided cancers have increased from 7 to 22 percent of the total cases, whereas sigmoid, rectosigmoid, and rectal cancers fell from 80 to 62 percent. The group from St. Mark's Hospital, London, have noted a decreasing percentage (not statistically significant) of cancers of the middle and lower third of the rectum, with a concomitant rise in the percentage of cases in the rectosigmoid, or upper third, of the rectum. This is considered to be one of the reasons proposed for the increasing numbers of sphincter-sparing operations (compared with abdomino perineal resection) performed at that institution.[11] At one major institution between 1939 and 1953, the incidence of rectal and sigmoid cancers was 51 percent and 13 percent, respectively, whereas during the period between 1959 and 1977, the incidence at the same sites was 32 percent and 31 percent, respectively.[7] These findings speak for the inadequacy of the rigid sigmoidoscope in the screening of patients and point to the necessity of using the longer flexible fiberoptic sigmoidoscope and/or colonoscope. Interestingly, it has been noted that in areas where the incidence of large bowel cancer is low, the neoplasms tend to be concentrated in the cecum and ascending colon.[10]

A sex difference exists in the incidences carcinoma of the rectum and carcinoma of the other segments of the large bowel. Wood and co-workers[12] reported that among 924 cases of colon cancer, 47 percent were in males and 53 percent were in females, whereas among 902 cases of rectal cancer, 59 percent were males and 41 percent were females. In a study of 2,313 cases of colorectal cancer from the Charity Hospital, New Orleans, comparison of rectal and sigmoid cancers revealed a statistically significant difference between males and females, with males more frequent in the former group and females in the latter.[13] Wynder notes that the sex ratio of colon cancer is near unity, whereas rectal cancer is mainly a male disease. Before the age of 60, however, colon cancer is more common in females, whereas later in life it is more common in males.[2]

In the United States the mean and median ages for the onset of colorectal cancer are 63 and 67 years.[12] In underdeveloped countries with a low incidence of colorectal cancer the average age of onset is at least 15 years earlier.[14] In the Western world colorectal cancer does occur in children, adolescents, and young adults, but rarely. Among 2,156 patients with colorectal cancer seen at Roswell Park Memorial Institute in Buffalo, New York, the incidence of this neoplasm in patients below the age of 35 years was 1.85 percent.[15] Of 2,600 patients treated for colorectal carcinoma at the Montpelier Cancer Institute in France between 1966 and 1983, 93 were younger than 40 years of age, an incidence of 3.6 percent.[16] These patients ranged in age from 18 to 40 years, with a mean age of 32 years. The male to female sex ratio was 1.05. Using 40 years of age as a cutoff, one notes an extremely high incidence of poorly differentiated or mucinous cancers in this age group.[15–19] In the usual adult population, mucinous and poorly differentiated cancers occur at an incidence of 15 percent and 20 percent, respectively,[11, 20, 21] whereas in young patients, 41.5 to 87 percent of cancers are of these types.[15–19] The prognosis in this young age group is very poor, and this may be due to the fact that most of these cancers present at an advanced stage.[15–19] In their series, Mills and Allen[17] noted that these tumors occurred mainly in young black females ($P < 0.001$). It is of interest that in countries where the incidence of colorectal cancer is low and the disease occurs in a younger age group, the great majority of tumors are mucoid or undifferentiated.[14] Some have noted an increased incidence of right-sided lesions in contrast to the more common rectal and sigmoid lesions noted in the normal older age population,[18, 19] whereas others have reported a distribution similar to that of the usual adult population.[15, 17] Again, it is to be noted that right-sided lesions predominate in low-incidence populations.[2, 14]

PATHOLOGY

Survival of colorectal cancer is dependent on a number of factors, including resectability, histopathologic characteristics, stage, and degree of vascular invasion of the tumor; bowel obstruction or perforation, and lymphatic infiltration.

GROSS MORPHOLOGY

Macroscopically, most colorectal adenocarcinomas may be classified as either polypoid or ulcerative infiltrating. Some studies have suggested that polypoid tumors have a much better prognosis than ulcerating lesions,[22–24] although others fail to support this contention.[25] Using the gross configuration in macro-whole-mount sections, Montessori and Donald[26] developed a tumor invasion profile that corresponded closely to the polypoid/ulcerative infiltrating categorization. They found that tumors with a "low invasion profile" had a much better prognosis than those with a "high invasion profile." Steinberg et al.[24] took into consideration tumor morphology (exophytic versus nonexophytic) and concluded that those with large nonexophytic tumors fared worse than those with large exophytic tumors. The extent of circumferential bowel wall involvement should be noted, as those patients with involvement of greater than three-fourths of the bowel wall circumference have significantly lower 5-year survival rates.[27]

Spratt and Spjut[28] found that prognosis was independent of size if the tumor was resectable.

They grouped cancers by size at 1-cm intervals (range, 1 to 23 cm) and found that the incidence of metastasis was constant for each group. Thus, they concluded that any large colorectal cancer that could be mobilized with adequate margins should be resected. Wolmark and co-workers[25] found tumor size to be unrelated to the presence of or number of lymph nodes containing metastatic cancer, indicating that tumor size is not a prognostic discriminant. Most colorectal cancers are well circumscribed and show little propensity for submucosal spread beyond their macroscopic borders; one should, however, always measure the length between tumor and gross surgical margins. Various studies have measured intramural tumor spread. Black and Waugh[29] concluded that 2 cm is an adequate margin of resection for tumors of the left colon, whereas Grinnell[30] concluded that 5 cm is an adequate margin of resection for tumors of the rectum and rectosigmoid. Copeland and co-workers[31] found that of those patients with rectal carcinoma who underwent curative resection, those with a 5 cm or more free margin had a 51 percent 5-year survival rate, whereas of those with margins less than 5 cm, only 38 percent were free of disease at 5 years. Similar findings were noted with suture line recurrence. More recent data, however, reveals that among those patients with rectal carcinoma who have microscopic distal spread of tumor, the vast majority will have tumor spread of 2 cm or less.[32] Patients with microscopic carcinoma that has spread beyond 2 cm nearly always have a poorly differentiated Dukes' stage C cancer.[32] The survival of these patients is not altered with abdominoperineal resection as opposed to low anterior resection since death is due to distant metastasis.[32, 33] Pollett and Nicholls[34] divided a group of patients undergoing low anterior resection for carcinoma of the rectum into three groups: 55 patients with distal margins of 2 cm or less (group 1), 177 patients with distal margins of 2 to 5 cm (group 2), and 102 patients with distal margins of 5 cm or more (group 3). These three groups were very similar with respect to Dukes' classification, extent of local spread, and histologic grade. The overall crude 5-year survival rates for groups 1, 2, and 3 were 69.1 percent, 68.4 percent, and 69.6 percent, respectively. Corresponding cancer-specific death rates of 25.5 percent, 23.2 percent, and 21.6 percent were recorded. Recurrence rates for the three groups were very similar. This information is reassuring in those surgical situations in which it is not possible to obtain 5 cm of distal bowel, such as with low rectal lesions (5 to 10 cm from the anal verge) in which sphincter preservation is desired. Low anterior resection with a distal margin of 1.5[35] to 2.0 cm[32, 34] will remove the entire tumor in the vast majority of these cases without adverse effect on survival and local recurrence patterns.

A new method of assessing the adequacy of surgical resection of rectal cancers has been proposed by Chan, Boey, and Wong.[36] These investigators suggest the use of a three-dimensional measurement of tumor growth, which they describe as *radial invasion* combined with an evaluation of *radial surgical clearance* to describe the margin of resection. Radial surgical clearance is essentially a measurement of the distance between the deepest point of tumor penetration and the "deep" plane of excision. This technique may provide data that are of value in designing adjuvant therapy.

PATHOLOGY OF LOCAL RESECTION

An alternative to radical surgery in the treatment of rectal carcinoma is the technique of local excision. In this procedure, the tumor is excised with a narrow margin of grossly normal tissue, either endoscopically or via transanal surgical intervention. Perirectal lymph nodes remain in situ.[37] Local excision was employed in the past to excise rectal cancers in patients who were deemed to represent a poor surgical risk for more radical surgery, for patients who absolutely refused a permanent colostomy, and as a palliative measure for patients who were believed to have incurable tumors.[38] In 1977, Morson and co-workers[39] proposed the idea that local excision of rectal cancers should be viewed as a "total biopsy." According to this concept, the adequacy of excision and potential need for

further definitive surgery could be determined through complete histopathologic examination of the excised tissue. The carcinoma was judged to be adequately excised if (1) the deep and lateral margins of resection were uninvolved by tumor, (2) the tumor was not a high-grade or poorly differentiated subtype, and (3) the tumor did not penetrate through the muscularis propria.

Certain clinical characteristics must be evaluated when deciding which patients might benefit from local excision. York Mason[40] has developed a clinical staging system (CS) for carcinoma of the rectum that is based on tumor mobility, since mobility represents a rough approximation of depth of invasion. According to this system, CS I tumors which are "freely" mobile, CS II tumors are mobile, CS III tumors are tethered but still mobile, CS IV tumors are fixed, and CS V tumors represent disseminated disease. Mason[40] states that patients with cancers designated CS I and CS II are candidates for local excision unless the surgeon detects firm, enlarged, fixed lymph nodes in the pararectal soft tissue. Some[37, 41] recommend that only patients with tumors measuring 3 cm or less should have their cancers excised locally, whereas others[38–40] do not consider this size a limitation. Tumor ulceration has been described as a contraindication to local excision by Hager et al.,[37] however, Whiteway et al.[38] do not consider ulceration in and of itself to be an adverse factor.

Once a patient has fulfilled the clinical criteria and undergone local excision of a rectal tumor, the histopathologic features of the excised specimen must be carefully evaluated. The criteria for adequacy of excision as proposed by Morson et al.[40] and described previously (i.e., negative margins, tumor confined to bowel wall, and grade I or II cancer) have been found to be useful by other investigators.[37, 38, 41, 42] If these histopathologic criteria are not met, or if the carcinoma is grade III, of the mucinous subtype, or displays lymphatic invasion, further radical surgery is indicated.[37, 42]

Whiteway and co-workers[38] studied 24 patients who underwent local excision for carcinoma of the rectum. Nineteen of these patients fulfilled the clinical and histologic criteria for local excision and therefore did not need to undergo further surgery. Of these 19 patients, 3 subsequently died of other causes, whereas 16 remained alive with no evidence of recurrence of cancer. Thus, the corrected 5-year survival rate was 84.5 percent with a cancer-specific death rate of 0 percent. Five patients required further surgery because they did not fulfill the histologic criteria for adequacy of excision; of these five, two died from poorly differentiated carcinoma, a cancer-specific death rate of 8.3 percent. Hager et al.[37] report an age-corrected 5-year survival rate of 90 percent for patients undergoing adequate local excision in whom the tumor was limited to the submucosa; local recurrence occurred in 8 percent of these patients. These workers also report an age-corrected 5-year survival rate of 78 percent for patients undergoing local excision in whom the tumor invaded into but did not penetrate through the muscularis propria. In these patients, local recurrence occurred in 17 percent and distant metastases occurred in 6 percent. Whiteway et al.[38] did not note a decrease in survival for patients with tumor invading the muscularis propria. Similarly, DeCosse et al.[42] found that the level of invasion was not an adverse factor unless the tumor invaded perirectal soft tissue. These investigators studied 57 patients with rectal carcinoma who underwent local excision and found an overall 5-year survival rate of 83.4 percent with a cancer-specific death rate of 10.5 percent. Willett and co-workers,[43] however, recommend postoperative radiation therapy for patients with tumor invasion into muscularis propria. Radiation may also be adjuvantly employed if sphincter preservation is desired or when the risk of surgery is high in patients whose tumors are judged to be inadequately excised.[43]

TUMOR SITE

The importance of tumor site with respect to survival and patterns of recurrence has been disputed.[28, 44–48] Eisenberg et al.[48] showed that patients with left-sided colon cancers tended to do worse than patients with right-sided cancers, especially after 5 years, since the majority of late cancer deaths were among patients with rectal and distal left colon cancers. These findings were particularly true for Dukes stage B and C lesions. The National Surgical Adjuvant Breast and Bowel Project (NSABP) data,[47] however, revealed that the worst prognosis was among patients with tumors of the rectum and rectosigmoid, whereas patients with left colon tumors had a better prognosis than those with tumors in any other site. The relative risk of treatment failure in rectal cancers was three times worse than the risk for left colon cancers, according to this study.

Colorectal cancer can present with a linitis plastica-type gross appearance, but this is rare. Grossly one sees a diffusely scirrhous infiltration of the bowel wall similar to that seen in linitis plastica of the stomach (Fig. 8-1). It should be kept in mind that most cases of linitis plastica of the colon are not primary lesions but metastases from other sites, although a case of primary linitis plastica of the colon with metastasis to the stomach has been reported.[49] The prognosis of primary linitis plastica is extremely poor.[49, 50]

HISTOPATHOLOGY

When we speak of epithelial neoplasms of the colon and rectum (excluding carcinoids) we essentially are referring to adenocarcinoma. Other forms, such as squamous carcinoma, adenosquamous carcinoma, adenocarcinoid, and small cell carcinoma do exist, but are uncommon.

The great majority of adenocarcinomas (85 percent) show relatively small amounts of mucin production, whereas approximately 10 to 15 percent of cases produce sufficient mucin to be categorized as mucinous or colloid adenocarcinoma. Colorectal adenocarcinoma (excluding mucinous or colloid type) is usually divided into three histologic grades, well differentiated (grade I), average grade (grade II), and poorly differentiated (grade III), based on the degree of differentiation of gland or tubule formation and individual cytologic features[21] (Figs. 8-2

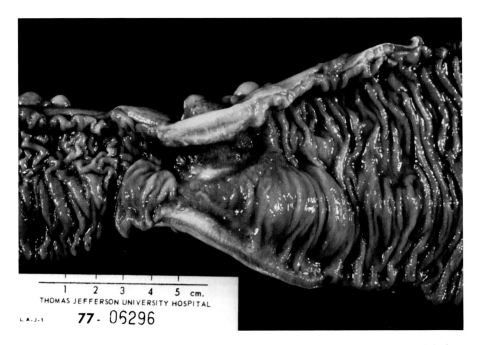

Fig. 8-1. Primary linitis plastica-type adenocarcinoma of the large bowel. The growth is mainly intramural with a localized diffuse thickening of bowel wall similar to that seen in linitis plastica of the stomach.

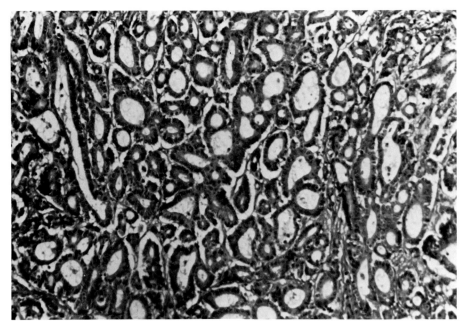

Fig. 8-2. Low-grade (grade I) adenocarcinoma of the large intestine. The glands are well formed. Nuclei are basally placed and do not show stratification. (Cf. Figs. 8-3 and 8-4. H&E, × 100.)

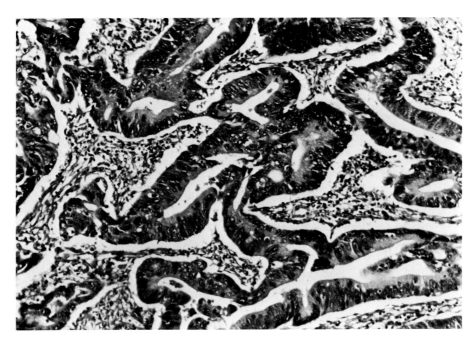

Fig. 8-3. Average-grade (grade II) adenocarcinoma of the rectum. One can identify gland formation, however, it is not as orderly as in Fig. 8-2. There is stratification of nuclei and some nuclear atypia. (H&E, × 100.)

to 8-4). Traditional teaching, based on data from St. Marks Hospital, has held that the majority of colorectal cancers (60 percent) fall into the average-grade category, whereas approximately 20 percent are well differentiated and 20 percent are poorly differentiated.[11, 21] One must realize, however, that there is great interobserver variation in assigning tumor grades.[51] Grading of colorectal cancers provides a good key to biologic behavior and prognosis. It has been shown that as the stage of spread advances, a progressive increase occurs in the proportion of histologically high-grade tumors and a decline occurs in the number of low-grade tumors.[21, 52] Correlating survival to grade, Dukes and Bussey[21] found that the 5-year survival in grades I, II, and III rectal cancer was 77 percent, 61 percent, and 29 percent, respectively. More recent studies of colorectal carcinoma have demonstrated 5-year survival rates of 62 to 83 percent for grade I, 43 to 63 percent for grade II, and 11 to 42 percent for grade III.[53–57] Grade has also been correlated to the incidence of lymph node

metastases, with low, average, and high-grade tumors showing a 30 percent, 47.1 percent, and 81.3 percent incidence of metastases, respectively.[21] Higher-grade tumors tend to have elevated serum carcinoembryonic antigen (CEA) levels, compared with low-grade tumors.[58] In looking at prognosis, one obviously must also consider stage, however; studies have shown that within the same stage, histopathologic grading plays an important part. This is most obvious in Dukes C lesions and those with extensive extramural spread, where combined grades I and II show statistically significant greater 5-year survival rates than in those with grade III adenocarcinoma.[21, 52]

Traditionally, carcinomas are classified as mucinous or colloid if 50 percent or greater of tumor area consists of mucin, although some restrict this term to tumors with at least 75 percent mucin.[59] These tumors can also be classified into the more common "extracellular" type and the rarer signet ring cell or "intracellular" type[20, 60] (Figs. 8-5 and 8-6). Mucinous carcino-

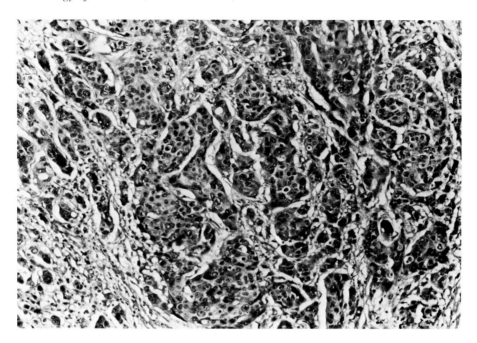

Fig. 8-4. High-grade (grade III) adenocarcinoma of the colon. The tumor infiltrates in sheets without evidence of gland formation. One can appreciate occasional "giant" hyperchromatic nuclei. (H&E, × 100.)

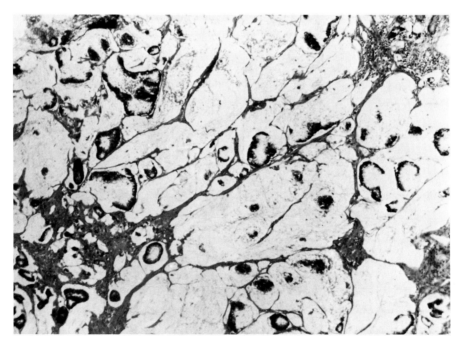

Fig. 8-5. Colloid or mucinous carcinoma (extracellular type). Large pools of mucin with free-floating clumps of tumor cells may be noted. (H&E, × 100.)

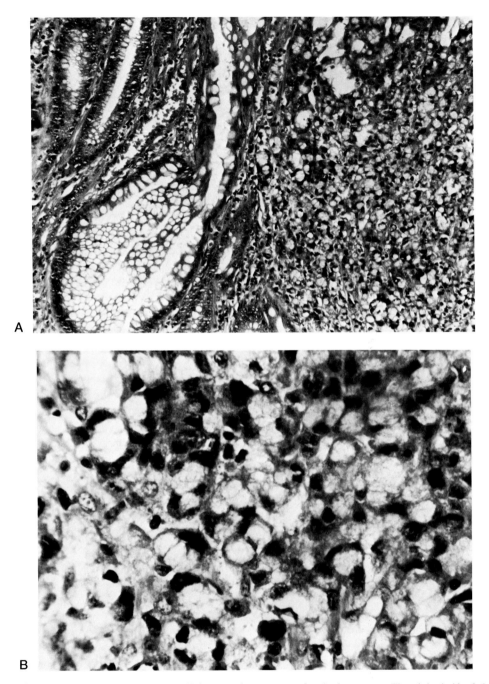

Fig. 8-6. (**A**) Signet ring cell (intracellular) mucinous type of colonic cancer. The right half of figure shows sheets of signet cells within the mucosa, while non-neoplastic colonic mucosa is to the left. (**B**) High-power view of signet ring cell cancer (H&E, Fig. A × 100, Fig. B × 400.)

mas have been associated with certain clinical and pathologic settings: young adults and children, male sex, villous adenomas, cancers arising secondary to therapeutic irradiation, ulcerative colitis, and cancers in low-incidence undeveloped countries.[14, 20] Symonds and Vickery[20] studied 132 cases of mucinous carcinoma of the colon and rectum, which accounted for 15 percent of colorectal cancers seen at their institution between 1955 and 1959. Looking at these tumors as a group (irrespective of site) they found that the 5-year survival for nonmucinous and mucinous cancers was 53 percent and 34 percent, respectively ($P < 0.005$).[20] However, when one looks at survival between mucinous and nonmucinous cancers with regard to site, there is no difference in survival, except for cancers of the rectum. Rectal mucinous cancers had an 18 percent 5-year survival rate, compared with 49 percent for rectal nonmucinous tumors ($P < 0.005$). Stage for stage, there was no difference in survival among mucinous cancers, except for those of the rectum. Sasaki et al.[59] investigated 316 mucinous and 45 signet ring cell carcinomas of the rectum, comparing these lesions with 413 nonmucinous tumors. Stage for stage, nonmucinous tumors and mucinous tumors were similar in terms of 5-year survival. These workers found that mucinous tumors tend to present at a more advanced stage, but that the presence of large mucinous areas was not significant as an independent prognostic variable. These observations are similar to those reported by Halvorsen and Seim.[61]

In their study of mucinous cancers, Pihl and co-workers[60] showed that the difference in survival between mucinous and nonmucinous tumors may be related to stage. They found a statistically significant difference in survival between these two histologic types in stage A and C lesions, mucinous tumors having a worse prognosis. There was no survival difference in stage B and D lesions for the two tumor subtypes.

In general, grading of mucinous tumors is difficult and unrewarding. One must, however, take note of the rare signet ring cell type, which is considered to be the "poorly differentiated"

variant of mucinous carcinoma. In a study of 426 mucinous adenocarcinomas of the rectum and rectosigmoid, Bonello and co-workers[62] found 17 (4 percent) to be of the signet ring cell type. Eighty-two percent of these signet ring cell cancers were stage C, and the overall 5-year survival of this group was 24 percent, compared with 55 percent for the "extracellular" mucinous type. In the study of Symonds and Vickery,[20] all patients with signet ring cell cancer died early. Sasaki et al.[59] report an overall 5-year survival of 13 percent for signet ring cell cancers; 91 percent of their cases (41 of 45 patients) had Dukes' C lesions. The lethality of signet ring cell cancer is also emphasized in children and young adults; there is, however, some suggestion that the rare cases of less-advanced disease (stages A and B) may not carry the ominous connotation of signet ring cell cancer in general.[18, 59, 62]

Squamous carcinoma and adenosquamous carcinoma of the colon and rectum are rare. Approximately 63 cases of the former have been reported in the English-language literature.[63] Before one can make a diagnosis of primary squamous carcinoma of the colon or rectum, certain criteria must be met: (1) There must be no other site of squamous cancer in the body and (2) no involvement with cloacogenic or squamous-lined mucosa. Several theories have been proposed to explain these unusual neoplasms, including (1) proliferation of uncommitted reserve cells, (2) squamous metaplasia, and (3) embryonic rests.[64] These lesions have also been reported in a background of ulcerative colitis, schistosomiasis, and pelvic irradiation.[63] Austin[65] suggested that anal-receptive intercourse may play a role in the development of rectal squamous carcinoma via a virally transmitted agent or some secondary effect of treatment for a sexually transmitted disease, but substantial evidence to support this theory is lacking. More likely, the recognition of a striking similarity between reported cases of primary squamous carcinoma and adenosquamous carcinoma with adenocarcinoma supports a theory that these lesions have a similar histogenesis, namely, pre-existing colorectal adenomas. The

Mayo Clinic study[66] found associated benign adenomas in the resected specimens of 7 of 20 cases. The finding of adenosquamous carcinomas adds support to this, and one could envision a squamous cancer arising from total metaplasia of one such lesion. Williams and co-workers,[64] in a study of 75 consecutive adenomas with invasive cancer, found one case that could be classified as an adenosquamous carcinoma. The same group found an incidence of 0.4 percent squamous metaplasia in benign adenomas. More evidence of such a theory is suggested by findings that the age, sex, and site distribution are similar to colorectal adenocarcinoma.[64, 66] Comer and co-workers[66] reported a 5-year survival rate of 30 percent in squamous cancers and adenosquamous carcinomas, compared with 50 percent for "garden-variety" adenocarcinomas. They explained this by the fact that the majority of their cancers were high grade. They also commented that survival did correlate with Dukes' staging. Michelassi et al.[63] report that among patients with primary squamous cell and adenosquamous carcinoma of the colon, the 5-year survival is 50 percent for Dukes B lesions and 33 percent for Dukes C lesions.

Small cell undifferentiated carcinoma is an uncommon neoplasm comprising less than 1 percent of colorectal cancers.[67–69] Although they grossly may resemble routine adenocarcinoma, these tumors are histologically identical to small cell (oat cell) carcinoma of the lung and behave in a similarly aggressive fashion (Fig. 8-7). The majority of cases present with metastatic disease involving the liver and lymph nodes.[67–69] Approximately one-third of small cell carcinomas are associated with an adenoma,[70] but even when the cancer is a small focus within an adenoma, it has the potential to metastasize widely.[67, 68] Small cell carcinoma may arise in association with adenocarcinoma[68, 69] or show areas of squamous differentiation.[67] Electron microscopic studies have disclosed neurosecre-

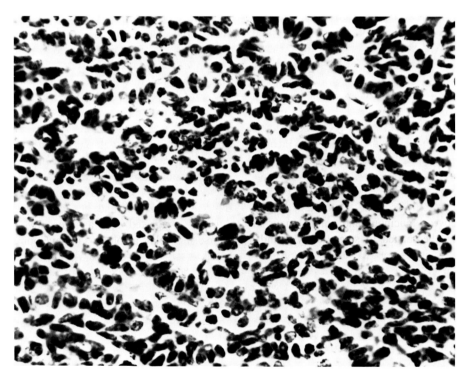

Fig. 8-7. Small cell undifferentiated cancer. Undifferentiated tumor cells with focal pseudorosette formation. Similarity to oat cell carcinoma of the lung may be noted. (H&E, × 400.)

tory granules within tumor cells[67–69, 71] and, in one report, neurosecretory granules and intracytoplasmic tonofilaments were present within the same cell.[71] These findings suggest that the cells of small cell undifferentiated carcinoma are capable of divergent differentiation.

Small biopsies of the rectum (and occasionally the colon) may conceivably present a dilemma in distinguishing small cell carcinoma from poorly differentiated (grade III) adenocarcinoma, lymphoma, cloacogenic carcinoma, and malignant melanoma. Wick and co-workers[69] have studied the immunohistochemical properties of colorectal small cell undifferentiated carcinoma and cloacogenic carcinoma. They have found that the former will express epithelial membrane antigen (EMA), neuron-specific enolase (NSE), chromogranin, neurofilaments, and Leu 7 (CD57), but will be negative for CEA and blood group antigens (BGAgs), whereas the latter will express EMA, CEA, and BGAgs, but not NSE, chromagranin, neurofilaments, or Leu 7. Poorly differentiated adenocarcinoma expresses an antigenic profile that is similar to cloacogenic carcinoma but expresses Leu-M1 (CD15), which is negative in cloacogenic carcinoma.[69] Although these workers did not specifically examine primary colorectal malignant lymphoma, they point out that of 113 noncolonic lymphomas studied, 100 percent expressed leukocyte common antigen (LCA) (CD 45), and all failed to express EMA, CEA, BGAgs, NSE, chromogranin, neurofilaments, or Leu-7. All of the nonlymphomatous tumors were negative for LCA (Table 8-1). Distinguishing features of malignant melanoma include immunoreactivity for S-100 protein and NSE with negative reactivity for EMA and LCA.[72] In addition, a monoclonal antibody, HMB45, which recognizes melanoma and neurocytic lesions with a high degree of sensitivity and specificity, has recently been developed.[73]

A few other unusual colorectal tumors warrant mention. Weidner and Zekan[74] have described a case of carcinosarcoma arising in the colon. This lesion contained areas of typical adenocarcinoma and squamous carcinoma admixed with a sarcomatous component composed of osteosarcoma, chondrosarcoma, and spindle cell sarcoma. Both the carcinoma and sarcoma portions of this tumor disclosed immunoreactivity for cytokeratin, indicating epithelial differentiation. There have been reports of patients with poorly differentiated colorectal cancers in whom elevated serum levels of human chorionic gonadotropin (hCG) have been detected.[75, 76] Choriocarcinoma differentiation has been observed in the primary colonic tumor[76] as well as in hepatic metastases,[77] and immunohistochemical studies have revealed the expression of hCG by both the colorectal tumors[75] and metastases.[77] Goblet cell carcinoid tumor, also known as adenocarcinoid tumor or crypt cell carcinoma, has been described in the colon and rectum and is similar to its counterpart in the appendix.[78] This lesion appears as an ulcerating or fungating mass. Histologically the cells are arranged in nests and trabecular cords with abundant intracellular mu-

Table 8-1. Differential Diagnosis of Undifferentiated Colorectal Tumors via Immunohistochemistry

Diagnosis	CK	EMA	LCA	NSE	S-100	CRG	NF	CEA	BGAgs	Leu-M1	Leu-7	HMB-45
Small cell carcinoma	+[a]	+	−	+	−	+	+	−	−	−	+	−
Poorly differentiated adenocarcinoma	+[a]	+	−	−	−	−	−	+	+	+	−	−
Cloacogenic carcinoma	+[b]	+	−	−	−	−	−	+	+	−	−	−
Lymphoma	−	−	+	−	−	−	−	−	−	+	−	−

[a] Low-/medium-molecular-weight cytokeratin.

[b] Low-/medium-/high-molecular-weight cytokeratin.

CK, cytokeratin; EMA, epithelial membrane antigen; LCA, leukocyte common antigen; NSE, neuron-specific enolase; CRG, chromogranin; NF, neurofilaments; CEA, carcinoembryonic antigen; BGAgs, blood group antigens.

(Data from Wick et al[69] and Gown et al.[73])

Table 8-2. Dukes' Staging System for Rectal Carcinoma

Stage A	Tumor confined to wall of rectum
Stage B	Tumor penetrates bowel wall (muscularis propria) to involve extrarectal tissues but without metastasis to regional lymph nodes
Stage C	Metastases present in regional lymph nodes
Modification of Stage C	
Stage C_1	Metastasis confined to regional lymph nodes
Stage C_2	Metastasis present in lymph nodes at mesenteric artery ligature (apical nodes)

(Data from Dukes[79] and Gabriel et al[80] (modification of stage C).)

cin, tubular differentiation, and in some cases, extracellular mucin.[78] Ultrastructural examination may reveal mucin granules (as seen in normal goblet cells) and occasional cells with cytoplasmic granules similar to those seen in Paneth or other endocrine cells.[78]

STAGING

Proper staging of neoplasms provides the clinician with the information necessary for optimal patient care. It also provides some indication of the expected course of that neoplasm. In 1932, Dukes[79] devised a staging system for rectal carcinoma that is still used today (Table 8-2). This staging classification is based on the degree of direct extension of the tumor through the bowel wall and the presence or absence of lymph node metastases. In this system, a Dukes A tumor is one in which the lesion is still confined within the bowel wall proper, a Dukes B lesion is one in which the tumor has spread through the entire bowel wall thickness and into the fat or beyond, and a Dukes C tumor is one that has metastasized to regional lymph nodes. Dukes originally reported 3-year survival rates of 80 percent, 73 percent, and 7 percent for his stages A, B, and C, respectively, whereas Whittaker and Goligher,[27] studying rectal cancers operated on between 1955 and 1968, found corrected 5-year survival rates of 91.9 percent, 71.3 percent, and 37.7 percent for Dukes' A, B, and C lesions, respectively. In 1935, Gabriel,

Dukes, and Bussey[80] modified this system slightly by subdividing stage C lesions into C_1 and C_2 (Table 8-2), where C_1 denotes lymph node metastases in the region of the cancer and C_2 includes lymph node metastases at the point of mesenteric blood vessel ligature (the reader should note the distinction between the Dukes and the Astler-Coller definitions of C_1 and C_2 lesions). In 1958 Dukes and Bussey[21] described a corrected 5-year survival of 40.9 percent for C_1 tumors and 13.6 percent for C_2 tumors. More recent studies of rectal carcinoma have disclosed stage-specific 5-year survivals of 88 to 99 percent for A, 71 to 79 percent for B, 40 to 45 percent for C_1 (Dukes'), and 10 to 14 percent for C_2 (32 to 41 percent overall for stage C).[27, 53, 59, 81, 82] Although the Dukes' staging system was originally described for rectal carcinoma, it is also of value in the staging of colon cancer.

Dukes acknowledged a fourth stage of rectal carcinoma defined by distant (i.e., hepatic) metastasis,[83] but it was Turnbull et al.[84] who designated this as stage D. Unfortunately, Turnbull considered direct extension of carcinoma into pelvic organs to be an example of stage D, whereas Dukes labelled those as B cases if the lymph nodes were negative. This lack of uniformity in the definition of stage D persists in the literature.[27, 48, 81] Pihl et al.[81] carefully defined their D cases in accordance with Whittaker and Goligher[27] as those in which there was visceral (e.g., hepatic) metastasis or in which the tumor had invaded adjacent pelvic organs (with or without lymph node metastases). Of 150 patients studied by these workers, 4 percent survived 5 years. Eisenberg and co-workers[48] found a 5-year survival of 4.1 percent in 488 patients classified as stage D (defined as those cases with distant metastasis and excluding cases with local contiguous organ involvement only).

The Astler-Coller[85] staging system is as follows: stage A represents intramucosal cancer only, stage B_1 represents tumor invading into the muscularis propria and no further (note that there is no provision for tumors limited to the submucosa), in stage B_2 the cancer directly extends beyond the bowel wall, stage C_1 represents

Table 8-3. Astler–Coller Staging System for Colorectal Carcinoma

Stage A	Tumor confined to mucosa
Stage B$_1$	Tumor invades muscularis propria but does not penetrate through to involve extramural tissues
Stage B$_2$	Tumor penetrates through muscularis propria to involve extramural tissues
Stage C$_1$	Metastases in regional lymph nodes; tumor does not penetrate through muscularis propria (limited to bowel wall)
Stage C$_2$	Metastasis in regional lymph nodes; tumor penetrates through muscularis propria into pericolorectal soft tissue

(From Astler and Coller,[85] with permission.)

lesions with positive regional lymph nodes, but the tumor proper is limited within the confines of the bowel wall, and stage C$_2$ represents lesions with positive lymph nodes and the tumor proper extending through the entire bowel wall thickness (Table 8-3). In this staging system, C$_1$ and C$_2$ lesions had 43 percent and 23 percent 5-year survival rates, respectively.

A universal staging system for colorectal carcinoma using TNM criteria has been jointly proposed by the American Joint Commission of Cancer (AJCC) and the Union Internationale Contre le Cancer (UICC).[86] (Tables 8-4 and 8-5). The TNM stages are designed to correspond directly to Dukes' stages while providing a more precise description of the extent of tumor growth. This system takes into consideration the number of lymph nodes containing metastatic carcinoma, an issue not addressed in the Astler-Coller and Dukes' systems. The clinical significance of the number of positive lymph nodes was appreciated by Dukes and Bussey in 1958,[21] when they noted that the corrected 5-year survival rate in patients with only one positive lymph node was 67.6 percent, compared with 36.1 percent and 2.1 percent for those with two to five and more than 10 positive lymph nodes, respectively. Spratt and Spjut[28] noted that the 5-year survival rate was less than 10 percent if more than six lymph nodes contained metastatic cancer.

Recent reports by the Gastointestinal Tumor Study Group (GITSG)[24, 87] have suggested the designations C$_1$ for patients with one to four positive lymph nodes and C$_2$ for patients with more than four lymph nodes containing cancer. Investigators with the National Surgical Adjuvant Breast and Bowel Projects (NSABP)[88] demonstrated that patients with more than four positive lymph nodes were 1.9 times as likely to die as patients with one to four positive nodes, regardless of depth of tumor invasion in the bowel wall ($P < 0.00001$, an independent variable), whereas Astler-Coller C$_2$ patients with one to four positive nodes were 2.5 times as likely to die as C$_1$ patients with one to four positive nodes ($P = 0.002$). Perhaps most interesting is the finding that patients with tumor confined to the bowel wall and one to four positive lymph nodes have a 5-year survival rate that is at least as favorable as the 5-year survival rate for patients with classic Dukes B lesions.[88, 89] Those cancers with lymph node metastases and tumor limited to the bowel wall

Table 8-4. TNM Designations in the AJCC/UICC Staging System for Colorectal Carcinoma

Designation	Description
T$_x$	The primary tumor cannot be evaluated
T$_0$	No evidence of primary tumor
T$_{is}$	Carcinoma in situ
T$_1$	Tumor invades into the submucosa
T$_2$	Tumor invades into muscularis propria
T$_3$	Tumor penetrates through muscularis propria into subserosa or into nonperitonealized pericoloic or perirectal tissue
T$_4$	Tumor perforates the visceral peritoneum or invades directly into other organs or tissues
N$_x$	The regional lymph nodes cannot be evaluated
N$_0$	No lymph node metastasis
N$_1$	Metastatic tumor in one to three pericolic or perirectal lymph nodes
N$_2$	Metastatic tumor in four or more pericolic or perirectal lymph nodes
N$_3$	Metastatic tumor in any lymph node along the course of a major named blood vessel
M$_x$	The presence of distant metastasis cannot be evaluated
M$_0$	No distant metastasis
M$_1$	Distant metastasis present

(From Hutter and Sobin,[86] with permission.)

Table 8-5. AJCC/UICC Staging System for Colorectal Carcinoma[a]

	TNM Designation	Dukes' Stage
Stage 0	T_{is}, N_0, M_0	—
Stage I	T_1, N_0, M_0	A
	T_2, N_0, M_0	
Stage II	T_3, N_0, M_0	B
	T_4, N_0, M_0	
Stage III	Any T, N_1, M_0	C
	Any T, N_2 or N_3, M_0	
Stage IV	Any T, any N, M_1	

[a] See Table 8-4 for TNM descriptions.
(From Hutter and Sobin,[86] with permission.)

had a 5-year survival rate of 70 percent, whereas those with lymph node metastases and tumor through the bowel wall had a 5-year survival rate of 30 percent.[89] The NSABP researchers also demonstrated that depth of tumor penetration is a significant independent variable.[89]

Studies from the NSABP[89] also suggest that prognosis based on the site of positive lymph nodes is less dependent on site per se than on the number of positive nodes. Finally, the presence of retrograde lymphatic spread of tumor to lymph nodes distal to the tumor portends a very poor prognosis.[90]

A recent staging system for rectal carcinoma has been developed by Jass et al.[53] following investigation of various grade- and stage-related parameters. This system is based on assigning numerical values to (1) number of lymph nodes containing metastatic tumor, (2) degree of lymphocytic infiltration at the advancing edge of tumor, and (3) extent of tumor spread through the intestinal wall (Table 8-6). Lymphocytic infiltration is graded as little, moderate, or marked. Tumor extension through intestinal wall is evaluated as none, slight to moderate, or extensive (tumor spread greater than 5 mm beyond the rectal wall). Five stages are then defined according to the sum of the numerical values; each stage has a statistically significant difference in corrected percent 5-year survival (Table 8-7). This system has recently been modified into four prognostic stages based on total

Table 8-6. Jass Classification of Rectal Carcinoma

Pathologic Variable	Score Value
Lymphocytic infiltration	
Marked	0
Moderate	3
Little	6
Lymph node metastases	
None	0
1–4	4
5 or more	8
Spread through bowel wall	
None	0
Slight to moderate	3
Extensive	6

Stage	Total Score
I	0
II	1–6
III	7–11
IV	12–16
V	17–20

(From Jass et al,[53] with permission.)

scores from four parameters: (1) tumor limited to bowel wall (yes or no); (2) character of invasive margin (expanding vs. infiltrating); (3) number of lymph nodes with metastases (0, 1 to 4, more than 4), and (4) peritumoral lymphocytic infiltrate (yes or no). The scores are summed (see Table 8-8) into group I (score 0 to 1), group II (score 2), group III (score 3), and group IV (score 4 to 5), whose corrected 5-year survivals are 94, 83, 56, and 27 percent respectively.[54]

Of all the staging methods available, the Dukes, Astler-Coller, and TNM systems are probably the most widely used. Table 8-9 lists

Table 8-7. Jass Classification of Rectal Carcinoma: Corrected 5-Year Survival

Stage	Corrected 5-Year Survival (%)
I	100
II	88
III	72
IV	32
V	6

(From Jass et al,[53] with permission.)

Table 8-8. Updated Jass Classification of Rectal Cancer

Pathologic Variable	Score
Tumor limited to bowel wall	
Yes	0
No	1
Invasive margin	
Yes	0
No	1
Number of lymph nodes	
containing metastases	
0	0
1–4	1
>4	2
Lymphocytic infiltrate	
Yes	0
No	1

Group	Total Score	Corrected 5-Year Survival (%)
I	0–1	94
II	2	83
III	3	56
IV	4–5	27

(From Jass et al,[54] with permission.)

5-year survival data for each system for comparison. In an attempt to evaluate the relative merits of these three sytems in the staging of rectal cancer, Fisher et al.[89] utilized data from the National Surgical Adjuvant Breast and Bowel project (NSABP) and found all three methods to be highly interrelated. The consistency and magnitude of prognostic discrimination among stages was, however, best demonstrated by the Dukes and TNM systems. These workers failed to find an advantage for the TNM system in precision of prognostication. They confirmed the independent prognostic value of depth of tumor penetration and thus recommended use of the Dukes staging system, but with subclassification of stage C cases according to the methods of Astler and Coller.[85]

VASCULAR INVASION

Following the first report by Brown and Warren,[91] numerous studies have sought to clarify the influence of vascular invasion by tumor on prognosis.[45, 92–97] When evaluating colorectal cancer for vascular invasion, one must be cognizant that the prognosis for survival depends not only on the presence of vascular invasion, but on the type of vessel involved and its location. Khankhanian and co-workers[92] studied vascular invasion (venous or lymphatic) of intramural vessels in cases of Dukes B colorectal cancer. They found intramural vascular invasion in 27 of 143 cases (18.8 percent), however, they found no difference in survival between those patients with or without vascular invasion. Talbot and co-workers[93] undertook a histopathologic study of 703 rectal cancers to establish guidelines for practicing pathologists, surgeons, and oncologists concerning the clinical significance of venous invasion by carcinoma of the rectum. They studied (1) intramural venous invasion versus extramural venous invasion, (2) size of the vein involved (thick or thin walled),

Table 8-9. Comparison of Percentages of 5-Year Survival Among Various Colorectal Carcinoma Staging Systems

AJCC/UICC[a]		Dukes'	Astler-Coller[b]	
Stage 0	(100%)		A	(100%)
Stage I (T$_1$)	(100%)	A (82–99%)[c, d]		
		(88–99%)[e, f]		
(T$_2$)	(85%)		B$_1$	(67%)
Stage II (T$_3$)	(70%)	B (65–78%)[c, d]	B$_2$	(54%)
		(71–79%)[e, f]		
(T$_4$)	(30%)			
Stage III (N$_1$)	(60%)	C (32–49%)[c, d]		
		(32–41%)[e, f]		
(N$_2$[g])	(30%)	C$_1$ (46–54%)[c, d]	C$_1$	(43%)
		(40–45%)[e, f]		
		C$_2$ (22–26%)[c, d]	C$_2$	(22%)
		(10–14%)[e, f]		
Stage IV (M$_1$)	(3%)			

[a] Data from Hutter and Sobin.[86]
[b] Data from Astler and Coller.[85]
[c] Data from Jass et al[53, 54] and Newland et al.[82]
[d] Colon and rectum combined.
[e] Data from Dukes and Bussey,[21] Whittaker and Goligher,[27] Jass et al,[53] Sasaki et al,[59] and Pihl et al.[81]
[f] Rectum only.
[g] Although AJCC/UICC N$_2$, Dukes' C$_1$/C$_2$, and Astler–Coller C$_1$/C$_2$ are not directly comparable, they are included as a point of referral.

(3) aneurysmal dilatation of the vein wall, (4) perivenous inflammation with damage to the vein wall and replacement with granulation tissue, and (5) tumor permeation of capillary channels in the vein wall itself. Only those cases with definite evidence of tumor spread into veins were classified as venous invasion, whereas cases with doubtful or possible venous spread were included in the negative or noninvasive group. Venous invasion was found in 52 percent of cases (16 percent intramural and 36 percent extramural). The corrected 5-year survival rate for cases with intramural venus invasion was 66 percent (which was almost identical to the rate for those cases without vascular invasion), whereas for those cases with extramural venous invasion, the 5-year survival rate was 33 percent (these figures are similar to those reported by Jass et al.,[53] who showed a 5-year survival rate of 41 percent for tumors invading veins and 67 percent for tumors that did not invade veins or that invaded submucosal veins only). In the group with extramural venous invasion, the 5-year survival rate for those with involvement of thick-walled versus thin-walled veins was 19 percent and 41 percent, respectively. Aneurysmal dilatation of the vein wall, inflammatory damage to the wall of the invaded vein, and formation of an endothelial mantle over intravascular tumor growth were favorable findings, whereas spread of tumor cells in capillary channels within the vein wall worsened the prognosis.

Minsky et al.[95, 96] retrospectively examined the influence of blood vessel invasion in 294 patients with colon carcinoma[95] and 168 patients with carcinoma of the rectum/rectosigmoid[96] who were resected for cure. Blood vessel invasion (BVI) was defined as the presence of tumor within an endothelium-lined channel surrounded by a wall of smooth muscle. In addition to hematoxylin and eosin (H & E) staining, sections were prepared with the Verhoeff elastic stain; this was done to distinguish BVI from lymphatic vessel invasion (LVI), in which tumor is present in an endothelium-lined channel without a muscular wall, and to correct for a false-negative detection rate of 84 percent for BVI in H & E-stained sections alone.[96] The overall inci-

dence of BVI was 42 percent in the colon and 48 percent in the rectum and rectosigmoid. No cases of arterial invasion were noted. The incidence of BVI was noted to increase with increasing stage and grade in the colon and rectum/rectosigmoid. In the rectum and rectosigmoid, there was a significant decrease in survival in patients with extramural BVI compared with those with intramural BVI or no BVI when not corrected for stage.[96] In the colon, a trend toward decreased survival was observed in patients with extramural BVI versus intramural BVI or no BVI when all stages were combined,[95] and combining patients with extramural and intramural BVI produced a significant decrease in survival compared with patients without BVI. Analysis of data from patients with colon and rectal/rectosigmoid cancers using a proportional hazards model, however, disclosed that BVI per se is not an independent prognostic variable.

LYMPHATIC INVASION

In a separate study to assess the prognostic importance of LVI, Minsky et al.[97] reviewed the records of 462 patients who underwent potentially curative surgery for carcinoma of the colon and rectum/rectosigmoid. H & E- and Verhoeff elastic-stained slides were examined; LVI was identified if tumor was seen within endothelium-lined channels without a wall of smooth muscle. Sixty-one patients (13 percent) were noted to have tumors with LVI and these were compared to the LVI-negative group. LVI was associated with a significant increase in the incidence of positive lymph nodes (59 percent versus 25 percent; $P = 0.0004$) and with an increased number of positive nodes (4.8 versus 2.2; $P = 0.0003$). Patients with LVI-positive colon cancer had a lower 5-year survival rate than LVI-negative patients (57 percent versus 84 percent, all stages); reduced survival rates were also noted for tumors of the rectum/rectosigmoid (38 percent versus 71 percent, all stages). These differences were statistically significant. LVI was found to be an independent prognostic variable by proportional hazards analysis.

Although much has been learned about the

influence of BVI and LVI on prognosis, much work still remains to be done. At least for the time being, it seems reasonable to conclude that LVI and extramural BVI (especially among thick-walled veins) significantly worsen the prognosis in patients with colorectal carcinoma.

BOWEL OBSTRUCTION AND PERFORATION

Bowel obstruction and perforation (often with abscess formation) reduce survival and disease-free survival.[44, 47, 98] Although these features may be detected clinically by radiologic examination or at the time of surgery, the pathologist can provide useful information by commenting on these findings during examination of the gross specimen. At the very least, this will provide confirmation of the clinical impression. It has also been suggested that tumor invasion of the free mesothelial surface is associated with a significant reduction in survival among patients with potentially curable cancers.[82]

LYMPHOCYTIC INFILTRATION

Lymphocytic infiltration of the primary colorectal cancer had been regarded as a measure of host response to tumor by some.[28, 53, 58] A sparse lymphocytic infiltrate has been associated with a worse prognosis by these workers. Jass et al.[53] have claimed that lymphocytic infiltration is a statistically significant variable in predicting patient outcome, and they have incorporated a semiquantitative appraisal of this feature into a multiparameter staging system (see the discussion on staging, above).

EARLY COLORECTAL CARCINOMA/MALIGNANT POLYP

Pathologists, like most physicians, seek to make a difference in the outcome of a patient's illness. One area in which the surgical pathologist plays an extremely important role in therapeutic management decisions is the evaluation of "early" colorectal carcinoma. Morson et al.[99] have defined *early colorectal cancer* as carcinoma that has spread beyond the muscularis

mucosa into the submucosa proper. This description does not encompass a stage in the histogenesis of colorectal cancer, but rather is a purely morphologic assessment. Many of these early carcinomas are detected following endoscopic removal of a colorectal polyp. Thus, a "malignant polyp" may be viewed as a polyp containing cancer that invades into the submucosa. Malignant polyps may be composed predominantly of adenoma with only a focus of carcinoma, or the entire polyp may be carcinomatous (a polypoid carcinoma). It follows from what has already been stated that a polyp with cancer limited to the mucosa is not considered to be a malignant polyp, for it lacks the biologic potential to metastasize.

In order to determine whether polypectomy has been curative in a particular case, the pathologist must take great care to ensure that the polyp is processed and examined properly. Improper handling can lead to erroneous interpretation, which may cause the patient to undergo unneeded surgery. Before the pathologist issues a final diagnostic report, it is essential that the technical aspects of specimen handling are conducted carefully, and that the method and completeness of tissue removal are confirmed. The latter requirement may necessitate consultation with the clinician, and this must be done without hesitation in order to resolve discrepancies and provide the best possible treatment and care to the patient.

The technical aspects of specimen preparation are very important and include fixation, sectioning, and proper specimen orientation. Without proper fixation, the polyp may crumble when cut, or may be difficult to assess histologically. Opinions vary concerning optimal formalin fixation time, with some workers[100, 101] recommending overnight fixation and others[102] recommending 2 to 6 hours of fixation. For polyps that are 1.5 cm or smaller, we believe that 2 to 3 hours of fixation of the whole specimen followed by 2 hours of fixation of the cut specimen is adequate, provided that large volumes of formalin are employed (10 vol. formalin to 1 vol. tissue). Larger polyps should fix overnight prior to cutting.

Proper cutting of the polyp requires participation of a pathologist to ensure that the pertinent histologic parameters can be evaluated. Before the polyp is cut, either a stalk or a diathermy mark (an area of grey to whitish discoloration) must be identified. The polyp is then cut sagittally through the stalk or diathermy mark so that the relationships of the elements (head, neck, stalk, etc.) are apparent and will be assessable histologically. Most polyps will require only a single cut, bisecting the polyp, although occasionally more than one cut will be necessary. All tissue is submitted for processing, and three levels should be cut per block. An alternative method is the one employed at the St. Mark's Hospital.[100] These pathologists prefer to embed the fixed uncut polyp whole on its side. The block is then trimmed until sections can be cut through the head and stalk of the polyp in continuity.

Frequent and cooperative communication between pathologist and edoscopist cannot be overemphasized if the patient is to receive optimal care. The pathologist should be informed as to whether the polyp was removed intact or in a piecemeal fashion, and whether any of the lesion was left behind. Polyps that have been removed in multiple fragments may be impossible to evaluate with respect to the margin of resection. At times, a fragment of a large adenoma may be submitted to pathology and a small focus of carcinoma within this fragment may be misinterpreted as having been curatively excised when, in fact, carcinoma remains behind in the patient. It is not uncommon for these types of specimens to be accompanied by a clinical history sheet containing only the description "colon polyp." Clearly, the best therapeutic decision-making occurs following unfettered interaction between the endoscopist and pathologist, a scenario strongly endorsed by the physicians at St. Mark's Hospital.[100]

There are several features inherent in the morphology of malignant polyps that should draw the attention of the pathologist. These features include (1) the configuration of the polyp, (2) the extent of the carcinoma, (3) the grade of carcinoma, and (4) the status of lymphatics

(Figs. 8-8 to 8-10). Polyp configuration may be described as pedunculated, semipedunculated, or sessile; these terms correspond to long stalk, short stalk, and sessile, respectively, as described by Cooper previously.[103] Although these descriptions are convenient, they may not be relevant when deciding on the adequacy of polypectomy, as is discussed below.

Pedunculated polyps are composed of a head, a neck, and a stalk. The stalk is separated from the head by the neck, which is the point at which adenomatous epithelium meets nonadenomatous epithelium. The margin of transection is usually identified by the coagulative necrosis characteristic of diathermy injury. When judging the extent of carcinoma in a malignant polyp, many[100, 102–107] examine whether or not the carcinoma invades the submucosa, and if so, whether the cancer involves the head, the stalk, and the margin of resection. Tumor at or within 1 to 2 mm of the resection margin is a more critical factor in determining adequacy of polypectomy than presence of tumor in the head or stalk. If the margin is positive or tumor is within 1 to 2 mm of the margin, further surgical resection is warranted.

Haggitt and co-workers[108] employ a somewhat different approach. These investigators divide the extent of cancer within the polyp according to the following levels: level 1, carcinoma invading the submucosa but limited to the head of the polyp; level 2, carcinoma invading to the neck of the polyp; level 3, stalk invasion by cancer; level 4, cancer into the submucosa of the bowel wall, below the stalk of the polyp, but above the muscularis propria. By this system, all sessile malignant polyps are level 4. In the absence of lymphatic invasion and grade III histology, these investigators believe that further surgery is only necessary for level 4 lesions.

Morson et al.[100] describe the excision of carcinomas as complete, doubtfully complete, and incomplete. Doubtfully complete excisions are those cases in which carcinoma is present within the coagulated tissue at the diathermy margin; incomplete excisions occur when histologic (tumor actually at the resection margin) and/or

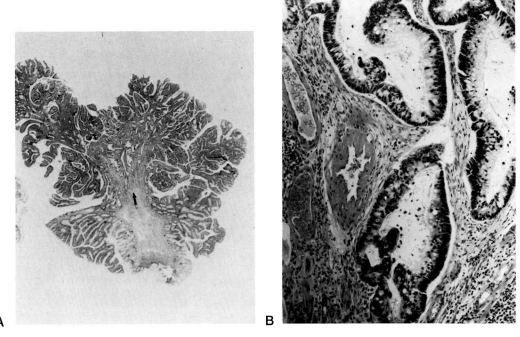

A   B

Fig. 8-8. (A) Pedunculated tubulovillous adenoma with focus of invasive carcinoma involving head of polyp only (arrow). The tumor invades into the submucosa of the polyp, but the stalk is free of tumor. The patient underwent polypectomy only and was free of disease 6 years later. **(B)** Higher-power view of invasive cancer. (H&E, × 100.)

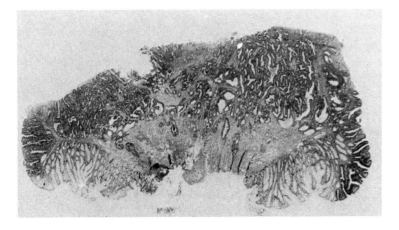

Fig. 8-9. Malignant polyp with short stalk. The great majority of the lesion is carcinoma, with the tumor invading into the stalk and near the margin of resection. This patient underwent a definitive colon resection and had metastases in one regional lymph node.

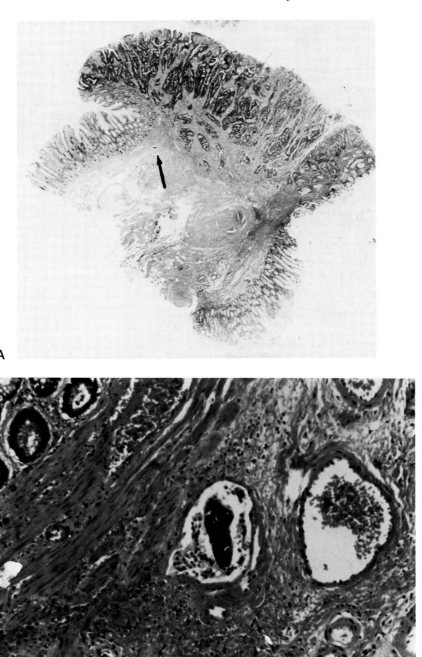

A

B

Fig. 8-10 **(A)** Malignant polyp with focus of lymphatic invasion (arrow). **(B)** Higher-power view of Fig. A showing tumor emboli within submucosal lymphatic. (H&E, × 100.)

Table 8-10. Findings in Surgically Resected Large Bowels Following Removal of Malignant Polyp with Carcinoma At or Near the Resection Margin

Study	No. Polyps with Carcinoma At or Near (within 1 to 2 mm) the Resection Margin	Lymph Node Metastases	Residual Carcinoma
Morson et al.[100]	20	0(0%)	2(10%)
Cooper[103]	24	5(20.8%)	1(4.1%)
Cranley et al.[102]	22	4(18.2%)	6(27.7%)
Wolff and Shinya[104]	24	1(4.1%)	6(25%)
Langer et al.[105]	6	0(0%)	4(66.6%)
Nivatvongs and Goldberg[107]	8	2(25%)	0(0%)
Total	104	12(11.5%)	19(18.3%)

(From Cooper,[109] with permission.)

endoscopic evidence indicates that cancer may have been left behind in the patient. These workers recommend further surgery for all incomplete excisions and in those doubtfully complete excisions where other clinical factors such as age and overall health of the patient are favorable for additional surgery. Morson and co-workers[100] support these recommendations with data from 20 patients with doubtfully complete or incomplete excisions, 11 of whom underwent definitive bowel resection. Nine of the resected patients were free of residual cancer, residual cancer was present at the polypectomy site in two patients, and no patient was found to have metastatic cancer in lymph nodes. All of the nine patients undergoing polypectomy only were alive and well at least 5 years after excision.

Various investigators[100, 102–105, 107] have provided data indicating that in cases in which carcinoma is at or near the margin of resection (including Morson's doubtfully complete excision), the incidence of lymph node metastasis varies from 0 to 25 percent. These patients also have residual carcinoma at an incidence of 3.3 to 66.6 percent (Table 8-10). When the resection margin is free of cancer (or cancer is more than 1 to 2 mm from the resection margin), the incidence of lymph node metastasis is 0 percent, as culled from acceptable cases in the literature (Table 8-11).

Poorly differentiated (grade III) carcinomas tend to behave in an aggressive fashion; these tumors should be treated with surgical resection even if the polyp margin is free of cancer.

Table 8-11. Findings in Surgically Resected Large Bowels Following Removal of Malignant Polyp with Negative Resection Margin

Study	No. of Polyps with Negative Resection Margin	Lymph Node Metastases	Residual Carcinoma
Morson et al.[100]	40	0	0
Cooper[103]	32	0	0
Cranley et al.[102]	18	0	0
Wolff & Shinya[104]	17	0	0
Langer et al.[105]	13	0	1(7.6%)[a]
Nivatvongs & Goldberg[107]	15	0	0
Total	135	0	1(0.74%)

[a] This case reportedly had a free margin, however, no data is provided regarding distances from margin, lymphatic invasion, or tumor grade.

(From Cooper,[109] with permission.)

Table 8-12. Outcome in Patients with Malignant Polyps Containing Grade III Carcinoma[a]

Study	No. of Polyps with Grade III Cancer	No. Residual Carcinoma	No. Lymph Node Metastases	No. Distant Metastases	No. DOD
Morson et al.[100]	3	0	0	NS	1(33.3%)
Haggitt et al.[108]	2	0	0	1(50%)	1(50%)
Cooper[103]	3	0	2(66.6%)	2(66.6%)	3(100%)
Cranley et al.[102]	4	2(50%)	0	1(25%)	2(50%)
Colacchio et al.[110]	2	NS	1(50%)	NS	NS
Total	14	2(14.2%)	3(21.4%)	4(28.5%)	7(50%)

[a] Every patient with grade III cancer and an adverse outcome had other negative parameters such as lymphatic invasion or tumor close to or at the resection margin.
NS, not stated; DOD, dead of disease.
(From Cooper,[109] with permission.)

These high-grade cancers have an incidence of lymph node metastasis that varies between 0 and 66.6 percent; the incidence of local recurrence is 0 to 50 percent.[100, 102, 103, 108–110] Death with local or distant disease has been reported, but these cases had other features (such as positive resection margins or LVI) that in all likelihood contributed unfavorably to the outcome.[100, 102, 103, 108–110] Patients with grade III cancers who were alive and well did not have these additional unfavorable variables (Table 8-12).

The presence of LVI by tumor in a malignant polyp is a feature that generates controversy when one is contemplating the need for further surgery. LVI not initially apparent may appear on deeper sections or, conversely, readily identifiable LVI may disappear upon serial sectioning. Is it possible that LVI is present in most polyps? One of the two cases of Haggitt et al.[108] in which lymphatic vessel invasion was noted developed local recurrence and distant metastasis. Lipper and co-workers[101] identified a single patient with LVI who was free of residual disease at colectomy. Of the four patients noted to have LVI by Cranley et al.,[102] one was discovered to have unresectable grade III cancer at surgery and died in less than a year. One of us[103] identified six patients with LVI, of whom only one (16.6 percent) had lymph node metastasis. This patient had a grade III carcinoma. It seems that the majority of cases with LVI and a poor outcome also had grade III histology[100–103, 108, 110] (Table 8-13).

Table 8-13. Outcomes in Patients with Malignant Polyps Containing Lymphatic Tumor Invasion

Study	No. of Polyps with Lymphatic Invasion	Local Recurrence	Lymph Node Metastases	DOD
Morson et al.[100]	0	NS	NS	NS
Haggitt et al.[108]	2	1(50%)[a]	0	1(50%)
Cooper[103]	6	0	1(16.6%)[b]	1(16.6%)[b]
Cranley et al.[102]	4	0	0	1(25%)
Colacchio et al.[110]	4	NS	2(50%)[c]	NS
Lipper et al.[101]	1	0	0	0
Total	17	1(5.8%)	3(17.6%)	3(17.6%)

[a] Patient also had distant metastases and was DOD; carcinoma was of an intermediate grade.
[b] Grade III carcinoma.
[c] One patient had grade III carcinoma.
NS, not stated; DOD, dead of disease.
(From Cooper,[109] with permission.)

Occasionally, polyps removed in endoscopy will prove to be composed entirely of carcinomatous epithelium without any residual adenoma. Many clinicians believed that these carcinomas were biologically more aggressive than cancers arising in a background of adenoma, and therefore recommended further definitive surgery in these cases. Thoughtful examination of available data would suggest that these tumors can be treated effectively via polypectomy if attention is paid to those parameters governing the management of adenomas with invasive cancer.[100, 101, 103, 108] There is support in the literature for the conclusion that those polypoid carcinomas demonstrating metastatic behavior have other poor prognostic features such as grade III histology, tumor at or near the transection margin, or LVI. Thus, polypoid carcinomas are no more aggressive per se than adenomas containing carcinoma.

The three important indicators of the therapeutic adequacy of polypectomy are (1) status of the resection margin, (2) presence or absence of LVI, and (3) histologic grade. Polypectomy can be considered curative when the resection margin is free of cancer (or cancer is more than 1 to 2 mm from the margin), no LVI is present, and the cancer is grade I or II. Definitive surgical resection should follow polypectomy when cancer is at or near (within 1 to 2 mm from) the margin because the incidence of lymph node metastasis and residual tumor are 11.5 and 18.3 percent, respectively (Tables 8-10 and 8-11). Whether surgery should be performed if LVI is noted is controversial. In these patients with LVI, the incidence of lymph node metastasis approaches 18 percent (Table 8-13). Although it is true that most patients with LVI and metastasis had grade III cancers, LVI by grade I or II cancers should probably be considered an unfavorable prognostic feature until more data on these types of cases are available. Grade III malignant polyps should be considered an indicator for further surgery, regardless of the status of other parameters (Table 8-12). Polypoid carcinomas should be evaluated with the same criteria as adenomas containing cancer.

Although the discussion above contains the generally accepted criteria for postpolypectomy bowel resection, the reader should be made aware of a few parting caveats. Even when criteria for further surgery are met, 50 to 80 percent of patients will have no evidence of residual carcinoma (either local or within lymph nodes) after radical bowel resection.[100, 102–105, 107] This is to be expected by the clinician and pathologist, and the patient should be so informed. A few investigators have described false negatives in which resected bowel contained residual cancer following polypectomy with negative margin, low grade (I or II) cancer, and no evidence of LVI. Langer and co-workers[105] reported residual cancer in a colon resection specimen in 1 of 13 cases in which the malignant polyps appeared to have been completely removed. These workers do not, however, describe the grade of the cancer, the distance of cancer from the margin of resection, or presence or absence of LVI. Colacchio et al.[110] claim a false-negative rate of 33 percent and advise resection for all patients found to have carcinoma within a polyp, but this report is exceptional to most of the studies reported in the literature.

Patients who have undergone bowel resection following polypectomy and in whom no evidence of residual carcinoma or lymph node metastases is detected should not automatically be considered cured. Morson[100] describes a patient with grade II carcinoma and a negative resection who later died from metastatic cancer. Similarly, Cooper[103] has reported two patients without cancer in their resection specimens who later developed liver metastases.

Although considerable discussion has been devoted to early colorectal cancer, the pathologist must be aware of those cases showing "pseudoinvasion" (PI) (Fig. 8-11). Although 5 percent of adenomas have invasive cancer, the incidence of PI varies from 2.5 percent to 10 percent.[111, 112] These lesions mimic invasive cancer by the presence of tongues of mucosa herniating into the submucosa through gaps or defects in the muscularis mucosa. In distinguishing PI from an adenoma with invasive cancer, several important facts should be kept in mind. Proper orientation is extremely important, and

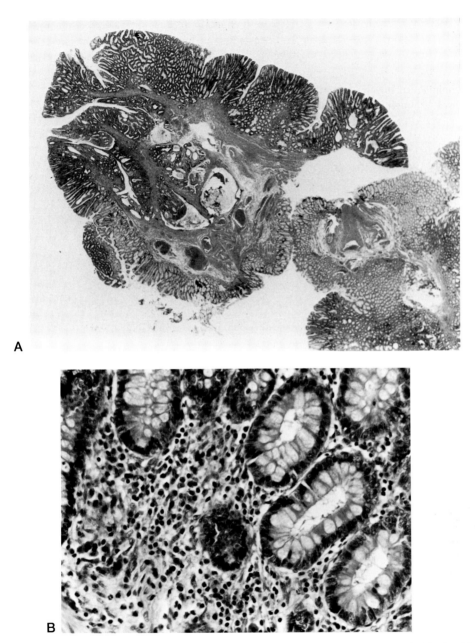

Fig. 8-11. (A) Adenoma showing pseudoinvasion. One can appreciate an "invagination" of epithelium and accompanying lamina propria into the submucosa, and not invasion by cancer. (Cf. Fig. 8-8, 8-9, and 8-10.) The somewhat characteristic cystically distended glands within the submucosa may also be noted. **(B)** Higher-power view of submucosal "inclusions," showing non-neoplastic epithelium by "lamina propria-supporting" tissue. (H&E, × 250.)

serial and deeper sections can be helpful in arriving at the proper diagnosis. If one examines a polyp with epithelial structures within the submucosa and no cancer in the mucosa itself, one should be very hesitant about making a diagnosis of invasive carcinoma. In PI polyps, another helpful finding is the presence of "lamina propria-supporting tissue" surrounding the epithelial submucosal inclusions. This suggests "herniation" of mucosal elements into the submucosa, and not invasion by carcinoma. Finally, benign-appearing epithelium in the submucosa should suggest a PI polyp. The treachery of these lesions is exemplified in the study by Greene,[113] in which 18 of 21 PI polyps had been initially misdiagnosed as invasive carcinoma.

MOLECULAR GENETICS OF COLORECTAL CARCINOMA

The past decade has been a period of rapid growth in our understanding of certain molecular aspects of cancer. The discovery of cellular oncogenes and antioncogenes combined with increasingly sensitive methods for studying DNA and RNA have provided a glimpse into the fundamental mechanisms of neoplastic transformation in a variety of cancers. Cytogenetic studies have progressed from such relatively straightforward procedures as karyotyping to the identification of allelic deletions, which occur with some frequency in certain tumors. It is not surprising that colorectal cancers have been the subject of research into the role of oncogenes, antioncogenes, and allelic deletions in carcinogenesis.

Of all the oncogenes studied thus far, the *ras* oncogenes have generated the most interest since they are the transforming genes most frequently detected in human cancers, including tumors of the colon and rectum.[114] There are three *ras* proto-oncongenes: H-*ras,* K-ras (first detected as viral oncogenes in the Harvey and Kirsten rat sarcoma viruses), and N-*ras.* These functional cellular proto-oncogenes encode for very similar 21-kD proteins (p21), which are membrane bound proteins that bind guanine nucleotides and possess intrinsic GTPase activity.[115, 116] These proteins are thought to possess signal-transduction properties. Single-point mutations in codons 12, 13, and 61 within *ras* proto-oncogenes convert them into active oncogenes, providing the capacity for malignant transformation.[116] Early studies of the presence of mutated *ras* genes revealed a high percentage (40 to 50 percent) of these mutations (particularly c-K-*ras*) in both colorectal carcinomas and adenomas.[117, 118] Vogelstein et al.[115] found mutated *ras* genes in 47 percent of the carcinomas studied, with 88 percent of the mutated genes being of the c-K-*ras* type. There was no apparent correlation between the presence of a *ras* oncogene and tumor location, depth of penetration, level of differentiation, or age or sex of the patient. Small tubular adenomas from patients with familial adenomatous polyposis (FAP) contained *ras* oncogenes in only 13 percent of polyps studied. Approximately 50 percent of adenomas from patients without FAP as well as adenomas containing invasive adenocarcinoma exhibited *ras* oncogene mutations. Adenomas larger than 1 cm contained *ras* mutations more frequently than adenomas smaller than 1 cm (58 percent vs. 9 percent, respectively; $P < 0.0001$). To determine whether certain patients were predisposed to developing *ras* mutations because of an environmental or genetic factor, multiple polyps from patients with familial adenomatous polyposis were analyzed, as were lesions from patients without FAP. In both groups, the presence of *ras* mutations in one tumor was not associated with an increased frequency of *ras* mutations in other tumors from the same patient.

Kerr et al.[119] compared the levels of c-*ras*-related cellular RNA in colorectal cancers with conventional staging criteria and clinical outcome in these neoplasms. These workers found that neither the presence of c-*ras* oncogene expression nor variations in the level of c-*ras* expression could be used to predict differences in the clinical behaviors of colorectal carcinomas.

Another oncogene that has been studied is c-*myc,* a cellular homologue of the transforming sequence present in the avian myelocytomatosis virus.[120] These gene codes for production of a 62-kD protein (p62^c-*myc*) that has been detected in significantly elevated levels in malignant colorectal tumors versus normal colonic mucosa.[121, 122] Sikora and co-workers[123] report a good correlation between p62^c-*myc* content and histologic grade of colorectal cancers. Erisman et al.[124] found no significant difference in survival between patients with high c-*myc* RNA levels and those with low c-*myc* RNA levels. Imaseki and co-workers[122] reported that the levels of c-*myc* expression in colorectal polyps were associated with malignant potential since adenomas with carcinoma in situ or high-grade dysplasia displayed high levels of expression compared to adenomas without dysplasia or carcinoma in situ. Thus, according to these investigators, the expression of c-*myc* oncogene may serve as a useful marker for evaluating the potential malignancy of colorectal polyps.

Deletions of specific chromosomal regions have been detected in colorectal neoplasms, and these allelic deletions have been studied via restriction fragment length polymorphism analysis of DNA.[115, 125, 126] The long arm (q) of chromosomes 5 and 18, as well as the short arm (p) of chromosome 17, have been identified as regions wherein allelic deletions occur. These regions are thought to contain tumor suppressing genes, or *antioncogenes,* which, when inactivated via deletion or mutation, allow malignant transformation to proceed.[125] Patients with FAP develop hundreds of colorectal adenomas following inheritance of this autosomal-dominant disorder.[127] A gene locus designated as *fap* is known to segregate with this disease and has been mapped to the long arm of chromosome 5 (5q). Twenty to 35 percent of colorectal cancers and 29 percent of adenomas in patients without FAP show 5q allelic deletions, but adenomas from FAP patients do not show this deletion.[115, 126, 128] Thus, the tumor-supressing role proposed for this gene is not yet clearly elucidated. Other allelic deletions studied by Vogelstein and co-workers[115] involve the long arm of chromosome 18; these deletions were seen in 73 percent of carcinomas, 47 percent

of adenomas containing invasive cancer, and to a lesser extent (11 to 13 percent) in pure adenomas. Allelic deletions of the short arm of 17 (17p) were noted in 75 percent of carcinomas, 24 percent of adenomas containing invasive cancer, and only 6 percent of benign adenomas.[115] A 53-kD protein (p53) that is believed to suppress neoplastic growth has been localized to a gene on the short arm of chromosome 17.[129] Evidence indicates that loss of p53 gene function through mutation or deletion results in loss of tumor suppression. Thus, although the p53 gene has been considered an oncogene by some workers,[130, 131] it is more accurately characterized as an antioncogene.

The early appearance of *ras*-gene mutations followed by allelic deletions in chromosomes 17 and 18 as reported by Vogelstein et al.[115] in the adenoma-carcinoma sequence of tumorigenesis points to a model of accumulated genetic alterations in the development of colorectal carcinoma. This model encompasses a growth-promoting oncogene combined with alterations in tumor suppressor genes that outline a progressive series of molecular changes in the development of colorectal cancer. Investigations have been undertaken to assess the possible clinical implications of chromosomal changes in 17p and 18q. Allelic deletions have been quantified and the *fractional allelic loss* (FAL) has been calculated to represent the fraction of chromosomal arms on which deletions are found.[125, 126] Kern et al[125] noted an association between FAL of 17p and 18q with lower survival rates and death from metastatic colorectal cancer, however, it is not clear whether this is a causal relationship or a sensitive marker of multifactorial chromosomal changes in aggressive tumors. These workers also noted a strong association between high FAL and family history of cancer as well as a lower rate of 17p and 18q allelic deletions in mucin-producing and right-sided cancers. Vogelstein et al.[126] calculated the median percentage of FAL in a group of patients with colorectal carcinoma in whom 17p and 18q deletions were observed. Patients with greater than the median FAL were more likely to develop recurrent disease and to die of their cancer than patients with less than the median FAL ($P < 0.01$) despite equal numbers of *ras*-gene mutations in both groups. These patients were similar with respect to age, sex, size of tumor, and depth of invasion. A subset of patients with less advanced tumors (Dukes A and B) was also studied; of 14 patients with greater than the median FAL, 11 developed recurrent disease (i.e., distant metastasis); of 14 patients with less than the median FAL, only 2 developed recurrent disease ($P < 0.0001$).

TUMOR ANTIGENS

The literature regarding colorectal cancer and tumor associated antigens (TAA) is voluminous. Many of these studies have employed immunohistochemistry using lectins, polyclonal, and monoclonal antibodies. Unfortunately, to date no TAA has been found to be specific for cancer, shown to be of prognostic significance, or to be site specific when it comes to colorectal cancer. These TAA have taught us about basic biochemical differences between non-neoplastic and neoplastic colonic epithelium. These TAA may play a role as receptors for growth factors or relate to cell to cell interaction and signaling. Most of the TAA studied are against carbohydrate moities, many with blood group specificity. These TAA can be classified into three major groups: (1) TAA that are absent in the normal colon, but present in fetal colon, adenomas, cancers, and reactive non-neoplastic epithelium (Fig. 8-12); (2) TAA that are normally present in specific subcellular compartments, but show cytostructural rearrangement upon neoplastic transformation (Fig. 8-13); and (3) TAA that are markers for specific enterocyte differentiation at different levels of the normal colon crypt. Examples of these are noted in Table 8-14.[132–158]

CYTOMETRIC DNA ANALYSIS IN COLORECTAL CARCINOMA

Pathologists use various criteria when examining tissues for histologic evidence of malignancy. Among these criteria are nuclear enlarge-ment and increased nuclear affinity for hematoxylin (hyperchromasia). Since DNA is the substance largely responsible for nuclear staining by hematoxylin and similar dyes, it is reasonable to assume that hyperchromasia may be a reflection of increased nuclear DNA content. In addition, cells synthesize DNA prior to dividing and thus rapidly growing tumors might be expected to contain numerous cells with increased amounts of DNA. These presumptions provide incentive for the quantitation of DNA content in various tumors, including those of the colon and rectum.[159]

The analysis of cellular DNA content has evolved into two distinct methodologies: image cytomorphometry and flow cytometry. The former technique involves the preparation of cells on glass slides with Feulgen stain, which binds stoichiometrically to DNA. Cells are then analyzed with the aid of a video image-based cytometer, which provides data based on the optical density of selected nuclei. Integrated software enables the cell analyzer to generate DNA histograms from which the DNA index of each peak is calculated.[160] Flow cytometry utilizes a device in which a stream of cells or cell nuclei are directed in single file past a light beam that produces fluorescence proportional to the amount of fluorochrome dye present in the cell. These fluorochromes (propidium iodide, acridine orange, and others) stain cell nuclei in a proportionate fashion similar to the Feulgen stain used in image cytometry, enabling the flow cytometer to produce DNA histograms.[159] Optimal histograms can also provide data for mathematic models, which then allow for calculation of the percentage of cells in the DNA synthesis phase, the so-called S phase fraction.[161]

Video cytometry and flow cytometry can both be performed on formalin-fixed paraffin embedded tissue as well as fresh material.[162] This enables investigators to assess a wealth of archival material with these instruments. Some have compared the results obtained by video-image cytomorphometry with those obtained by flow cytometry and most have reported a good correlation between these techniques for various tumors.[160] Aneuploid populations of tumor cells detected by image cytometry are occasionally missed by flow cytometry, however, and may

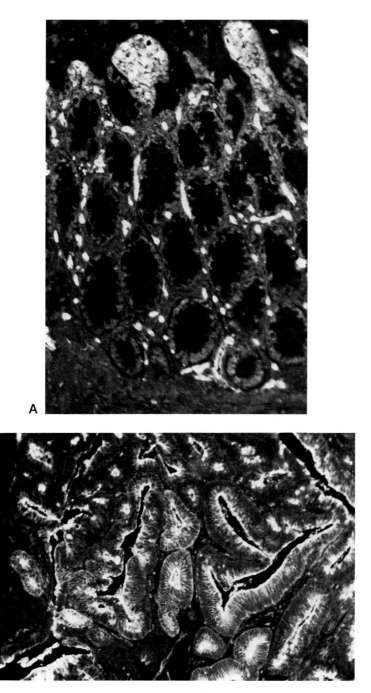

Fig. 8-12. **(A)** Section of normal sigmoid colon with bright fluorescence localized to capillaries but absent in the goblet cells. This indicates the absence of A blood group substance in the goblet cells. Section treated with anti-A as primary antibody. **(B)** Adenocarcinoma showing presence of A blood group substance as evidenced by fluorescence localized to ''glycocalyx'' and/or apical portion of acini. Section treated with anti-A as primary antibody. (Fig. A × 250, Fig. B × 100.)

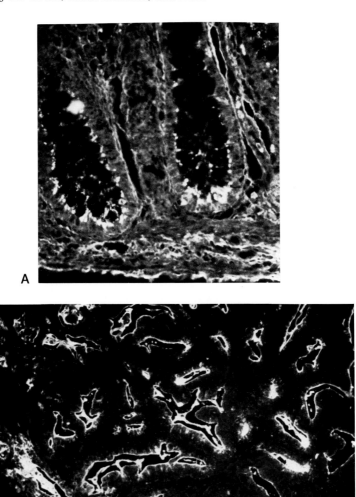

Fig. 8-13 (A) Sigmoid colon showing fluorescence (T antigen or PNA binding sites) localized to the supranuclear portion of cells, whereas the goblet cells are a negative. **(B)** Colonic adenocarcinoma showing bright fluorescence in region of the glycocalyx indicating presence of T blood group antigens. Note the cytologic rearrangement of T antigen in the colon cancer compared to normal colon (Fig. A). (PNA-Anti PNA-FITC, Fig. A × 250, Fig. B × 100.)

reflect "contamination" of the flow cytometry cell study population by inflammatory or non-neoplastic cells.[160]

A number of investigators[163–174] have studied the implications of flow cytometric DNA analysis on various pathologic and clinical facets of colorectal carcinoma. Crissman et al.[161] have provided a very interesting review of these published series. By combining data from published reports and extrapolating survival data when necessary from published survival curves in prospective studies with less than 5 years' follow

Table 8-14. Blood Group-Related Tumor-Associated Antigens

Group[a]	Antigen	Normal Colon	Fetal Colon	Adenoma	Carcinoma	IBD	References
I	A	$-(+^b)$	+	+	+	ND	132–134, 138, 140
	B	$-(+^b)$	+	+	+	ND	132–134, 138, 140
	H	$-(+^b)$	+	+	+	ND	132–134, 138, 140
	Leb	$-(+^b)$	ND	+	+	ND	135–138
I & II	Sial TN (B72.3)	$-(+^c)$	+	+	+	+	141–144
II	T antigen	$+^c$	+	+	+	+	141, 145–148
III	Sial-Le a	$+^d$	+	+	+	+	136, 159–152
	Le y	$+^e$	+	+	+	+	136, 139, 149, 153, 154
	Le x	+	+	+	+	ND	136, 155, 156
	Le a	$+^f$	ND	+	+	ND	138, 140, 157
	Sial-Le x	$+^e(-)$	ND	+	+	ND	156, 160

[a] See text under Tumor Antigens for explanation of group.
[b] Proximal colon.
[c] Golgi-like expression.
[d] Expressed by cells at the surface of the crypt.
[e] Expressed by cells at the base of the crypt.
[f] Expressed by cells throughout the entire length of the crypt.
IBD, Inflammatory bowel disease; ND, No data.

up, Crissman and co-workers found overall 5-year survival rates of 65 and 43 percent for diploid and aneuploid tumors, respectively. These data reflect all stages combined, and were obtained from both retrospective and prospective studies. The data suggest a survival advantage for patients with diploid cancers versus those with aneuploid cancers of the colorectum. When analyzing survival by stage, it was noted that stage A diploid tumors had a 5-year survival rate of 84 percent versus 67 percent for aneuploid stage A tumors. The 5-year survival rate for the latter group is a variance with conventional historical stage A cancers, however, this may be due to the small number of cases studied. Stage B colorectal cancers had 5-year survival rates of 63 percent and 38 percent for diploid and aneuploid tumors, respectively. Stage C tumor survival rate was 50 percent for diploid cancers and 13 percent for aneuploid cancers.

Attempts to correlate DNA content as measured by flow cytometry and such histologic parameters as extent of differentiation and pattern of invasion have not been too successful. Several studies have been unable to demonstrate correlation between DNA content and tumor grade.[103, 164, 168, 170–174] It has been noted, however, that vascular invasion is more likely to occur with abnormal DNA content,[164, 171] although one published report[174] disputes this. The value of DNA aneuploidy as a prognostic variable is a topic of controversy, with some investigators concluding that aneuploidy is independently associated with a poor prognosis[163, 165, 169] and others believing that is it not significant or that it is not an independent variable.[166–168, 170, 173] As Crissman et al.[161] mention in the summary of their review, it is difficult to draw conclusions regarding the prognostic value of flow-cytometric DNA analyses because of patient selection biases (particularly in retrospective studies) and variations in technique in cell sample preparation. Nonetheless, it seems reasonable to point out that higher-stage tumors have proportionately more aneuploid cancers, aneuploid tumors tend to have a poorer survival compared with diploid tumors, and, although unrelated to tumor grade, aneuploidy correlates with such poor prognostic parameters as vascular invasion.[161] Finally, although Bauer et al.[168] reported that the proportion of colorectal carcinoma cells in S phase correlated independently with poor prognosis, this S phase fraction represents a calculation based on a mathematical model that lacks standardization and should probably be considered an indirect measurement of tumor proliferative activity.

Only a few reports[172, 176] have described the use of image cytometry in the analysis of colorectal tumors. These investigators have shown results similar to those obtained via flow cytometry and have indicated a worse prognosis for aneuploid colorectal cancer. Emdin et al.[172] used static cytometry and flow cytometry on several tumors and found good correlation between the results of each method.

ACKNOWLEDGMENT

The authors would like to express their sincere appreciation for the excellent secretarial assistance provided by Ms. Mary Jo Marchionni.

REFERENCES

1. Silverberg E, Boring CC, Squires TS: Cancer statistics, 1990. Ca 40: 9, 1990
2. Wynder EL: The epidemiology of large bowel cancer. Cancer Res 35:3388, 1975
3. Berg JW, Howell MA: The geographic pathology of bowel cancer. Cancer 34:807, 1974
4. Correa P: Comments on the epidemiology of large bowel cancer. Cancer Res 35:3395, 1975
5. Wynder EL, Kajitani T, Ishikawa S, et al: Environmental factors of cancer of the colon and rectum. Cancer 23:1210, 1969
6. Stemmerman GN, Mandel M, Mower H: Colon cancer: its precursors and companions in Hawaii Japanese. Natl Cancer Inst Monogr 53:175, 1979
7. Rosato FE, Marks G: Changing site distribution patterns of colorectal cancer at Thomas Jefferson University Hospital. Dis Colon Rectum 24:93, 1981
8. Welch JP: Trends in the anatomic distribution of colorectal cancer. Conn Med 43:457, 1979
9. Rhodes JB, Holmes FF, Clark GM: Changing distribution of primary cancers in the large bowel. JAMA 238:1641, 1977
10. Cady B, Persson AV, Monson DO, Mauz DL: Changing patterns of colorectal carcinoma. Cancer 33:422, 1974
11. Lockhart-Mummery HE, Ritchie JK, Hawley PR: The results of surgical treatment for carcinoma of the Rectum at St. Mark's Hospital from 1948 to 1972. Br J Surg 63:673, 1976
12. Wood DA, Robbins GF, Zippin C, et al: Staging of cancer of the colon and cancer of the rectum. Cancer 43:961, 1979
13. Falterman KW, Hill CB, Markey JC, et al: Cancer of the colon, rectum, and anus: a review of 2313 cases. Cancer 34:951, 1974
14. Elmasri SH, Boulos PB: Carcinoma of the large bowel in the Sudan. Br J Surg 62:284, 1975
15. Recalde M, Holyoke ED, Elias EG: Carcinoma of the colon, rectum, and anal canal in young patients. Surg Gynecol Obstet 139:909, 1974
16. Domerque J, Ismail M, Astre C, et al: Colorectal carcinoma in patients younger than 40 years of age. Cancer 61:835, 1988
17. Mills SE, Allen MS Jr: Colorectal carcinoma in the first three decades of life. Am J Surg Pathol 3:443, 1979
18. Odone V, Chang L, Caces J, et al: The natural history of colorectal carcinoma in adolescents. Cancer 49:1716, 1982
19. Simstein NL, Kovalcik PJ, Cross GH: Colorectal carcinoma in patients less than 40 years old. Dis Colon Rectum 21:169, 1978
20. Symonds DA, Vickery AL Jr: Mucinous carcinoma of the colon and rectum. Cancer 37:1891, 1976
21. Dukes CE, Bussey HJR: The spread of rectal cancer and its effects on prognosis. Br J Cancer 12:309, 1958
22. Rankin FW, Olson PF: The hopeful prognosis in cases of carcinoma of the colon. Surg Gynecol Obstet 56:366, 1933
23. Grinnel RS: The grading and prognosis of carcinoma of the colon and rectum. Ann Surg 109:500, 1939
24. Steinberg SM, Barwick KW, Stablein DM: Importance of tumor pathology and morphology in patients with surgically resected colon cancer. Findings from the Gastrointestinal Tumor Study Group. Cancer 58:1340, 1986
25. Wolmark N, Fisher ER, Wieand HS, Fisher B: The relationship of depth of penetration and tumor size to the number of positive nodes in Dukes' C colorectal cancer. Cancer 53:2707, 1984

26. Montessori GA, Donald JC: Invasion profile of colorectal carcinoma. Dis Colon Rectum 21:26, 1978

27. Whittaker M, Goligher JC: The prognosis after surgical treatment for carcinoma of the rectum. Br J Surg 63:384, 1976

28. Spratt JS Jr, Spjut HJ: Prevalence and prognosis of individual clinical and pathologic variables associated with colorectal carcinoma. Cancer 20:1976, 1967

29. Black WA, Waugh JM: The intramural extension of carcinoma of the descending colon, sigmoid, and rectosigmoid. A pathologic study. Surg Gynecol Obst 87:457, 1948

30. Grinnell RS: Distal intramural spread of carcinoma of the rectum and rectosigmoid. A pathologic study. Surg Gynecol Obstet 87:457, 1948

31. Copeland EM, Miller LD, Jones RS: Prognostic factors in carcinoma of the colon and rectum. Am J Surg 116:875, 1968

32. Williams NS, Dixon MF, Johnston D: Reappraisal of the 5 cm rule of distal excision for carcinoma of the rectum: A study of distal intramural spread and of patients' survival. Br J Surg 70:150, 1983

33. Penfold JC: A comparison of restorative resection of carcinoma of the middle third of the rectum with abdominoperineal excision. Aust NZ J Surg 44:354, 1974

34. Pollett WG, Nicholls RJ: The relationship between the extent of distal clearance and survival and local recurrence rates after curative anterior resection for carcinoma of the rectum. Ann Surg 198:159, 1983

35. Madsen PM, Christiansen J: Distal intramucosal spread of rectal carcinomas. Dis Colon Rectum 29:279, 1986

36. Chan KW, Boey J, Wong SKC: A method of reporting radial invasion and surgical clearance of rectal carcinoma. Histopathology 9:1319, 1985

37. Hager T, Gall FP, Hermanek P: Local excision of cancer of the rectum. Dis Colon Rectum 26:149, 1983

38. Whiteway J, Nicholls RJ, Morson BC: The role of surgical local excision in the treatment of rectal cancer. Br J Surg 72:694, 1985

39. Morson BC, Bussey HJR, Samoorian S: Policy of local excision for early cancer of the colorectum. Gut 18:1045, 1977

40. Mason AY: Malignant tumors of the rectum: local excision. Clin Gastroenterol 4:582, 1975

41. Biggers OR, Beart RW, Ilstrup DM: Local excision of rectal cancer. Dis Colon Rectum 29:374, 1986

42. DeCosse JJ, Wong RJ, Quan SHQ, et al: Conservative treatment of distal rectal cancer by local excision. Cancer 63:219, 1989

43. Willett CG, Tepper JE, Donnelly S, et al: Patterns of failure following local excision and postoperative radiation therapy for invasive rectal adenocarcinoma. J Clin Oncol 7:1003, 1989

44. Steinberg SM, Barkin JS, Kaplan RS, Stablein DM: Prognostic indicators of colon tumors. The Gastrointestinal Tumor Study Group experience. Cancer 57:1866, 1986

45. Rich T, Gunderson LL, Lew R, et al: Patterns of recurrence of rectal cancer after potentially curative surgery. Cancer 52:1317, 1983

46. Minsky BD, Mies C, Rich T, et al: Potentially curative surgery of colon cancer: Patterns of failure and survival. J. Clin Oncol 6:106, 1988

47. Wolmark N, Wieand HS, Rockette HE, et al: The prognostic significance of tumor location and bowel obstruction in Dukes' B and C colorectal cancer. Ann Surg 198:743, 1983

48. Eisenberg B, DeCosse JJ, Harford F, Michalek J: Carcinoma of the colon and rectum. The natural history reviewed in 1704 patients. Cancer 49:1131, 1982

49. Stevens WR, Ruiz P: Primary linitis plastica carcinoma of the colon and rectum. Mod Pathol 2:265, 1989

50. Almagro UA: Primary signet-ring carcinoma of the colon. Cancer 52:1453, 1983

51. Thomas GDH, Dixon MF, Smeeton NC, Williams NS: Observer variation in the histological grading of rectal carcinoma. J Clin Pathol 36:385, 1983

52. Newland RC, Chapuis PH, Pheils MT, MacPherson JG: The relationship of survival to staging and grading of colorectal cancer—a prospective study of 503 cases. Cancer 47:1424, 1981

53. Jass JR, Atkin WS, Cuzick J, et al: The grading of rectal cancer: historical perspectives and a multivariate analysis of 447 cases. Histopathology 10:437, 1986

54. Jass JR, Love SR, Northover JMA: A new prognostic classification of rectal cancer. Lancet 1:1303, 1987

55. Phillips RKS, Hittinger R, Blesovsky L, et al: Large bowel cancer: surgical pathology and its

relationship to survival. Br J Surg 71:604, 1984

56. Cohen JR, Theile DE, Evans EB, et al: Colorectal cancer at the Princess Alexandria Hospital: a prospective study of 729 cases. Aust NZ J Surg 53:113, 1983

57. Chapuis PH, Deut OF, Fisher R, et al: A multivariate analysis of clinical and pathological variables in prognosis after resection of large bowel cancer. Br J Surg 72:698, 1985

58. Zamcheck N, Doos WG, Prudente R, et al: Prognostic factors in colon carcinoma. Correlation of serum carcinoembryonic antigen level and tumor histopathology. Hum Pathol 6:31, 1975

59. Sasaki O, Atkin WS, Jass JR: Mucinous carcinoma of the rectum. Histopathology 11:259, 1987

60. Pihl E, Nairn RC, Hughes ESR, et al: Mucinous colorectal carcinoma: immunopathology and prognosis. Pathology 12:439, 1980

61. Halvorsen TB, Seim E: Influence of mucinous components on survival in colorectal adenocarcinomas: a multivariate analysis. J Clin Pathol 41:1068, 1988

62. Bonello JC, Sternberg SS, Quan SHQ: The significance of signet cell variety of adenocarcinoma of the rectum. Dis Colon Rectum 23:180, 1980

63. Michelassi F, Mishlove LA, Stipa F, Block GE: Squamous cell carcinoma of the colon. Experience at the University of Chicago, review of the literature, report of two cases. Dis Colon Rectum 31:228, 1988

64. Williams GT, Blackshaw AJ, Morson BC: Squamous carcinoma of the colorectum and its genesis. J Pathol 129:139, 1979

65. Austin DE: Etiological clues from descriptive epidemiology: squamous carcinoma of the rectum and anus. Natl Cancer Inst Monogr 62:89, 1982

66. Comer TP, Beahrs OH, Dockerty MB: Primary squamous cell carcinoma and adenoacanthoma of the colon. Cancer 28:1111, 1971

67. Mills SE, Allen MS, Cohen AR: Small cell undifferentiated carcinoma of the colon. A clinicopathological study of five cases and their association with colonic adenomas. Am J Surg Pathol 7:643, 1983

68. Schwartz AM, Orenstein JM: Small cell undifferentiated carcinoma of the rectosigmoid colon. Arch Pathol Lab Med 109:629, 1985

69. Wick MR, Weatherby RP, Weiland LH: Small cell neuroendocrine carcinoma of the colon and rectum: clinical, histological, and ultrastructural comparison with cloacogenic cancer. Hum Pathol 18:9, 1987

70. Cooper HS: Intestinal neoplasms. p.1032 In Sternberg S (ed.):Diagnostic Surgical Pathology. Raven Press, New York, 1989

71. Petrelli M, Tetangco E, Reid JD: Carcinoma of the colon with undifferentiated, carcinoid, and squamous cell features. Am J Clin Pathol 75:581, 1981

72. Werdin C, Limas C, Knodell RG: Primary malignant melanoma of the rectum. Evidence for origination from rectal mucosal melanocytes. Cancer 61:1361, 1988

73. Gown AM, Vogel AM, Hoak D, et al: Monoclonal antibodies specific for melanocytic tumors distinguish subpopulations of melanocytes. Am J Pathol 123:195, 1986

74. Weidner N, Zekan P: Carcinosarcoma of the colon. Report of a unique case with light microscopic and immunohistochemical studies. Cancer 58:1126, 1986

75. Hainsworth JD, Greco TA: Human chorionic gonadotropin production by colon cancer. Cancer 56:1337, 1985

76. Nguyen GK: Adenocarcinoma of the sigmoid colon with focal choriocarcinoma metaplasia. Dis Colon Rectum 25:230, 1982

77. Park CH, Reid JD: Adenocarcinoma of the colon with choriocarcinoma in its metastases. Cancer 46:570, 1980

78. Watson PH, Alguacil-Garcia A: Mixed crypt cell carcinoma. A clinicopathological study of the so-called goblet cell carcinoid. Virchows Arch A 412:175, 1987

79. Dukes CE: The classification of cancer of the rectum. J Pathol Bacteriol 35:323, 1932

80. Gabriel WB, Dukes C, Bussey HJR: Lymphatic spread in cancer of the rectum. Br J Surg 23:395, 1935

81. Pihl E, Hughes ESR, McDermott FT, et al: Carcinoma of the rectum and rectosigmoid: cancer specific long-term survival. Cancer 45:2902, 1980

82. Newland RC, Chapuis PH, Smyth EJ: The prognostic value of substaging colorectal carcinoma. Cancer 60:852, 1987

83. Dukes CE: The surgical pathology of rectal cancer. J Clin Pathol 2:95, 1949

84. Turnbull RB, Kyle K, Watson FR, Spratt J: Cancer of the colon: the influence of the no-

touch isolation technique on survival rates. Ann Surg 166:420, 1967

85. Astler VB, Coller FA: The prognostic significance of direct extension of carcinoma of the colon and rectum. Ann Surg 139:846, 1954

86. Hutter RVP, Sobin LH: A universal staging system for cancer of the colon and rectum. Arch Pathol Lab Med 110:367, 1986

87. Lessner HE, Mayer RJ, Ellenberg SS: Adjuvant therapy of colon cancer: results of a prospectively randomized trial. N Engl J Med 310:737, 1984

88. Wolmark N, Fisher B. Wieand HS: The prognostic value of the modifications of the Dukes' C class of colorectal cancer. Ann Surg 203:115, 1986

89. Fisher ER, Sass R, Palekar A, et al: Dukes' classification revisited. Cancer 64:2354, 1989

90. Grinnell RS: Lymphatic block with atypical and retrograde lymphatic metastases and spread in carcinoma of the colon and rectum. Ann Surg 163:272, 1966

91. Brown CF, Warren S: Visceral metastasis from rectal carcinoma. Surg Gynecol Obstet 66:611, 1938

92. Khankhanian N, Mavligit GM, Russell WD, Schimek M: Prognostic significance of vascular invasion in colorectal cancer of Dukes' B class. Cancer 39:1195, 1977

93. Talbot IC, Ritchie S, Leighton MH, et al: Spread of rectal cancer within veins. Histologic features and clinical significance. Am J Surg 141:15, 1981

94. Grinnell RS: The lymphatic and venous spread of carcinoma of the rectum. Ann Surg 116:200, 1942

95. Minsky BD, Mies C, Rich TA, et al: Potentially curative surgery of colon cancer: the influence of blood vessel invasion. J Clin Oncol 6:119, 1988

96. Minsky BD, Mies C, Recht A, et al: Resectable adenocarcinoma of the rectosigmoid and rectum II: the influence of blood vessel invasion. Cancer 61:1417, 1988

97. Minsky BD, Mies C, Rich TA, Recht A: Lymphatic vessel invasion is an independent prognostic factor for survival in colorectal cancer. Int J Radiat Oncol Biol Phys 17:311, 1989

98. Willett C, Tepper JE, Cohen A, et al: Obstructive and perforative colonic carcinoma: patterns of failure. J Clin Oncol 3:379, 1985

99. Morson BC, Dawson IMP, Day DW, et al: Malignant epithelial tumors. p.604. In Morson BC, Dawson IMP, Day DW, et al: Morson and Dawson's Gastrointestinal Pathology. 3rd Ed. Blackwell Scientific Publishers, Oxford, 1990

100. Morson BC, Whiteway JE, Macrae FA, Williams CB: Histopathology and prognosis of malignant colorectal polyps treated by endoscopic polypectomy. Gut 25:437, 1985

101. Lipper S, Kahn LB, Ackerman LV: The significance of microscopic invasive cancer in endoscopically removed polyps of the large bowel: a clinicopathologic study of 51 cases. Cancer 52:1691, 1983

102. Cranley JP, Petras RE, Carey WD, et al: When is endoscopic polypectomy adequate therapy for colonic polyps containing invasive carcinoma? Gastroenterology 91:419, 1986

103. Cooper HS: Surgical pathology of endoscopically removed malignant polyps of the colon and rectum. Am J Surg Pathol 7:613, 1983

104. Wolff WI, Shinya H: Definitive treatment of ''malignant'' polyps of the colon. Ann Surg 182:516, 1975

105. Langer JC, Cohen Z, Taylor BR, et al: Management of patients with polyps containing malignancy removed by colonoscopic polypectomy. Dis Colon Rectum 27:6, 1984

106. Coutsoftides T, Sivak MV, Benjamin SP, Jagelman D: Colonoscopy and the management of polyps containing invasive cancer. Ann Surg 188:638, 1978

107. Nivatvongs S, Goldberg SM: Management of patients who have polyps containing invasive carcinoma removed via colonoscope. Dis Colon Rectum 21:8, 1978

108. Haggitt RC, Golzbach RE, Soffer EE, Wruhle LD: Prognostic factors in colorectal carcinomas arising in adenomas: implications for lesions removed malignant colorectal polyps. Gastroenterology 89:328, 1985

109. Cooper HS: The role of the pathologist in the management of patients with endoscopically removed malignant colorectal polyps. Pathol Annu 23:25, 1988

110. Colacchio TA, Forde KA, Scantlebury VP: Endoscopic polypectomy. Inadequate treatment for invasive colorectal carcinoma. Ann Surg 194:704, 1981

111. Muto T, Bussey JH, Morson BC: Pseudo-carcinomatous invasion in adenomatous polyps of the colon and rectum. J Clin Pathol 26:25, 1973

112. Qizilbash AH, Meghji M, Castelli M: Pseudo-carcinomatous invasion in adenomas of the colon and rectum. Dis Colon Rectum 23:529, 1980

113. Green FL: Epithelial misplacement in adenomatous polyps of the colon and rectum. Cancer 33:206, 1974

114. Bos JL: The *ras* gene family and human carcinogenesis. Mutat Res 195:255, 1988

115. Vogelstein B, Fearon ER, Hamilton SR, et al: Genetic alterations during colorectal tumor development. N Eng J Med 319:525, 1988

116. Bos JL: *ras* Oncogenes in human cancer: A review. Cancer Res 49:4682, 1989

117. Bos JL, Fearon ER, Hamilton SR, et al: Prevalence of *ras* gene mutations in human colorectal cancers. Nature 327:293, 1987

118. Forrester K, Almoguera C, Han K, et al: Detection of high incidence of k-*ras* oncogenes during human colonic turmorigenesis. Nature 327:298, 1987

119. Kerr IB, Spandidos, DA, Finlay IG, et al: The relation of *ras* family oncogene expression to conventional staging criteria and clinical outcome in colorectal carcinoma. Br J Cancer 53:231, 1986

120. Colby WW, Chen EY, Smith DH, Levinson AD: Identification and nucleotide sequence of a human locus homologue to the v-*myc* oncogene of avian myelocytomatosis virus MC29. Nature 301:722, 1983

121. Erisman MD, Rothberg PG, Diehl RE, et al: Deregulation of c-*myc* gene expression in human colon carcinoma is not accompanied by amplification or rearrangement of the gene. Mol Cell Biol 5:1969, 1985

122. Imaseki H, Hayashi H, Taira M, et al: Expression of c-*myc* oncogene in colorectal polyps as a biological marker for monitoring malignant potential. Cancer 64:704, 1989

123. Sikora K, Chan S, Evan G, et al: c-*myc* oncogene expression in colorectal cancer. Cancer 59:1289, 1987

124. Erisman MD, Litwin S, Keidan RD, et al: Non-correlation of the expression of the c-*myc* oncogene in colorectal carcinoma with recurrence of disease or patient survival. Cancer Res 48:1350, 1988

125. Kern SE, Fearon ER, Tersmette KWF, et al: Allelic loss in colorectal carcinoma. JAMA 261:3099, 1989

126. Vogelstein B, Fearon ER, Kern SE, et al: Allelotype of colorectal carcinomas. Science 244:207, 1989

127. Haggitt RC, Reid BJ: Hereditary gastrointestinal polyposis syndromes. Am J Surg Pathol 10:871, 1987

128. Solomon E, Voss R, Hall V, et al: Chromosome 5 allelic loss in human colorectal carcinomas. Nature 328:616, 1987

129. Baker SJ, Fearon ER, Nigro JM, et al: Chromosome 17 deletions and p53 gene mutations in colorectal carcinomas. Science 244:217, 1989

130. Wolf D, Harris N, Rotter V: Reconstitution of p53 expression in a non-producer Ab-MuLV-transformed cell line by transfection of a functional p53 gene. Cell 38:119, 1984

131. van de Berg FM, Tigges AJ, Schipper MEI, et al: Expression of the nuclear oncogene p53 in colon tumours. J Pathol 157:193, 1989

132. Cooper HS, Haesler WH: Blood group substances of tumor antigens in the distal colon. Am J Clin Pathol 69:594, 1978

133. Cooper HS, Cox J, Patchefsky, AS: Immunohistochemical study of blood group substances in polyps of the distal colon. Am J Clin Pathol 73:345, 1980

134. Dabelsteene E, Graemn N, Claussen H, Hakomori SI: Structural variations of blood group A antigens in human normal colon and carcinomas. Cancer Res 48:181, 1988

135. Cooper HS, Marshall C, Ruggerio F, Steplewski Z: Hyperplastic polyps of the colon and rectum. An immunohistochemical study with monoclonal antibodies against blood group antigens (Sialosyl-Lea, Lea, Leb, Lex, Ley, A, B, H). Lab Invest 57:421, 1987

136. Ruggerio F, Cooper HS, Steplewski Z: Immunohistochemical study of colorectal adenomas with monoclonal antibodies against blood group antigens (Sialosyl-Lea, Leb, Lex, Ley, A, B, H). Lab Invest 59:96, 1988

137. Itzkowitz SH, Yuan M, Ferrell D, et al: Cancer associated alterations of blood group antigen expression in human colorectal polyps. Cancer Res 46:5976, 1986

138. Yuan M, Itzkowitz SH, Palekar A, et al: Distribution of blood group antigens A, B, H, Lea, and Leb in human normal, fetal, and malignant colonic tissue. Cancer Res 45:4499, 1985

139. Brown A, Ellis IO, Embleton MJ, et al: Immunohistochemical localization of Y-hapton and

the structurally related H-type 2 blood group antigen on large bowel tumors and normal adult tissue. Int J Cancer 33:727, 1984

140. Shoentag, Primus FJ, Kuhns SW: ABH and Lewis blood group expression in colorectal carcinoma. Cancer Res 47:1695, 1987
141. Itzkowitz SH, Yuan M, Montogomery CK, et al: Expression of Tn, sialosyl-Tn, and T antigens in human colon cancer. Cancer Res 49:197, 1989
142. Thor A, Itzkowitz SH, Schlom J, et al: Tumor associated glycoprotein (TAG-72) expression in ulcerative colitis. Int J Cancer 43:810, 1989
143. Thor A, Ohuchi N, Szpak CA, et al: Distribution of oncofetal antigen tumor associated glycoprotein 72 defined by monoclonal B 72.3. Cancer Res 46:3118, 1986
144. Listrom MB, Little JV, McKinley M, Fenoglio-Preiser CM: Immunoreactivity of tumor associated glycoprotein (TAG-72) in normal, hyperplastic, and neoplastic colon. Hum Pathol 20:994, 1989
145. Cooper HS, Reuter BE: Peanut lectin binding sites in polyps of the colon and rectum: adenomas, hyperplastic polyps, and adenomas with in-situ carcinoma. Lab Invest 49:655, 1983
146. Cooper HS: Peanut lectin binding sites in large bowel carcinoma. Lab Invest 47:33, 1982
147. Cooper HS, Farano P, Coapman RA: Peanut lectin binding sites in colons of patients with ulcerative colitis. Arch Pathol Lab Med 111:270, 1987
148. Coapman RA, Cooper HS: Peanut lectin binding sites in human fetal colon. Arch Pathol Lab Med 110:124, 1986
149. Cooper HS, Steplewski Z: Immunohistochemical study of ulcerative colitis with monoclonal antibodies against tumor associated and/or differentiation antigens. Gastroenterology 95:686, 1988
150. Atkinson BF, Ernst CF, Herlin M, et al: Gastrointestinal cancer associated antigen in immunoperoxidase assay. Cancer Res 42:4820, 1982
151. Bara J, Zabaleta EH, Mollicone R, et al: Distribution of GICA in normal intestinal and endocervical mucosa and in mucinous ovarian cysts using antibody NS 19-9. Am J Clin Pathol 85:152, 1986
152. Gong EC, Hirohashi S, Shimosato Y, et al: Expression of carbohydrate antigen 19-9 in stage specific embryonic antigen 1 in non-tu-

morous and tumorous epithelium of the human colon and rectum. J Natl Cancer Inst 7:447, 1985
153. Abe K, Hakomori SI, Oshiba S: Differential expression of difucosyl type 2 chain (Ley) defined by monoclonal antibody AH6 in different locations of colonic epithelia, various histological types of colonic polyps, and adenocarcinoma. Cancer Res 46:2639, 1986
154. Kim YS, Yuan M, Itzkowitz SH, et al: Expression of Ley and extended Ley blood group related antigens in human malignant, pre-malignant, and non-malignant colonic tissue. Cancer Res 46:5985, 1986
155. Shi ZR, McIntyre LJ, Knowles BB, et al: Expression of a carbohydrate differentiation antigen, stage specific embryonic antigen 1, in human colonic adenocarcinoma. Cancer Res 44:1141, 1984
156. Yuan M, Itzkowitz SH, Ferrell LD, et al: Expression of Lex and sialylated Lex antigens in human colorectal polyps. J Natl Cancer Inst 78:479, 1987
157. Sakamoto J, Furukawa K, Cordone-Cardo C, et al: Expression of Lea, Leb, X, and Y blood groups antigens in human colonic tumors and normal tissue and human derived cell lines. Cancer Res 46:1553, 1986
158. Fukushima K, Hirota M, Terasaki PI, et al: Characterization of sialosylated Lex as a new tumor associated antigen. Cancer Res 44:5279, 1984
159. Gansler T: Applications of flow cytometric DNA quantitation in tumor pathology. J Clin Immunoassay 12:30, 1989
160. Bauer TW, Tubbs RR, Edinger MG, et al: A prospective comparison of DNA quantitation by image and flow cytometry. Am J Clin Pathol 93:322, 1990
161. Crissman JD, Zarbo RJ, Ma CK, Visscher DW: Histologic parameters and DNA analysis in colorectal adenocarcinomas. Pathol Annu 24:103, 1989
162. Crissman JD, Zarbo RJ, Neibylski CD, et al: Flow cytometric DNA analysis of colon adenocarcinomas: a comparative study of preparatory techniques. Mod Pathol 1:198, 1988
163. Armitage NC, Robins RA, Evans DF, et al: The influence of tumor cell DNA abnormalities on survival in colorectal cancer. Br J Surg 72:828, 1985

164. Wolley RC, Schreiber K, Koss LG, et al: DNA distribution in human colon carcinoma and its relationship to clinical behavior. J Natl Cancer Inst 69:15, 1982

165. Kokal WA, Gardine RL, Sheibani K, et al: Tumor DNA content in resectable primary colorectal carcinoma. Ann Surg 209:188, 1989

166. Jass JR, Mukawa K, Goh HS, et al: Clinical importance of DNA content in rectal cancer measured by flow cytometry. J Clin Pathol 42:254, 1989

167. Jones DJ, Moore M, Schofield PF: Prognostic significance of DNA ploidy in colorectal cancer: a prospective flow cytometric study. Br J Surg 75:28, 1988

168. Bauer KD, Lincoln ST, Vera-Roman JL, et al: Prognostic implications of proliferative activity and DNA aneuploidy in colonic adenocarcinoma. Lab Invest 57: 329, 1987

169. Quirke P, Dixon MF, Clayden AD, et al: Prognostic significance of DNA aneuploidy and cell proliferation in rectal adenocarcinoma. J Pathol 151:285, 1987

170. Fischer ER, Siderits RH, Sass R, Fisher B: Value of assessment of ploidy in rectal cancers. Arch Pathol Lab Med 113:525, 1989

171. Scott NA, Rainwater LM, Wieand HS, et al: The relative prognostic value of flow cytometric DNA analysis and conventional clinicopathologic criteria in patients with operable rectal carcinoma. Dis Colon Rectum 30:513, 1987

172. Emdin SO, Sterling R, Roos G: Prognostic value of DNA content in colorectal carcinoma. A flow cytometric study with some methodologic aspects. Cancer 60:1282, 1987

173. Melamed MR, Enker WE, Banner P, et al: Flow cytometry of colorectal carcinoma with three year follow up. Dis Colon Rectum 29:184, 1986

174. Kokal W, Shiebani K, Terz J, Harada JR: Tumor DNA content in the prognosis of colorectal carcinoma. JAMA 255:3123, 1986

175. Schutte B, Reynders MM, Wiggers T, et al: Retrospective analysis of the prognostic significance of DNA content and proliferative activity in large bowel carcinoma. Cancer Res 47:5494, 1987

176. Forsslund G, Cedermark B, Ohman U, et al: The significance of DNA distribution pattern in rectal carcinoma. A preliminary study. Dis Colon Rectum 27:579, 1984

9

Epithelial Neoplasia of the Appendix

Henry D. Appelman

It is not surprising that epithelial proliferations in the appendix challenge the surgical pathologist only infrequently, when one considers that the appendix is the smallest part of the gastrointestinal tract. Most of these proliferations are carcinoid tumors with typical patterns that are readily identified. Noncarcinoid epithelial appendiceal neoplasms are so unusual that very few pathologists, even those in the largest centers, have had much experience with them. At the same time, appendectomy specimens removed for acute appendicitis are a standard and very common part of the daily surgical pathology workload. Also, there are very few clearcut data in the literature or in the textbooks to assist the surgical pathologist in making confident diagnoses of noninflammatory appendiceal disease, or even in understanding them. What literature exists is cluttered with terms, often appendiceal site-specific ones, such as *mucocele, pseudomyxoma peritonei, microglandular carcinoma, adenocarcinoid,* and *cystadenoma,* yet it is currently not clear how these conditions are or are not related, and what exactly they mean. This review is intended to identify the specific, mainly neoplastic and proliferative, appendiceal lesions, and to define what relationships exist among them. Carcinoid tumors of usual or common types are not discussed.

To begin, a series of questions can be posed, which this chapter attempts to answer:

1. What is the cause of the appendiceal mucocele?
2. Do the data support the existence of the dilated, mucus-filled appendix known as the *retention cyst?*
3. What is the natural history of mucous extrusion into the peritoneal cavity, the disease designated *pseudomyxoma peritonei?*
4. Does carcinoma of the appendix evolve through the same adenoma-to-carcinoma sequence that seems to explain the genesis of ordinary large bowel carcinoma?
5. Do colonic-type hyperplastic polyps occur in the appendix?
6. Is the peculiar appendiceal tumor composed of well-differentiated goblet-type cells, Paneth cells, and endocrine cells—variably termed *goblet cell carcinoid, adenocarcinoid,* or *crypt cell carcinoma*—a specific entity?

THE STATUS OF THE LITERATURE

The published experiences with abnormal appendiceal mucosal proliferations are limited, in terms of both number and length of follow-up.

Most of the clinicopathological studies of appendiceal neoplasia in the English-language literature have been published in the past 30 years. During this time, by combining the largest series and including most case reports, there have been a total of only about 700 cases published, including all entities.[1-34] These can be separated into specific categories, as indicated in Table 9-1. Even the largest series have only about 30 cases in any category.

Therefore, the information that forms the basis of this review is, by necessity, a tabulation

Table 9-1. Noncarcinoid Epithelial Proliferations of the Appendix

Hyperplastic mucosa or polyp[a]
Adenomas
  Colonic-type (localized tubular, tubulovillous, villous)
    adenoma
  Mucinous cystadenoma (circumferential)[a]
Carcinomas
  Colonic-type adenocarcinoma
  Mucinous carcinoma and cystadenocarcinoma[a]
  Signet ring cell carcinoma
  Adenocarcinoid tumor (mucinous carcinoid tumor, crypt
    cell carcinoma, etc.)

[a] Reported to cause a mucocele.

of the experiences of many investigators, including that of this chapter's author. A data compendium of this kind is fraught with imperfections. It is necessary to rely on the diagnostic histologic interpretations of many different pathologists, which may or may not be uniform. Unfortunately, all too often the diagnostic criteria are not rigidly stated in the various papers. As a result, it is not always clear whether the cases truly belong in the categories in which they are reported. For instance, the distinction between noncystic and cystic adenomas may be artificial (probably in most cases), as is the distinction between noncystic and cystic carcinomas (discussed later).

HYPERPLASTIC (METAPLASTIC) POLYPS—MUCOSAL HYPERPLASIA OR METAPLASIA

Hyperplastic (metaplastic) polyps are typically small sessile lesions (up to 0.5 cm) that occur in the colon but predominate in the rectum, apparently as an accompaniment of aging. Microscopically, they are seen as plaque-like thickenings of mucosa, containing elongated tubules with serrated lumens produced by alternating foci of stratified and nonstratified epithelium. There is a distinct change in the crypt cell population, with a diminution in the number of goblet cells and a marked increase in the number of absorptive cells. Highly characteristic is the basement membrane beneath the surface epithe-

lium, which is strikingly thickened compared with the normal.[35]

Hyperplastic or metaplastic mucosa or polyps have been described in the appendix in three papers covering a total of 59 cases.[13, 36, 37] Fifty-four, or 92 percent, were found in incidentally removed appendices, 10 of which were in patients with colonic carcinoma. A few were considered to be associated with small mucoceles. About 70 percent occurred in women—an expected result, because of the very high number of incidental appendectomies in women. About three-fourths of the patients were over the age of 40 years, although it is difficult to get a clear picture of the age distribution from these studies.

These lesions are considered to be comparable to the hyperplastic polyps in the colon, by virtue of their expanded mucosae and crypt luminal serrations. However, there are several peculiarities that raise doubts about how many reported cases really were typical colonic-style hyperplastic polyps in the appendix. First, many of the illustrations of the appendiceal lesions picture an increase in the mucous or goblet cell population in the so-called hyperplastic crypts, not the decrease so characteristic of their colonic counterparts, and, as mentioned above, a few were even thought to cause mucoceles. Second, in only one of the studies is there mention of a thickened basement membrane beneath the surface epithelium, and the highest-power photomicrograph in that paper does not demonstrate this.[13] In the other studies, there is no mention of the subsurface basement membrane, and it does not stand out in any of the illustrations. Finally, in this author's experience with about 200 mucosal proliferations in the appendix, only a few suggestive examples of a colonic-type hyperplastic polyp with a slightly thick subsurface basement membrane occurred (Fig. 9-1). The rest of the appendiceal lesions examined in our institution that resembled those reported as hyperplastic polyps have not simply serrated lumens, but actually small villi projecting into the lumens (Fig. 9-2), usually accompanied by infolding of the outer crypt contours, an indistinct basement membrane, and pseudostratified,

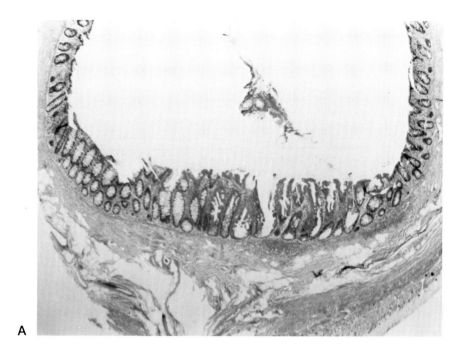

A

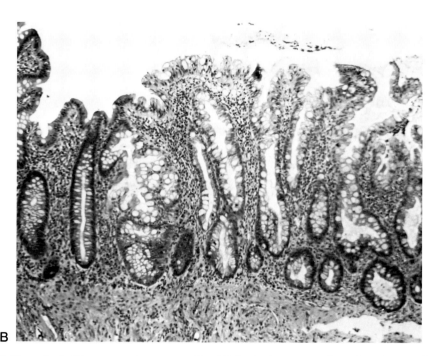

B

Fig. 9-1 Hyperplastic-like mucosa in an appendix. (**A**) In the low-power view, there is a sessile mucosal expansion in the center. (**B**) In the higher-power view, the mucosa is thick, the central and right-side lumens have partly serrated outlines, and the subsurface basement membrane is visible and, thus, possibly thick. (Fig. A × 25, Fig. B × 106.)

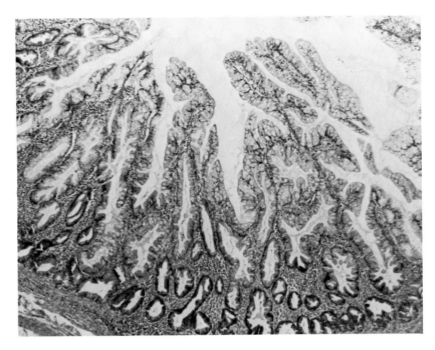

Fig. 9-2. Circumferential appendiceal villous adenoma with serrated crypt lumens, resembling a hyperplastic polyp, but with villiform surface. (× 53.)

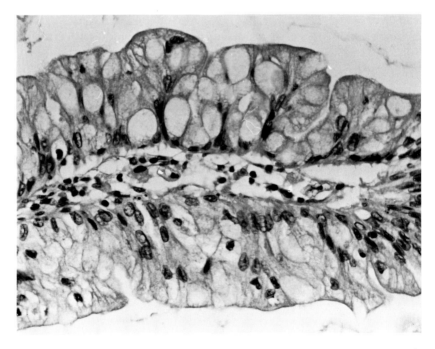

Fig. 9-3. The same adenoma as in Figure 9-2. The epithelium is stratified with piled-up disoriented goblet cells and columnar cells. The subsurface basement membrane is not visible. (× 424.)

predominantly mucinous epithelium (Fig. 9-3) that also occurs in various adenomas and that can be found even in pseudomyxomas. Hyperplastic polyps do occur in the appendix, however, the published reports exaggerate their existence.

COLONIC-TYPE NONCYSTIC LOCALIZED ADENOMAS

Only rarely will appendiceal mucosa produce localized nodular adenomas of virtually the same spectrum as those encountered in the colon.[13, 20] When they do occur, the adenomatous epithelium is identical to that seen in colonic adenomas, with cellular crowding and elongation, elongation and hyperchromatism of the nuclei with various amounts of stratification or piling up, increased numbers of mitotic figures, and mucus depletion (or, more appropriately, lack of mucus production) (Figs. 9-4 and 9-5). Also, they may have tubular, villous, or mixed features. However, they are hardly ever pedunculated. Occasional adenomas may project as bulbous lumps into the appendiceal lumen, but it is rare for them to have a stalk. This probably relates somehow to the limited size they can attain in the small appendiceal lumen, so that the size of a localized adenoma may be inhibited spatially by the wall on the side opposite its point of origin. If a localized adenoma ever grows large enough to fill the lumen and even bulge the appendiceal contour, it certainly will be an unusual event. Colonic-type appendiceal adenomas may occur in adenomatosis coli (familial adenomatous polyposis).[25]

THE USUAL APPENDICEAL MUCINOUS CIRCUMFERENTIAL ADENOMA OR CYSTADENOMA OF VILLOUS OR UNDULATING PATTERNS

Whereas localized colonic-type adenomas with mucus-depleted, compacted, elongated epithelium are extremely rare in the appendix,

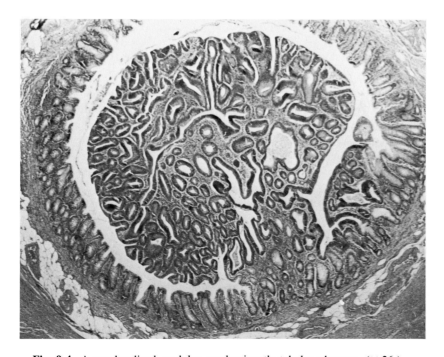

Fig. 9-4. A rare localized, nodular, predominantly tubular adenoma. ($\times$ 26.)

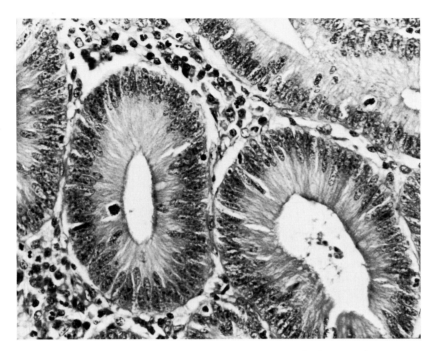

Fig. 9-5. The adenoma in Figure 9-4 contains tubules lined by colonic-type adenomatous epithelium, with tall, crowded columnar cells, slightly stratified elongated nuclei, mitoses, and little cytoplasmic mucin. (× 424.)

more diffuse, usually circumferential, adenomas are relatively common. Appendiceal adenomas tend to be sessile. Sessile colonic adenomas appear to grow peripherally by progressive recruitment of adjacent or marginal mucosa. In a hollow tube with the great diameter of the colon, this can result in large, plaque-like lesions, but only infrequently do they become large enough to encircle the lumen. In the appendix, by contrast, with its narrow lumen, such progressive recruitment early on may lead to complete lumenal encirclement. Thus, most appendiceal adenomas may be classified as circumferential adenomas or cystadenomas. Some are associated with virtually no lumenal dilatation, whereas others produce huge thin-walled cysts. In the colon the vast majority of adenomas, especially the small ones of 2 cm or less in diameter, have the predominately tubular pattern. In contrast, in the appendix, most adenomas of comparable size are mainly villous or undulating, and many of them may be found in the appendiceal literature under the designa-

tion *villous adenoma*. In the colon, the villous pattern in adenomas appears to be an expression of an enhanced growth potential, as compared with the tubular pattern. It is quite likely, although statistically unproven, that a comparable situation occurs in the appendix.

By the time they are discovered, many appendiceal adenomas have ruptured, extruding mucus into the abdominal cavity; thus, they are also lost in the bulk of case reports and short series dealing with the entity classically entitled *pseudomyxoma peritonei*.

There have been four relatively large published series of adenomas, covering 35, 42, 42, and 46 cases, and a large number of adenomas also are found in single case reports or small series of up to 8 cases.[13–15, 18, 20]

In both the large series and the combined case reports, the age of the patients with these adenomas covers the interval from the second through the ninth decades, with a median in the mid-sixth decade. However, the peak occurs in the seventh decade, and the age distribution resembles that for carcinoma and pseudomyxoma. In the large series, females are about twice as commonly effected as males. This striking female predominance in the large series may relate to the high (over 50 percent) incidence of asymptomatic lesions discovered during laparotomies for nonappendiceal diseases, although the cases are not broken down by sex and symptomatology. In contrast, in the combined case reports and small series, there is a slight male predominance, about 4:3. This more equal sex incidence may be explained by a tendency by investigators to report symptomatic cases. Asymptomatic cases are evenly split between the sexes, whereas reported adenomas with associated symptoms have been shown to be twice as likely in men as in women. Since data such as these are based on chance reporting, editorial tolerance for case reports, and presentation of cases by virtue of some fact interesting to the investigators, the preceding clinical features are likely to be a rough estimate of the truth. However, this is a typical indication of the inconsistencies in the appendiceal neoplastic literature.

Certain clinical features do become repetitive in both the larger series and in the case reports. Symptoms associated with appendiceal cystadenomas have tended to be those of acute appendicitis, including right lower quadrant pain, with or without fever, nausea, vomiting, and leukocytosis. However, almost all of these appendices had histologic acute appendicitis, suggesting that it was not the adenomas at all that were symptomatic; rather, the appendicitis called attention to the appendix, and the adenomas were merely incidental findings. It is possible that an adenoma in the proximal appendix can obstruct the lumen, much like a fecalith, and lead to acute appendicitis distally.

A smaller number of patients, generally about 15 percent, present with a palpable abdominal mass, usually in the right lower quadrant. These are probably the patients who have the largest cystic adenomas and those whose adenomatous appendices have ruptured, extruding mucus into the periappendiceal area.

It also is obvious that although some adenomas are found in inflamed appendices or in patients with masses, most adenomas are incidental findings in appendices removed during hysterectomies, colectomies, oophorectomies, and cholecystectomies. This fact undoubtedly accounts for the somewhat high frequency of associated neoplasia in other sites, especially in colon and ovary, that has been said to accompany appendiceal neoplasms. However, this association with extra-appendiceal neoplasia is totally unpredictable and varies from one extreme to the other, depending on the series. Thus, the incidence of associated ovarian neoplasms varies from 11 of 46 (24 percent) in one series to one of 42 (2 percent) in another.[15, 20] Similarly, the incidence of associated colorectal neoplasia varies from 0 of 35 cases (0 percent) to 9 of 42 cases (21 percent).[13, 18] The reader can pick and choose the desired association, depending on preference or favorite investigator.

For most reported cases, the part of the appendix involved was not specified. For the 33 reported cases in which the location was identified, 21 percent were in the proximal appendix, 10 percent were in the middle, 39 percent were near the tip, and 30 percent were defined as diffuse, involving most of the appendix.

Microscopically, there are two types of adenomatous epithelium that occur in the setting of the circumferential adenoma. The first is a crowded, thin, tall columnar epithelium with large apical mucin vacuoles and elongated, but generally basally positioned, nuclei (Fig. 9-6). The second is a more disorganized epithelium, with small, generally round to oval nuclei that may be positioned at the base of the cell or toward the lumenal surface. The cells are either compressed, with little eosinophilic cytoplasm, or distended, with a large mucus droplet that sits on the side of the cell opposite the nucleus (see Fig. 9-3). As a result, this epithelium often appears to contain stratified goblet cells, similar in orientation to those found in some forms of dysplasia associated with long-standing ulcerative colitis. This latter form of adenomatous epithelium is likely to occur in a villous circumferential adenoma that contains serrated crypt outlines, both lumenal and exter-

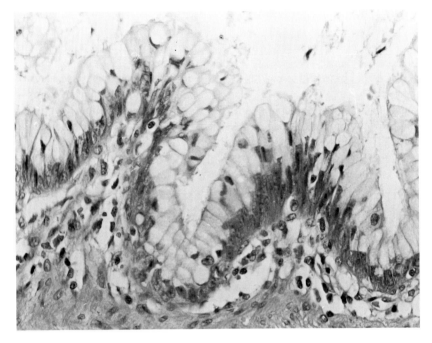

Fig. 9-6. The most common type of appendiceal adenomatous epithelium contains basal, elongated nuclei and apical mucin droplets. (× 424.)

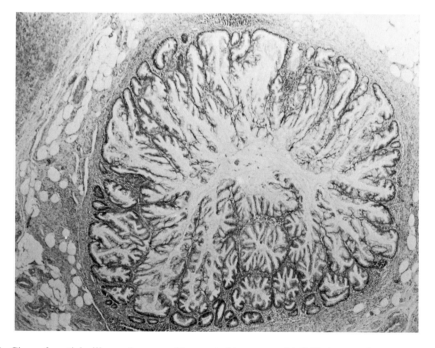

Fig. 9-7. Circumferential villous adenoma with serrated lumens and infolded external crypt contours. The epithelium is mucinous and of the type illustrated in Figure 9-3. The appendiceal lumens is not dilated (not a mucocele). (× 33.)

nal, mimicking somewhat the appearance of the hyperplastic colonic polyp, but more closely resembling some of the borderline malignant mucinous ovarian tumors (Figs. 9-2, 9-3, and 9-7). The subsurface basement membrane is never thickened.

The first type of adenomatous epithelium is by far the more common type. It can be seen in several settings. First, it is the typical epithelium in the dilated, mucus-filled appendix known as the *mucocele,* where it is found in the flat mucosa. Second, it is the epithelium of most circumferential or localized villous adenomas of the appendix (Figs. 9-8 and 9-9). Third, it is the epithelium that lines the undulating mucosa in what may be one of the early stages of the circumferential adenoma or cystadenoma. In this lesion, the mucosa is neither flat nor clearly villous, but is thrown into short folds or minivilli, producing a wavy or undulating mucosal pattern that may be designated as *undulating cystadenoma* (Fig. 9-10). Finally, both types of mucus-producing adenomatous epithelium may become progressively more dysplastic, with gradual loss of mucus production,

increasing stratification of nuclei, and increases in nuclear pleomorphism and mitotic figures (Fig. 9-11). Either or both of these epithelia are commonly found adjacent to invasive appendiceal adenocarcinoma, and may be the precursor adenomatous epithelia, comparable to the adenomatous epithelium that is the precursor of ordinary large bowel carcinoma.[19, 38, 39] In occasional adenomas, both epithelia may exist in the same lesion (Fig. 9-12). Sometimes the two types of adenomatous epithelium will exist in the same adenoma. Some investigators refer to this as a *mixed adenoma/hyperplasia.*

THE RELATION BETWEEN CYSTADENOMA AND MUCOCELE

The appendix mucocele is a dilated, usually thin-walled and mostly uniloculated sac filled with thick tenacious mucus (Figs. 9-13 to 9-15). Occasionally, it is multiloculated (Fig. 9-16). In order for such a phenomenon to occur, several conditions must be met. First, the outflow of lumenal contents must be obstructed.

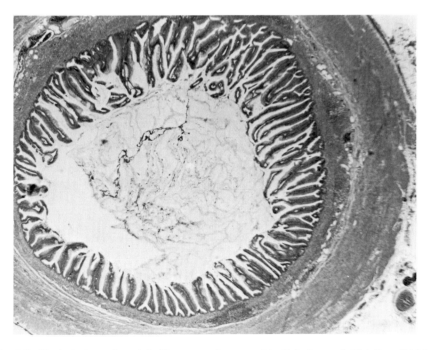

Fig. 9-8. Typical circumferential villous cystadenoma with slight lumenal dilatation. (× 16.)

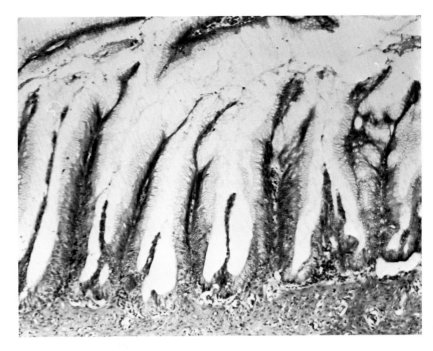

Fig. 9-9. Higher-power view of the tall villi in Figure 9-8. These are covered by mucinous epithelium similar to that in Figure 9-6. (× 106.)

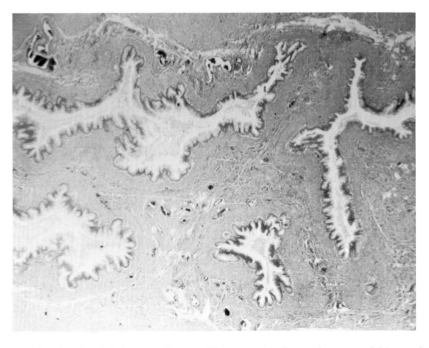

Fig. 9-10. Multiloculated undulating cystadenoma. The mucosa is thrown into wavy folds or minute villi. The epithelium is the same as that in Figure 9-6. (× 26.)

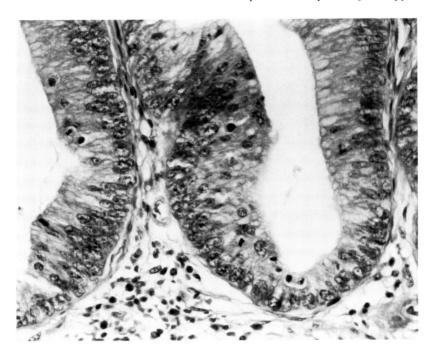

Fig. 9-11. Villous cystadenoma. In this field the epithelium is more dysplastic, with greater crowding of cells, more nuclear stratification with many nuclei at the lumenal face, and increased mitoses and nuclear hyperchromatism. (× 424.)

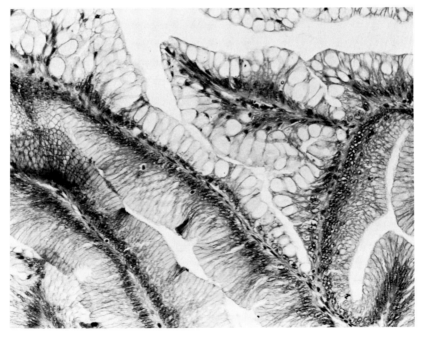

Fig. 9-12. Cystadenoma. Both types of mucinous adenomatous epithelium are present in this field; the common form with the apical mucin is at the bottom, and the serrated type is on the top. (× 212.)

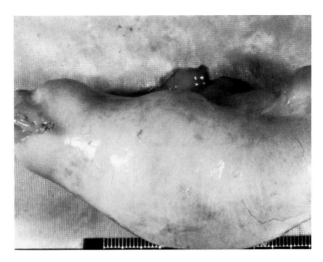

Fig. 9-13. External surface of a large, bulging mucocele formed by a cystadenoma.

This may be by a plug of some kind, such as a fecalith, the thick mucus mass itself, a scar, or even a tumor, but, just as successfully, a malfunctioning muscularis incapable of squeezing appendiceal contents into the cecum may produce the same degree of obstruction. Second, there can be no pyogenic bacterial contamination, since that would stimulate an acute inflammatory reaction with pus; a classical mucocele contains only mucin without pyogenic inflammation. Third, some epithelium must be present that is capable of excessive mucus production. It is certainly not clear whether normal appendiceal epithelium has this capacity. Finally, the wall must contain the increased mucus under increasing intralumenal pressure, because once it ruptures and spills mucus outside the appendix, cystic dilatation is no longer a consideration.

Mucoceles have been subdivided by virtue of their lining epithelium into non-neoplastic and neoplastic types. The non-neoplastic form,

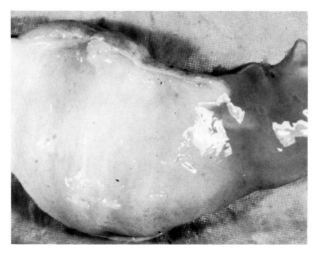

Fig. 9-14. The mucocele in Figure 9-13 opened. The mass of mucin has flowed onto the background at the right. Note the thin wall, seen best at the top center.

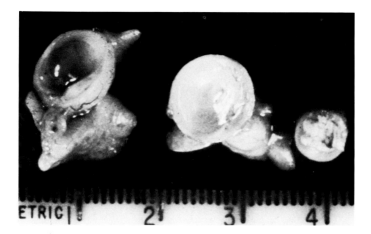

Fig. 9-15. A mucinous cystadenoma producing a 1-cm mucocele in the middle third.

also called *retention cyst, simple mucocele,* or *ectasia,* is considered to result from a sterile obstruction of the appendiceal outflow, with accumulation of material in the lumen, mild dilatation, and subsequent flattening of the mucosa.[15] Such slightly dilated appendices can be found in any large collection of incidentally removed appendices, but it is our experience that these dilatations are never large, probably no more than 1 cm, certainly not of the size encountered in the neoplastic lesions, which at times may measure 6 cm or more in diameter.

The neoplastic nucoceles come in benign and malignant varieties, and are called *mucinous cystadenoma* or *cystadenocarcinoma.*

Mucinous cystadenomas are dilated variants of either the undulating or villous circumferential adenomas. Careful review of a series of mucoceles suggests they may evolve in the following manner. The undulating or villous cystadenomas gradually dilate as a result of mucus accumulation, leading to progressive flattening of the epithelium with subsequent loss of mucus production (Fig. 9-17 A-F). On occasion, partial

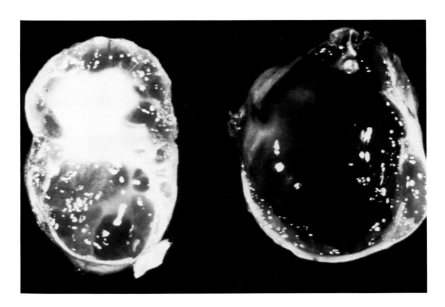

Fig. 9-16. This mucocele is the result of a multiloculated cystadenoma.

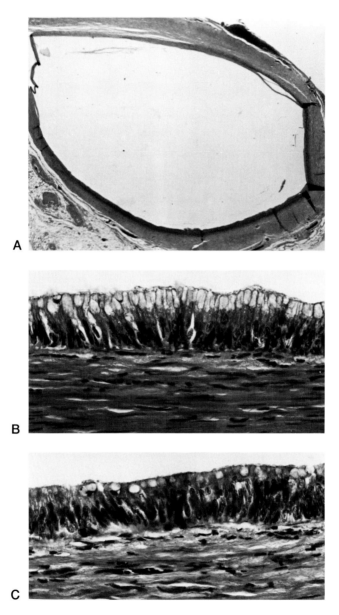

Fig. 9-17. (**A–G**) Sequential views of progressively flattened epithelium in a cystadenoma seen at low power in Fig. A, beginning with typical mucinous adenomatous epithelium in Fig. B and ending with the surface granulomatous reaction to the lumenal mucus in Fig. G. (*Figure continues.*)

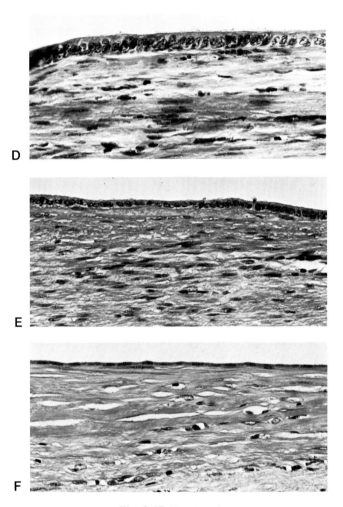

Fig. 9-17 (*Continued*).

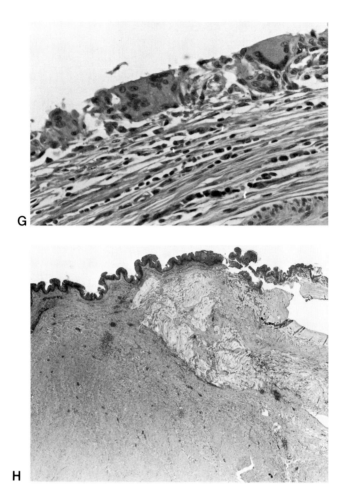

Fig. 9-17 *(Continued)*. (**H**) Loss of epithelium in this cystadenoma resulted in intramural mucus extravasation on the right. (Fig. A × 13. Figs. B–G × 424, Fig. H × 32.)

to total loss of epithelium occurs (ulceration), leading to direct contact of the intralumenal mucus with the mural stroma and a resultant granulomatous or mucous extravasation reaction on the lumenal surface to this mucus (Fig. 9-17G).

In some mucoceles, scattered remnants of well-developed villi covered by mucinous adenomatous epithelium may be found, which apparently are gradually spread further and further apart as the wall is stretched by the accumulating mucus in the lumen (Fig. 9-18).

Most peculiar is what occurs in the appendiceal wall during the evolution of cystadenomas. Even in the predilated stage, there is a gradual loss of the appendiceal lymphoid tissue and muscularis mucosae, with progressive scarring of the submucosa (Fig. 9-19). This seems to be followed by a gradual loss of mucularis propria and conversion of the entire wall to collagen, a substance that has no resiliency and that can be progressively stretched (Fig. 9-17). In general, the collagenization and loss of smooth muscle coexists with the dilatation and stretching, but the degree of smooth muscle loss is not related necessarily to lumenal diameter, since some small mucoceles have no residual smooth muscle, whereas in some large ones many smooth muscle bundles persist. Occasionally, the collagenous wall will become secondarily calcified.

On occasion the adenomatous epithelium seems to dissect or herniate into the collagenous wall, presumably through some points of weakness. It has been suggested that these weakened areas are the result of prior inflammation, but many such herniations or extensions seem to be into pre-existing diverticula, which are fairly common in appendices (Figs. 9-20 and 9-21). Most likely, continued extension of adenomatous epithelium with mucus accumulation in these foci can lead to rupture and spillage of mucus, and possibly even of neoplastic epithelium, into the peritoneal cavity, where a fibrosing reaction results. This peritoneal mucous extravasatium has been called *pseudomyxoma peritonei.* Periodically, this herniation of adenomatous epithelium and rupture can occur even in the absence of overt dilatation, so that localized mucus extrusions can develop from appendices that are not truly mucoceles. Sometimes, only the mucus appears to dissect into the wall, so that finding pools of mucus without epithelium, deep in the wall, is not unusual. Herniated mucinous adenomatous epithelium should not be confused with invasive carcinoma, but at times the distinction may be a difficult morphologic diagnostic problem, especially since some carcinomas may also produce mucoceles.

Finally, a simple anatomic question should be posed here. How dilated must an appendiceal lumen be to qualify as a mucocele? For instance, does an appendix that contains a circumferential mucin-producing adenoma but no dilated lumen qualify as a cystadenoma? Such a lesion is probably a precursor of an adenoma with a dilated lumen. But is there a lower limit on the size of an acceptable mucocele? It would be presumptuous of any one to arbitrarily define such a limit, and probably silly. We can leave the designation of *mucocele,* therefore, to those appendices that the observer thinks are dilated enough.

INVASIVE CARCINOMA OF THE APPENDIX

It is now generally accepted that the ordinary forms of carcinoma of the human colon develop through the adenoma-carcinoma sequence, with first the formation of a neoplastic epithelium with low-grade dysplastic features (adenomatous epithelium) followed by higher grades of dysplasia, including intramucosal carcinoma and eventually invasive carcinoma.[38, 39] Such an epithelial sequence may occur in pedunculated polypoid adenomas, but more commonly it occurs in flat or sessile adenomatous foci, especially in large ones and in those that have a predominantly villous architecture. In the appendix, the same adenoma-carcinoma sequence seems to be operative.[19] Careful sampling of appendices containing carcinomas usually reveals adenomatous foci, which are also mainly villous, at the edge of the carcinomas (Figs. 9-22 and 9-23).

Clinically, carcinoma of the appendix, as reported in the literature, is a disease with a slight male predominance, with four cases in males reported for every three in females (4:3), and an age distribution covering mainly the fifth through the seventh decade, with a median of about 60 years. In the reported cases, about three-fourths of the patients had symptoms possibly referable to their tumors, which included those of appendicitis, palpable masses, or complications of carcinomatous spread in the abdomen, such as intestinal obstruction. Both sexes had the same symptoms with much the same frequency. Carcinomas discovered in incidental appendectomies compose only about a quarter of the cases.

Grossly, the appearance of appendiceal carcinoma is probably a function of its stage. Low-stage lesions, namely those confined to the appendiceal wall, are seen as thickenings. High-stage lesions, those extending beyond the wall, are likely to present to the surgeon as masses, often inflammatory looking, with the appendix buried somewhere in the middle or even obliterated completely. In most reported cases, the location of the tumor within the appendix has not been identified, but in those cases in which the site has been specified, peculiarly, 43 percent occurred in the proximal segment, 14 percent occurred in the middle, and 39 percent were found in the distal part. This contrasts with the location of adenomas, of which proximal lesions were half as common as lesions in the other locations. Perhaps the discrepancy here may

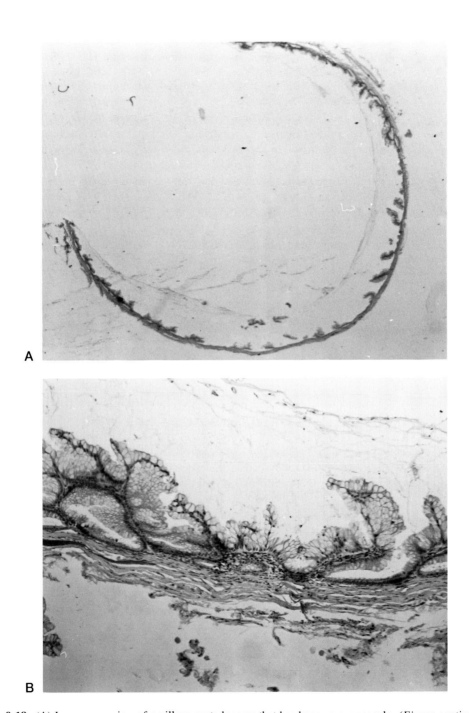

Fig. 9-18. (A) Low-power view of a villous cystadenoma that has become a mucocele. (*Figure continues.*)

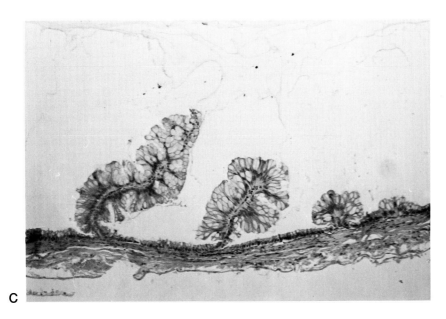

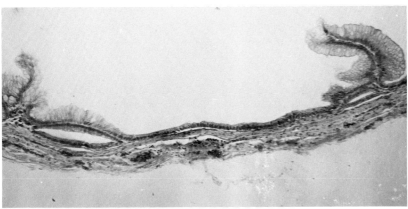

Fig. 9-18 (*Continued*). (**B–D**) Samples of the wall in different areas with progressive separation of remaining villi. (Figs. B–D × 106.)

be explained by the large number of reported cases of appendiceal carcinomas whose locations have not been described, many possibly because of diffuse destruction of the appendix by tumor. Nevertheless, the unusual frequency of proximal tumors raises one interesting issue, namely, whether some of these reported proximal lesions were really cecal carcinomas extending secondarily into the appendix.

About a quarter of the cases have been described as cystadenocarcinomas, which have presented as mucoceles that were indistinguishable grossly from the cystadenomas. Since the remainder were not specified as being cystic, they are grouped under the broad heading of *mucinous* or *colonic-type carcinomas* in this discussion. This separation may be artificial, since typical colonic-style adenocarcinomas are quite rare in the appendix.[13]

The single microscopic prerequisite for the diagnosis of appendiceal carcinoma is invasion by neoplastic cells through the muscularis muco-

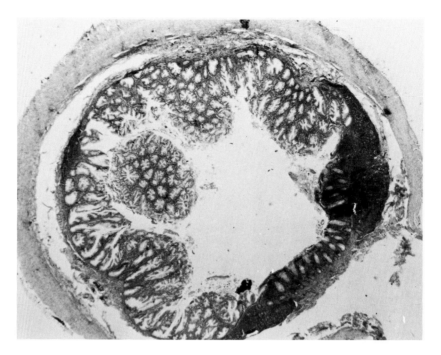

Fig. 9-19. Villous cystadenoma covering about two-thirds of the mucosa. The lymphoid tissue has been lost almost totally from the areas covered by the tumor, but lymphoid tissue persists where the normal mucosa remains, in the lower right corner. (× 22.)

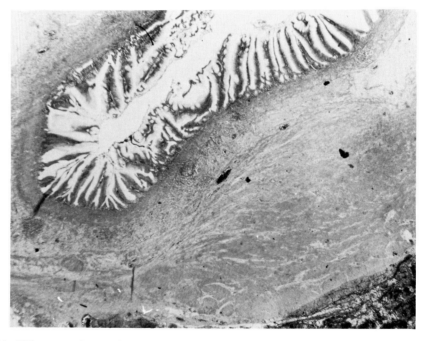

Fig. 9-20. Villous cystadenoma in which there is a herniation of mucosa into the wall in the lower left corner. The thick muscularis propria on the right, which thins to the lower left, suggests that this herniation is really a diverticulum. (× 22.)

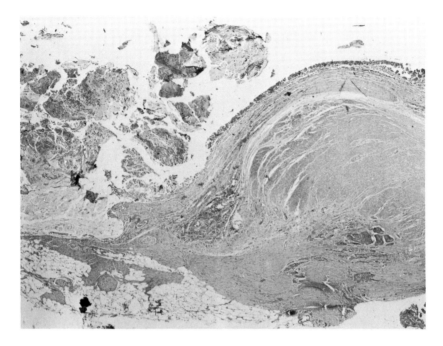

Fig. 9-21. Mucinous cystadenoma with mucus penetrating the wall through a defect in the muscularis propria; at the left of center, which is also probably a diverticulum. ($\times$ 33.)

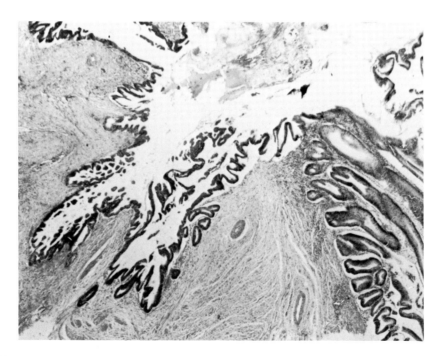

Fig. 9-22. High-grade dysplastic or carcinomatous epithelium covering a similar diverticulum on the left with villous adenoma containing low-grade dysplastic epithelium at its margin on the right. ($\times$ 33.)

sae (Figs. 9-23 and 9-24). The noninvasive lesions, namely the adenomatous mucosae and high-grade intramucosal dysplasias, including intramucosal carcinomas, have been discussed previously.

Peculiar to the appendix is the tendency for invasive carcinoma to produce dilated mucus-filled tubular structures as the tumor works its way through the wall (Figs. 9-24 to 9-27). The small tubule- or gland-forming carcinomas seen

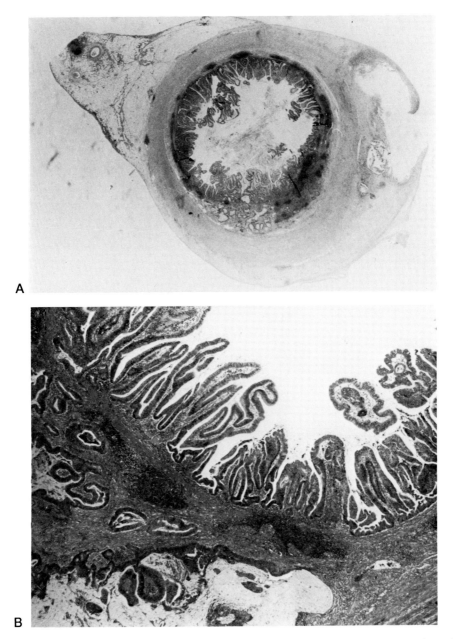

Fig. 9-23. (**A & B**) Superficially invasive cystadenocarcinoma arising from the base of a circumferential villous adenoma. (Fig. A × 10, Fig. B × 26.)

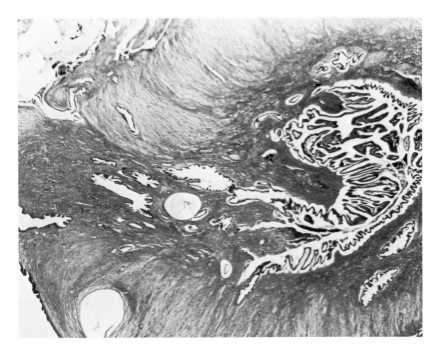

Fig. 9-24. Invasive adenocarcinoma of the appendix (on the left) extending into the wall from a circumferential in situ lesion resembling a nondilated villous cystadenoma (on the right). (× 14.)

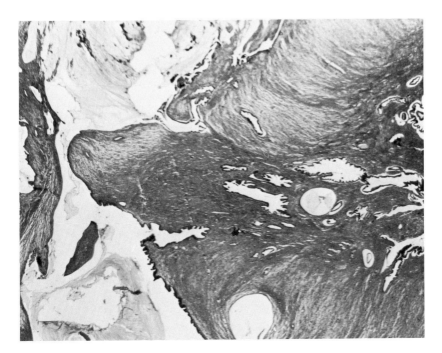

Fig. 9-25. Where the tumor in Figure 9-24 extends completely through the appendiceal wall, it becomes a cystic, mucus-filled compartment (mucinous cyst adenocarcinoma). (× 14.)

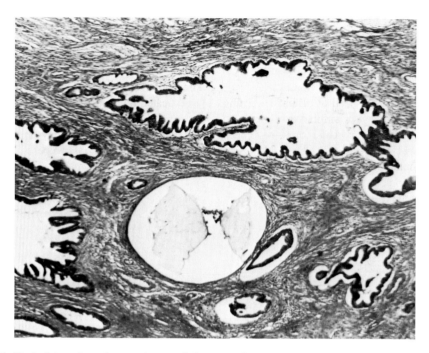

Fig. 9-26. Typical invasive adenocarcinoma of the appendix produces dilated mucus-filled tubules in the wall. (× 53.)

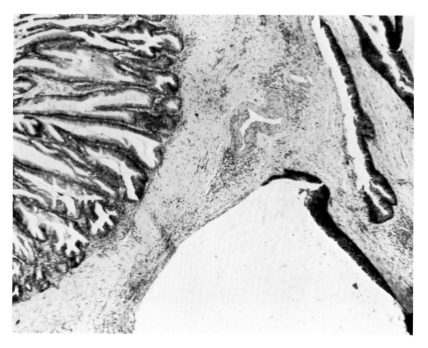

Fig. 9-27. Invasive adenocarcinoma deep in the wall of the right, producing cystic structures. Note the adjacent lesion on the left, which is a villous adenoma with serrated crypts. (× 53.)

so commonly in the colon are quite unusual in the appendix. Many of the microglandular appendiceal carcinomas that have been described in the literature appear to be variants of adenocarcinoid tumor, which is discussed later.[19]

Cases of signet ring cell or diffuse spreading appendiceal carcinoma, similar to one of the common forms of gastric carcinoma, have been described, but are so rare that further discussion of them would be superfluous.

As the tumors extend beyond the confines of the appendix, they often produce large quantities of mucus, resulting in another variant of pseudomyxoma peritonei, in this case a variant comparable to peritoneal carcinomatosis.

There has been some debate concerning the proper treatment for invasive appendiceal carcinoma. The optimal treatment obviously is total removal of the neoplasm. Since many tumors involve the proximal appendix near its junction with the cecum, and since many also have extended beyond the appendix to produce mixed neoplastic and inflammatory masses that also involve the cecal tip, most appendiceal carcinomas are best treated by right hemicolectomy. For very low-stage lesions, appendectomy alone may be sufficient treatment if the margin of resection at the cecal tip is free of tumor. It is the very low-stage lesions that are discovered

incidentally only after histologic study of the appendix. Actuarial analysis of reported cases, regardless of gross appearance and histologic features and based solely on the surgical procedure, indicates that the 5-year survival rate for those treated by appendectomy alone is 54 percent, and the 10-year rate is 41.5 percent. For those treated by hemicolectomy, the 5- and 10-year survival rates are both 66 percent, a significant difference, compared with the rates for appendectomy. However, such data are uncontrolled and apparently result from a choice of procedure that depends on the findings of the surgeon at the time of the laparotomy.

Survival also depends to a minor extent on the presence or absence of symptoms referable to the tumor at the time of presentation. The 5- and 10-year actuarial survival rates for asymptomatic appendiceal carcinomas are 65 percent and 54 percent. Those for symptomatic tumors are 57 percent and 41 percent, respectively.

If all cases reported as invasive appendiceal adenocarcinoma, regardless of symptoms or treatment, are examined collectively, the 5- and 10-year actuarial survival rates are 61 percent and 46 percent, respectively (Fig. 9-28). For noncystic lesions (i.e., those not specifically designated as cystic), the rates are 62 percent and 55 percent compared to 59 percent and 37

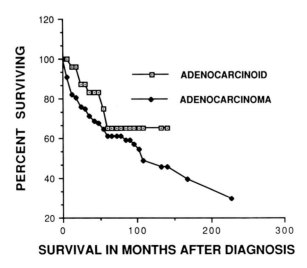

Fig. 9-28. Actuarial survival curves of reported cases of appendiceal carcinoma and adenocarcinoid tumors.

percent, respectively, for cystic lesions. Superficially, this suggests that cystadenocarcinoma is associated with a delayed mortality; this rarely occurs with noncystic lesions. However, too few cystic carcinomas have been followed beyond 5 years for these 10-year survival rates to be considered significant. Also, as mentioned previously, the distinction between cystic and noncystic lesions may be arbitrary; they may not be separate phenomena.

PSEUDOMYXOMA PERITONEI

The extravasation of mucous material into the peritoneal cavity has been designated as *pseudomyxoma peritonei*. It is almost always secondary to some type of mucinous neoplasm, usually either of the ovary or of the appendix. In this discussion, only its relation to a precursor appendiceal tumor will be considered.

The two appendiceal neoplasms associated with excessive production and accumulation of mucus are the mucinous cystadenoma, the basis for the most common type of appendix mucocele, and its malignant counterpart, the mucinous cystadenocarcinoma. Once the cystadenoma ruptures or dissects through the wall, or once the cystadenocarcinoma either ruptures or invades beyond the confines of the appendix to implant on the peritoneal surfaces, the mucus contents contact the peritoneum, inciting a fibrotic reaction identical to that which occurs when the cystadenomas ulcerate, causing mucus to come in contact with the appendiceal mural stroma.

Some cases of pseudomyxoma are localized, and generally are limited to the right lower quadrant around the appendix. In other cases, progressively larger accumulations of mucus and the ensuing fibrosing reaction involve more and more of the peritoneal surfaces, sometimes filling the entire abdominal cavity and turning it into a mass of matted loops of bowel, other viscera, mucus, and scar.

There are examples of pseudomyxomas of various extent that have been successfully treated by gross total removal of the mucus, a process quaintly spoken of as the "bailing-out procedure."[5] There are also cases in which, after gross removal of the mucus, the mucus reaccumulates and additional operative removals (perhaps several) are attempted; on occasion continued recurrance may eventually cause death of the patient, usually as a result of irreparable intestinal obstruction.

In some pseudomyxomas, no neoplastic epithelium can be found even after fastidious histologic sampling, whereas in others neoplastic columnar epithelium of various degrees of dysplasia is present, mixed with the mucus and scar (Figs. 9-29).

In some cases when epithelium is present in the mucinous implants, surgical removal results in no further mucus accumulation. In other cases, the epithelium continues to grow and produce mucus, and even eventually metastasizes, usually to lymph nodes.

There is no conflict among these bits of information if they are examined in terms of the biologic propensities of the neoplastic epithelium in question. As was mentioned in the preceding discussion of mucoceles, it appears obvious that the initial accumulation of mucus in the appendiceal lumen is the result of overproduction by the epithelium and failure of clearance from the appendix into the cecum.

If the mucocele ruptures and no neoplastic epithelium is released from the appendix into the peritoneal cavity, it is unlikely that mucus will reaccumulate once the extravasated mucus is surgically removed and the appendix, the site of overproducing epithelium, is also removed. In fact, the extruded mucin might even be reabsorbed spontaneously. Thus, pseudomyxoma with no epithelium in the peritoneal implants is likely to be a benign disease.

If adenomatous epithelium with no invasive capabilities is seeded onto the peritoneal surfaces with the mucus, continued growth of this epithelium and continued production of excessive mucus may be limited. Also, the spread of such mucus-producing epithelium is most often localized. In this case, careful gross removal of both the peritoneal mucinous implants and the appendiceal adenoma is likely to achieve

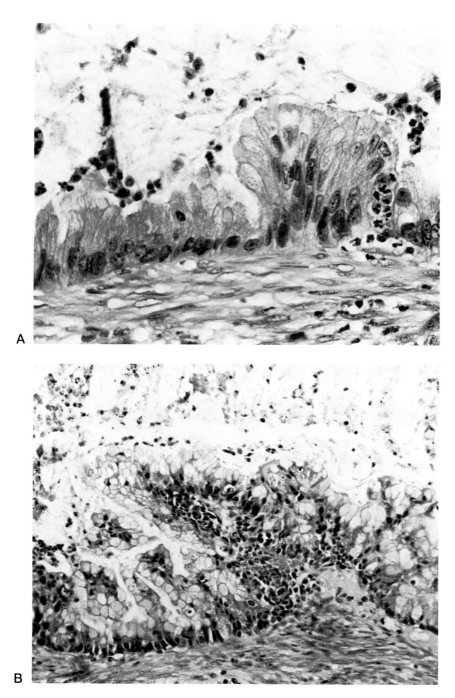

Fig. 9-29. Various types of epithelium encountered in pseudomyxoma. (**A**) Resemblance to a typical mucinous adenomatous epithelium. (**B**) Looks the same but has serrated lumens. (*Figure continues.*)

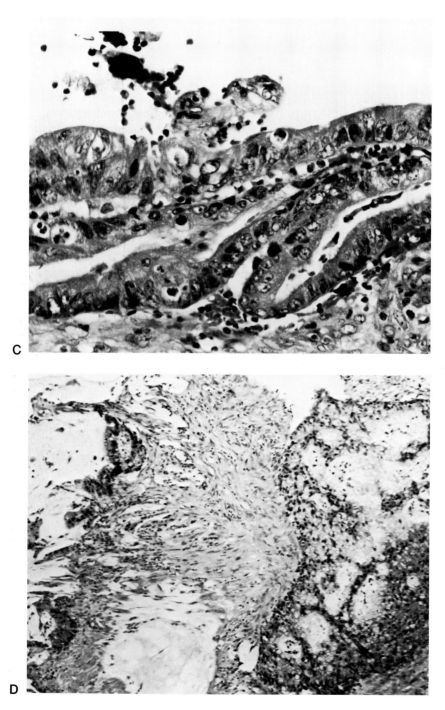

Fig. 9-29 (*Continued*). (**C**) More dysplastic. (**D**) Resemblance to colonic carcinoma with an epithelial mass forming secondary lumens. Mucus and scar to the left and center (Fig. A × 424, Fig. B × 212, Fig. C × 424, Fig. D × 106.)

cure. It has been suggested that a cystadenoma that has ruptured may continue to extrude viable mucus-producing epithelium into the peritoneal cavity. If the appendix is removed, the source of this constant seeding is lost, and no further mucus accumulation will be possible.

If *carcinomatous* epithelium has been extruded from the appendix into the peritoneal cavity, then, true to its capability of uncontrolled growth, this epithelium may spread, involve more and more peritoneal surface, and produce more and more mucus. Complicating this situation is the fact that the cytologic features of the epithelium in the peritoneal implants are not always clear predictors of its biologic capabilities of continued growth. Carcinomatous epithelium arising in many sites appears deceptively bland from time to time, even in its metastases. There is no reason to expect that appendiceal carcinomatous epithelia are any different.

Some information concerning the behavior of pseudomyxoma can be gleaned from actuarial survival analysis of the reported cases. First, if all cases of pseudomyxoma are analyzed together, it is clear that the survival curve is quite similar to that for all cases of invasive adenocarcinoma of the appendix. The 5- and 10-year survival rates for pseudomyxoma are 69 percent and 41 percent, respectively, virtually identical to those for adenocarcinoma in general. These data suggest that pseudomyxoma and adenocarcinoma behave in much the same way, and may even represent slight variations of the same disease.

The reported cases can be analyzed even further. It seems that no case of localized pseudomyxoma, namely, that limited to the right lower quadrant, has even been followed by extension, metastasis, and death after initial diagnosis and treatment. Therefore, the survival of patients with pseudomyxoma depends on clinical stage. At the same time, diffuse pseudomyxoma, that involving extensive peritoneal surface, has a 3-year actuarial survival rate of 73 percent and a 9-year rate of 34 percent. (The 10-year rate is impossible to calculate because of the limited periods of follow-up of reported cases.) This can be compared with all reported cases of appendiceal carcinoma with extra-appendiceal spread at the time of diagnosis, for which the 3-year survival rate is only about 29 percent. (Further survival rates are again impossible to determine because of the limited follow-up.) Thus, if diffuse pseudomyxoma is a form of appendiceal carcinoma with peritoneal carcinomatosis, it is a much less aggressive disease than other forms of carcinoma of the appendix that have already spread beyond the appendix at the time of diagnosis.

Analysis of age and sex incidence rates based on reported cases of pseudomyxoma introduces some conflicting data regarding its association with, or even identity with, appendiceal carcinomas. The peak and median ages of occurence are identical for pseudomyxoma and both types of appendiceal carcinoma. At the same time, pseudomyxoma has a striking male predominance, with about five males reported for every two females (5:2). Appendiceal carcinomas are split more evenly between the sexes. This sex difference suggests that there is some not-yet explained factor or factors that either make men more susceptible to the peritoneal mucous extravasation from mucinous appendiceal tumors or that confer immunity to this phenomenon in women.

GOBLET CELL CARCINOID TUMOR (MUCINOUS CARCINOID TUMOR, ADENOCARCINOID, OR CRYPT CELL CARCINOMA)

In 1969, in the French-language pathology literature, a peculiar appendiceal tumor was described that contained both endocrine cells and mucus-containing cells.[40] However, not until 1974 did this neoplasm achieve prominence in the English-language pathology literature, in a paper by Klein, who reported three cases, and termed the lesion a *mucinous carcinoid tumor*.[41] Later in 1974, Subbuswamy and co-workers reported 12 more cases under the designation *goblet cell carcinoid*.[42] In 1978, Warkel and co-workers published the results of their study of 39 cases from the Armed Forces Institute of Pathology (AFIP).[43] They changed the name again, this time to *adenocarcinoid,* and even were able to recognize two variants. In 1981, Isaacson reported four more cases and added still a fourth designation, *crypt cell carcinoma.*[44] Since the publication of Klein a number of small series and single case reports have appeared, bringing the total number of cases in the literature to about 150.[45–62] It also appears that similar cases have been described as types of adenocarcinoma of the appendix, especially *microglandular carcinoma.*[48, 20] Most likely a large number of cases, scattered among various institutions, have not yet made their way into print (perhaps fortunately). For instance, we have meticulously avoided publishing our 12 cases. As a result, the reader probably has been saved the frustration of having to confront still additional designations for this entity, distinctive and unusual as it may be. It is intriguing when as few as 150 cases of anything result in five different names. In this discussion, *adenocarcinoid* will be used simply because it is the shortest designation.

Whatever the name (and it is not the purpose of this chapter to choose a favorite) there is a unique appendiceal epithelial neoplasm that seems to arise from the base of the mucosa, infiltrate to various depths of the wall, and contain a mixture of rather mature-appearing intestinal cells, including goblet cells, Paneth cells, and endocrine cells. What makes this tumor so unusual is that it seems to be almost totally confined to the appendix, with only rare tumors of similar appearance reported as arising in other parts of the gut.

As described in the published accounts of these tumors, the gross appearances are disappointing. Usually they are not even grossly apparent and are discovered by accident on microscopic examination. Much of the explanation for this lies in the fact that these tumors often occur in appendices that are sites of severe acute suppurative inflammation, with all the discoloration and thickening inherent in that type of appendicitis. Nevertheless, these tumors do not produce a distinct mass or lump. Rather, since

they infiltrate diffusely over a fairly broad front, they are likely to appear only as a thickening and/or induration of various parts of the appendix, if they can be recognized at all. As a result of these gross subtleties, very few tumors have been accurately measured and their sizes recorded. The smallest probably are a few millimeters; the largest recorded tumor was 2.5 cm in maximum dimension.[45] About three-fourths occur in the distal appendix, often at or near the tip, with the remaining one-fourth involving either the middle third or the base near the cecum, or infiltrating the appendix diffusely.

The microscopic features constitute the distinguishing characteristics of adenocarcinoid tumor. The tumor is composed mainly of goblet cells or signet ring cells, often huge and over distended, with crescent-shaped nuclei compressed at the cell periphery by the large mucus blobs (Fig. 9-30). These goblet cells are arranged in clusters or strands containing various numbers of cells. Occasionally, single goblet cells can be found separate from clusters. These cellular collections tend to have smooth or knobby surfaces, the latter corresponding to the bulging mucus globules. Lumens occasionally can be found, but most clusters do not have them (Fig. 9-31). The nuclei tend to be peripherally oriented in the clusters, but occasionally are located centrally. The goblet cell mucus is mainly acidic and takes the Alcian blue stain when the combined periodic acid-Schiff (PAS)-Alcian blue technique is used. In the only extensive study of the mucus in adenocarcinoid tumor, the author concluded that the mucin was nonsulfated and probably a sialomucin.[44]

Mixed with the goblet cells are unpredictable numbers of Paneth cells with large, brightly eosinophilic granules (depending on the fixative), which can be brought out further by PAS and Masson trichrome stains (Fig. 9-32). Also present are endocrine cells, which can often be recognized in hematoxylin and eosin preparations by a finely granular eosinophilic cytoplasm, but which are more easily appreciated using argyrophilic stains, such as the Grimelius and Cherukian-Schenk or immunohistochemical stains for endocrine markers, such as neurone-

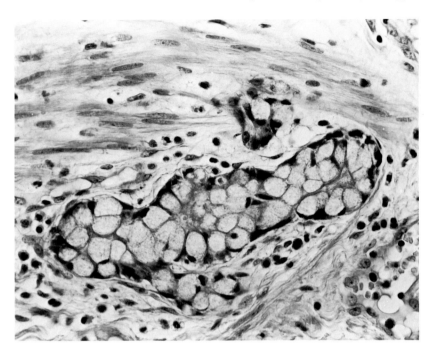

Fig. 9-30. Adenocarcinoid tumor. A typical nest of goblet or signet ring cells with their nuclei mostly peripheral. The nest has no lumen. (× 424.)

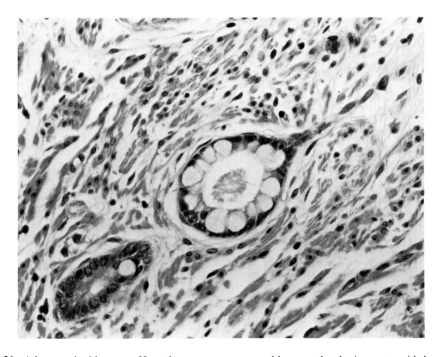

Fig. 9-31. Adenocarcinoid tumor. Here the tumor nests resemble normal colonic crypts with lumens and alternating goblet cells and tall columnar cells. (× 424.)

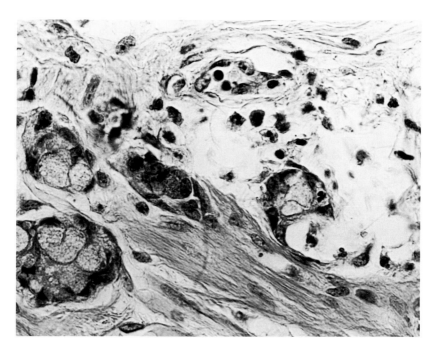

Fig. 9-32. Adenocarcinoid tumor at the base of the mucosa. In the center there is a small nest of granular Paneth cells; to the left are clusters of goblet cells. ($\times$ 678.)

specific enolase or chromogranin. (Fig. 9-33). Some tumors contain large numbers of either or both Paneth and endocrine cells, whereas in other tumors there may be none. Finally, there are some cells that are neither goblet, Paneth, or endocrine, and may be more like primitive cells of the intestinal crypts. In general, in the typical areas, the nuclei are not pleomorphic, mitotic figures are rare, and cytoplasmic differentiation is dominant.

The tumor nests, or clusters, arise in the basalar part of the mucosa, presumably from some precursor mucosal aberration; unfortunately, as of this writing, the precursor lesion has not been convincingly identified (Fig. 9-34). In occasional tumors, the basal crypt epithelium adjacent to the intramucosal tumor nests may appear dysplastic, with enlarged nuclei, and may have an increased number of overdistended and disoriented goblet cells. However, it is difficult in such situations to be certain if these dysplastic crypts are truly altered normal crypts or if they are tumor-derived crypt-like structures. What

is accepted is that the appendiceal mucosa usually does not have any of the in situ neoplastic alterations characteristic of the usual forms of adenomas and carcinomas. Even when the base of the mucosa is filled with tumor nests, the surface epithelium and luminal half of the crypts are either normal or have regenerative changes, possibly secondary to the accompanying acute appendicitis that occurs in over two-thirds of the cases. In two cases mucoceles were reported to occur in conjunction with acute appendicitis,[46, 20] and in two other cases a villous adenoma occurred[43]; whether these lesions presumably were in direct continuity with the adenocarcinoid tumor and were precursor mucosal dysplasias is not known (Fig. 9-35).

The cell nests fan out from the mucosa and infiltrate to variable depths, often through the wall and even into the mesoappendix and subserosa (Fig. 9-36). There is surprisingly little tumor-associated stroma; in fact, the tumor nodules seem to lie within the tissues of the appendiceal wall as if they were haphazardly

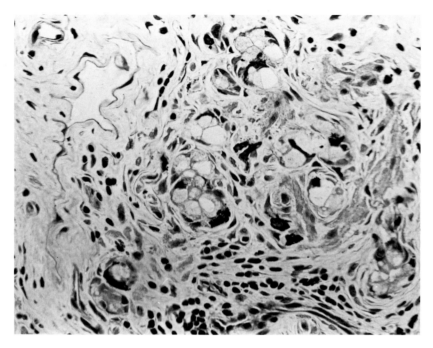

Fig. 9-33. In this area, endocrine cells with darkly stained granules are present in the epithelial nests. (Churukian-Schenk, × 424.)

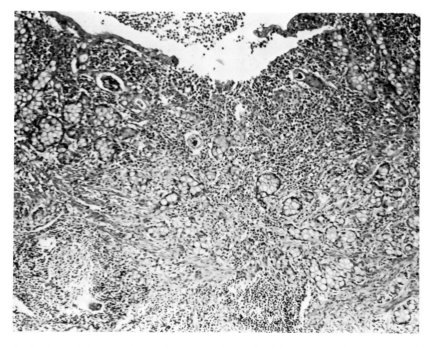

Fig. 9-34. In the base of the mucosa are the nests and strands of the adenocarcinoid tumor, which extend into the superficial submucosa at the lower right. The mucosal surface has no in situ neoplastic changes. (× 106.)

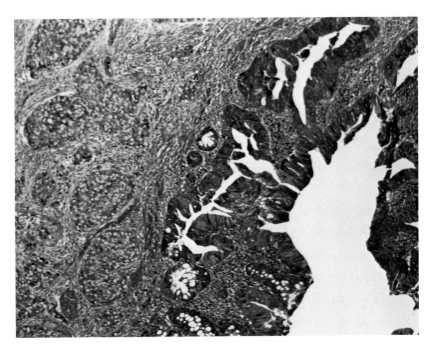

Fig. 9-35. Nests of adenocarcinoid tumor (left) extend from the base of a cystadenoma (center and right). (× 106.)

dropped there. As they extend through the muscularis propria, there is a tendency for the clusters and cords to be oriented in the same direction as the muscle fibers (Fig. 9-36). Also, quite often the goblet cells in the muscularis appear to enlarge even further and coalesce, creating large pools of mucus that sometimes surround the entire appendiceal submucosa and mucosa (Fig. 9-37).

In the subserosa, perineural infiltration is frequently found, as is lymphatic permeation by tumor nests (Fig. 9-38).

Up to this point, the description has focused on the differentiated adenocarcinoid, which is the most common pattern. There are, however, a few modifications. In the AFIP series, a second type of tumor was identified, the tubular adenocarcinoid, characterized by tubules with lumens that were sometimes filled with inspissated mucus (Fig. 9-31). The tumor cells tended to be columnar and oriented toward the lumens, with the nuclei lying peripherally. Another variation involves increasing degrees of dysplasia with

the addition of mitoses and pleomorphism to the typical picture, so that the tumor appears more and more like an adenocarcinoma forming small aggregates (Fig. 9-39). In fact, in one study it seems that the investigators grouped all of their cases of adenocarcinoid tumors under the heading of *microglandular carcinoma*.[20] Finally, some tumors have been described as containing nests of cells that resemble those of typical carcinoid tumor.[35] Interestingly, in the cases in which metastases have been studied, the metastases appeared as various patterns of adenocarcinoma, carcinoid tumor, or even typical adenocarcinoid.[32]

In virtually every paper on adenocarcinoid tumors, the investigators have worried about the histogenesis of these lesions. Here is a tumor that makes several types of highly differentiated, highly sophisticated cells, arises somewhere in the base of the mucosa, infiltrates in a strange pattern reminiscent of some type of carcinoid tumor, avoids just about every part of the gut except the appendix, and, at least as far as the

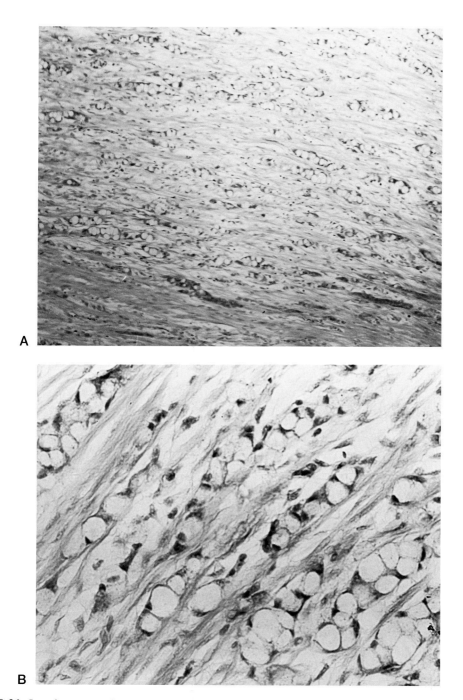

Fig. 9-36. Invasive nests of adenocarcinoid tumor lie between, and parallel to, bundles of muscularis propria. There is virtually no tumor-associated stroma. (Fig. A, low power, × 120, Fig. B, high power, × 424.)

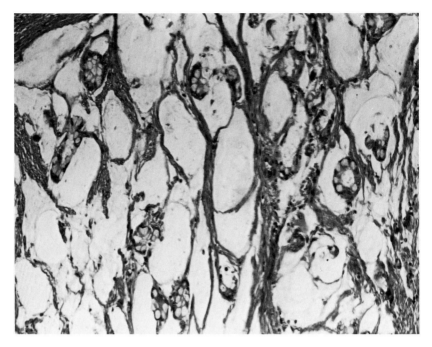

Fig. 9-37. Large mucin pools are formed deep in the muscularis propria, apparently by the coalescence of goblet cells and their contents. Well-differentiated tumor tubules may be seen. (× 212.)

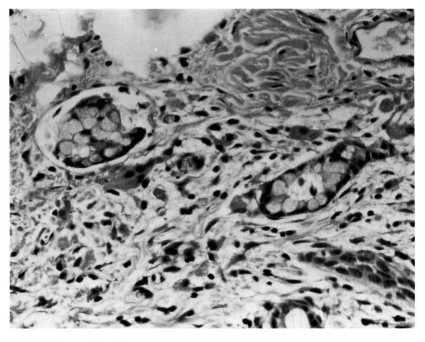

Fig. 9-38. Periappendiceal lymphatic permeation by a nest of adenocarcinoid tumor. (× 424.)

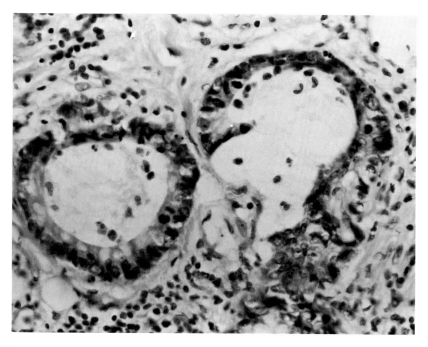

Fig. 9-39. An adenocarcinoid tumor containing an area with increased mitoses and nuclear hyperchromatism and pleomorphism. (× 424.)

early papers were concerned, had remarkable survival rates and low metastatic potential. Ultrastructural studies have reported conflicting data. In some studies, the investigators believed they could identify tumor cells that contained both mucous granules and neurosecretory granules, suggesting that a common precursor cell gave rise to both the endocrine cells and the goblet cells, and presumably to the Paneth cells as well.[49, 50] Other studies have failed to find cells with both mucous and endocrine granules and have suggested that the tumors are derived from proliferation of independent cells of different types.[51, 52] One immunohistochemical study suggested that the tumors were derived from lysozyme-producing cells comparable to those found in the normal small intestine crypts, presumably a metaplastic phenomenon peculiar to the appendix, since adenocarcinoid tumors do not seem to occur in the small bowel, where such precursor cells are ordinarily found.[49] The data are too muddled at present to allow a clearcut histogenetic theory to emerge. Whether this

peculiar tumor is derived from one precursor or from several it is obvious that multidirectional differentiation occurs. On rare occasions, one of the differentiated cell types may become dominant, thus explaining those cases that look more like adenocarcinomas and those that contain carcinoid tumor foci. Although initially the adenocarcinoid tumor was thought to be a part of the carcinoid spectrum, we now recognize that it is not an endocrine tumor at all, but a type of adenocarcinoma.

To a great extent, the adenocarcinoid tumors are fairly predictable in their clinical characteristics. The disease shows a predilection for persons in their sixth decade of life. Both sexes are affected equally. Peculiarly, the median age for men at the time of diagnosis is 10 years greater than that for women. About 75 percent of the patients with this tumor come to medical attention because of symptoms identical to those of acute appendicitis. Whether the association between adenocarcinoids and acute appendicitis is causally related is not clear. In a few reported cases, there was a suggestion that tumor situated proximally in the appendix obstructed the lumen partially, and that inflammation resulted secondarily. However, since the tumors are so small, in general, they are incidental findings in acutely inflamed appendices.

The most controversial aspect of this tumor relates to its biologic behavior. Initially, the adenocarcinoid tumor was thought to be a tumor of very low malignant potential. In fact, of 38 cases reported in a variety of early small series, only two metastasized: one at 5 years after treatment and the other at 6 months after treatment.[42, 47] However, for this entire group the median duration of follow-up was only 24 months. In the first large series, which involved 39 cases from the AFIP, six tumors metastasized, with the metastases being found up to 2 years after initial diagnosis and treatment.[43] In this study, the 5-year actuarial survival rate was about 80 percent, with only a slight decline to about 73 percent at 10 and 15 years. If those tumors reported as "microglandular carcinomas" of appendix are really the same as the adenocarcinoid tumors and are included with them for the purpose of calculating survival data, then the actuarial 5- and 10-year survival rates for the non-AFIP-reported tumors becomes 65 percent, somewhat lower than the figure reported in the AFIP series (Fig. 9-28). What these survival figures indicate is that the adenocarcinoid tumor is not harmless, as first was thought. Its behavior during the first 5 years after diagnosis is similar to that of other forms of appendiceal carcinoma. However, it seems not to cause late mortality after 5 years (Fig 9-28).

Metastases frequently involve the peritoneal surfaces, where, on occasion, they may produce a pseudomyxoma (Fig. 9-40).[55] They also have been reported as the cause of ovarian Krukenberg tumor, where the goblet cells become signet ring cells mixed with the hyperplastic ovarian stroma.[56, 57, 61]

With respect to recommended therapy, the data are also not conclusive. However, this is true for malignant appendiceal tumors in general. The most commonly recommended treat-

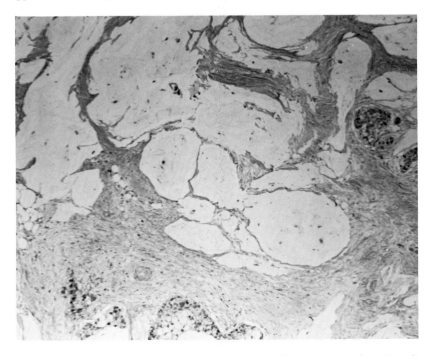

Fig. 9-40. Pseudomyxoma secondary to metastastic adenocarcinoid tumors to peritoneal surfaces. There are mucus pools in upper right and center and tumor nests in lower left and right center. (× 106.)

ment is total removal. If the appendectomy alone has achieved this, then probably nothing further is required. If the tumor extends to the proximal margin or has metastasied to nodes, something further is required, probably some form of right colonic resection. It is unlikely that this approach will be modified for many years to come, since no single institution has enough cases to carry on a carefully controlled therapeutic trial.

Are there any morphologic hints that suggest an adenocarcinoid tumor is malignant? Size is no help. As mentioned earlier, size is difficult to determine in these tumors because they tend to produce a diffuse thickening instead of a lump. In the AFIP series, the tumors that metastasized were quite small, between 0.9 and 1.2 cm in greatest dimension.[43] There is a suggestion that metastasizing tumors tended to occur in noninflamed appendices, so that the lack of inflammation may cause suspicion of malignancy. Perineural infiltration and lymphatic permeation are not useful indications of malignancy, since they occur so commonly that they are almost an accepted part of the typical tumor anatomy. Warkel and co-workers concluded that the most useful parameters in predicting malignancy were evidence of extension beyond the appendix at the time of the initial operative procedure, foci of dedifferentiation (such as areas resembling anaplastic carcinoid or mucinous cystadenocarcinoma), and a mitotic count of two or more per 10 high-power fields (exact microscopic type and size of field are not stated in their paper).[43] Whether these features will hold up as prospective predictors of aggressive behavior remains to be seen.

The latest word on the adenocarcinoid tumor again comes from investigators at the AFIP, who found that they could tell the metastasizing from the nonmetastasizing tumors.[63] The non-metastasizing ones they now call "goblet cell carcinoids," although "adenocarcinoid tumor" was originally the AFIP designation. These are confined to the appendix and mesoappendix, are grossly subtle, and contain the small well-developed goblet cell-rich clusters and tubules, as described above, with scattered serotonin-containing endocrine cells. The metastasizing tumors are called "mixed carcinoidadenocarci-

nomas." These have extra-appendiceal spread, such as into cecum or adjacent viscera, at the time of diagnosis and contain an adenocarcinomatous component that can be mucous or signet ring cell, in addition to the goblet cell or typical carcinoid tumor pattern. They are probably correct. In our experience, the aggressive tumors always have had some histologic changes beyond what the nonaggressive ones possessed, such as mucinous areas, pleomorphism, or solid cellular foci.

SUMMARY

At the beginning of the discussion, six questions were posed that defined the controversies that have frequently muddied our knowledge of appendiceal epithelial proliferations. These can now be answered in the same order.

1. The mucinous cystadenoma is the common cause of the appendix mucocele.

2. The appendiceal retention cyst, a non-neoplastic mucocele, namely one resulting from obstruction of a sterile appendix with accumulation of mucus produced by normal mucosa, may exist; but the data suggest that, at best, the retention cyst will be nothing more than a slight dilatation.

3. Pseudomyxoma peritonei, the phenomenon of mucous extravasation into the peritoneal cavity, is comparable in its behavior to adenocarcinoma of the appendix, although it is a less aggressive disease than carcinoma of the appendix with extra-appendiceal spread at the time of diagnosis. Survival seems to be stage dependent. The biologic behavior of the lesion is most dependent on the presence of carcinomatous epithelium in the peritoneal implants.

4. Carcinoma of the appendix seems to evolve through an adenoma-carcinoma sequence comparable to that for ordinary large bowel cancer.

5. At the moment, it appears that colonic style hyperplastic polyps, with the typical mucus cell depletion and thick subsurface basement membrane, occur in the appendix only rarely. Most of the reported cases seem to be examples of adenomas with serrated crypt lumens.

6. The adenocarcinoid tumor of the appendix (and its four or more synonyms) is a specific entity with a clearly distinctive microscopic anatomy, but it behaves much like other appendiceal carcinomas. It should be recognized as an adenocarcinoma and not as an endocrine tumor or carcinoid tumor.

Finally, the reader is reminded that most of the information described in this discussion is based on reported cases, which have been published with remarkably limited clinical follow-up and imperfectly defined diagnostic criteria. Only when large series of these lesions with appropriately lengthy follow-up are analyzed can we be certain whether these conclusions are valid.

REFERENCES

1. Sieracki JC, Tesluk H: Primary adenocarcinoma of the vermiform appendix. Cancer 9:997, 1956
2. Wilson R: Primary carcinoma of the appendix. Am J Surg 104:238, 1962
3. Hellsten S: Mucocele and carcinoma of the appendix. Acta Path Microbiol Scand 60:473, 1964
4. Totten JC, Bernhardt H, Young JM: Primary adenocarcinoma of the appendix. South Med J 58:76, 1965
5. Bernhardt H, Young JM: Mucocele and pseudomyxoma peritonei of appendiceal origin. Am J Surg 109:235, 1965
6. Das Gupta TK, Paglia MA: Primary malignant tumors of the appendix. NY J Med 66:890, 1966
7. Hellsten S, Giores JE: Mucocele of the appendix. Acta Chir Scand 133:491, 1967
8. Edmonson HT, Hobbs ML: Primary adenocarcinoma of the appendix. Am Surgeon 33:717, 1967
9. Parson J, Gray GF, Thorbjarnarson B: Pseudomyxoma peritonei. Arch Surg 101:545, 1970
10. Broders CW, Miranda R: Mucocele of the appendix: review of eleven cases and report of two cases. Am Surgeon 37:434, 1971
11. Ghosh BC, Huvos AG, Whiteley HW: Pseudomyxoma peritonei. Dis Colon Rectum 15:420, 1972
12. Limber GK, King RE, Silverberg SG: Pseudomyxoma peritonei: a report of ten cases. Ann Surg 178:587, 1973
13. Higa E, Rosai J, Pizzimbono CA, Wise L: Mucosal hyperplasia, mucinous cystadenoma and mucinous cystadenocarcinoma of the appendix. Cancer 32:1525, 1973
14. Gibbs NM: Mucinous cystadenoma and cystadenocarcinoma of the vermiform appendix with particular reference to mucocele and pseudomyxoma peritonei. J Clin Pathol 26:413, 1973
15. Aho AJ, Heinonen R, Lauren P: Benign and malignant mucocele of the appendix. Acta Chir Scand 139:392, 1973
16. Cohen SE, Wolfman EF Jr: Primary adenocarcinoma of the vermiform appendix. Am J Surg 127:704, 1974
17. Qizilbash AH: Primary adenocarcinoma of the appendix. A clinicopathological study of 11 cases. Arch Pathol 99:556, 1975
18. Qizilbash AH: Mucoceles of the appendix. Their relationship to hyperplastic polyps, mucinous cystadenomas, and cystadenocarcinomas. Arch Pathol 99:548, 1975
19. Wolff M, Ahmed N: Epithelial neoplasms of the vermiform appendix (exclusive of carcinoid). Pt. I. Adenocarcinoma of the appendix. Cancer 37:2493, 1976
20. Wolff M, Ahmed N: Epithelial neoplasms of the vermiform appendix (exclusive of carcinoid). Pt. II. Cystadenomas, papillary adenomas, and adenomatous polyps of the appendix. Cancer 37:2511, 1976
21. Jones RA, MacFarlane A: Carcinomas and carcinoid tumors of the appendix in a district general hospital. J Clin Pathol 29:687, 1976
22. Gamble HA: Adenocarcinoma of the appendix: an unusual case and review. Dis Colon Rectum 19:621, 1976
23. Chang P, Attiyeh FF: Adenocarcinoma of the appendix. Dis Colon Rectum 24:176, 1981
24. Munk JF: Villous adenoma causing acute appendicitis. Br J Surg 64:593, 1977
25. Mibu R, Itoh H, Iwashita A, et al: Carcinoma in situ of the vermiform appendix associated with adenomatosis of the colon. Dis Colon Rectum 24:482, 1981
26. Baeta B, Barnes WH, Desa DJ: Adenocarcinoma of the appendix. Can J Surg 25:553, 1982
27. Panton ON, Bell GA, Owen DA: Adenocarcinoma of the vermiform appendix: retrospective study and literature review. Can J Surg 26:276, 1983
28. Wackym PA, Gray GF, Jr.: Tumors of the appendix. I. Neoplastic and non-neoplastic mucoceles. South Med J 77:283, 1984
29. Ferro M., Anthony PP: Adenocarcinoma of the appendix. Dis Colon Rectum 28:457, 1985

30. Williams RA, Whitehead R: Non-carcinoid epithelial tumours of the appendix—a proposed classification. Pathology 18:50, 1986

31. Schlatter MG, McKone, TK, Scholten DJ, et al: Primary appendiceal adenocarcinoma. Am Surg 53:434, 1987

32. Cerame MA: A 25-year review of adenocarcinoma of the appendix. A frequently perforating carcinoma. Dis Colon Rectum 31:145, 1988

33. Lyss AP: Appendiceal malignancies. Semin Oncol 15:129, 1988

34. Burgess P, Done HJ: Adenocarcinoma of the appendix. J R Soc Med 82:28, 1989

35. Lane N, Kaplan H, Pascal RR: Minute adenomatous and hyperplastic polyps of the colon: divergent patterns of epithelial growth with specific associated mesenchymal changes. Contrasting roles in the pathogenesis of carcinoma. Gastroenterology 60:537, 1971

36. MacGillivray JB: Mucosal metaplasia in the appendix. J Clin Pathol 25:809, 1972

37. Qizilbash AH: Hyperplastic (metaplastic) polyps of the appendix: report of 19 cases. Arch Pathol 97:385, 1974

38. Fenoglio CM, Lane N: The anatomical precursor of colorectal carcinoma. Cancer 34:819, 1974

39. Muto T, Bussey HJR, Morson BC: The evolution of cancer of the colon and rectum. Cancer 36:2251, 1975

40. Gagne F, Fortin P, Dufour V, Delage C: Tumeurs de l'appendice associant des caracteres histologiques de carcinoide et d'adenocarcinome. Ann Anat Pathol (Paris) 14:393, 1969

41. Klein HZ: Mucinous carcinoid tumor of the vermiform appendix. Cancer 33:770, 1974

42. Subbuswamy SG, Gibbs NM, Ross CF, Morson BC: Goblet cell carcinoid of the appendix. Cancer 34:338, 1974

43. Warkel RL, Cooper PH, Helwig EB: Adenocarcinoid, a mucin-producing carcinoid tumor of the appendix. Cancer 42:2781, 1978

44. Isaacson P: Crypt cell carcinoma of the appendix (so-called adenocarcinoid tumor). Am J Surg Pathol 5:213, 1981

45. Haqqani MT, Williams G: Mucin producing carcinoid tumors of the vermiform appendix. J Clin Pathol 30:473, 1977

46. Chen V, Qizilbash AH: Goblet cell carcinoid tumor of the appendix. Arch Pathol Lab Med 103:180, 1979

47. Olsson B, Ljungberg O: Adenocarcinoid of the vermiform appendix. Virchows Arch [A] 386:201, 1980

48. Wood DA: Tumors of the intestines. pp. 177, 190–191. In Atlas of Tumor Pathology. Section 6, fascicle 22. Armed Forces Institute of Pathology, Washington, DC, 1967

49. Abt AB, Carter SL: Goblet cell carcinoid of the appendix. An ultrastructural and histochemical study. Arch Pathol Lab Med 100:301, 1976

50. Warner TFCS, Seo IS: Goblet cell carcinoid of appendix. Ultrastructural features and histogenetic aspects. Cancer 44:1700, 1979

51. Cooper PH, Warkel RL: Ultrastructure of the goblet cell type of adenocarcinoid of the appendix. Cancer 42:2687, 1978

52. Rodriguez, FH Jr, Sarma DP, Lunseth JH: Goblet cell carcinoid of the appendix. Hum Pathol 13:286, 1982

53. Wolff M: Crypt cell carcinoma. Letter to the Editor. Am J Surg Pathol 6:188, 1982

54. Hofler H, Kloppel G, Heitz PU: Combined production of mucus, amines and peptides by goblet-cell carcinoids of the appendix and ileum. Pathol Res Pract 178:555, 1984

55. Edmonds P, Merino MJ, LiVolsi VA, Duray PH: Adenocarcinoid (mucinous carcinoid) of the appendix. Gastroenterology 86:302, 1984

56. Hirschfield LS, Kahn LB, Winkler B, et al: Adenocarcinoid of the appendix presenting as bilateral Krukenberg's tumor of the ovaries. Arch Pathol Lab Med 109:930, 1985

57. Hood IC, Jones BA, Watts JC: Mucinous carcinoid tumor of the appendix presenting as bilateral ovarian tumors. Arch Pathol Lab Med 110:336, 1986

58. Bak M, Jorgensen LJ: Adenocarcinoid of the appendix presenting with metastases to the liver. Dis Colon Rectum 30:112, 1987

59. Watson PH, Alguacil-Garcia A: Mixed crypt cell carcinoma. A clinicopathological study of the so-called "Goblet cell carcinoid." Virchows Arch [A] 412:175, 1987

60. Bak M, Asschenfeldt P: Adenocarcinoid of the vermiform appendix. A clinicopathologic study of 20 cases. Dis Colon Rectum 31:605, 1988

61. Miller RT, Sarikaya H, Jenison EL: Adenocarcinoid tumor of appendix presenting as unilateral Krukenberg tumor. J Surg Oncol 37:65, 1988

62. Berardi RS, Lee SS, Chen HP: Goblet cell carcinoids of the appendix. Surg Gynecol Obstet 167:81, 1988

63. Burke AP, Sobin LH, Federspiel BH, et al: Goblet cell carcinoids and related tumors of the vermiform appendix. Am J Clin Pathol 94:27, 1990.

10

Neuroendocrine Cells and Their Proliferative Lesions

Yogeshwar Dayal

It is now clearly established that the gastrointestinal tract and its glandular derivatives are richly endowed with a variety of different endocrine cell types that are inconspicuously dispersed along the mucosa. This population of intraepithelial cells with granular or clear cytoplasm distinct from other mucosal epithelial elements was first recognized by Heidenhain.[1] However, these cells have been referred to as *Kultschitzky cells* because of the mistaken belief that they were first observed by him.[2] These cells closely resemble the chromaffin cells of the adrenal medulla, and consequently are also referred to as *enterochromaffin cells;* and, because of their morphologic uniformity (triangular to oval shape and clear to faintly eosinophilic granular cytoplasm) under conventional light microscopy, these cells were initially believed to represent a homogeneous population that served an ill-defined endocrine function.[3]

Despite their morphologic uniformity, these endocrine cells display significant histochemical variability with respect to autofluorescence,[4] masked metachromasia,[5] argyrophilia, and argentaffinity after formaldehyde fixation.[6] This histochemical heterogeneity is now known to be due to intracellular stores of certain polypeptides and biogenic amines that are the specific secretory products of these cells. Thus, the initial concept of a morphologically homogeneous endocrine cell population of the gut has now evolved into one in which the gut represents a dispersed endocrine system (DES) consisting of a constellation of functionally heterogeneous cell types, each with a specific secretory product.

Each endocrine cell type synthesizes, stores, and secretes a specific polypeptide hormone and/ or biogenic amine that acts as a chemical messenger in orchestrating the various secretory, motor, and absorptive functions of the gut.[7] Because of the multiplicity of functionally distinct cell types dispersed along the mucosa, the mammalian gut is now regarded as the most complex, and perhaps the largest, endocrine organ of the body.

GENERAL CHARACTERISTICS

The endocrine cells of the gut are generally seen to have a triangular or pyramidal shape, with a broad base and a narrow apical pole that insinuates itself between the adjacent epithelial cells to communicate with the lumen (Fig. 10-1). A majority of endocrine cells show such luminal communications, and are referred to as *open-type endocrine cells,* whereas those few cells (such as those in the oxyntic mucosa of the stomach) that lack this feature are designated as *closed-type endocrine cells.*[8] This feature explains how the open cells can monitor minor changes in the pH or the composition of the luminal contents and release their secretory products either locally or into the circulation. Some workers have proposed that the luminal communications can also act as conduits for the release of secretions directly into the lumen,

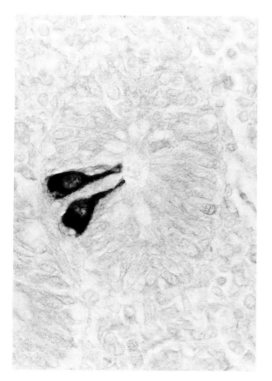

Fig. 10-1. Normal human colonic mucosa showing two EC cells in a transverse section of a crypt. The flask-shaped cells abut on the basement membrane and have narrow apical processes that insinuate themselves between the lateral borders of the adjacent epithelial cells to communicate with the lumen. Such processes are characteristic of open-type gastrointestinal endocrine cells. (Peroxidase-antiperoxidase technique using a rabbit antibody against serotonin, 1:1000; methyl green counterstain, × 813.)

as has been shown to be the case with the gastrin-producing G cells of the antral mucosa.[9] The closed cells presumably respond to distension or humoral stimulation. In addition to their apical processes, some open cells, such as the somatostatin-producing D cells of the antropyloric mucosa, also show elaborate neuronal-like cytoplasmic processes that extend laterally from their basal portions to envelop and terminate around neighboring exocrine and endocrine cells, whose functions they then effectively modulate.[10] Since these cells release secretory products that act on adjacent target cells (in

addition to their endocrine secretions), they are said to also have a paracrine function.

Ultrastructurally, these cells are characterized by the presence of numerous membrane-bound secretory granules, abundant endoplasmic reticulum, and a prominent Golgi apparatus. The broad basal pole of the cell rests directly on the basal lamina, whereas the narrow apical pole (in the open-type cells only) terminates in the lumen in a tuft of microvilli. At their apical pole, these cells are anchored to the adjacent epithelial cells by junctional complexes, whereas laterally they are separated from adjacent epithelial cells by a narrow interstitial space. The intracytoplasmic secretory granules are preferentially clustered in the perinuclear area and in the basal pole of the cell. The secretory product of the cells is synthesized in the endoplasmic reticulum, processed in the Golgi apparatus, and stored within the secretory granules until released into the circulation, interstitial space, or the lumen. Since the ultrastructural morphology of the secretory granules of each individual cell type is sufficiently characteristic with respect to size, shape, electron density, and the like, this feature is extensively used for the ultrastructural identification of the various cell types (Table 10-1).

It should be noted, however, that although the secretory granules of each cell type are sufficiently characteristic ultrastructurally, they normally show minor morphologic deviations.[11] For example, three subpopulations of secretory granules—one large (220 to 240 mn in diameter) electron lucent, another small (150 to 170 nm in diameter) electron dense, and an intermediate-sized (200 to 220 nm in diameter) pale-cored—have been observed in the human antral G cells.[12] Variations in the relative proportions of the different types of granules have been attributed to fixation artifacts,[13, 14] differences in the functional status of the cell,[15, 16] co-existence of multiple secretory products such as adrenocorticotropic hormone (ACTH) and gastrin,[14, 17] or the presence of different molecular forms (G_{34}, G_{17}, G_4, etc.) of gastrin.[16, 18] Recent studies have shown that these subpopulations actually represent a continuum within a homoge-

Table 10-1. Ultrastructural Characteristics of Secretory Granules

Cell Type	Secretory Product(s)	Size	Granule Characteristics
			Morphology and Histochemistry
G	Gastrin, ACTH, [Met]enkephalin, GAWK	150–400 nm	Round, moderate but variably electron-dense cores with a fuzzy content; argyrophil[a]
IG	Gastrin	150–220 nm	Round, small, and dark granules; argyrophil[a]
D	Somatostatin	250–400 nm	Variably sized round granules with moderate to weakly electron-dense cores and a tight limiting membrane; argyrophil only by the Hellerstrom-Hellman technique
S	Secretin	180–220 nm	Small, round to somewhat irregular granules with intensely osmiophilic cores and a thin but distinct peripheral halo. Weakly argyrophil.[a] The granules are closely similar to those of D_1 cells but are more electron dense.
I	Cholecystokinin	240–300 nm	Intermediate-sized round granules with moderately electron-dense cores that are morphologically similar to those of L cells; nonargyrophil
K	GIP	200–350 nm	Large round or irregular granules with dense eccentric cores and a less dense granular matrix that is argyrophil by the Sevier-Munger technique
N	Neurotensin	up to 300 nm	Round, moderately electron-dense cores that are variably argyrophil[a]
L	Enteroglucagon	250–300 nm	Small (in colon) or intermediate-sized (in ileum), round to slightly irregular granules. Identical to the I cells but readily distinguishable from them by the characteristic peripheral localization of the silver granules around the rim[a]
EC_1	5-HT, Substance P, [Leu]enkephalin	200–300 nm	Pleomorphic, elongated, reniform, round, oval or pear-shaped, medium to large granules with highly electron-dense cores and a thin peripheral halo; argentaffin
EC_2	5-HT, Motilinlike, [Leu]enkephalin	200–400 nm	Pleomorphic, large, round to irregular granules, similar to those of EC_1-type cells, but somewhat angulated; variably electron-dense; argentaffin
EC_n	5-HT, unknown	200–300 nm	Small to medium-sized, elongated or oval granules with moderate but variable electron density and argentaffinity
ECL	Unknown		Large vacuolated granules with an eccentric, coarse textured electron-dense core surrounded by a thin halo and bounded by a delicate wavy membrane
D_1	VIP-like	140–200 nm	Small, round, pleomorphic granules with moderate to highly electron-dense cores and a narrow halo. Granules resemble those of S cells. May represent a consortium of several functionally different cell types; argyrophil[a]
P	Bombesinlike	90–150 nm	Very small, round secretory granules with moderately electron-dense cores and a narrow peripheral halo. Closely resemble those of D_1 and S cells; poorly argyrophil[a]
PP	Pancreatic polypeptide	150–170 nm	Small, round electron-dense granules that are only inconstantly argyrophilic[a]
X	Unknown	up to 250 nm	Small to medium-sized round granules with moderately electron-dense and argyrophil cores[a]

[a] Argyrophilia, except when specified, refers to Grimelius positivity.

neous population, and that different molecular forms of gastrin are preferentially localized in specific subpopulations of these granules. Thus, G_{34} is chiefly localized in the small electron-dense granules, whereas G_{17} is seen chiefly in the pale intermediate-sized granules and in only some of the smaller granules. Neither G_{17} nor G_{34} are seen in large electron-lucent granules.[12] Since G_{17} is normally derived by tryptic cleavage of its precursor G_{34} molecule, the normal variations in granule morphology correlate with various stages of intracellular processing of the gastrin molecule, and could therefore also reflect different phases in their maturational sequence.

IDENTIFICATION AND NOMENCLATURE

Exponential advances in the field of gut endocrinology have recently led to the identification, purification, chemical characterization, and sequencing of numerous gut hormones. The availability of potent antibodies to these hormones have provided morphologists with a specific and sensitive means of immunohistochemically identifying different cell types and have led to the mapping of their anatomic distribution in the gut. A working classification of the gastrointestinal endocrine cells, based on the ultrastructural and immunohistochemical characteristics, was formulated in 1977 at a meeting in Lausanne, Switzerland.[19] A revised and updated version of the nomenclature, secretory profile, and anatomic distribution of the various endocrine cells currently known to populate the gut is summarized in Fig. 10-2. In the Lausanne classification, while the nomenclature of the enterochromaffin (EC) cells and the enterochromaffin like (ECL) cells was retained because of its familiarity, the alphabetical designations of the other cells were derived from the first letters of the hormones that the cells were known or presumed to secrete. This classification, originally based on a "one cell, one hormone" concept, has had to be modified in light of subsequent developments. When it was shown that the same peptide (gastrin) is secreted by two ultrastructurally different cell types, the cell type that was identified later was given a new designation—the IG cell (intestinal gastrin-producing cell)—to distinguish it from the G cell (antropyloric gastrin-producing cell). In other instances when a given cell type (e.g., the EC_1 cell) has been found to secrete an amine (5-hydroxytryptamine [5-HT]) along with one or more peptides, the peptide localized first (substance P) has been used as the point of reference, since the same

amine (5-HT) can be localized in ultrastructurally different cells (EC_1, EC_2, and EC_n) that produce other hormones. It is anticipated that further modifications of this classification will be required periodically as newer secretory products are identified and ascribed either to existing cell types or to others yet to be described.

PEPTIDERGIC INNERVATION OF THE GUT

In addition to its adrenergic and cholinergic innervation, the gastrointestinal tract also contains an intramural network of peptidergic nerve fibers. When visualized immunocytochemically, the peptidergic nerve fibers typically show a beaded appearance, and their secretory granules are closely similar to those of peptide-containing endocrine cells. Several peptides, including somatostatin, substance P, vasoactive intestinal polypeptide (VIP), cholecystokinin (CCK), [Met]- and [Leu]enkephalins, bombesin, calcitonin gene-related peptide (CGRP), galanin, and neuropeptide Y (NPY), have been immunocytochemically localized in these enteric nerves.[20–23] It is now established that most, if not all, enteric neurons contain more than one peptide or a combination of peptides and amines,[24] and that each type of neuronal population has a characteristic distributional pattern.[25–30] Some types project preferentially into the muscle coats (inhibitory/excitatory fibers), others run between ganglia (interneuronal fibers), while still others are prominently localized around blood vessels, sphincters, and epithelial cells in the mucosa. Such a distributional pattern suggests that they have a variegated role in regulating blood flow, sphincter tone, and absorptive functions.[30] The presence of identical peptides in both endocrine cells and peptidergic nerves of the gut indicates that some of these peptides are capable of not only acting as true hormones but also functioning as classic neurotransmitters and paracrine messengers. In view of the multifaceted regulatory efforts that these peptides exert on the integrated secretory, absorptive, and motor functions of the gut, they

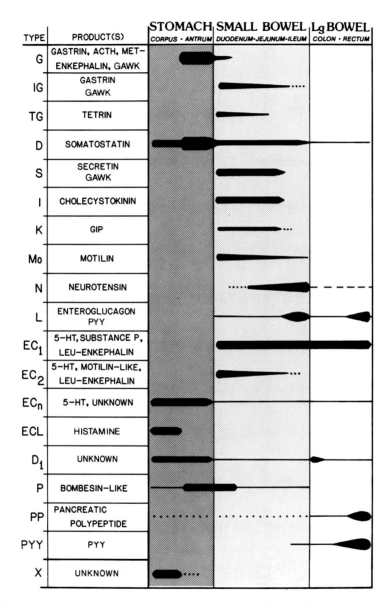

Fig. 10-2. The anatomic distribution of the various endocrine cell types in the human gastrointestinal tract. The nomenclature corresponds to the Lausanne classification updated in light of subsequent developments. The extent of the solid lines indicates the presence of specific cell types at different levels in the gut, whereas the width reflects their relative numbers at each site. The interrupted lines indicate the presence of very few cells. (ACTH, adrenocorticotrophic hormone; GH, growth hormone; GIP, gastric inhibitory peptide; 5-HT, 5-hydroxytryptamine; VIP, vasoactive intestinal peptide.) (From Dayal,[160] with permission.)

are now more accurately referred to as *regulatory peptides* rather than hormones, neurotransmitters, or neuromodulators. Such refinements in our thinking have gradually eroded the functional distinctions between the "true hormones" and the neurotransmitters held by earlier physiologists and are more in tune with the *paraneuron concept,* which holds that the gut endocrine cells are both functionally and morphologically closely related to the neurons.[31-33]

HISTOGENESIS OF ENDOCRINE CELLS OF THE GUT

Although the gut endocrine cells represent at least 19 distinct cell types, they share a number of histochemical and ultrastructural characteristics not only among themselves, but also with other endocrine cell types such as the C cells of the thyroid; the chromaffin cells of the adrenal medulla; the islet cells of the pancreas; the corticotrophs and melanotrophs of the pituitary; and certain cells in the carotid body, the bronchi, the hypothalamus, and the sympathetic ganglia, among others.[34, 35] The most important histochemical property common to several of these cells is their capacity for uptake and decarboxylation of a number of aromatic amines or their precursors. The term *APUD,* an acronym for this characteristic, was, therefore adopted as a generic name for the entire family of these widely dispersed endocrine cells.[35, 36] The occurrence of histochemical properties such as argyrophilia, masked metachromasia, and APUD characteristics in such widely dispersed endocrine cell populations was originally explained on the basis of their presumed common origin in the neural crest, the neuroendocrine-programmed ectoblast, or the primitive epiblast.[36-39] Although such a histogenetic origin appears to be true for such endocrine cells as the thyroidal C cells, the type 1 cells of the carotid body, the cells of the anterior pituitary, and those in the adrenal medulla, experimental evidence indicates that gastrointestinal endocrine cells are endodermal in origin.[40-42] Recent ultrastructural

studies conducted in humans and in neonatal mice have demonstrated that immature mucous cells of the stomach are pluripotent and capable of differentiating into mucous, parietal, chief, or endocrine cells.[43, 44] A similar histogenetic origin has been demonstrated by others for endocrine cells of the small and large intestines.[45] Perhaps the local tissue microenvironment may have a regulatory role in this regard.[46] Thus, in the developing human fetus, because antropyloric differentiation and the appearance of uncommitted endocrine cells within the gastric mucosa are both seen to precede antral G cell differentiation by at least 8 weeks,[47] it has been surmised that the antropyloric milieu somehow induces G- cell differentiation. In postnatal life, too, the appearance of G cells within ectopically situated gastric mucosa (e.g., in Meckel's diverticula and small bowel duplications) is seen only in areas of antropyloric differentiation.[48] Additional support for a common mode of origin of the endocrine cells and the nonendocrine mucosal epithelial cells may also be derived from such clinical observations that tumors show a spectrum of overlapping morphologic features, such as the production of periodic acid-Schiff (PAS) positive mucinous material by carcinoid tumors and the presence of endocrine cells in otherwise well-differentiated adenocarcinomas.[49]

IDENTIFICATION OF NEUROENDOCRINE CELLS

A number of histochemical staining reactions were developed and refined to gain insight into the chemical composition of the secretory products of the endocrine cells: these stains were very popular until the early seventies. However, some of them were of rather limited usefulness since they neither stained all of the various cell types nor characterized the secretory products of the positively stained cells. Nonetheless, some of these procedures have remained useful for the visualization of these cells and for the broad categorization of tumors (carcinoids) arising from these cells. Thus, although silver stains for argyrophilia and argentaffinity are widely used in surgical pathology practice, their current utility lies more in the detection of endocrine cells and their tumors than in their ability to identify the secretory products elaborated by them. This latter task is currently more or less exclusively achieved by immunocytochemical methods. A brief account of some of the more important histochemical stains and immunocytochemical markers of neuroendocrine cells is given below for their diagnostic importance in surgical pathology.

HISTOCHEMICAL STAINS FOR
NEUROENDOCRINE CELLS

Formalin-Induced Fluorescence

Several biogenic amines, including tryptamine, 5-hydroxytryptamine (5-HT), and 5-hydroxytryptophan (5-HTP), among others, when exposed to specific aldehydes, yield condensation products that not only have strong reducing properties but also exhibit a specific fluorescence under ultraviolet (UV) light. The fluorescent technique of Falk and co-workers[50] and its subsequent modifications[51, 52] utilize the fluorogenic properties of these condensates for the identification of specific amines within the intracytoplasmic granules of normal and neoplastic endocrine cells. This technique is both highly sensitive and specific for decarboxylated amines, such as serotonin (5-HT). Cells containing 5-HT can be readily visualized by their strong yellow fluorescence when deparaffinized unstained tissue sections obtained from formalin-fixed paraffin-embedded material are examined under UV light. Alternatively, air-dried cryostat sections obtained from fresh unfixed tissues or air-dried touch preparations, exposed to gaseous formaldehyde for 1 to 2 hours under carefully regulated conditions of temperature and humidity, and examined under UV light will also yield the characteristic granular bright yellow intracytoplasmic fluorescence.[53] Such fluorescence needs to be distinguished from the orange-yellow autofluorescence of lipofuscin-

containing cells. Since the formaldehyde-induced fluorescence technique represents a relatively simple and reliable method for detecting the 5-HT-containing EC cells, several modifications of this technique involving exposure of tissue sections to ozone or hydrochloric acid were subsequently developed for visualization of the gastrin-containing G cells.[51, 52] However, with the availability of potent and specific antisera to a variety of peptide hormones, these methods have been more or less completely supplanted by immunocytochemical methods for the localization of these secretory products. In a study comparing the results of formaldehyde-induced fluorescence, argentaffin stains, and the immunocytochemical technique for localization of 5-HT-containing cells, we found excellent correlation between the autofluorescence of 5-HT-containing cells, the results of argentaffin stains (Masson-Fontana technique), and the immunocytochemical method (Dayal Y, Wolfe HJ: Unpublished observations). However, because of the greater sensitivity of the immunocytochemical technique, 5-HT could be identified in a greater number of cells by that method than by the fluorescence method.

Silver Staining Techniques

Silver staining techniques were originally evolved as substitutes for chromaffin reactions. A number of techniques using a variety of silver salts under different conditions were developed in an effort to characterize the secretory products in various endocrine cells. Broadly speaking, these histochemical reactions are designated as *argentaffin* and *argyrophil* reactions. In the argentaffin reaction (Masson-Fontana technique) reduction of the ammoniacal silver nitrate is brought about primarily by the reducing capacity of intracellular components themselves, whereas in the argyrophil reaction (Sevier-Munger, Hellerstrom-Hellman, Bodian, and Grimelius techniques) the silver salts in an aqueous or alcoholic solution attach themselves to the intracytoplasmic secretory granules and are then reduced to metallic silver by exposure to an exogenous reducing substance.[54–56] In the endocrine cells of the normal gut as well as in carcinoids arising from them, a positive argentaffin reaction shows a strong correlation with their 5-HT content, as demonstrated by formaldehyde-induced fluorescence and immunoreactivity for 5-HT.[50, 53, 57] Perhaps the argentaffinity is related to the strong reducing properties of the condensates that 5-HT forms after formaldehyde fixation. In our experience, both the intensity of the argentaffin reaction itself and the number of cells that show argentaffinity are invariably less than that demonstrated by immunocytochemical techniques. Further, whereas only a faint argentaffinity may be demonstrable in suboptimally fixed autopsy material that has undergone advanced autolysis, immunoreactivity for 5-HT is still preserved. At the ultrastructural level, too, argentaffinity is displayed only by the 5-HT-containing EC_1 and EC_2 type cells, and the silver grains are selectively clustered over the pleomorphic secretory granules that represent the intracellular storage sites for serotonin.[58]

Although the vast majority of gut endocrine cells are known to be nonargentaffin, they are argyrophil when stained by the Grimelius, Sevier-Munger, Davenport, or Hellerstrom-Hellman technique.[57] However, despite the widespread use of argyrophil procedures for the visualization of gut endocrine cells, the exact cytochemical basis for this reaction remains unclear, although a possible relationship to the presence of sialoglycopeptides with a β_{1-4}-glycosidic linkage has been suggested.[59] These newer techniques for the demonstration of argyrophilia have been very useful in the identification of specific subpopulations of gut endocrine cells.[57] Thus, the Grimelius technique stains all cells except the somatostatin-producing D cells. The Sevier-Munger method stains only the serotonin-producing EC cells, the glucose-dependent insulinotropic peptide (GIP)-producing K cells, the CCK-producing I cells, the D_1 cells (storing a VIP-like peptide), and the ECL cells (which are now known to produce

histamine).[57, 58] The Hellerstrom-Hellman modification of Davenport's technique selectively demonstrates the somatostatin-producing D cells.[57] Since the argentaffin reaction involves the reduction of ionic silver to its metallic form by endogenous reducing substances, whereas argyrophilia requires the exogenous addition of similar agents, all argentaffin (serotonin-producing) cells in the gut also give a positive argyrophil reaction. However, since the argyrophil stains identify a much larger population of endocrine cell types (including the serotonin-producing EC cells), not all argyrophil cells give a positive argentaffin reaction.

The various argyrophil stains have also been adapted for use at the electron microscopic level.[60] Thus, the argentaffinity and argyrophilia of the various cells, as observed by the Masson-Fontana, Grimelius, Davenport, or Sevier-Munger technique, have proven to be very useful adjuncts to granule morphology toward an ultrastructural classification of these endocrine cells.[57, 58] Although in general the small grains of oxidized metallic silver are seen to be selectively peppered over the central cores of the secretory granules, in some cells (such as the enteroglucagon-producing L cells of the midgut) these silver grains are seen to concentrate on the peripheral halo between the core and the limiting membrane of the granules.[60]

IMMUNOCYTOCHEMICAL MARKERS OF NEUROENDOCRINE CELLS

Immunocytochemical staining techniques using antibodies against various regulatory substances have significantly enhanced our ability to identify the various functionally distinct endocrine cell types in tissue sections. Under light microscopy these techniques are therefore being used extensively to visualize these cells in both normal and abnormal tissues. At the ultrastructural level, these techniques have not only enabled us to localize specific secretory products within individual secretory granules, but have also helped in the localization of different molecular forms of the secretory product in the maturing secretory granules.[12] Several procedural modifications are currently available, but the use of the colloidal gold technique is particularly advantageous. Since the highly electron-dense gold spheres are available in different sizes, multiple antibodies labeled with gold particles of different sizes can be used to co-localize different products or molecular variants of the same product on a single tissue section.[12, 61]

Neuron-Specific Enolase

Neuron-specific enolase (NSE) is an isoenzyme of the glycolytic enzyme enolase, which is ubiquitously present in a variety of tissues. Immunohistochemical studies have localized NSE in both neural and endocrine components of the DES. In the gastrointestinal tract, NSE has been localized in all endocrine cell types and in the myenteric nerves.[62] In the pancreas, NSE has been similarly localized in the insular and extrainsular endocrine cells, the peptidergic nerves, and the neuroinsular complexes.[62] NSE is thus a useful generic marker for both neuroendocrine cells and myenteric nerves of the gut and pancreas as well as for neuroendocrine tumors that arise in these organs. Since it is present in functionally mature cells, immunostaining for it is characteristically faint in certain types of tumors. Because NSE is a cytosolic enzyme not related to neurosecretory granules, staining for NSE is characteristically nongranular in type, and is frequently demonstrable even in sparsely granulated cells, where silver stains and immunohistochemical staining for (granule-related) markers such as chromogranins is either faint or undetectable. Despite these advantages, the specificity of NSE as a marker for neuroendocrine differentiation has been disputed, since NSE has been demonstrated in a variety of non-neuroendocrine cells and in such non-neuroendocrine tumors as malignant melanoma and malignant lymphoma.[63–65] In view of these short-

comings, immunoreactivity of NSE should be interpreted with caution and only in light of other ancillary information.[66]

Chromogranins

Chromogranins constitute a family of highly acidic soluble glycoproteins that was first identified in chromaffin granules of adrenal medullary cells.[67] This family is composed of at least three related molecular forms, designated as A, B, and C.[68] Chromogranin A is by far the most abundant, and is structurally related to parathyroid secretory protein 1. Chromogranin B is a higher-molecular-weight protein that is identical to secretogranin I. Chromogranin C (secretogranin II) has a molecular weight intermediate between the other two forms, and corresponds to the pituitary tyrosine sulfated protein (TSP) 86/84.[69, 70] Immunohistochemical studies have localized chromogranins in secretory granules of a variety of neuroendocrine cell types including those in the gastrointestinal tract, lung, pancreas, parathyroid, thyroid, pituitary, and paraganglia.[69, 71] In the gut, immunoreactivity for chromogranins has been localized in practically all of the endocrine cell types.[69, 71, 72] In the pancreas, it has been localized in insular and extrainsular endocrine cells. Since the presence of chromogranins in endocrine cells correlates strongly with some of the histochemical reactions (i.e., metachromasia, masked metachromasia, and argyrophilia) used for identification of such cells, it is possible that chromogranins may indeed be the uncharacterized "acidic proteins" responsible for those reactions.[69, 73, 74]

In view of their presence in a variety of neuroendocrine cells, chromogranins are now extensively used as a generic marker for the immunohistochemical demonstration of these cells. On account of their intragranular location, it has been suggested that these proteins have a role in hormone storage and release. Because chromogranins are co-liberated with the primary secretory product(s) of the secretory granules they may also have a role in stabilization of the soluble secretory product. More recently, chromogranins have been recognized to be the precursor for pancreastatin, and possibly for other peptides as well.[75, 76] Furthermore, it is quite likely that chromogranins additionally exert their action *after* exocytosis, either by serving as a carrier protein or as a regulatory peptide acting on target cells in the immediate vicinity (paracrine effect), or after gaining access into the circulation (endocrine function). Be it as it may, since circulating levels of chromogranins are elevated in patients with neuroendocrine tumors, it has been suggested that such elevations can be helpful both in diagnosing such tumors and in monitoring their course following surgical extirpation or chemotherapy.[77, 78]

Synaptophysin

Synaptophysin, a glycoprotein originally isolated from presynaptic vesicles of bovine neurons, is a major calcium-binding protein of the synaptic vesicle membrane.[79] It has now also been localized in adrenal medullary cells, the paraganglia, and the neuroendocrine cells of the gut, pancreas, lung, and pituitary.[80]

Synaptophysin has been found to be a valuable adjunct to NSE and chromogranins as a generic marker not only for neuroendocrine cells in the gut, pancreas, and elsewhere but for neuroendocrine tumors as well. It has been identified in such neuroendocrine tumors as pituitary and parathyroid adenomas, medullary carcinomas of thyroid, gastrointestinal carcinoids, and endocrine tumors of the pancreas, lung, and skin, as well as in neuroblastomas, ganglioneuroblastomas, ganglioneuromas, pheochromocytomas, and paragangliomas,[81–83] but not in normal exocrine glands and non-neuroendocrine tumors.[82] Such a widespread but selective distribution of synaptophysin in neuroendocrine cells is to be expected, since it is an integral constituent of the membrane surrounding neurosecretory granules. Although synaptophysin antibodies work quite satisfactorily on routinely fixed tissues processed for light microscopy, staining is more consistent, crisper, and more intense in Bouin's-fixed tissues.

In addition to the above-mentioned generic markers of neuroendocrine cells, several others, such as PGP 9.5, Leu 7, 7B2, and cytochrome b561, are also available. However, their diagnostic utility, dependability, and reliability need to be more adequately evaluated before they find general acceptability.

ENDOCRINE CELL HYPERPLASIAS

Hyperplasia signifies a non-neoplastic (nonautonomous) proliferation of a given cell type that results in an increase in its total cell mass. It is a morphologic phenomenon that requires morphologic criteria for its recognition and confirmation, and implies the presence of increased numbers of cells per unit area of mucosa. A diagnosis of gastrointestinal endocrine cell hyperplasia relies primarily on the identification of increased numbers (beyond twice the standard deviation (SD) in age- and sex-matched controls) of cells per unit area of mucosa.[84]

Our knowledge of the basic mechanisms responsible for endocrine cell hyperplasia is rather fragmentary. Whereas earlier studies had indicated that the neuroendocrine cells, the absorptive columnar cells, and the mucin-producing goblet cells were all derived from a common pluripotent progenitor cell and had a similar turnover rate,[85–88] subsequent workers have demonstrated that although a small proportion of cells of each type may indeed be derived from pluripotent stem cells, the majority of gastrointestinal endocrine cells are obtained by self-replication of mature endocrine cells and have half-lives and turnover rates different from those of nonendocrine epithelial cells.[89–93] Cumulative evidence indicates that endocrine cell hyperplasias in the gut result from a combination of a number of different mechanisms, such as prolongation of the half-life of these cells, augmented self-replication of mature cells, and differentiation of a larger fraction of uncommitted stem cells into specific neuroendocrine cell types. Each mechanism may be triggered by a release from the normal restraining influence of an inhibitor of neuroendocrine cell proliferation, a lack of the normal negative feedback mechanism, or the trophic influence of certain peptides or secretagogues.[92–98] Perhaps the trophic effects of hormonal influences and the local tissue microenvironment also have a significant role to play, and could explain not only the appearance of appropriate endocrine cell types in areas of antropyloric and intestinal metaplasia but also the appearance of specific endocrine cell increases in different types of hyperplasias.[99–101]

Since endocrine cell hyperplasias generally lack a clear-cut correlation with specific clinical or biochemical abnormalities they often remain clinically unsuspected. This is chiefly because hyperplastic cells usually do not release enough secretions into the blood to produce significant elevations in their circulating basal levels. Thus, although endocrine cell hyperplasia may occasionally have significant functional implications, hyperplasia does not necessarily imply a concomitant hyperfunctioning state. Even when they are present, endorcine cell hyperplasias generally do not produce recognizable lesions that can be biopsied.

Morphologically, too, hyperplasias of gastrointestinal endocrine cells are difficult to recognize and document, primarily because of (1) the heterogeneity of the endocrine cell population and the dispersed nature of its distribution in the gut, (2) the normal variability in the numbers of a given cell type in different segments of the gut, and (3) the elaborate morphometric analyses required for quantitating cell numbers. Some of the difficulties in the morphologic documentation of endocrine cell hyperplasias also relate to the fact that in certain conditions associated with such increases (e.g., chronic atrophic gastritis, pernicious anemia, and gluten sensitive enteropathy), the involved gastric or intestinal mucosa is significantly atrophied. It is therefore difficult to establish whether the observed increase represents a genuine hyperplasia or a mere overcrowding related to decreased mucosal

volume. Similarly, considerable controversy has resulted from differences in the morphometric methodologies and the frames of reference employed by various workers to document endocrine cell hyperplasias. Thus some workers have counted individual cells, others have chosen sophisticated computer-assisted methods and point-counting techniques, and still others have used scanning integrating image analyzers and quantitated the positively stained cells by measuring absorbance of light by different tissue components.[102, 103] Results, too, have been expressed in a variety of different ways, with some using absolute cell counts per unit area of mucosa and others using cells per unit length of mucosa, high-power field, gland, or crypt as their frame of reference.[94, 104, 105] Although these different frames of references may have been adopted to avoid some of the pitfalls referred to earlier, they often make comparisons between different reports difficult, especially since diametrically opposite results have occasionally been arrived at.[94, 106–110]

With gradual improvements in our understanding of the normal physiologic role of various endocrine cell types, their interrelationships with other endo- and exocrine types and their status in various diseases, we have also come to realize that hyperplasias of gut endocrine cells can not only be the primary cause of some clinical syndromes, but may also occur secondarily in certain conditions. Endocrine cell hyperplasias of the gut are therefore categorized as *primary* and *secondary,* and although either form can theoretically affect any cell type, this has so far been reported in a few cell types only.

HYPERPLASIAS OF ANTROPYLORIC G CELLS

Primary Antral G Cell Hyperplasia

Primary antral G cell hyperplasia is a clinical entity in which G cell hyperplasia occurs without a known predisposing cause. The disease has in the past been variously referred to as pseudo-Zollinger-Ellison syndrome, Zollinger-Ellison syndrome type 1, nontumorous hypergastrinemic hyperchlorhydria (NTHH), antral gastrinosis, or primary antral G cell hyperplasia (PAGCH).[111–113] Of these, PAGCH is the currently preferred term because it most accurately reflects the pathophysiologic mechanism responsible for the clinical symptoms. Patients present with clinical and biochemical features similar to those seen in duodenal ulcer disease and Zollinger-Ellison syndrome.[114–116] Although some workers have observed an autosomal-dominant inheritance of this disease,[104, 105] others have not encountered a familial tendency, indicating that PAGCH can occur on a sporadic basis as well.[114–116] A distinction between patients with PAGCH, those with duodenal ulcer disease, and those with classic Zollinger-Ellison syndrome is critical for clinical management, and is essentially achieved through certain provocative tests (Table 10-2). When clinically suspected, a diagnosis of PAGCH should always be confirmed by demonstrating G cell hyperplasia in endoscopically obtained antral mucosal biopsies.

Secondary Antral G Cell Hyperplasia

Antropyloric G cell hyperplasia (AGCH) has been observed to occur secondarily in a variety of clinical conditions (Table 10-3). The AGCH seen in gastric outlet obstruction and pyloric stenosis is believed to be secondary to the intragastric retention of food and the resultant gastric distension. The AGCH in patients with atrophic gastritis, pernicious anemia, and retained excluded antrum syndrome is secondary to a decrease or absence of hydrochloric acid bathing the antral mucosa.[99, 117] The AGCH seen in Zollinger-Ellison syndrome type 1 is a primary event, whereas in acromegaly it could either be a part of the multiple endocrine neoplasia (MEN) syndrome or secondary to the effect of an as yet unidentified trophic factor secreted by the pituitary.[118] In hyperparathyroidism, although a subsidiary parathyroid hormone effect cannot be completely excluded, the AGCH appears to be most likely due to hypercalcemia since it has also been observed in a variety of other chronic hypercalcemic states, including multiple myeloma, sarcoidosis, generalized carcinomatosis, and MEN syndrome type I.[94, 119]

The G cell hyperplasia that follows truncal vagotomy is due to a combination of chronic antral distension, decreased luminal acidity, and release from a vagally mediated inhibitor of G cell proliferation.[120] The AGCH observed in chronic uremia is most likely related to the chronic atrophic (uremic) gastritis that these patients develop.[121] Some, but not all, workers have demonstrated AGCH in stomachs resected

Table 10-2. Differential Diagnosis of Primary Antral G Cell Hyperplasia (PAGCH)

	PAGCH Syndrome	Duodenal Ulcer	Zollinger-Ellison Syndrome
BAO:MAO ratio	Variable	Under 60%	Over 60%
Meal stimulation test	Marked hypergastrinemia	Mild hypergastrinemia	
Secretin stimulation test	No response	Fall in serum gastrin levels	Rise in serum gastrin levels
Calcium stimulation test	No response	No response	Rise in serum gastrin levels
Antropyloric G cell, population	Diffusely hyperplastic	Normal or moderately hyperplastic	Within normal limits

BAO, basal acid output; MAO, maximal acid output.
(From Dayal & Wolfe,[240] with permission.)

**Table 10-3. Clinical Conditions Associated with
Antropyloric G Cell Hyperplasia**

Primary antral G cell hyperplasia (Zollinger-Ellison syn-
drome type 1)
Gastric outlet obstruction
Chronic atrophic gastritis
Pernicious anemia
Retained excluded antrum syndrome
Multiple endocrine neoplasia syndrome type 1 (Sipple)
Acromegaly
Chronic hypercalcemic states
   Multiple myeloma
   Sarcoidosis
   Disseminated carcinomatosis
Duodenal ulcer disease
Postvagotomy state
Pluriglandular autoimmune syndrome
Longterm therapy with
   H$_2$-receptor blockers (cimetidine, ranitidine, etc.)
   Proton-pump inhibitors (omeprazole)
   Cyprofibrate
Chronic uremia
?Cirrhosis

(From Dayal & Wolfe,[240] with permission.)

from patients with recalcitrant duodenal ulcer disease.[106–110] More recently, AGCH has been reported in patients receiving such H$_2$-receptor antagonists as cimetidine.[122] The increase in G cell numbers in these patients is secondary to the inhibition of acid secretion and has been implicated as a possible mechanism for the recurrence of ulcers after cessation of therapy.[122]

The distributional pattern of the G cells in both primary and secondary antral G cell hyperplasias is identical, and is characterized by the presence of increased numbers of immunocytochemically identifiable G cells in each antropyloric gland (Fig. 10-3). In sharp contrast to the random and irregular spatial distribution of the G cells in the lower third of the normal antral mucosa, the hyperplastic population spans both the lower and middle thirds of the mucosal thickness. In longstanding cases, the diffuse AGCH may also be associated with formation of numer-

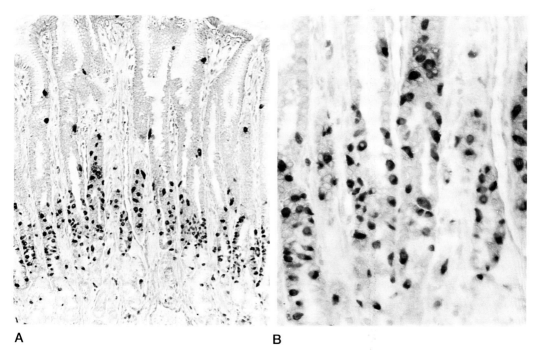

A   B

Fig. 10-3. Hyperplasia of antropyloric G cells in a patient with pernicious anemia. **(A)** In sharp contrast to the irregular and sparse distribution of the normal G cells in the lower third of the mucosa thickness, the hyperplastic G cells are present in practically all antral glands, occupy both the lower and intermediate thirds of the mucosa, and focally even extend into the superficial mucosa as well. **(B)** Higher-power magnification showing the basal location of the positively stained intracytoplasmic secretory granules. (Immunoperoxidase technique using antigastrin antibodies; methyl green counterstain, ×128.) (From Dayal et al.,[102] with permission.)

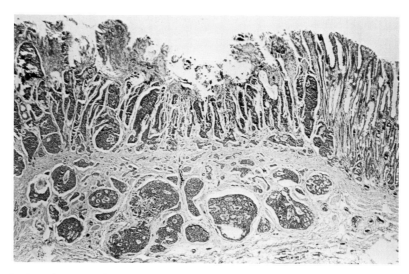

Fig. 10-4. Section of gastric antrum showing a carcinoid tumor with superficial ulceration of the overlying mucosa. This 12-year-old boy with Zollinger-Ellison syndrome had diffuse hyperplasia of the antropyloric G cells and multiple "microcarcinoids" in the antral mucosa. (Courtesy of Dr. Belur Bhagavan, Mt. Sinai Hospital, Baltimore. From Dayal et al.,[102] with permission.)

ous, small, micronodular clusters of G cells in the lamina propria. These micronodular clusters are capable of progressing to G cell carcinoid tumors (gastrinomas)[111, 123] (Fig. 10-4). This progression of G cell hyperplasia to G cell carcinoids is analogous to the hyperplasia–neoplasia sequence described for ECL cells in the oxyntic mucosa of patients with chronic atrophic gastritis or pernicious anemia.[84, 99, 124–126] Both chronic atrophic gastritis and pernicious anemia, long known to predispose to the development of gastric cancer, are now also being implicated as signalling a high risk for the development of gastric carcinoids.[99, 124–131]

HYPERPLASIA OF ENTEROCHROMAFFIN-LIKE CELLS

One of the most significant characteristics of the ECL cells is that they are under the trophic influence of gastrin. These cells therefore undergo a secondary hyperplasia in chronically hypergastrinemic states.

Hyperplastic and neoplastic ECL cell proliferation have been best documented in rodents, most notably in the *Mastomys* sp., in which they give rise to histamine-induced gastric and duodenal ulcers.[132] More recently, ECL cell hyperplasias (and occasionally even ECL cell carcinoids) have been observed in rats following the long-term administration of various H_2-receptor blockers (e.g., ranitidine or cimetidine) and omeprazole (an inhibitor of the H^+-K^+-ATPase proton pump in parietal cells).[92, 97, 133–138] The ECL cell hyperplasia in such instances is due to the hypergastrinemia induced secondarily by the marked suppression of acid secretion.[97, 98, 137–139] Gastrin has a well-known trophic influence on the oxyntic epithelial cells.[139–142] Cell kinetic studies have shown that since the increase in the labelling index of ECL cells in hypergastrinemic states is more pronounced than that of the uncommitted stem cells and other self-replicating functionally mature cells,[92, 93, 139] the ECL cells are particularly sensitive to the mitogenic effects of gastrin, and that the hyperplastic ECL cells are predominantly, if not completely, derived from replication of mature ECL cells rather than an augmented differentiation of the stem cells into ECL cells.

In humans, ECL cell hyperplasias and ECL cell carcinoids (composed predominantly or exclusively of ECL cells) are most often observed in patients with chronic atrophic gastritis, pernicious anemia, or Zollinger-Ellison syndrome.[126, 127, 143–149] Hyperplasias and tumors of ECL cells have also been observed in patients receiving antisecretory therapy with H_2-blockers or omeprazole[150, 151] and are believed to be related to hypergastrinemia induced secondarily by these agents.[143] In the oxyntic mucosa of these patients, argyrophil stains have shown a spectrum of hyperplastic lesions ranging from a diffuse increase in argyrophil cell numbers through linear and nodular aggregates, to intramucosal and frank carcinoids.[99, 102, 125, 152, 153] Such a progression has recently been formalized into a hyperplasia–neoplasia sequence.[84] In this scheme, the earliest stage, *simple hyperplasia,* is characterized by increased numbers of positively stained cells scattered singly or in clusters of up to three or four cells per gland deep in the oxyntic mucosa (Fig. 10-5). The number of such cells per unit measure of the oxyntic mucosa should exceed 2 SD over the normal range in age- and sex-matched controls. When such proliferating endocrine cells are seen arranged in a linear or a daisy-chain-like arrangement along the basement membrane of the gland, the lesion is designated as *linear hyperplasia* (Fig. 10-6). The next recognizable stage, *micronodular hyperplasia,* is characterized by the presence of endocrine cell clusters that do not exceed the diameter of a gastric gland (100 to 150 μm) in size (Fig. 10-7). This is the earliest stage that can be seen under the hematoxylin and eosin (H&E) stain; and the clusters, bounded by an intact basement membrane, are characteristically located in the basiglandular portion of the mucosa. Aggregates of several such micronodular lesions, each with its intact basement membrane, constitutes the stage of *adenomatoid hyperplasia* (Fig. 10-8). Enlargement of each micronodule, with breakdown of its basement membrane, presence of cytologic atypia, increased nuclear:cytoplasmic ratio, and a reduction in the intensity of argyrophilia is the hallmark of the

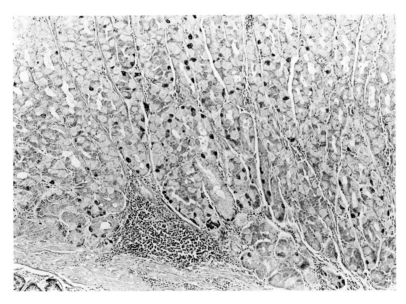

Fig. 10-5. Simple hyperplasia of argyrophil endocrine cells in the oxyntic mucosa of a patient with chronic atrophic gastritis type 1. Note the increased numbers of argyrophil cells dispersed singly or in small clusters of up to three or four cells in the closely packed glands. (Grimelius stain with methyl green counterstain.) (From Dayal & Wolfe,[240] with permission.)

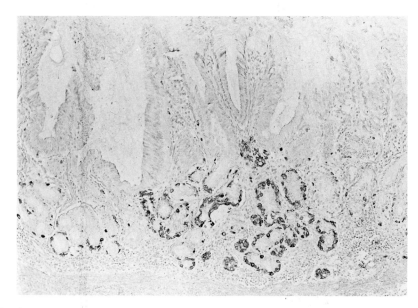

Fig. 10-6. Linear hyperplasia of argyrophil endocrine cells in the oxyntic mucosa of a patient with chronic atrophic gastritis type 1. The markedly increased numbers of argyrophil cells are arranged in a linear daisy-chain-like fashion along the basement membrane of the glands. (Grimelius stain with methyl green counterstain.) (From Dayal & Wolfe,[240] with permission.)

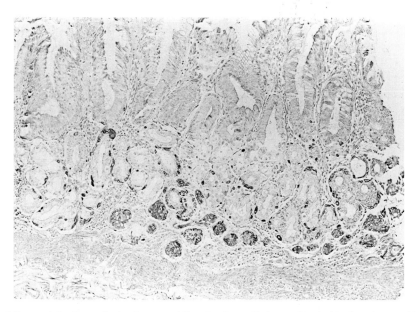

Fig. 10-7. Micronodular hyperplasia of argyrophil endocrine cells in a patient with chronic atrophic gastritis type 1. Focal nodular clusters of 5 to 25 endocrine cells up to 100 μm in size but not exceeding the diameter of the gastric glands are seen deep in the lamina propria abutting the muscularis mucosae. A few glands also show linear hyperplasia of the endocrine cells. (Grimelius stain with methyl green counterstain.) (From Dayal & Wolfe,[240] with permission.)

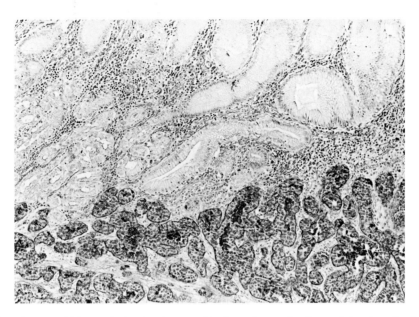

Fig. 10-8. Adenomatoid hyperplasia showing a collection of several micronodules deep in the oxyntic mucosa of a patient with chronic atrophic gastritis type 1. Although the micronodules are in close proximity to each other, their basement membranes are still intact. (Grimelius stain with methyl green counterstain.) (From Dayal & Wolfe,[240] with permission.)

dysplastic (precarcinoid) lesions. The dysplastic stage marks the borderline between the clearly hyperplastic stages preceding it and the neoplastic stage (carcinoid) following it in the sequence. These lesions, ranging between 150 μm and 0.5 mm in diameter, can show such morphologic variations as enlarging micronodules (nodular aggregates more than 150 μm in diameter), fusing micronodules (formed by coalescence of several adjacent micronodules), microinvasive lesions (clusters of atypical cells infiltrating the lamina propria between the glands), or nodules with newly formed stroma (when the nodules acquire a lobular or trabecular pattern) (Fig. 10-9). The *carcinoid stage* is characterized by nodular infiltrating growths more than 0.5 cm in diameter. Lesions are completely intramucosal at first, but gradually extend intramurally, and invade vascular or lymphatic channels to produce nodal and distant metastases (Fig. 10-10). This classification has particular relevance for its implication in assessing the neoplastic potential of ECL cell hyperplasias in different

clinical conditions and for the evaluation of their risk of developing into gastric carcinoids.

The co-existence of ECL cell carcinoids with varying grades of ECL cell hyperplasias in the oxyntic mucosa of hypergastrinemic patients strongly reinforces the belief that the different hyperplastic lesions represent sequential steps in the evolution of gastric ECL cell carcinoids (Fig. 10-11). Whereas ECL cell carcinoids and the hyperplastic lesions preceding it are most often seen in patients with chronic atrophic gastritis and pernicious anemia,[99, 124–131, 145, 154] these tumors are very uncommon in Zollinger-Ellison syndrome even though these patients have more severe hypergastrinemia and are known to also have endocrine cell hyperplasia in the oxyntic mucosa.[124, 148, 154, 155] The few Zollinger-Ellison syndrome patients in whom ECL cell carcinoids have developed have all had the MEN type 1 syndrome.[154, 156] It is quite likely that either the genetic make-up of these patients predisposes them to develop ECL cell hyperplasia,[156] or that the hypercalcemia and

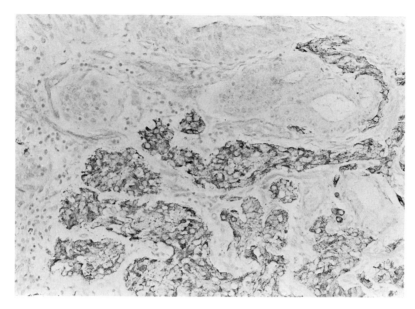

Fig. 10-9. Dysplastic lesion showing large irregular clusters of proliferating endocrine cells deep in the lamina propria. These clusters lack a basement membrane; the cells are only faintly argyrophil and show nuclear atypia. (From Dayal & Wolfe,[240] with permission.)

antral G cell hyperplasia present in these patients together induce hypergastrinemia and secondary ECL cell hyperplasia even prior to the development of gastrinomas.[157] Since nonfamilial Zollinger-Ellison syndrome patients have normal antropyloric G cell counts,[158] they do not develop ECL cell hyperplasia until several years after the appearance of a gastrinoma and the onset of the resultant hypergastrinemia. The relative infrequency of ECL cell carcinoids in patients with nonfamilial Zollinger-Ellison syndrome is therefore related first to the long time it takes such hyperplasias to develop and progress to the carcinoid stage, and second to the fact that a significant number of these patients undergo a gastrectomy in the interim. Nevertheless, the occasional reports of such tumors developing in patients with the non-familial form of Zollinger-Ellison syndrome indicate that ECL cell carcinoids can occasionally develop in these patients as well.[129, 149, 154, 159] This has considerable clinical relevance since the number of Zollinger-Ellison syndrome patients undergoing long-term gastric acid blockade therapy with agents that induce secondary hypergastrinemia

is increasing. It is also quite likely that in the future, ECL cell hyperplasias and ECL cell carcinoids will also be detected in a variety of other chronic hypergastrinemic states as well.[160]

Although ECL cell hyperplasia is seen in nearly 10 percent of patients undergoing endoscopy for upper gastrointestinal symptoms,[125] its clinical significance is currently unclear. Because these hyperplastic lesions have the ability to develop into potentially malignant carcinoid tumors, it has been suggested that ECL cell hyperplasias should be regarded as preneoplastic lesions.[84] However, the clinical risk is not so much in having the lesions as in their progression to invasive carcinoids. It is important to bear in mind that not all hyperplasias progress to carcinoids, and that even the few that do are perhaps slow to do so. In the absence of radiologically or endoscopically detectable carcinoid tumors, these lesions should be managed conservatively by periodic endoscopy and biopsy to monitor their progression. It should be noted however, that the early hyperplastic lesions are radiologically and endoscopically undetectable.[128] Even the earliest lesions (mi-

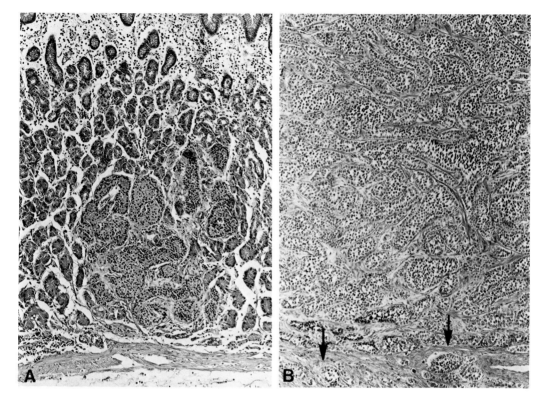

Fig. 10-10. (**A**) Intramucosal carcinoid located deep within the oxyntic mucosa of a patient with Zollinger-Ellison syndrome and possibly also MEN syndrome type 1. Note the trabecular arrangement of the tumor cells. (**B**) Higher-power magnification of another tumor showing the closely packed trabecular arrangement of the tumor cells and their extension into the superficial submucosa (arrows). (H&E.) (From Dayal & Wolfe,[240] with permission.)

cronodular hyperplasia) visible on routine light microscopy are located deep within the mucosa and are covered by an intact epithelium (Fig. 10-7). Quite often they are not even included in mucosal biopsies obtained with the usual 2 to 3 mm size biopsy forceps. It is therefore important that multiple full-thickness mucosal biopsies with ''jumbo'' biopsy forceps be obtained when patients at risk for endocrine cell hyperplasia are being evaluated or followed up. When a carcinoid tumor develops, management should·be dictated by clinical symptomatology and tempered by such pathologic features as size, number, and location of the tumor(s) as well as the absence or the presence of cytologic atypia, increased nuclear:cytoplasmic ratio, local invasion, and metastases of the tumors.

HYPERPLASIA OF ENTEROCHROMAFFIN CELLS

Although the term *enterochromaffin cell* has been used generically for all endocrine cells of the gut, its current usage is limited to indicate the serotonin-producing endocrine cells. Dispersed throughout the gastrointestinal mucosa, the EC cells constitute the largest single endocrine cell population in the gut.

EC cell hyperplasia has been observed in small bowel biopsies from both children and adults with untreated celiac disease[161, 162] (Fig. 10-12). Such hyperplasias appear to be related to the severity of the enteropathy and are associated with a concomitant increase in the serotonin concentration per EC cell, a raised serotonin

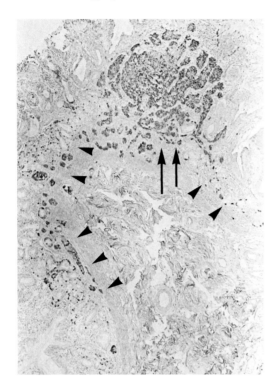

Fig. 10-11. Scanning photomicrograph view of oxyntic mucosa of a patient with chronic atrophic gastritis type 1 showing a small carcinoid tumor with early submucosal invasion (arrows) arising in a background of argyrophil endocrine cell hyperplasia in adjacent mucosa (arrowheads). (Grimelius stain with methyl green counterstain.) (From Dayal & Wolfe,[240] with permission.)

to chronic mucosal inflammation since similar increases in EC cell numbers also occur in chronic gastritis, appendicitis, and cholecystitis, as well as in areas close to intestinal strictures.[155, 166] Morphologically, the hyperplastic EC cells are restricted to the basal portion of the crypts and have occasionally been associated with micronodular clusters similar to those observed with G and ECL cell hyperplasias. Unlike their gastric counterparts, ileal, appendiceal, and colorectal carcinoids do not appear to arise from such hyperplasias.[167–169] Focal areas of EC cell hyperplasia with microadenomatous clusters have been reported as a fortuitous association of unknown significance in a solitary case report of a patient with megacolon.[170]

content in the intestinal mucosa, modest elevations of serotonin levels in the blood, and increased urinary excretion of 5-hydroxyindole acetic acid (5-HIAA).[163–165] Thus, the hyperplastic EC cells in celiac disease are hyperfunctioning, and show increased serotonin synthesis and release.[164, 165] Since all of these abnormalities revert back to normal shortly after gluten withdrawal, the morphologic and functional EC cell abnormalities in celiac disease appear to be an integral part of the disease and related to the reparative regeneration following gluten-induced mucosal cell injury.[163–165] Such EC cell hyperplasias appear to be a nonspecific response

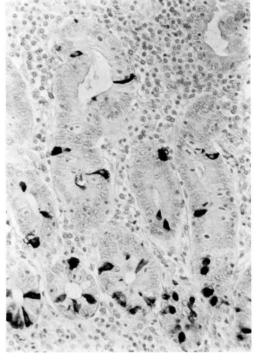

Fig. 10-12. Jejunal mucosa of a child with untreated gluten-sensitive enteropathy showing severe villous atrophy and increased numbers of EC cells in the hyperplastic crypts. (Immunoperoxidase technique using antiserotonin antibody; methyl green counterstain.)

HYPERPLASIA OF D CELLS

Hyperplasia of the antral D cells has been observed in duodenal ulcer disease.[85, 110, 171–173] However, since this hyperplasia is not a universal finding in these patients but is seen only in those with a concomitant AGCH, it has been suggested that D cell hyperplasia in duodenal ulcer patients occurs secondarily to the AGCH and a hypersecretory state.[171, 173] However, antral D cell hyperplasia in the absence of AGCH has been observed in such hypersecretory states as Zollinger-Ellison syndrome.[172]

Hyperplasias of intestinal D cells, in association with a similar increases in EC, K, Mo, and L cell numbers, have been reported in patients with celiac disease. These hyperplastic increases are all believed to be a nonspecific regenerative response to the gluten-induced mucosal injury.[163–165]

Primary hyperplasia of the antral D cells has so far been reported in one patient only. This patient, a 37-year-old woman with pituitary dwarfism, obesity, and goiter, had a marked D cell hyperplasia diffusely involving the fundic, antral, and duodenal mucosa. The investigators speculated that the short stature and the other endocrine abnormalities in this patient had resulted from a life-long hypersomatostatinemia.[174]

HYPERPLASIAS OF OTHER ENDOCRINE CELL TYPES

More recently, hyperplasias of endocrine cells have been identified by argyrophil stains in colonic mucosa of patients with idiopathic ulcerative colitis or Crohn's disease.[175–178] Although the specific cell type(s) involved in such proliferations have not been histochemically investigated in detail, it has been reported that the bulk of such an increase is due to EC cell hyperplasia. While this may merely be a reflection of the larger number of EC cells present in the colorectal mucosa, this needs to be studied further. In view of the extensive involvement of the various bowel segments in patients with inflammatory bowel disease, it is likely that more than one cell type may be involved. Although the precise reason for such a hyperplasia is unknown, it appears to be a nonspecific response to inflammation and tissue repair, or a relative "sparing" of the endocrine cells by the tissue destructive process. Such a mechanism has been proposed for the endocrine cell hyperplasia observed in graft-versus-host disease,[179] and may not only be operative in inflammatory bowel disease but in other conditions such as enterocolitis due to food allergies as well.[180]

CARCINOID TUMORS

GENERAL CHARACTERISTICS

Gastrointestinal carcinoids are neoplasms that arise from endocrine cells or their precursors, which are normally dispersed throughout the mucosa of the gut. They can arise anywhere in the gastrointestinal tract, and have been classified conventionally into the foregut, midgut, and hindgut categories, based on the embryologic derivation of their site of origin.[181] Approximately 60 to 80 percent of these tumors arise in the midgut, with the appendix and distal ileum as their most common sites of origin.[182] Although an additional 10 to 25 percent arise from hindgut-derived structures, the majority of hindgut carcinoids are rectal in origin.[182, 183] In the foregut, the stomach is the site of greatest predilection, followed by the duodenum and esophagus.[182] Gastrointestinal carcinoids are frequently multicentric in origin,[184–189] and patients with carcinoids have also been shown to have a higher frequency of developing other primary tumors both in the gastrointestinal tract and elsewhere.[188–191] Carcinoid tumors were originally distinguished from adenocarcinoma on account of their histologic features and their relatively indolent clinical behavior. Since the presence of local intramural invasion in these slowly growing tumors does not have the same ominous connotation as in adenocarcinomas, the distinction between "benign" and "malignant" carcinoids has been traditionally based on the absence or presence of demonstrable metastases. It has now become increasingly clear that all carcinoids are potentially malignant lesions, and that this tendency for aggressive behavior is related to a number of factors, such as the anatomic site of origin, the extent of intramural penetration by the tumor cells, and the size of the tumor.[182, 184, 187, 189, 192–194] Thus, appendiceal and rectal carcinoids are seldom malignant, and even though a majority of them show extensive local spread, metastatic dissemination is relatively infrequent.[182, 184] Ileal and colonic carcinoids, in contrast, are frequently malignant, and a high proportion of these tumors have already metastasized by the time they are first detected.[182, 184]

A significant majority of gastrointestinal carcinoids are clinically silent and are first discovered incidentally during surgery or autopsy. A smaller proportion are symptomatic, and give rise to rather nonspecific symptoms related to their anatomic location in the gut. Thus the polypoid gastric carcinoids present with gastrointestinal bleeding or gastric outlet obstruction. Duodenal, ampullary, and periampullary tumors may additionally lead to jaundice owing to obstruction of bile flow. Intestinal carcinoids give rise to gastrointestinal obstruction, infarction, or bleeding. Since most carcinoids appear as nodular mucosal or submucosal tumors rather than as annular growths, obstruction is usually due to intussusception or to a sharp angulation and fixation of the bowel loop at the site of the tumor.[188, 195–197] This kinking is related to a desmoplastic fibrosis involving the mesentery, and is frequently accompanied by a sharply localized area of muscular hypertrophy underlying the tumor.[197] Blood vessels caught in this mesenteric fibrosis may be secondarily compressed, and may produce an ischemic necrosis in the involved segment of the bowel. Bowel infarctions associated with ileal carcinoids may also be caused by a peculiar concentric thickening of the vessel walls that is most likely produced by increased local concentrations of 5-HT released by the tumor cells.[188, 198, 199] The mural

thickening is seen as an increased deposition of elastic tissue in the intima of the afferent vessels and the adventitial coat of the efferent veins draining the tumor.[198, 199] Rectal carcinoids most often give rise to bleeding and passage of bright red blood per rectum.

Although appendiceal carcinoids are occasionally detected incidentally in appendices removed for appendicitis, this association is usually fortuitous. Since the tumors are most commonly located in the distal third, or the tip of the appendix, they are unlikely to have caused the appendicitis. It is interesting to note that in extra-appendiceal locations, symptomatic carcinoids show a strong association with deep intramural invasion of the tumor cells. Thus, whereas 74 to 82 percent of symptomatic tumors had invaded up to or beyond halfway through the wall, less than 13 percent of asymptomatic carcinoids did so.[189, 192] Although local tissue invasion by carcinoid tumors does not in itself imply malignancy, deep local penetration by tumor is associated with aggressive behavior and a high incidence of metastatic spread to regional nodes and distant sites.[189, 192] In one series, 90 percent of the deeply invasive tumors had already metastasized when first detected, whereas none of the superficially invasive tumors had done so.[192] A similar association has been noted between the size of the primary tumor and the incidence of metastases. More than two-thirds of the tumors greater than 2 cm in diameter show metastases when first discovered, whereas those under 1 cm in size show metastases in less than 5 percent of instances; aggressive potential of tumors 1 to 2 cm in size closely approximates that of the larger lesions.[187, 188, 193, 194]

SECRETORY PRODUCTS

Since each of the various endocrine cell types dispersed in the gastrointestinal mucosa can give rise to carcinoids upon neoplastic transformation, these tumors may be expected to reflect the hormonal program of their putative parent cell. It is now well recognized that carcinoid tumors can produce a variety of secretory products (biogenic amines or polypeptides), either singly or in concert, and in amounts that may produce clinical manifestations. Thus, these tumors are also associated with certain clinically recognizable syndromes, such as carcinoid syndrome, Zollinger-Ellison syndrome, somatostatinoma syndrome, and Cushing's syndrome, that are directly attributable to biogenic amine or peptide overproduction. Such tumors are, therefore, designated as *hormonally functional* in nature, whereas others are, by the same token, regarded as *nonfunctional*. It is important to bear in mind that by radioimmunoassay (RIA) and immunocytochemical techniques, even "nonfunctional" carcinoids can be frequently shown to contain one or several of these amines and peptides.[200, 201] That these tumors do not produce biochemically detectable or clinically recognizable abnormalities may be due to a number of factors, such as the small amounts of the products being produced, intermittent release of these products into the circulation, rapid degradation of the product(s) in the peripheral circulation, and the molecular heterogeneity and relative biological potency of the secretory product. As a corollary, therefore, *only those tumors that synthesize biologically active materials and release them in amounts sufficient to overwhelm their normal degradative mechanisms produce biochemical and clinical abnormalities of hormonal excess.*

Although carcinoid tumors have been conventionally subclassified into *argentaffin* and *nonargentaffin* categories on the basis of their reactivity to silver stains, neither of these types is ever purely one or the other. Argentaffin tumors contain a dominant population of cells that are argentaffin (i.e., both argentaffin and argyrophil positive), a minor population of argyrophil cells (that are argentaffin negative), and nonreactive cells that are both argentaffin and argyrophil negative. Similarly, nonargentaffin tumors show a majority of argyrophil cells, with some nonreactive cells also present. Additionally, tumor cells in carcinoids frequently show disparities between their amine or peptide content on the one hand and their anticipated histochemical reactions on the other. Thus, although argentaf-

finity is normally a characteristic of the normal EC cells, some of which produce both 5-HT and substance P, tumor cells in argentaffin carcinoids do not always contain substance P within them. Neither are the tumor cells containing substance P always argentaffin. Similarly, whereas the gastrin-producing tumors (gastrinomas) are argyrophil by the Grimelius technique and show large numbers of cells immunoreactive for gastrin, not all tumor cells show these properties: not all argyrophil cells show immunoreactivity for gastrin, nor are all such immunoreactive cells argyrophil in nature.[7, 200, 201]

HISTOLOGIC FEATURES

Histologically, carcinoid tumors show a variety of architectural patterns. Commonly referred to as the *insular, trabecular, glandular, mixed,* or *undifferentiated* patterns, they have also been designated as types A to E.[202] More recently, other histologic patterns such as the *psammomatous* and *goblet cell* varieties have also been recognized.[203–205]

The pure *insular* pattern (type A of Soga and Tazawa[202]) is the most common histologic pattern for gastrointestinal carcinoids, and is most frequently observed in ileal and appendiceal carcinoids. Since these two anatomic locations together account for the vast majority of gastrointestinal carcinoids, the insular pattern is regarded as characteristic, if not pathognomonic, of midgut carcinoids. It is characterized by solid islands of closely packed monomorphic tumor cells separated by variably thick septa (Fig. 10-13A). The tumor cells are usually small, round to oval, and uniform in size, with scant, faintly granular eosinophilic cytoplasm. The nuclei are uniform in morphology but may show considerable pleomorphism and even bizarre forms (Fig. 10-13B). Mitotic activity is seldom prominent. Occasionally, the islands show a peripheral rim of palisaded cells with densely eosinophilic granular cytoplasm (Fig. 10-13C). In some instances, tumor cells within the islands may show pseudoglandular structures around thin-walled vessels, or glandular areas

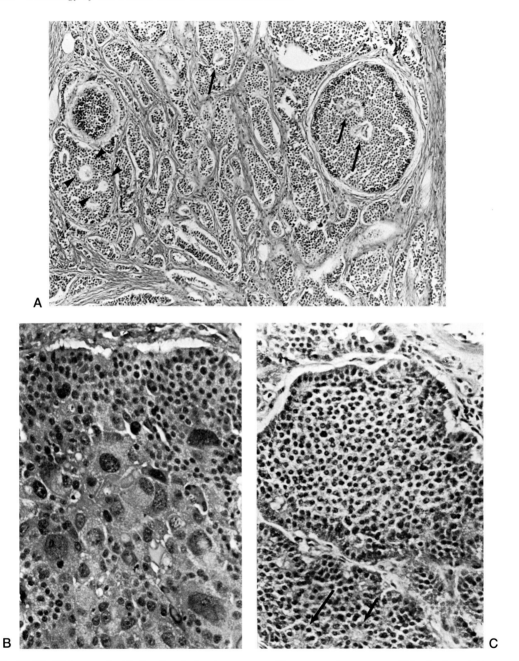

Fig. 10-13. Midgut carcinoids showing the insular pattern and its commonly encountered histologic variations. **(A)** Islands of tumor cells are separated by variably thick connective tissue septa, and contain glandular (arrowheads) and pseudoglandular (arrows) structures entrapped in the islands. The glandular structures contain pale eosinophilic secretions in their lumina, whereas the pseudoglandular areas contain delicate vascular channels. **(B)** Portion of an island of tumor cells from a different ileal carcinoid showing cellular pleomorphism, nuclear atypism, variations in nuclear size, and presence of numerous bizarre giant nuclei. **(C)** Insular area from another ileal carcinoid showing peripheral palisading by a row of darker-staining cells with granular cytoplasm. Two rosettelike structures are also present (arrows). (H&E, Fig. A × 128, Fig. B × 325, Fig. C × 325.)

with luminal spaces that may contain a homogeneous pale pink secretion within them.

The *trabecular* pattern (type B of Soga and Tazawa[202]) is characterized by anastomosing cords or ribbons of tumor cells separated from each other by collagenous stroma. The cords are usually 1 to 2 cells thick, and the cells themselves may either be small and spindle-shaped with scanty cytoplasm or larger with abundant cytoplasm. The nuclei are elongated and oriented with their long axis at right angles to the axis of the cords (Fig. 10-14). A pure trabecular arrangement is most often encountered in hindgut carcinoids, although it may also be seen as part of a mixed architectural pattern (type C of Soga and Tazawa[202]) in carcinoids arising in foregut-derived structures.[7, 183, 202]

The *glandular* pattern (type C of Soga and Tazawa[202]) characterized by the presence of "tubular, acinar, or rosette like structures" is uncommon for carcinoid tumors. This pattern was seen in only two of the 62 carcinoids in Soga's original series.[202] Although we have seen an occasional pancreatic endocrine tumor with a pure glandular pattern, we have not encountered it in gastrointestinal carcinoids. In their series of 109 endocrine tumors of the gut, pancreas, and lung, Jones and Dawson found only two (one pancreatic tumor and one bronchial tumor) with a pure glandular pattern.[206] In another series of 138 gastrointestinal and extraintestinal carcinoids, a pure glandular pattern was encountered in only three instances.[207] In our own material, glandular differentiation in gastrointestinal carcinoids has only been observed in association with an insular pattern, that is, in tumors with a mixed architectural pattern (Fig. 10-15).

The *undifferentiated* pattern (type D of Soga and Tazawa[202]) is a relatively uncommon histologic pattern, and is characterized by small, medium, or large undifferentiated cells lying in sheets, with very little intervening stroma (Fig. 10-16). The tumor cells may be small and spindle-shaped with elongated compact hyperchromatic nuclei, scanty cytoplasm, indistinct outlines, and few mitoses or may have abundant cytoplasm, large nuclei, and prominent nucleoli with variable pleomorphism and mitotic activity. Individual tumors can contain

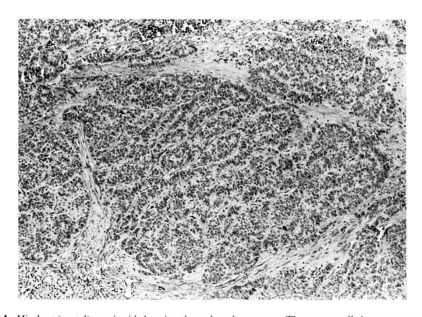

Fig. 10-14. Hindgut (rectal) carcinoid showing the trabecular pattern. The tumor cells have scanty cytoplasm, elongated nuclei, and are arranged in cords one to two cells thick separated by a delicate stroma that is rich in capillaries. (H&E, × 128.)

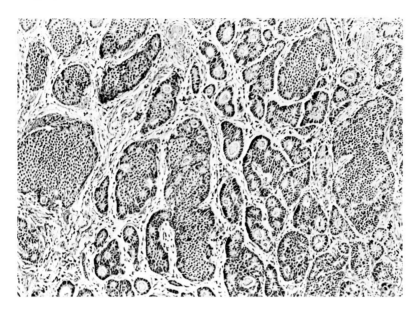

Fig. 10-15. Ileal carcinoid showing areas of well-formed glandular structures in a background of a typical insular architectural pattern. Although several glandular structures are seen as distinctly separate from the larger solid insular areas, others are located within such islands. Serial sections frequently disclose a continuity between such separate glandular structures and the adjacent solid islands. This pattern is believed to be a variant of the insular pattern. (H&E, × 128.)

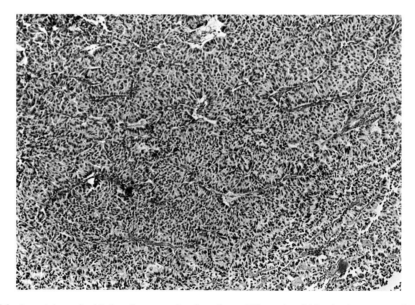

Fig. 10-16. A rectal carcinoid showing a predominantly undifferentiated histologic pattern. Such a tumor may not even be suspected to be a carcinoid. However, trabecular areas such as those seen in the top right quadrant of the photomicrograph were helpful in making the correct diagnosis. Tumor cells in both the trabecular and the closely packed undifferentiated areas were argyrophilic. (H&E, × 128.)

both patterns within them and, with more thorough sampling, may even show areas of acinar, insular, or trabecular differentiation. Although tumors with such areas can be easily identified as carcinoids, it is easy to understand how a diagnosis of carcinoid tumor may not be entertained if the area sampled is composed entirely of spindle-shaped, poorly differentiated cells. Such neoplasms frequently retain some histochemical characteristics, such as argyrophilia and argentaffinity, that help establish their endocrine origin. Undifferentiated tumors of the gut should, therefore, be routinely screened for argentaffinity, argyrophilia and immunoreactivity for chromogranins, and NSE, etc. In the truly nonargentaffin (non-reactive) carcinoids, transmission electron microscopy can be helpful in demonstrating intracytoplasmic secretory granules and in clinching the diagnosis.

The *mixed* pattern (type E of Soga and Tazawa[202]) is characterized by the presence of any two or more of the architectural patterns already described. The component patterns either may be intimately blended or may exist side by side as a mosaic with only minimal intermingling (Fig. 10-17). This pattern characterizes a majority of foregut and a small proportion of hindgut lesions, but may be observed in occasional midgut carcinoids as well. Differences in the relative frequency of the mixed pattern in relation to anatomic distribution (as reported in the various series) may depend on both the histologic criteria adopted by the various workers and whether the series of cases includes pancreatic, bronchial, and extraintestinal lesions.[202, 206] The various architectural components in a mixed histologic pattern may be present in variable proportions, and several areas may need to be sampled before the mixed character of a given tumor can be established. Mixed tumors metastasize true to type, and can be shown to preserve their architectural characteristics if adequately sampled.

Psammomatous Carcinoids

A psammomatous pattern, characterized by the presence of numerous concentrically lamellated and calcified structures, is a rare histologic variant of carcinoid tumors. In our experience this occurs in less than 1 percent of all carcinoids (Dayal Y, Wolfe HJ: Unpublished obser-

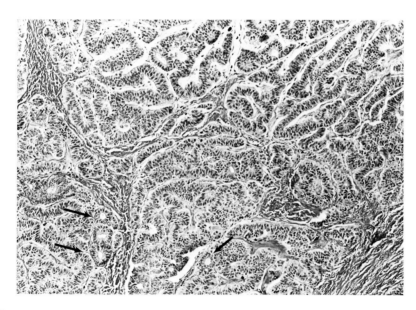

Fig. 10-17. Rectal carcinoid showing a mixed architectural pattern with an intimate blending of predominantly trabecular areas with those showing well-formed glandular structures (arrows). (H&E, × 128.)

vations). In our own cases, as well as in those reported by other workers, these tumors have arisen in the duodenum, ampulla of Vater, or the periampullary region.[203, 208–215] These tumors are usually small and always solitary.

Histologically, they are characterized by a mixed architectural pattern (A + C or B + C) with a predominant glandular (type C) component. Although the presence of psammoma bodies and the numerous gland like structures may initially suggest the diagnosis of an adenocarcinoma, the mixed histologic pattern of these lesions should permit them to be recognized as carcinoid tumors. As opposed to carcinomas of the thyroid, ovary, or endometrium, where psammoma bodies are associated with a predominantly papillary pattern, the psammoma bodies in carcinoids are associated with predominantly glandular areas in a tumor with a mixed architectural pattern (Fig. 10-18). The tumor cells are fairly monomorphic, with abundant cytoplasm, round nuclei, and minimal to no detectable mitotic activity. Cellular pleomorphism and atypia have not been observed with this histologic variant. The tumor cells are nonargentaffin (by the Masson-Fontana technique), strongly argyrophil (by the Hellerstrom-Hellman technique), and may show focal Grimelius positivity.[201–203]

The psammoma bodies, varying from 5 to 30 μm in diameter and strongly birefringent under polarized light, stain a strong bluish-pink with H&E stain, and are mostly located in the glandular lumina. They stain weakly within the von Kossa stain but show a strong diastase-resistant PAS positivity. They do not stain with any of the argentaffin or argyrophil techniques, and also fail to stain with toluidine blue or Congo red.[201–203]

Goblet Cell Carcinoids

Although goblet cell carcinoids most commonly occur in the appendix, similar tumors have also been described elsewhere in the gut.[49, 204, 205, 216–218] Originally referred to as *mucinous* or *goblet cell carcinoid*, these tumors have also been designated as *mucus-secreting*

carcinoid, adenocarcinoid, and *crypt cell carcinoma of the appendix.*[219–223] The appendiceal tumors show small clusters of well-differentiated tumor cells in a solid insular or glandular arrangement. There is a variable admixture of cells with copious mucin and eccentrically located nuclei (signet ring forms), and cells with abundant pale eosinophilic cytoplasm containing numerous subnuclear granules. Variable numbers of cells with features intermediate between these two forms are also present. The tumor cells appear well differentiated and uniform in size, with minimal nuclear-atypia and scarce mitoses. Occasional tumors have also shown Paneth cell differentiation in focal areas.[204] Tumor cells frequently show lymphatic and vascular invasion and prominent areas of local intramural or even transmural extension into the periappendiceal fat.[205, 217] Regional nodal metastases are present at diagnosis in a significant proportion of cases.[221]

Histochemically, tumor cells show presence of neutral and acid mucopolysaccharides (PAS and Alcian blue stains at pH 2.5), and both argentaffin as well as argyrophil granules have been demonstrated in a variable proportion of tumor cells.[217] Whereas some workers have reported the presence of such granules within the mucin-producing cells,[216, 220] others have been unable to demonstrate this despite a detailed study at both the light and electron microscopic levels.[205, 222] Thus, since these tumors share features common to both adenocarcinomas and carcinoids, they were originally thought to be variants of carcinoid tumors.[216, 220] However, a gradually enlarging body of evidence now indicates that histogenetically, goblet cell carcinoids are *not* true endocrine cell tumors but are derived from an immature crypt cell that is normally present in the gastrointestinal mucosa.[218, 223]

HISTOGENESIS

Although certain tumors designated as *argentaffinomas, gastrinomas,* and *somatostatinomas* were initially believed to be derived from the

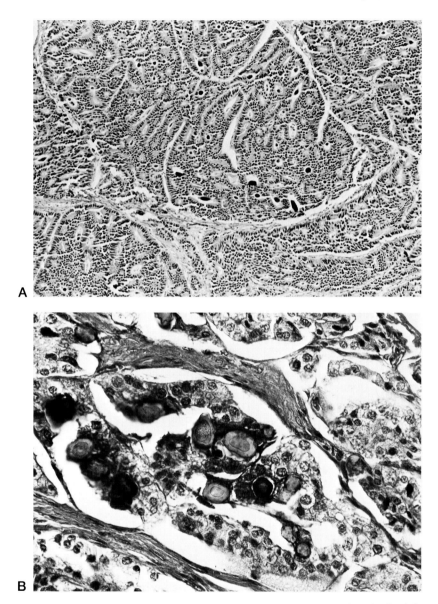

Fig. 10-18. (A) A psammomatous carcinoid of the duodenum showing a predominantly glandular architecture and numerous densely staining spherical or oval psammoma bodies in the glandular lumina. (B) Higher-power magnification of the same tumor showing a cluster of psammoma bodies. The concentric lamellations are clearly visible. Note that the tumor cells show minimal cytoplasmic atypia. (H&E, Fig. A × 128, Fig. B × 355.) (Fig. B from Dayal & Wolfe,[261] with permission.)

EC_1, G, and D cells, respectively, it was not possible to assign a similar lineage to other gastrointestinal carcinoids because of the heterogeneity in their various characteristics. Even argentaffinomas, gastrinomas, and somatostatinomas, each of which produces excessive amounts of a particular secretory product, are multihormonal in nature.[209, 224–232] Some of the other products (insulin, calcitonin, ACTH, nonepinephrine, and others) elaborated by the tumor cells are not even normally produced in the gut endocrine cells. Thus, it is more accurate to think of them as serotonin-producing, gastrin-producing, or somatostatin-producing tumors, rather than as neoplasms arising from cells from normally secrete these products.

Even at the ultrastructural level these tumors show considerable variability, and the morphologic characteristics of their secretory granules may or may not be identical to those of their normal counterparts.[227–232] Gastrinomas, at least, have been shown to contain several different types of secretory granules.[228] Some of these granules are typical for antral G cells, whereas others designated as "atypical" do not resemble granules of any known endocrine cell type.[228] Such atypical granules have also been observed in a variety of other endocrine tumors and in immature, functionally uncommitted endocrine cells.[228, 233, 234] A growing body of evidence now indicates that carcinoids arise from immature, functionally uncommitted endocrine cells that subsequently undergo further differentiation along any one or more directions. The degree of differentiation and functional maturation of the neoplastic cells would then determine how closely the various histochemical, secretory, and ultrastructural characteristics of the neoplastic cells approximate those of the various normal endocrine cell types. Such a histogenetic origin explains not only the histochemical and functional heterogeneity of these tumors but their multihormonality as well. Further, a histogenetic origin of this kind would also account for the variability in the ultrastructural morphology of some of these tumors, as well as for the ability to produce mucin that is occasionally observed in others.

FOREGUT CARCINOIDS

Because the stomach and duodenum are embryologically derived from the foregut, gastroduodenal carcinoids were initially lumped together by earlier workers into the single category of foregut carcinoids.[181] Subsequent observations have shown that although these tumors share some common morphologic and histochemical features, gastric carcinoids differ significantly from their duodenal counterparts in their immunohistochemical and ultrastructural characteristics as well as their clinical and biologic behavior. Broad generalizations regarding this group of tumors made by earlier investigators are therefore no longer valid.

Gastric Carcinoids

Gastric carcinoids have generally been regarded as uncommon tumors that account for 3 to 5 percent of all gastrointestinal carcinoids and for up to 0.3 percent of all gastric tumors.[235] However, more recent studies indicate that they comprise between 11 and 30 percent of all gastrointestinal carcinoids.[236, 237] This increase in the overall incidence of gastric carcinoids may be multifactorial. Gastric carcinoids are frequently of the ECL cell type and arise in a background of chronic atrophic gastritis or pernicious anemia.[238] They therefore co-exist with the hyperplastic and adenomatous polyps that are so common in these conditions.[239, 240] It is quite likely that, because in the preendoscopy era such polyps were not biopsied, their true nature may never have been established. Moreover, gastric carcinoids often have a solid or trabecular architecture that is different from the insular pattern of the more common midgut carcinoids.[241] Some of these lesions may therefore have been misdiagnosed as poorly differentiated adenocarcinomas.[242, 243] In a retrospective analysis of 140 gastric tumors originally diagnosed as adenocarcinoma, 7 percent of the tumors were eventually reclassified as carcinoids.[244] More recently, the widespread use of immunohistochemical and ultrastructural methods has significantly improved our ability to diagnose these tumors more accurately. Last, but not the least important, is our increased awareness of the higher potential of these tumors to develop in a variety of hypergastrinemic states, and the emergence of an enlarging pool of patients at higher risk for developing gastric carcinoids (Table 10-4). Such a pool in-

Table 10-4. Conditions Associated with an Increased Risk for Developing Multicentric Gastric Carcinoids

Chronic atrophic gastritis (type A)
Pernicious anemia
Zollinger-Ellison syndrome (familial and nonfamilial)
Patients on pharmacologic gastric acid blockade (H_2-receptors, proton pump inhibitors)
Chronic renal failure (+/-hemodialysis)[a]
Autoimmune disorders[a]
  Polyglandular autoimmune syndrome[a]
  Sjögren's syndrome[b]
  Rheumatoid arthritis[b]
  Myxedema[c]
  Addison's disease[c]
  Diabetes mellitus type 1 (IDDM)[c]

[a] Chronic atrophic gastritis with hypergastrinemia.
[b] Antibodies to parietal cells and intrinsic factor.
[c] Achlorhydria, hypergastrinemia, and gastric carcinoids.

cludes patients with duodenal ulcer disease or Zollinger-Ellison syndrome who are on prolonged treatment with such gastric acid blockers as cimetidine, ranitidine, and omeprazole[150, 151, 245, 246]; patients with chronic renal failure; and those with such autoimmune disorders as diabetes mellitus type 1, Addison's disease, Sjögren's syndrome, rheumatoid arthritis, autoimmune thyroiditis, and the polyglandular autoimmune syndrome. A high proportion of patients with some of these disorders have chronic atrophic gastritis and hypergastrinemia,[121, 144, 146, 247–251] whereas others additionally have antiparietal cell and/or anti-intrinsic factor antibodies in their circulation.[248, 249, 252, 253] In fact, patients with diabetes mellitus and Addison's disease have been shown to have achlorhydria, hypergastrinemia, and gastric carcinoids.[144, 146, 250, 254] It is very likely, therefore, that in the future, as more of those at risk are carefully screened, both ECL-cell hyperplasias and ECL-cell carcinoids will be encountered with greater frequency.

Gastric carcinoids are commonly classified on cytologic grounds into ECL cell, non-ECL cell, and mixed cell types. The ECL cell carcinoids arise in a background of ECL cell hyperplasia and chronic hypergastrinemia. They are therefore multicentric in origin and are mostly confined to the oxyntic mucosa. The non-ECL cell carcinoids arise sporadically, most often in normogastrinemic patients; these tumors are unassociated with any pre-existing endocrine-cell hyperplasia, are usually single, and may arise anywhere in the stomach. The mixed cell carcinoids arise in foci of intestinal metaplasia and are similar to the midgut carcinoids in their immunohistochemical and ultrastructural characteristics. They may arise anywhere in the stomach and are not derived from an antecedent endocrine cell hyperplasia.

Despite similarities in their clinical, histologic, histochemical, and immunohistochemical profiles, ECL cell carcinoids differ significantly from non-ECL cell carcinoids in their biologic behavior and ultimate outcome (Table 10-5). Thus, the incidence of regional lymph node metastasis (55 percent) and hepatic metastasis (24 percent) and the overall 5-year survival figure of 50 percent seen in gastric carcinoids in general[255] is in sharp contrast to the corresponding figures of 16 and 4 percent for the ECL cell tumors.[154] Although survival figures for this latter group are not yet available, all reports indicate that their prognosis, even in the presence of metastasis, is superior to that of the non-ECL cell group.[123, 127, 146, 152, 256, 257] Even when such tumors have been incompletely excised, they have been seen at re-exploration several years later not to have grown or metastasized.[123] In general, tumors greater than 2 cm in diameter are more likely to be associated with both intramural invasion and metastatic spread. Although gastric carcinoids less than 1 cm in size may rarely metastasize,[258] tumors smaller than 2 cm are generally not associated with metastases. Features adversely influencing long-term survival include such variables as a large size of the individual tumors, presence of extensive local invasion, and nodal or distant metastases. Microscopic features such as nuclear atypia, pleomorphism, increased nuclear : cytoplasmic ratio, variability in nuclear size, and increased mitotic activity indicate aggressive biologic behavior and a poorer prognosis.

When stained for argyrophilia the ECL cell tumors stain only with the Sevier-Munger tech-

Table 10-5. Comparative Profile of Gastric Carcinoids in Hyper- and Normogastrinemic Patients

	Hypergastrinemia-Associated Gastric Carcinoids	Sporadically Occurring Gastric Carcinoids
Number	Usually multicentric	Invariably single
Size	Usually small (<2 cm)	Usually large (>3 cm)
Endocrine cell hyperplasia	Present	Absent
Argyrophilia		
Grimelius	Diffusely positive	Diffusely positive
Sevier-Munger	Diffusely positive	Variably positive
Neuroendocrine markers (NSE, chromogranins, etc.)	Diffusely positive	Diffusely positive
Regulatory peptides	Usually negative	Heterogeneous
	Most cells negative, some positive for 5-HT, gastrin, etc.	Variably positive for 5-HT, 5-HTP, ACTH, and β-MSH, etc.
Ultrastructure	Secretory granules	Very variable
	Vacuolated with large halo and small eccentric core	
	Granulated core with thin halo	
	Agranulated cells with few D_1- or P-type cells	
Clinical	Endocrinologically "silent" "atypical carcinoid syndrome" in 7%	Atypical carcinoid syndrome (histamine, 5-HTP, 5-HT) Cushing's syndrome
Biologic behavior	Less aggressive	More aggressive
Nodal metastasis	16%	55%
Liver metastasis	4%	24%
5-year survival	NA	50%

(From Dayal & Wolfe,[240] with permission.)

nique, whereas the non-ECL and the mixed cell carcinoids show moderately intense staining with the Grimelius technique, although a few nonreactive cells are invariably seen interspersed between the argyrophil cells (Dayal Y, Wolfe HJ: Unpublished observations).[259–261] In our own series of 45 gastrointestinal carcinoids, all of the 10 foregut (3 gastric and 7 duodenal) were argyrophil and nonargentaffin in nature (Table 10-6). Five tumors (three gastric and two duodenal) showed strong Grimelius positivity, whereas four duodenal tumors were argyro-

Table 10-6. Silver Staining in 45 Gastrointestinal Carcinoids

Staining Property	Foregut (10)	Midgut (27)	Hindgut (8)	% Positive
Argyrophilia				
Grimelius	5	27	6	96
Hellerstrom-Hellman	5			
Argentaffinity				
Masson-Fontana		18		40
Nonreactivity			2	

(From Dayal & Wolfe,[261] with permission.)

phil only by the Hellerstrom-Hellman technique. One of these tumors also contained some Grimelius-positive cells scattered within it. The relatively high frequency (52 percent) of nonreactive tumors in Soga and Tazawa's series is most likely due both to the fact that these workers did not use the Sevier-Munger stain and to differences in the sensitivity of the argyrophil stains that were employed by them.[202] Except for the occasional goblet cell carcinoid arising in the stomach, gastric carcinoids do not show evidence of mucin production. Both gastric and duodenal carcinoids produce a number of secretory products, including amines such as histamine and serotonin and peptides such as somatostatin, gastrin, glucagon, substance P, ACTH, and calcitonin,[208, 209, 261, 262] and a majority of these show the presence of multiple secretory products.[259–161]

In our own series of 45 gastrointestinal carcinoids that included 10 tumors of foregut origin, we could demonstrate somatostatin in 8 tumors (80 percent), and serotonin and gastrin in 3 each. ACTH was present in two, whereas glucagon, gastrin, and substance P was present in one each[261] (Table 10-7). Three of the tumors were multihormonal, and one such tumor contained cells immunoreactive for as many as six products (Fig. 10-19). Some of these were present in a high proportion of tumor cells (dominant population), whereas others were detected only in small, randomly dispersed clusters that in aggregate amounted to no more than 15 percent of the tumor cells (minority population). Thus, although somatostatin immunoreactive cells were detected in 8 of the 10 foregut carcinoids, only in 5 duodenal tumors did they constitute the dominant population.

In each of these tumors, since somatostatin was localized in over 90 percent of the cells, these duodenal carcinoids would, by immunohistochemical criteria, be designated as somatostatinomas, although none of these would have been otherwise identified as such since they had not produced the somatostatinoma syndrome. It is of interest that four of these duodenal tumors characterized by a psammomatous pattern were immunoreactive exclusively for somatostatin. These tumors were nonargentaffin and showed argyrophilia only by the Hellerstrom-Hellman technique. Ultrastructurally, these cells showed numerous intracytoplasmic secretory granules similar to those of normal D cells. Immunoelectron microscopic studies showed somatostatin to be localized exclusively in the electron-dense cores of the secretory granules. Thus, although the psammomatous pattern represents an uncommon histologic variant of carcinoid tumors, it is a feature of duodenal somatostatinomas.[208, 209] The immunocytochemical demonstration of serotonin in three of six nonargentaffin foregut carcinoids is most

Table 10-7. Immunocytochemical Profile of 45 Gastrointestinal Carcinoids

Regulatory Substance(s)	Foregut (10)	Midgut (27)	Hindgut (8)	Total (45)	% Positive
Serotonin	3	24	1	28	62
Somatostatin	8	1	5	14	31
Substance P	1	11		12	26
Pancreatic polypeptide			7	7	16
Glucagon	1		4	5	11
Calcitonin		3		3	7
ACTH	2	1		3	7
Gastrin	3			3	7
Insulin					
Growth hormone releasing factor					
Multisecretory	3	12	6	21	47

(From Dayal & Wolfe,[261] with permission.)

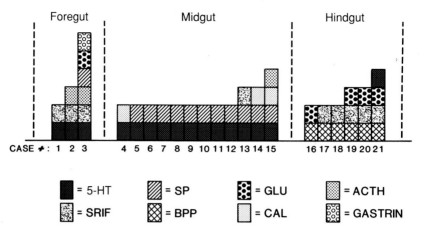

Fig. 10-19. The immunocytochemical profiles of 21 multihormonal carcinoids. Of the three such foregut tumors, one was immunoreactive for as many as six regulatory substances. Of the 12 multihormonal midgut carcinoids, serotonin and substance P were co-localized in 11. Multihormonality was seen in six of eight hindgut carcinoids. In this location, the commonest combination was that of PP and somatostatin. (From Dayal & Wolfe,[261] with permission.)

likely related to the greater sensitivity of the immunohistochemical techniques.

Ultrastructural appearances of gastric carcinoids can be quite variable. Tumor cells in ECL cell carcinoids that arise in a background of ECL cell hyperplasia (as in chronic atrophic gastritis, pernicious anemia, and other hypergastrinemic states) show morphologically heterogeneous secretory granules that either have a wide halo and small eccentric-electron-dense cores or show moderately electron-dense cores with a granular interior and a thin halo (Fig. 10-20). The non-ECL cell tumors, on the other hand, contain granules identical to those in normal D1 or P cells, whereas the mixed-type tumors arising from foci of pyloric or intestinal metaplasia may show a population of cells that are either agranular or contain granules similar to those in normal neoplastic EC and ECL cells[125, 144, 154, 263–265] (Fig. 10-20).

Although foregut carcinoids are invariably nonargentaffin, a few argentaffin tumors have been described arising in stomachs with intestinal metaplasia.[266] The argentaffinity of the tumor cells correlates well with their serotonin content, and in a few instances substance P has also been identified within them.[260] The

tumor cells, thus, closely recapitulate characteristics of the normal EC_1 cells.[266] Ultrastructurally, too, the tumor cells show pleomorphic granules of the EC_1 cell type. Since the gastric mucosa is normally devoid of EC_1-type cells, some workers have suggested that these argentaffin gastric carcinoids arise from the metaplastically derived EC_1 cells in areas on intestinalization.[266]

MIDGUT CARCINOIDS

Carcinoids arising in the midgut are easily recognized by their characteristic insular (type A) growth pattern. Although some tumors show a seemingly mixed (type A + C) architectural pattern, we and others regard this as a variant of the insular pattern.[206, 261] We have not observed this mixed pattern in tumors outside the midgut, and all carcinoids with this pattern have shown a co-existent insular architecture in other areas. Although nonargentaffin carinoids have been reported in the appendix,[267] most midgut lesions are of the argentaffin type and contain fair amounts of serotonin.[259, 261] In a series of 33 midgut carcinoids studied for their argen-

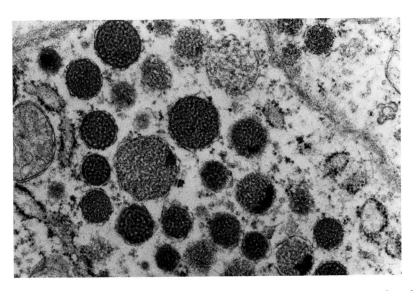

Fig. 10-20. Electron micrograph of an ECL cell carcinoid showing numerous large- and medium-sized, granular-cored, electron-dense secretory granules.(From Dayal & Wolfe,[240] with permission.)

taffin and argyrophil properties, 30 tumors (91 percent) were found to be argentaffin whereas 3 additional tumors were found to be argyrophil.[259] Our observations (Table 10-6) are very similar; 18 of 27 (66 percent) midgut carcinoids were argentaffin, whereas the remaining 9 tumors were seemingly made up of argyrophilic cells only. Since six of these nine tumors were incidentally discovered during autopsy, it is very likely that argentaffinity of the tumor cells may have been lost secondary to postmortem autolysis or suboptimal fixation.[7, 57] In all argentaffin tumors, and especially those of the midgut, where both the argentaffin and argyrophil reactions are usually strongly positive, there are always more argyrophil cells than argentaffin cells. This is mainly related to the fact that although the argentaffin stain selectively identifies serotonin-containing cells, the argyrophil stains additionally visualize other functional cell types.[7, 57] However, when allowance is made for the number of argentaffin cells, most midgut carcinoids are seen to have only a minority population of argyrophil cells. With each of these staining reactions, the intensity of cytoplasmic staining varies from area to area, presumably because the tumor cells are in different phases of their secretory cycle. Similarly the pattern of cytoplasmic staining also shows variability; individual tumor cells may show the silver granules either diffusely scattered throughout the cytoplasm or selectively clustered toward the peripheral pole of the tumor cells (Fig. 10-21). With the possible exception of goblet cell carcinoids of the appendix and those with areas of glandular differentiation, midgut carinoids generally do not show any evidence of mucin production. In tumors with glandular structures, mucicarmine or PAS positivity is usually confined to the luminal contents of the glands, and the lining cells show little or no cytoplasmic staining. In the goblet cell carcinoids, intracytoplasmic mucin is chiefly present in the signet ring-like cells. Although some workers have observed mucin globules in cells that also contained argyrophil granules, others have not been able to confirm this.[205, 216, 221, 222]

Immunocytochemical studies have demonstrated a variety of secretory products, including serotonin, gastrin, calcitonin, dopamine, norepinephrine, substance P, enteroglucagon, ACTH, calcitonin, motilin, neurotensin,

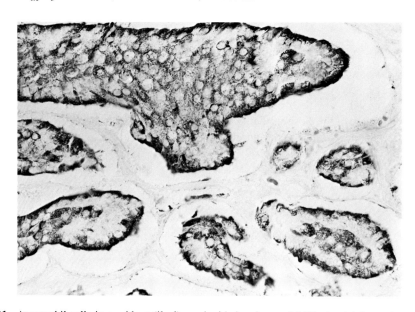

Fig. 10-21. Argyrophil cells in a midgut (ileal) carcinoid showing variability in staining patterns. Whereas cells in the center of the insular clusters show diffuse intracytoplasmic staining, those at the periphery show a preferrential clustering of the argyrophil granules toward their outer poles. (Grimelius stain using methyl green counterstain, × 813.)

and somatostatin, in midgut carcinoids.[200, 201, 227, 232, 268–270] Some of these studies were sharply focused on the demonstration of one or two particular products, and provided little information on the relative frequency with which some of the other products might be present.[268–270] In a study of 45 gastrointestinal carcinoids surveyed for the immunocytochemical localization of various secretory products (Table 10–7), 24 of 27 (89 percent) midgut carcinoids showed immunoreactivity for serotonin and 11 (47 percent) were positive for substance P. Among the products tested for, calcitonin was detected in three tumors, whereas somatostatin and ACTH were found in one tumor each. Immunoreactivity for serotonin correlated very well with the argentaffin nature of these tumors. Whereas all argentaffin tumors were immunoreactive for serotonin, serotonin was also demonstrated in six additional tumors that were argentaffin negative. All of these tumors were incidental findings at autopsy. It is of interest, therefore, that although postmortem autolysis may have led to the loss of argentaffinity in these tumors,[57] their immunoreactivity

for serotonin was still preserved. Although gastrin, glucagon, pancreatic polypeptide, and insulin were not present in any of our midgut carcinoids, other workers have demonstrated gastrin, enteroglucagon, and substance P in a high proportion of such tumors.[268–270] It has been shown that four out of every five midgut carcinoids secrete more than one secretory product.[268] Serotonin with substance P is the most common combination encountered (100 percent), followed by serotonin with substance P and enteroglucagon (88 percent). In our material, multihormonality was seen only in 12 tumors (44 percent); in addition to serotonin, substance P was present in 11, ACTH and somatostatin were present in 1 tumor each.

In all multihormonal tumors, the various secretory products were generally localized in different cells or in different areas. In contrast to this, substance P and serotonin were generally localized within the same cell. This is due to the fact that both the serotonin and substance P are stored together in the same secretory granules.[261, 270]

Ultrastructurally these tumors are a fairly homogeneous group, and are characterized by cells with large numbers of pleomorphic, relatively electron-dense secretory granules that are morphologically identical to those of intestinal EC_1 cells (Fig. 10-22). These granules, like those of the normal EC_1 cell, are both argentaffin and argyrophil. Because of the close similarities between the histochemical, functional, and ultrastructural characteristics of midgut carcinoids and those of EC_1-type cells, these tumors are commonly referred to as EC_1 cell tumors.[266]

HINDGUT CARCINOIDS

The vast majority of hindgut carcinoids are located in the rectum, and very few carcinoids normally arise in the descending or sigmoid colon.[182, 183, 271] The rectum, therefore, is the third most common site for gastrointestinal carcinoids. Histologically, these tumors show either a pure trabecular arrangement or a mixed pattern with a predominantly glandular component.[7, 202] Until recently, most hindgut carcinoids were thought to be nonreactive to the argentaffin and argyrophil staining techniques.[202, 259, 272] However, the majority of rectal carcinoids are argyrophil by the Grimelius technique. In the cases reported here (Table 10-6), six of eight rectal carcinoids (75 percent) were argyrophil. This figure compares favorably with the cumulative figure of 64 percent calculated from previously published series that employed the Grimelius silver stain.[273] Argentaffinity, on the other hand, is encountered only infrequently, and has been demonstrated in only 11 percent of the previously published cases.[273] Both argentaffinity and argyrophilia may involve extensive or focal clusters of tumor cells, but argentaffin-positive cells most often constitute a small minority of tumor cells. Hindgut carcinoids showing a predominant population of argentaffin cells have been described, but are rare.[273–275]

Immunocytochemical techniques have demonstrated an impressive array of secretory products in rectal carcinoids. Tumors systematically surveyed for the presence of various peptides

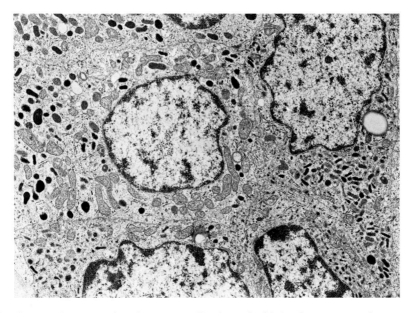

Fig. 10-22. Electronmicrograph of a midgut (appendiceal) carcinoid showing numerous dense core secretory granules that are morphologically identical to those seen in the normal intestinal EC_1 cells. The tumor cells showed diffuse argentaffinity and strong immunoreactivity for serotonin. (Glutaraldehydeformaldehyde fixation, × 8,200.)

and biogenic amines have been shown to contain pancreatic polypeptide, glucagon, somatostatin, substance P, insulin, β-endorphin, enkephalin, and serotonin.[183, 273, 274, 276] Pancreatic polypeptide, somatostatin, and glucagon were the three most commonly encountered secretory products in our own cases (Table 10-7) (Fig. 10-23), as well as in previously published reports.[183, 273, 276, 277] Multihormonality, observed in six of eight (75 percent) rectal carcinoids in our own material, has also been observed in nearly 50 percent of tumors in other series.[183, 277] Most multihormonal tumors produced two to three products, and various combinations of pancreatic polypeptide (PP), glucagon, somatostatin, and substance P have been domonstrated frequently in such tumors.[183, 273, 277] A review of the previously published cases shows that serotonin, insulin, β-endorphin, and enkephalin are only infrequently produced by rectal carcinoids, whereas other peptides, including gastrin, CCK, secretin, motilin, neurotensin, GIP, VIP, ACTH, and calcitonin, have not been detected in them.[183, 273]

Occasionally electron microscopic studies may be essential to establish the endocrine nature of these tumors, and are particularly crucial for this purpose when a nonreactive hindgut tumor is the object of investigation. Argentaffin rectal carcinoids show large number of pleomorphic electron-dense granules identical to those seen in the intestinal EC_1 cells.[274, 277] Tumor cells in the argyrophil and the nonreactive rectal carcinoids, on the other hand, are seen to contain numerous small to medium-sized granules ranging between 140 and 250 nm in size. These granules have moderately, but variable, electron-dense cores with closely approximated limiting membranes. These granules show morphologic characteristics closely similar to those of the D_1 cell, a cell type that has not yet been associated with any known secretory product,[273] although it is believed to produce a VIP-like peptide.

It is thus clear that the overwhelming majority of gastrointestinal carcinoids contain intracellular stores of one or more regulatory substances and frequently express considerable heterogeneity in this regard. The frequency of these findings

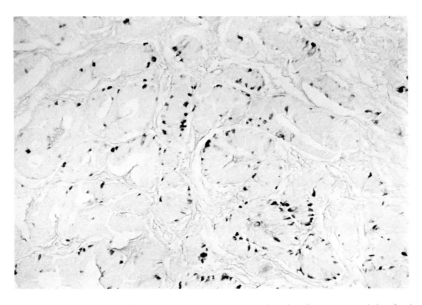

Fig. 20-23. Hindgut (rectal) carcinoid with a trabecular pattern showing immunoreactivity for bovine pancreatic polypeptide. The staining reaction is exclusively confined to the periphery of the tumor cell clusters. (Peroxidase-antiperoxidase technique, rabbit antibovine pancreatic polypeptide 1 : 10,000; methyl green counterstain, × 128.) (From O'Briain & Dayal,[7] with permission.)

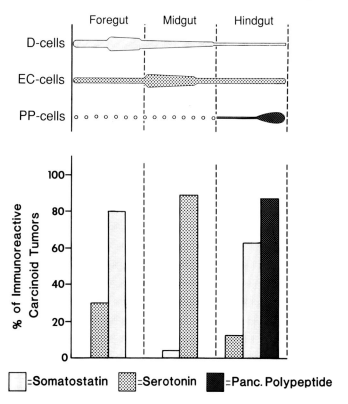

Fig. 10-24. Comparison between the frequency of immunoreactivity for somatostatin, serotonin, and pancreatic polypeptide in fore-, mid-, and hindgut carcinoids, respectively, and the relative frequency of the D, EC, and PP cells in the corresponding segments of the gut. (From Dayal & Wolfe,[261] with permission.)

will rise to even higher levels as these tumors are tested against antibodies to a wider panel of regulatory substances. Despite such heterogeneity, it is clear that carcinoids arising in a particular segment of the gut show a strong association with immunoreactivity for specific regulatory substances (Table 10-7). Thus 80 percent of foregut carcinoids in our series contained somatostatin immunoreactive cells, whereas nearly 90 percent of those in the midgut were positive for serotonin and hindgut tumors showed reactivity in an equally high frequency for PP. The presence of PP immunoreactive cells in seven of eight rectal carcinoids closely parallels the anatomic and density distributional pattern of PP cells in the normal rectal mucosa (Figure 10-24). Similarly, the presence of somatostatin in 8 of 10 foregut carcinoids corre-

lates very well with the large number of D cells normally present in the foregut. However, the presence of such cells in only 1 of 27 midgut carcinoids and 5 of 8 hindgut carcinoids is at variance with the size of the D cell population in each of these other two locations (Fig. 10-24). Immunoreactivity for serotonin, observed in 24 midgut carcinoids, correlated very well with the large normal EC cell population in this segment. However, despite the widespread distribution of these cells in the other two segments, serotonin reactivity was seen in only 3 of 10 foregut and 1 of 8 hindgut carcinoids. Differences between the frequency of somatostatin-and serotonin-positive cells normally present in a given segment of the gut and that seen in carcinoids in the same location remain unexplained.

BIOLOGICALLY FUNCTION-ING TUMORS

GENERAL CHARACTERISTICS

Gastrointestinal carcinoids are frequently associated with such clinical syndromes as the carcinoid syndrome, Zollinger-Ellison syndrome, and Cushing's syndrome, to each of which they are causally related. Although such "biologically functioning" or "hormonally active" tumors have been encountered only infrequently in the past, they are now being identified with increasing frequency, in some instances (e.g., Zollinger-Ellison syndrome) even before the clinical features characteristic of the syndrome have developed. This has largely been due to increased sophistication in our ability to correlate the tumor with elevated circulating levels of various peptides and their metabolities. However, the importance of increased clinical awareness and a thorough evaluation of these tumors by histochemical, immunocytochemical, and electron microscopic techniques can hardly be overemphasized. Nonetheless, one must bear in mind that the mere immunocytochemical demonstration of a particular product in a tumor, even in an overwhelming majority of tumor cells, does not necessarily imply that a tumor is biologically functioning. This appellation should be conferred on a tumor only after a thorough clinicopathologic evaluation of the entire case has been made and after it has been established that the tumor is secreting large amounts of the substance that is directly responsible for the clinical syndrome.

CARCINOID SYNDROME

The isolation of relatively large amounts of serotonin from ileal carcinoids[278] and the demonstration of elevated levels of 5-HT in the blood and urine of patients with these tumors[279] led to the recognitin of the functional nature of carcinoid tumors and the delineation of the carcinoid syndrome.[280, 281] The major clinical manifestations of this syndrome are paroxysms of flushing and wheezing or asthma-like attacks, diarrhea, and right-sided heart failure owing to stenosis of the tricuspid and pulmonary valves. Several minor features, such as abdominal pain, edema, pellagra-like skin lesions, peptic ulcers, and malabsorption are also occasionally present.[182, 282–284] Several peptides, such as gastrin, insulin, substance P, calcitonin, glucagon, somatostatin, and several biogenic amines, such as 5-HTP, serotonin (5-HT), histamine, and bradykinin, have been identified in these tumors.[200, 201, 232, 268, 269, 285, 286] However, serotonin is the principal agent responsible for the carcinoid syndrome. Normally less than 1 percent of the dietary tryptophan is converted into serotonin. This occurs in a variety of different anatomic locations, including the brain and the EC cells of the gastrointestinal mucosa. Serotonin from the EC cells is released into the portal circulation, where most of it is promptly mopped up by the platelets, while a small amount remains unbound (free) in the blood. The 5-HT is taken up by the liver and lungs, oxidatively deaminated into 5-HIAA and excreted in the urine.[287] On account of the APUD characteristics of their cells, both primary and metastatic carcinoid tumors take up excessive amounts of tryptophan (up to 60 percent of the dietary intake). In tumor cells, this is first 5-hydroxylated to form 5-HTP, which is then decarboxylated to yield 5-HT.

Whereas most carcinoid tumors associated with the malignant carcinoid syndrome (midgut carcinoids) are known to produce large quantities of 5-HT, they also elaborate significant but smaller amounts of 5-HTP and 5-HIAA. Due to a relative or absolute deficiency of the decarboxylating enzyme(s), foregut carcinoids are unable to decarboxylate all the 5-HTP formed by them; these tumors, therefore, produce large amounts of 5-HTP with relatively smaller amounts of 5-HT. The 5-HTP released into the circulation is converted into 5-HT by the decarboxylase in normal tissues. Since some of the clinical manifestations (such as flushing) of the histamine and 5-HTP-induced carcinoid syndrome are qualitatively different from those seen in the classic (5-HT-produced) syndrome, it has also been designated as the *atypical syndrome*. As opposed to patients with the *classic syndrome,* whose blood and urine contains elevated levels of 5-HT and 5-HIAA, those with the atypical syndrome show excessive amounts of 5-HTP, 5-HT, and 5-HIAA in their circulation and urine.[283] A number of excellent reviews on the clinical, biochemical, metabolic, and other aspects of the carcinoids syndrome have been recently published,[182, 282, 283, 288] and may be referred to for further details.

Although the syndrome is classically associated with midgut carcinoids,[280, 281] it has also been described in association with gastric, pancreatic, appendiceal, cecal, colonic, and rectal carcinoids,[188, 189, 238, 284, 285, 288–294] as well as those in extraintestinal locations.[284, 293, 294] The syndrome occurs in 5 to 11 percent of patients with gastrointestinal carcinoids,[188, 189, 192] and has been estimated to occur in 1 percent of all patients with carcinoids and in 20 percent of those with distant metastases.[284]

In the case of gastrointestinal carcinoids, the development of the syndrome invariably, but not necessarily, requires the presence of hepatic metastases so that sufficient amounts of 5-HT and 5-HTP reach the systemic circulation without undergoing metabolic inactivation. Metastatic deposits in the liver attain sizes that, in aggregate, are much larger than the primary tumor, and frequently produce enormous amounts of 5-HT and 5-HTP. Further, hepatic metastases drain these products directly into the systemic circulation via the efferent hepatic veins, thereby sequestering them from hepatic degradation. A review of four previously published series[188, 189, 192, 288] reveals that of the 37 patients with malignant carcinoid syndrome attributable to gastrointestinal carcinoids, 35 had hepatic metastases, while 2 had extensive nodal and peritoneal implants.[188] Since the total mass of malignant tissue in these two patients was very large, it is likely that the amounts of 5-HT and 5-HTP liberated from the tumor cells may have overwhelmed normal degradative mechanisms to produce the syndrome.

On account of the rich vascular anastomoses between the portal and systemic circulations, the lower rectum normally drains into the inferior vena cava via the inferior hemorrhoidal veins. Secretory products of rectal carcinoids are, therefore, drained directly into the systemic circulation without being routed through the liver. These tumors can, therefore, produce the carcinoid syndrome, even in the absence of hepatic metastases.[188, 189, 192, 288]

Functioning tumors giving rise to the carcinoid syndrome are histologically indistinguishable from other functioning or nonfunctioning tumors arising in comparable sites. Their histochemical characteristics, too, usually conform to the patterns displayed by other carcinoids in that anatomic segment, and reflect their 5-HT and 5-HTP content. Tumors of midgut origin show strong argentaffinity and formaldehyde-induced fluorescence that correlates with their abundant 5-HT content demonstrable by RIA and immunocytochemical procedures. On the other hand, foregut carcinoids associated with the atypical carcinoid syndrome are nonargentaffin in nature because they produce histamine or 5-HTP rather than 5-HT. Most of the functioning tumors that have been studied ultrastructurally have arisen in the midgut and have demonstrated large numbers of pleomorphic secretory granules that characterize both the normal EC_1 cells and midgut carcinoids in general.[266]

GASTRINOMA SYNDROME

Zollinger and Ellison's original description of the Zollinger-Ellison syndrome in 1955[295] was soon followed by identification of gastrin as the active principle responsible for it.[7, 296–298] Since that time, refinements in RIA procedures for determining circulating levels of different molecular forms of gastrin and the development of provocative tests such as the calcium stimulation, secetin infusion, and protein-meal stimulation tests have not only improved our diagnostic capabilities but have almost revolutionized our entire concept of this syndrome.[7, 296–299] In contrast to the triad of fulminant peptic ulcer disease, copious gastric acid hypersecretion, and the presence of a pancreatic non-β islet cell tumor, it is now recognized that peptic ulcer disease is *not* essential for its diagnosis: the patients may have only mild to moderate hyperchlorhydria, and the associated gastrin-producing tumor (gastrinoma), if found, may be pancreatic, gastrointestinal, or extrapancreatic and extragastrointestinal in its location.[7, 233, 296–298, 300–304] For a diagnosis of the Zollinger-Ellison syndrome, therefore, emphasis is currently placed on (1) demonstration of significantly elevated basal serum gastrin levels; (2) results of provocative tests, especially demonstration of an increase in serum gastrin levels following secretin infusion; (3) localization of a pancreatic or extrapancreatic tumor; and whenever possible (4) preoperative or intraoperative demonstration of very high gastrin levels in the venous effluent from the tumor (thereby clearly establishing the tumor as a gastrinoma).[298]

Although the major molecular forms of gastrin normally present in the body, G_{17} and G_{34}; are the chief forms of gastrins produced by gastrinomas, small amounts of G_{13} and G_{45} may also be produced.[228, 305] Most tumors produce both G_{17} and G_{34}, although in varying proportions. The biologic potency and half-lives of these various molecular forms of gastrins vary considerably, and it is important to remember, therefore, that serum gastrin levels as usually determined by RIA procedures represent the sum total of the immunoreactivities of the various components present, and provide little or no insight into the circulating *biologic activity*. Since G_{17} is known to be about 6 to 8 times as potent as G_{34}, a blood level of 40 pg of G_{17} per milliliter would be as potent as about 300 pg of G_{34}. It is therefore easy to understand why some patients with flagrant clinical and biochemical manifestations of the Zollinger-Ellison syndrome may have only mild elevations in serum gastrin levels (if predominantly G_{17}), whereas others may show milder forms of the disease despite pronounced hypergastrinemia (if predominantly G_{34}).

Although gastrinomas, single or multiple, are most frequently encountered in the pancreas, nearly 15 percent of these are extrapancreatic in location.[233] Nearly 13 percent of all gastrinomas are located in the wall of the second portion of the duodenum,[300] and occasionally such tumors have also been identified in the stomach[306, 307] and biliary passages.[233] Whereas nearly 50 percent of duodenal gastrinomas are solitary, those arising in the stomach are frequently multiple and have occasionally been seen to arise in a background of pre-existing antral G cell hyperplasia (antral gastrinosis).[187, 308] Of the 103 duodenal gastrinomas reported from the Zollinger-Ellison Tumor Registry, nearly 40 percent already had demonstrable metastases at the time of diagnosis.[300] However, since gastrinomas tend to grow slowly, the presence of local and distant metastatic spread is not incompatible with prolonged survival.[296] An interesting feature of gastrinomas is the tendency of the tumors to regress (or at least to cease advancing) after total gastrectomy.[296]

Gastrinomas cannot be differentiated from other functional or nonfunctional carcinoids on the basis of morphology alone. Whereas pancreatic gastrinomas usually tend to show a trabecular pattern, duodenal and gastric gastrinomas show a mixed architectural arrangement, sometimes with a prominent glandular or pseudoglandular component. Local intramural invasion by tumor cells may occasionally extend to the muscularis or beyond. Vascular and lymphatic invasion by tumor cells is also frequently present. Tumor cells are consistently argyrophil by the Grimelius technique and show immunoreactivity for gastrin (Fig. 10-25). However, individual tumors may show considerable variations within them, not only in the number of cells that stain but also in the intensity of the staining reactions. Comparisons between parallel sections, one stained for argyrophilia and the other for localization of gastrin, show that not all argyrophil cells are immunoreactive for gastrin nor are all immunoreactive cells argyrophil. Further, the number of cells immunoreactive for gastrin in a given tumor fails to show a positive correlation with both the serum and

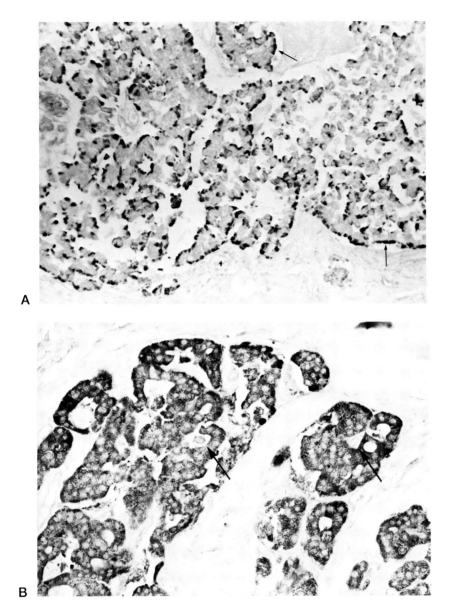

Fig. 10-25. **(A)** Duodenal gastrinoma associated with Zollinger-Ellison syndrome showing immunoreactivity for gastrin in the majority of tumor cells. Note that the gastrin immunoreactivity in the cells varies from area to area, and that the reaction product is mostly confined to the basal pole of the cells (arrows). (Peroxidase-antiperoxidase technique, rabbit antigastrin serum 1:1,000; methyl green counterstain, × 128.) **(B)** Somatostatinoma showing strong cytoplasmic staining for somatostatin. Note that although staining is seen in practically every tumor cell, there is considerable variation in staining intensity. The psammoma bodies in the lumina of the glandular structures (arrows) are completely nonimmunoreactive. (Fig. A from O'Briain & Dayal,[7] with permission; Fig. B from Dayal & Ganda,[315] with permission.)

tumor gastrin content as determined by RIA procedures. The former discrepancy may be related to the granule content of the tumor cells; tumors associated with very high blood levels of gastrin show a predominance of sparsely granulated cells, since the secretory product (gastrin) has already been released into the circulation. An analogous situation has also been observed frequently in prolactinomas of the pituitary.[309] The latter discrepancy may be related to problems inherent in the sampling of these tumors for the two procedures. Increasing numbers of gastrinomas are being regarded as multihormonal in nature, since a variety of polypeptides including glucagon, somatostatin, insulin PP, ACTH, and enkephalins have been localized within them.[228, 305, 307]

Ultrastructurally, gastrinomas show considerable heterogeneity in the morphology of their secretory granules. However, four major categories have been identified according to the presence of typical G cell type granules (type I), typical and atypical granules (type II), atypical granules only (type III), and granules characteristic of other endocrine cell types (type IV).[228, 305]

SOMATOSTATINOMA SYNDROME

Although small numbers of somatostatin-containing cells are present in up to one-third of nonfunctioning gastrointestinal carcinoids[261] (Table 10-3), tumors composed exclusively or predominantly of somatostatin immunoreactive cells are very rare, and account for less than 1 percent of the endocrine tumors of the gut and pancreas. Such tumors, referred to as *somatostatinomas*, arise almost exclusively from (and are almost evenly divided between) the pancreas and the duodenum.[203, 229, 310–315] Approximately 80 such tumors have been reported so far, and we have additionally studied five other unreported cases. However, in addition to the well-documented examples of duodenal somatostatinomas, there are many others buried in the literature under such terms as *foregut APUDomas, duodenal carcinoids,* and *carcinoid-islet cell tumors.*[316–326] Although it is difficult to assess the true incidence of somatostatinomas in previously published cases of duodenal carcinoids, it is of interest that a recent series of 65 duodenal carcinoids included 32 tumors (47 percent) with a significant population of somatostatin-containing cells.[321] Although relevant details were not reported, at least eight of these tumors would appear to be somatostatinomas on their morphologic and immunohistochemical characteristics alone. Similarly at least 2 additional somatostatinomas can be identified in the series of 12 duodenal carcinoids reported by Stamm et al.[320]

The somatostatinoma syndrome is most commonly observed in elderly individuals, and twice as often in females as in males. It is typically characterized by diabetes mellitus, diarrhea, steatorrhea, hypochlorhydria or achlorhydria, weight loss, and anemia.[310, 311] A high frequency of gallstones and biliary tract disease has also been observed in these patients. All of these features are due to the high circulating levels of somatostatin and can be reproduced by prolonged somatostatin infusion.[327] The abdominal pain could either be related to the biliary tract disease or to subacute intestinal obstruction produced by the exophytic intestinal tumors.

Current evidence indicates that intestinal tumors do not produce the full-blown picture of this syndrome (Dayal Y, Wolfe HJ: Unpublished observations),[203, 232, 314, 315] whereas pancreatic somatostatinomas are frequently associated with the somatostatinoma syndrome. This is perhaps because (1) these tumors lead to jaundice and intestinal obstruction early in their development, and therefore are resected before the syndrome can develop, (2) most duodenal somatostatinomas are small and do not produce sufficient somatostatin to give rise to the syndrome, and (3) the various molecular forms of somatostatin produced by the tumors perhaps lack the full potency and range of biologic activity. Quite often the true nature of these rare tumors is recognized only after appropriate histochemical, immunocytochemical, RIA, or ultrastructural studies have been performed.[203, 232, 314, 315] Although all previously published pancreatic somatostatinomas have been malignant tumors that had already metastasized when first discovered,[229–231, 310–313] the incidence of malignancy in duodenal somatostatinomas is perhaps just as high. Despite their small size (4 cm average diameter), these tumors show deep intramural invasion and metastases to paraduodenal nodes.[209–211, 328–333] Widespread metastases to the liver, lungs, kidneys, bones, skin, ovaries, adrenals, and thyroid have been reported.[332, 333]

Histologically, these tumors usually have a mixed architectural pattern with areas of trabecular, follicular, or acinar differentiation similar to those commonly seen in other endocrine tumors.[7, 297] The tumor cells are argyrophil only with the Hellerstrom-Hellman technique and are Grimelius negative. In seven duodenal somatostatinomas in our series, we observed small clusters of Grimelius-positive argyrophil cells that had failed to stain with the Hellerstrom-Hellman technique.

Immunocytochemical techniques show a pre-ponderance of somatostatin-positive cells. Occasional tumors have shown additional immunoreactivity in a small subpopulation of cells for ACTH (with features of Cushing's syndrome),[229] gastrin (with peptic ulceration),[232] and calcitonin (motor diarrhea).[231] Other secretory products such as insulin, glucagon, PP, CCK, secretinin, motilin, substance P, neurotensin, glicentin, GIP, VIP, [Met] enkephalin, and serotonin, among others, have been sought for unsuccessfully in these tumors.[230, 232, 310, 312, 314]

Ultrastructural studies performed on both pancreatic and duodenal tumors indicate that somatostatinomas are quite homogeneous in their composition. Almost all tumors have been described as containing round 250 to 400-nm secretory granules with variably electron-dense cores (Fig. 10-26).[203, 310–315] The minor differences noted in two tumors perhaps best correlate with the other secretory product (calcitonin) that each tumor was seen to be producing.[230, 231]

Since ultrastructural studies have shown that psammoma bodies in such tumors are products

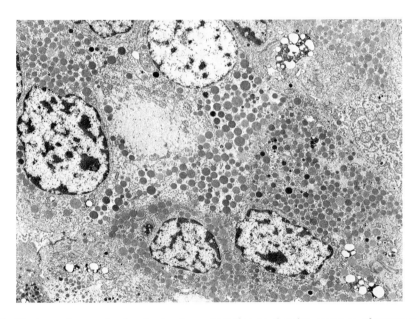

Fig. 10-26. Electron micrograph of a duodenal somatostatinoma showing presence of numerous variably electron-dense round secretory granules varying between 250 and 400 nm in diameter. This tumor contained abundant somatostatin immunoreactive cells. (Glutaraldehyde-formaldehyde fixation, × 18,200.)

of active secretion by the tumor cells,[203] their formation may be related to the synthesis of the somatostatin molecule in a manner analogous to the formation of amyloid in the calcitonin-producing medullary carcinoma of thyroid and the insulin-producing endocrine tumors of the pancreas.

Although only a few of the reported somatostatinomas have been evaluated for their secretory profile, quite a few have been shown to be multihormonal.[209, 229–232, 311, 315]

CUSHING'S SYNDROME

Whereas ACTH production can be frequently demonstrated in gastrointestinal carcinoids, in only rare instances is such ectopic ACTH production sufficiently excessive to cause clinical manifestations of Cushing's syndrome.[334–337] In all such cases, the carcinoids have reportedly arisen in foregut-derived structures (such as lungs and stomach). Although bronchial carcinoids (and oat cell carcinomas of the lung) are known to often give rise to Cushing's syndrome,[284, 338, 339] gastrointestinal carcinoids do so very infrequently. Only a handful of well-documented cases have been reported, and in all such instances the carcinoids were located in the stomach.[335–337] In each case, the tumors conformed to the usual histologic, histochemical, and ultrastructural characteristics of foregut carcinoids, and were malignant, having already metastasized to the regional nodes or the liver.[335–337] Two of these tumors, in addition to secreting large amounts of ACTH, were also shown to produce β-MSH[335] or β-LPH.[337] In the latter, both ACTH and β-LPH were localized within the same cells.

ASSOCIATION WITH OTHER CLINICAL CONDITIONS

Distinct from their relationship with Zollinger-Ellison, carcinoid, and Cushing's syndromes, an association has also been described between gastrointestinal carcinoids and other clinical conditions, such as MEN syndrome and von Recklinghausen's disease.[209, 224, 261, 328, 340–352]

MEN syndrome is a familial condition transmitted by a pleotropic, autosomal dominant gene with a high penetrance and variable phenotypic expressivity.[341, 346, 353] Patients with MEN type I (Wermer's) syndrome characteristically develop hyperplasia or endocrine tumors of the pancreas, the anterior pituitary, the parathyroids, the adrenal cortex, and the thyroid.[353] In addition, these patients are known to frequently develop carcinoid tumors, multiple subcutaneous and visceral lipomas, renal cortical adenomas and carcinomas, as well as villous adenomas and adenocarcinomas of the colon.[340, 341] The carcinoids may be located in the gut (most commonly in the jejunum and ileum) or in such extraintestinal locations as the lungs, the pancreas, and the thymus.[341] Irrespective of their locations, carcinoids in patients with Wermer's syndrome are identical in all respects to corresponding lesions seen in sporadic nonfamilial cases, and may even be hormonally functioning, producing the carcinoid syndrome.[341] Up to 20 percent of patients with this syndrome show evidence of gastric hypersecretion and peptic ulcer disease.[354] Such patients may present first with features of Zollinger-Ellison syndrome, and the underlying Wermer's syndrome may not be recognized until later. Similarly, since up to 40 percent of patients with Zollinger-Ellison syndrome may have other nonpancreatic endocrine tumors,[355] it is important that these patients also be evaluated for possible co-existent MEN syndrome.

The association of gastrointestinal carcinoids with von Recklinghausen's disease, recognized recently, appears to be an uncommon event.[342–345, 356] The tumors tend to be incidentally discovered and hormonally "silent," but may occasionally be functional, as in the case of a 13-year-old child reported by Garcia and co-workers.[344] In this patient, too, the clinical presentation was dominated by features of Zollinger-Ellison syndrome, whereas the familial neurofibromatosis (and the possible presence of MEN syndrome) was detected later. Although some of the patients reported in the literature with this association may represent genuine cases of von Recklinghausen's disease, others have shown clinical and biochemical features indicating that the neurofibromatosis itself may have been a component of the MEN syndrome type III (II$_B$).[343, 344] Quite a few of the more recently described cases have also had coexistent uni- or bilateral pheochromocytomas, duodenal paragangliomas, ganglioneuromas, or schwannomas.[224, 225, 315, 347, 348, 352] It is not clear, therefore, whether the reported cases represent an association of gastrointestinal carcinoids with familial neurofibromatosis per se or with MEN type III (II$_B$), of which neurofibromatosis is a component. Careful studies on all such cases (and their families) identified in the future are expected to elucidate this.

DIAGNOSIS OF CARCINOID TUMORS

Carcinoid tumors are most commonly diagnosed by their characteristic histopathologic features as visualized under the conventional H&E stain. However, although tumors exhibiting the common insular, trabecular, and mixed architectural patterns can be easily recognized as carcinoids, undifferentiated tumors and those with goblet cell or psammomatous features are quite often misdiagnosed as adenocarcinomas. This is specially true of gastric carcinoids since these tumors frequently exhibit a solid or mixed architecture that is different from the insular pattern seen in midgut carcinoids.[242, 243] In a retrospective analysis of 140 gastric tumors originally diagnosed as adenocarcinoma, 7 percent of the tumors were eventually reclassified as carcinoids.[244] Although the true endocrine nature of such neoplasms can be established easily by electron microscopic demonstration of typical membrane-bound secretory granules in the tumor cells, these granules are most conveniently visualized at the light microscopic level by their argentaffin (Masson-Fontana stain) or argyrophil properties (Grimelius, Sevier-Munger, or Hellerstrom-Hellman techniques).

Since the Grimelius technique demonstrates argyrophilia in a variety of different endocrine cell types,[57] it has proven very useful in detecting a high proportion of carcinoid tumors,[7, 200, 201–259, 273, 274, 297] and is therefore heavily relied on for the identification of these tumors in surgical pathology practice. However, it is important to bear in mind that the gastric ECL cell carcinoids require the Sevier-Munger stain for argyrophilia, whereas true nonreactive carcinoids and those with sparsely granulated cells would require electron microscopic studies for demonstration of the intracytoplasmic granules. Further, since argyrophil granules can occasionally be seen both in exocrine cells as well as in adenocarcinomas,[49, 297, 357–359] caution needs to be exercised in interpreting argyrophil stains in neoplastic lesions. Results of silver impregnation techniques should ideally be considered in the context of other morphologic findings. True carcinoid tumors, even those with prominent glandular areas, show minimal cytologic aberrations. Cellular pleomorphism and nuclear atypia, when present, is usually confined to small foci, and these tumors generally show large numbers of argentaffin or argyrophil cells. Although stray solitary argyrophil cells or small clusters of such cells frequently can be seen randomly scattered in adenocarcinomas, these cells are very few in number, and the tumor cells show the characteristic hallmarks of malignancy—cytologic atypia, nuclear pleomorphism, increased mitotic activity, and the like—which further distinguishes them from carcinoids. NSE, and other markers of neuroendocrine differentiation (e.g., chromogranins, pancreastatin, or synaptophy sin) associated with neurosecretory granules have also been demonstrated in the various gut endocrine cell types.[65, 72, 75–78] Their presence in tumor cells has now emerged as a reliable and diagnostically useful marker for carcinoids and other neuroendocrine cell tumors.

With the recognition that the vast majority of gastrointestinal carcinoids elaborate one or more polypeptide hormones or amines, there is an increasing need for an accurate characterization of the secretory repertoire of these tumors. This is especially so because a significant proportion of these are known to produce multiple secretory products. In our own series (Table 10-7), although all of the 42 tumors that were immunoreactive for one or more secretory products were argyrophil by the Grimelius technique, no consistent relationship emerged between argyrophilia on the one hand, and the demonstration of a particular secretory product on the other. Since argyrophil stains provide no insights into the functional characteristics of these tumors, they need to be supplemented by immunocytochemical studies for localization of the various secretory products within the tumor cells. Such analyses not only delineate the functional characteristics of these tumors, but also improve our understanding of other biologic features, enhance clinicopathologic correlations, and help define specific clinical syndromes attributable to overproduction of some of these secretory products.

ACKNOWLEDGMENTS

The author wishes to thank Sonia Alexander for preparation of photomicrographs; Rosalie Daly, Lorraine Duhamel, and Rahul Bhatnagar for technical assistance; and Lisa Hansbury for secretarial assistance.

REFERENCES

1. Heidenhain R: Untersuchungen uber den Bau der Labdrusen. Arch Mikr Anat 6:368, 1870
2. Kulschitzky N: Zuf frage uber den Bau des Darmkanals. Arch Mikrosk Anat 49:7, 1897
3. Masson MP: La glande endocrinaire de l'intestine chez l'home. CR Acad Sci (Paris) 158:59, 1914
4. Barter R, Pearse AGE: Mammalian enterochromaffin cells as the source of serotonin. J Pathol Bactol 69:25, 1955
5. Cecilia M, Rost M, Rost FWD: An improved method for staining cells of the endocrine polypeptide (APUD) series by masked metachromasia. Histochem J 8:93, 1976
6. Dawson I: The endocrine cells of the gastrointestinal tract. Histochem J 2:527, 1970
7. O'Briain DS, Dayal Y: The pathology of gastrointestinal endocrine cells. p. 75. In DeLellis RA (ed): Diagnostic Immunohistochemistry. Masson Publishing USA, New York, 1981
8. Fujita T, Kobayashi S: The cells and hormones of the GEP endocrine system. p. 1. In Fujita T (ed): Gastroenteropancreatic Cell System. A Cell-Biological Approach. Igaku-Shoin, Tokyo, 1973
9. Fiddian-Green RG, Farrell J, Havlichek D Jr, Kothary P, Pittenger G: A physiological role for luminal gastrin? Surgery 83:663, 1978
10. Larsson LI, Golterman N, DeMagistris L, et al: Somatostatin cell processes as pathway for paracrine secretion. Science 205:1393, 1979
11. Grube D, Aebert H: Immunocytochemical investigations of the gastroenteropancreatic endocrine cells using semi-thin and thin serial sections. p. 83. In Grossman M, Lechago J (eds): Cellular Basis of Chemical Messengers in the Digestive System. Academic Press, San Diego, 1981.
12. Varndell IM, Harris A, Tapia FJ, et al: Intracellular topography of immunoreactive gastrin demonstrated using electron immunocytochemistry. Experentia 39:713, 1983
13. Mortensen NJ McC, Morris JF: The effect of fixation conditions on the ultrastructural appearance of gastrin cell granules in the rat pyloric antrum. Cell Tissue Res 176:251, 1977
14. Larsson LI: Peptides of the gastrin cells. p. 85. In Amdrup E, Rehfeld, JF (eds): Gastrin and the Vagus. Academic Press, London, 1979
15. Forssmann WG, Orci L: Ultrastructure and secretory cycle of the gastrin-producing cell. Z Zellforsch Mikrosk Anat 101:419, 1969
16. Hakanson R, Alumets J, Rehfeld JF, et al: The life cycle of the gastrin granule. Cell Tissue Res 222:479, 1982
17. Larsson LI: Immunocytochemical characterization of ACTH-like immunoreactivity in cerebral nerves, and in endocrine cells of the pituitary and gastrointestinal tract by using region-specific antisera. J Histochem Cytochem 28:133, 1980
18. Vaillant C, Dockray G, Hopkins CR: Cellular origins of different forms of gastrin: the specific immunocytochemical localization of related peptides. J Histochem Cytochem 27:932, 1979
19. Solcia E, Polak JM, Pearse AGE, et al: Lausanne 1977 classification of gastroenteropan-

creatic endocrine cells. p. 40. In Bloom SR (ed): Gut Hormones. Churchill Livingston, Edinburgh, 1978

20. Goodrich JT: Serotonergic neurons in human bowel: distribution in congenital megacolon (Hirschsprung's disease) of man and mouse. Gastroenterology 73:A-2/868, 1977

21. Furness JB, Costa M: Types of nerves in the enteric nervous system. Neuroscience 5:1, 1980

22. Costa M, Furness JB: Neuronal peptides in the intestine. Br Med Bull 38:247, 1982

23. Griffith SG, Burnstock G: Serotonergic neurons in human fetal intestine: an immunohistochemical study. Gastroenterology 85:929, 1983

24. Costa M, Furness JB, Gibbins IL: Chemical coding of enteric neurons. Prog Brain Res 68:217, 1986

25. Schultzberg M, Hokfelt T, Nilsson G, et al: Distribution of peptide- and catecholamine-containing neurons in the gastrointestinal tract of rat and guinea pig: immunohistochemical studies with antisera to substance P, vasoactive intestinal peptide, enkephalins, somatostatin, gastrin/cholecystokinin, neurotensin and dopamine beta-hydroxylase. Neuroscience 5:689, 1980

26. Ferri GL, Botti PL, Vezzadini P, et al: Peptide-containing innervation of the human intestinal mucosa: An immunocytochemical study on whole-mount preparations. Histochemistry 76:413, 1982

27. Kurian SS, Ferri GL, DeMay J, Polak JM: Immunocytochemistry of serotonin-containing nerves in the human gut. Histochemistry 78: 523, 1983

28. Costa M, Furness JB, Smith IJ, et al: An immunohistochemical study of the projections of somatostatin-containing neurons in the guinea pig intestine. Neuroscience 5:841, 1980

29. Brodin E, Sjolund K, Hakanson R, Sundler F: Substance P-containing nerve fibres are numerous in human but not in feline intestinal mucosa. Gastroenterology 85:557, 1983

30. Sundler F, Hakanson R, Leander S: Peptidergic nervous systems in the gut. Clin Gastroenterol, No. 3:517, 1980

31. Fujita T: The gastroenteric endocrine cells and its paraneuronic nature. p. 191. In Coupland RE, Fujita T: (eds): Chromaffin, Enterochromaffin and Related Cells. Elsevier, Amsterdam, 1976

32. DeRobertis E: Histophysiology and Synapses and Neurosecretion. Pergamon Press, Oxford, 1964

33. Fujita T: Present status of paraneuron concept. Arch Histol Cytol 52:1, 1989

34. Pearse AGE: Common cytochemical properties of cells producing polypeptide hormones, with particular reference to calcitonin and the thyroid C cells. Vet Rec 79:587, 1966

35. Pearse AGE: The cytochemistry and ultrastructure of polypeptide hormone producing cells of the APUD series and the embryologic physiologic and pathologic implication of the concept. J Histochem Cytochem 17:303, 1969

36. Pearse AGE: The diffuse neuroendocrine system and the APUD concept; related "endocrine" peptides in brain, intestine, pituitary, placenta and the anuran cutaneous glands. Med Biol 55:115, 1977

37. Pearse AGE, Polak JM: Neural crest origin of the endocrine polypeptide (APUD) cells of the gastrointestinal tract and pancreas. Gut 12:783, 1971

38. Pearse AGE, Polak JM, Bloom SR: The newer gut hormones. Cellular sources, physiology, pathology and clinical aspects. Gastroenterology 72:746, 1977

39. Pearse AGE, Polak JM: Embryology of the diffuse neuroendocrine system and its relationship to the common peptides. Fed Proc 38:2288, 1979

40. Andrew A: A study of the developmental relationship between enterochromaffin cells and the neural crest. J Embryol Exp Morphol 11:307, 1963

41. Andrew A: Further evidence that the enterochromaffin cells are not derived from the neural crest. J Embryol Exp Morphol 31:589, 1974

42. LeDouarin NM: The embryological origin of the endocrine cells associated with the digestive tract: experimental analysis based on the use of a stable cell marking technique. p. 49. In Bloom SR (ed): Gut Hormones. Churchill Livingstone, Edinburgh, 1978

43. Nomura Y: On the submicroscopic morphogenesis of parietal cells in the gastric gland of the human fetus. Z Ant Entwickl 125:315, 1966

44. Matsuyama M, Suzuki H: Differentiation of immature mucus cells into parietal, argyrophil and chief cells in stomach grafts. Science 169:385, 1970

45. Leblonde CP, Cheng H: Identification of stem cells in the small intestine of the mouse. p. 7. In Carnie AB, Lala PK, Osmond DG (eds): Stem Cells of Renewing Cell Population. Academic Press, San Diego, 1976

46. Tischler A, Dichter MA, Biales B, et al: Neuroendocrine neoplasms and their cells of origin. N Engl J Med 296:919, 1977

47. Grand RF, Watkins JB, Torti FM: Development of the human gastro-intestinal tract: a review. Gastroenterology 70:790, 1976

48. Dayal Y, Wolfe HJ: Gastrin-producing cells in ectopic gastric mucosa of developmental and metaplastic origins. Gastroenterology 75:655, 1978

49. Sidhu GS: The endodermal origin of digestive and respiratory tract APUD cells: histopathologic evidence and review of the literature. Am J Pathol 96:5, 1979

50. Falck B, Owman C: A detailed methodological description of the fluorescence method for the cellular demonstration of biogenic monoamines. Acta Univ Lund II(7):5, 1965

51. Larsson LI, Sundler F, Hakanson R, et al: Immunofluorescent localization of gastrin in rabbit antropyloric mucosa to argyrophil cells exhibiting formaldehyde-ozone-induced fluorescence. Histochemie 37:81, 1973

52. Hakanson R, Larsson LI, Nishizaki H, et al: A new type of formaldehyde-induced fluorescence in a population of endocrine cells in cat antropyloric mucosa. Histochemie 34:1, 1973

53. DeLellis RA: Formaldehyde-induced fluorescence technique for the demonstration of biogenic amines in diagnostic histopathology. Cancer 28:1704, 1971

54. Sevier A, Munger B: A silver method for paraffin sections of neural tissue. J Neuropathol Exp Neurol 24:130, 1965

55. Hellerstrom C, Helman B: Some aspects of silver impregnation of the islet of Langerhans in the rat. Acta Endocrinol (Kbh) 35:518, 1960

56. Grimelius L: A silver nitrate stain for A₂ cells of human pancreatic islets. Acta Soc Med Upsala, 73:243, 1968

57. Grimelius L, Wilander E: Silver stains in the study of endocrine cells of the gut and pancreas. Invest Cell Pathol 3:3, 1980

58. Vassallo G, Capella C, Solcia E: Endocrine cells of the human gastric mucosa. Z Zellforsch 118:49, 1971

59. Solcia E, Capella C, Frigerio B: Histochemical and ultrastructural studies on the argentaffin and argyrophil cells of the gut. p. 223. In Coupland RE, Fujita T (eds): Chromaffin, Enterochromaffin and Related Cells. Elsevier, Amsterdam, 1976

60. Vassallo G, Capella C, Solcia E: Grimelius silver stain for endocrine cell granules as shown by electron microscopy. Stain Technol 46:7, 1971

61. Bendayan M, Nanci A, Herbener GH, et al: A review of the study of protein secretion applying the protein A-gold immunocytochemical approach. Am J Anat 175:379, 1986

62. Lloyd RV, Warner TF: Immunohistochemistry of neuron specific enolase. p. 127. In DeLellis RA (ed): Advances in Immunohistochemistry. Masson, New York, 1984

63. Haimoto H, Takahashi Y, Koshikawa T, et al: Immunohistochemical localization of gamma enolase in normal human tissues other than nervous and neuroendocrine tissue. Lab Invest 52:257, 1985

64. Gould VE, Fodstad O, Memoli VA, et al: Neuroendocrine cells and associated neoplasms of the skin. p. 545. In Evolution and Tumor Pathology of the Neuroendocrine system. Falkmer S, Hakanson R, Sundler F (eds): Elsevier, Amsterdam, 1984

65. Vinores SA, Bonnin JM, Rubinstein LJ, Marangos PJ: Immunohistochemical demonstration of neuron specific enolase in neoplasms of the CNS and other tissues. Arch Pathol Lab Med 108: 536, 1984

66. Schmechel D: Gamma subunit of the glycolytic enzyme enolase: non-specific or neuron specific. Lab Invest 52:239, 1985

67. Blaschko H, Comline RS, Schneider FH, et al: Secretion of a chromaffin granule protein, chromogranin, from the adrenal medulla after splanchnic nerve stimulation. Nature 215:58, 1967

68. Fischer-Colbrie R, Frischenschlager I: Immunological characterization of secretory proteins of chromogranins A, chromogranins B, and enkephalin-containing peptides. J Neurochem 44:1854, 1985

69. Rindi G, Buffa R, Sessa F, et al: Chromogranin A, B and C immunoreactivities of mammalian endocrine cells: Distribution, distinction from cultured hormones/prohormones and relationship with the argyrophil component of secretory granules. Histochemie 85:19, 1986

70. Rosa P, Hille A, Lee RWH, et al: Secretogranins I and II: two tyrosine-sulfated secretory proteins common to a variety of cells secreting peptides by the regulatory pathway. J Cell Biol 101:1999, 1985

71. Lloyd RV: Immunohistochemical localization of chromogranin in normal and neoplastic endocrine tissues. Pathol Annu 22:69, 1987

72. Facer P, Bishop AE, Lloyd RV, et al: Chromogranin: a newly recognized marker for endocrine cells of the human gastrointestinal tract. *Gastroenterology* 89:1366, 1985

73. Lloyd RV, Mervak T, Schmidt K, et al: Immunohistochemical detection of chromogranin and neuron specific enolase in pancreatic endocrine neoplasms. Am J Surg Pathol 8:607, 1984

74. Grube D, Aunis D, Bader F, et al: Chromogranin A (CGA) in the gastroentero-pancreatic (GEP) endocrine system: CGA in the mammalian endocrine pancreas. Histochemie 85, 441, 1986

75. Konecki DS, Benedum UM, Gerdes HH, Huttner WB: The primary structure of human chromogranin A and pancreastatin. J Biol Chem 262: 17026, 1988

76. Iacangelo AL, Fischer-Colbrie R, Koller KJ, et al: The sequence of porcine chromogranin A messenger RNA demonstrates that chromogranin A can serve as the precursor for the biologically active hormone pancreastatin. Endocrinology 122: 2339, 1988

77. O'Connor DT, Deftos LJ: Secretion of chromogranin A by peptide-producing endocrine neoplasms. N Engl J Med 314: 1145, 1986

78. Sobol RE, Memoli V, Deftos LJ: Hormone-negative, chromogranin-A-positive endocrine tumors. N Engl J Med 320: 444, 1989

79. Rehm H, Wiedemann B, Betz H: Molecular characterization of synaptophysin, a major calcium-binding protein of the synaptic vesicle membrane. EMBO J 5: 535, 1986

80. Gould VE, Wiedemann B, Lee I, et al: Synaptophysin expression in neuroendocrine neoplasms as determined by immunohistochemistry. Am J Pathol 126: 243, 1987

81. Wiedemann B, Franke WW, Kuhn C, et al: Synaptophysin: a marker protein for neuroendocrine cells and neoplasms. Proc Nat Acad Sci 83: 3500, 1986

82. Gould VE, Lee I, Wiedemann B, et al: Synaptophysin: a novel marker for neurons, certain neuroendocrine cells and their neoplasms. Hum Pathol 17: 979, 1986

83. Chejfec G, Falkmer S, Grimelius L, et al: Synaptophysin. A new marker for pancreatic neuroendocrine tumors. Am J Surg Pathol 11:241, 1987

84. Solcia E, Bordi C, Creutzfeldt W, et al: Histopathological classification of nonantral gastric endocrine growths in man. Digestion 41: 185, 1988

85. Leblond CP, Messier B: Renewal of chief cells and goblet cells in the small intestine as shown by radio-autography after injection of thymidine-H^3 into mice. Anat Rec 132: 247, 1958

86. Cheng H, Leblond CP: Origin and differentiation and renewal of the four main epithelial cell types in the mouse small intestine. I. Columnar cell. Am J Anat 141: 461, 1974

87. Cheng H: Origin and differentiation and renewal of the four main epithelial cell types in the mouse small intestine. II: Mucus cells. Am J Anat 141: 481, 1974

88. Cheng H, Leblond CP: Origin and differentiation and renewal of the four main epithelial cell types in the mouse small intestine. III. Entero-endocrine cells. Am J Anat 141: 503, 1974

89. Thompson EM, Price YE, Wright NA: Kinetics of enteroendocrine cells with implications for their origin: a study of the cholecystokinin and gastrin subpopulations combining tritiated thymidine labelling with immunocytochemistry in the mouse. Gut 31: 406, 1990

90. Lehy T: Self replication of somatostatin cells in the antral mucosa of rodents. Cell Tissue Kinet 15: 495, 1982

91. Deschner E, Lipkin, M: An autoradiographic study of the renewal of agentaffin cells in human rectal mucosa. Exp Cell Res 43: 661, 1966

92. Tielmans Y, Hakanson R, Sundler F, Willems G: Proliferation of enterochromaffin like cells in omeprazole treated hypergastrinemic rats. Gastroenterology 96: 723, 1989

93. Tielmans Y, Axelson J, Sundler F, et al: Serum gastrin concentration affects the self replication rate of the enterochromaffin like cells in the rat stomach. Gut 31: 274, 1990

94. Dayal Y, Wolfe, HJ: G-cell hyperplasia in chronic hypercalcemia: an immunocytochemical and morphometric analysis. Am J Pathol 116: 391, 1984

95. Dayal Y, Voelkel EF, Tashijian AH, Jr, et

al: Antropyloric G-cell hyperplasia in hypercalcemic rabbits bearing the VX_2 carcinoma. Am J Pathol 89: 391, 1977

96. Inokuchi H, Fujimoto S, Kawai K: Cellular kinetics of gastrointestinal mucosa with special reference to gut endocrine cells. Arch Histol Jpn 46, 137, 1983.

97. Larsson H, Carlson E, Mattson H, et al: Plasma gastrin and gastric enterochromaffin-like cell activation and proliferation: studies with omeprazole and ranitidine in intact and antrectomized rats. Gastroenterology 90: 391, 1986

98. Ryberg B, Mattson H, Sundler F, et al: Effects of inhibition of gastric acid secretion in rats on plasma gastrin levels and density of enterochromaffin-like cells in the oxyntic mucosa. Supplement: Sixth International Symposium on Gastrointestinal Hormones. Can J Physiol Pharmacol, 110: 34, 1986

99. Bordi C, Ravazzola M, DeVita O: Pathology of endocrine cells in gastric mucosa. Ann Pathol 3: 19, 1983

100. Dayal Y, Wolfe HJ: Gastrin-producing cells in ectopic gastric mucosa of developmental and metaplastic origins. Gastroenterology 75: 655, 1978

101. Dayal Y, Wolfe HJ: Endocrine cells in Barrett's epithelium. p. 59. In Spechler, SJ, Goyal, RK (eds): Barrett's Esophagus: Pathophysiology, Diagnosis and Management. Elsevier, New York, 1985

102. Dayal Y, DeLellis RA, Wolfe HJ: Hyperplastic proliferations of the gastrointestinal endocrine cells. Am J Surg Pathol 11: 87, 1987

103. Polak J, Pearse A, Gibson S: Cellular endocrinology of the gut and pancreas. p. 89. In Fujita T (ed): Endocrine, Gut and Pancreas. Elsevier, Amsterdam, 1976.

104. Lewin KJ, Yang K, Ulrich T, et al: Primary gastrin cell hyperplasia: report of five cases and a review of the literature. Am J Surg Pathol 8:821, 1984

105. Lewin KJ: The endocrine cells of the gastrointestinal tract: the normal endocrine cells and their hyperplasias, Part I. p. 1. In Sommers SC, Rosen PP (eds): Pathology Annual. Part 1. Vol. 21. Appleton-Century Crafts, East Norwalk, CT, 1986

106. Dayal Y, Wolfe, HJ: Antropyloric G-cell population in gastric and duodenal ulcer disease: a morphometric analysis. Lab Invest 38:341, 1978

107. Takahashi T, Shimazu H, Yamgishi T, Tani M: G-cell population in resected stomach from gastric and duodenal ulcer patients. Gastroenterology 78:498, 1980

108. Keuppens F, Willems G, Vansteen-Kistle Y, Woussen-Cole MD: Estimation of the antral and duodenal gastrin cell population removed by gastrectomy from patients with peptic ulcer. Surg Gynecol Obstet 146:400, 1978

109. Royston CMS, Polak JM, Bloom SR, et al: G-cell population of the gastric antrum, plasma gastrin and gastric acid secretion in patients with and without duodenal ulcer. Gut 19:689, 1978

110. Polak JM, Bloom SR, Bishop AE, McCrossan MV: D-cell pathology in duodenal ulcers and achlorhydria. Metabolism 27 (Supp. 1):1239, 1978

111. Bhagavan BS, Hofkins GA, Woel GM, Koss LG: Zollinger-Ellison syndrome. Ultrastructural and histochemical observations in a child with endocrine tumorlets of gastric antrum, Arch Pathol 98:217, 1974

112. Cowley DJ, Dymock IW, Boyes BE, et al: Zollinger-Ellison syndrome type 1: clinical and pathological correlations in a case. Gut 14:25, 1973

113. Friesen SR, Tomita T: Pseudo-Zollinger-Ellison syndrome: hypergastrinemia, hyperchlorhydria without tumor. Ann Surg 194:481, 1981

114. Polak JM, Stagg B, Pearse AGE: Two types of Zollinger-Ellison syndrome. Immunofluorescent, cytochemical and ultrastructural studies of the antral and pancreatic gastrin cells in different clinical states. Gut 13:501, 1972

115. Ganguli PC, Polak, JM, Pearse AGE, Elder JB: Antral gastrin-cell hyperplasia in peptic ulcer disease. Lancet i:583, 1974

116. Ganguli PC, Polak JM, Pearse AGE, et al: Antral G-cell hyperplasia with peptic ulcer disease: a new clinical entity. Gut 14:822, 1973

117. Walsh JH, Grossman MI: Gastrin. N Engl J Med 292:1324, 1975

118. Ivey JK: Current concepts of physiological control of gastric acid secretion: clinical applications. Am J Med 58:389, 1975

119. DeLellis RA, Dayal Y, Tischler AS, et al: Multiple endocrine neoplasia (MEN) syndromes: cellular origins and interrelationships. p. 163. In Richter GW, Epstein MA (eds): Review of Experimental Pathology. Vol. 28. Academic Press, San Diego, 1986

120. Magallanes F, Mulholland MW, Bonsack M, Delany JP: Does a non-acid lumen cause G-cell hyperplasia. Curr Surg 43:281, 1983

121. Muto S, Murayama N, Asano S, et al: Hypergastrinemia and achlorhydria in chronic renal failure. Nephron 40:143, 1985

122. Nielsen HO, Jensen KB, Christiansen LA: The antral gastrin-producing cells in duodenal ulcer patients: a density study before and during treatment with cimetidine. Acta Pathol Microbiol Immunol Scand [A] 88:383, 1980

123. Morgan JE, Kaiser CW, Johnson W, et al: Gastric carcinoid (gastrinoma) associated with achlorhydria (pernicious anemia). Cancer 51:2332, 1983

124. Bordi C, Cabrielli M, Missale G: Pathological changes in endocrine cells in chronic atrophic gastritis. Arch Pathol Lab Med 102:129, 1978

125. Bordi C, D'Adda T, Balato FT, Ferrari C: Carcinoid (ECL cell) tumor of the oxyntic mucosa of the stomach: A hormone dependent neoplasm: Prog Surg Pathol 9:177, 1988

126. Hodges JR, Isaacson P, Wright R: Diffuse enterochromaffin-like (ECL) cell hyperplasia and multiple gastric carcinoids: a complication of pernicious anemia. Gut 22:237, 1981

127. Borch K, Renval H, Liedberg H: Gastric endocrine cell hyperplasia and carcinoid tumors in pernicious anemia. Gastroenterology 88:638, 1985

128. Lehtola J, Karttunen T, Krekala I, et al: Gastric carcinoids with minimal or no macroscopic lesion in patients with pernicious anemia. Hepatogastroenterology 32:72, 1985

129. Carney JA, Go VLW, Fairbanks VF, et al: The syndrome of gastric argyrophil carcinoid tumors and non-antral gastric atrophy. Ann Intern Med 99:761, 1983

130. Moses RE, Frank BB, Leavitt M, Miller R: The syndrome of type A chronic atrophic gastritis, pernicious anemia, and multiple gastric carcinoids. J Clin Gastroenterol 8:61, 1986

131. Muller J, Kirchner T, Muller-Hermelin K: Gastric endocrine cell hyperplasia and carcinoid tumors in atrophic gastritis type A. Am J Surg Pathol 11:909, 1987

132. Soga J, Kohro T, Tazawa K, et al: Argyrophil cell microneoplasia in the Mastomys stomach—an observation on early carcinoid formation. J Nat Cancer Inst 55:1001, 1975

133. Havu N: Enterochromaffin-like cell carcinoids of gastric mucosa in rats after life-long inhibition of gastric secretion. Digestion 35 (Suppl 1):42, 1986

134. Poynter D, Pick CR, Harcourt RA, et al: Association of long lasting unsurmountable histamine H_2-blockade and gastric carcinoid tumors in the rat. Gut 26:1284, 1985

135. Betton GR, Dormer CS, Wells T, et al: Gastric ECL-cell hyperplasia and carcinoids in rodents following chronic administration of H_2-antagonists SK&F 93479 and oxmetidine and omeprazole. Toxicol Pathol 16(2):288, 1988

136. Ekman L, Hansson E, Havu N, et al: Toxicological studies on omeprazole. Scand J Gastroenterol 20 (Suppl 108):53, 1985

137. Sundler F, Hakanson R, Carlsson, E, et al: Hypergastrinemic after blockade of acid secretion in the rat: trophic effects. Digestion 35 (Suppl 1):56, 1986

138. Ryberg B, Bishop AE, Bloom SR, et al: Omeprazole and ranitidine, antisecretagogues with different modes of action, are equally effective in causing hyperplasia of enterochromaffin-like cells in rat stomach. Regul Pept 25:235, 1989

139. Blom H: Alterations in gastric mucosal morphology induced by longterm treatment with omeprazole in rats. Digestion 35 (Suppl 1):98, 1986

140. Ryberg B, Axelson J, Hakanson R, et al: Trophic effects of continuous infusion of $[Leu^{15}]$-gastrin-17 in the rat. Gastroenterology 98:33, 1990

141. Hakanson R, Oscarson J, Sundler F: Gastrin and the trophic control of gastric mucosa. Scand J Gastroenterol 21 (Suppl 118):18, 1986

142. Hakanson R, Blom H, Carlsson E, et al: Hypergastrinemia produces trophic effects in stomach but not in pancreas and intestines. Regul Pept 13:223, 1986

143. Bordi C, Ferrari C, D'Adda T, et al: Ultrastructural characterization of fundic endocrine cell hyperplasia associated with atrophic gastritis and hypergastrinemia, Virchows Arch [A] 409:335, 1986

144. Larsson LI, Rehfeld JF, Stockbrugger R, et al: Mixed endocrine gastric tumors associated with hypergastrinemia of antral origin. Am J Pathol 93:53, 1978

145. Wilander E: Achylia and the development of gastric carcinoids, Virchows Arch [A] 394:151, 1981

146. Harvey RF, Bradshaw MJ, Davidson CM, et al: Multifocal gastric carcinoid tumors, achlor-

hydria, and hypergastrinemia. Lancet 1:951, 1985

147. Bordi C, Pilato F, Carfagna G, et al: Argyrophil cell hyperplasia of fundic mucosa in patients with chronic atrophic gastritis. Digestion 35 (Suppl 1):130, 1986

148. Solcia E, Capella C, Buffa R, et al: Pathology of the Zollinger-Ellison syndrome. Prog Surg Pathol 1:119, 1980

149. Grigioni WF, Caletti GC, Gabrielli M, et al: Gastric carcinoids of ECL cells. Pathological and clinical analysis of eight cases. Acta Pathol JPN 35:361, 1985

150. Lehy T, Mignon M, Cadiot G, et al: Gastric endocrine cell behavior in Zollinger-Ellison patients upon long-term potent antisecretory treatment. Gastroenterology 96:1029, 1989

151. Lamberts R, Creutzfeldt W, Stockman F, et al: Long term omeprazole treatment in man: effects on grastric endocrine cell populations. Digestion 39:126, 1988

152. Borch K, Renvall H, Leidberg G, Anderson BN: Relations between circulating gastrin and endocrine cell proliferation in the atrophic gastric fundic mucosa. Scand J Gastroenterol 21:357, 1986

153. Dayal Y, Underwood K, Daly R: Is atrophic gastritis, intestinal metaplasia or endocrine cell hyperplasia causally related to gastric carcinoids? *Gastroenterology* 94:A89, 1988

154. Solcia E, Capella C, Sessa F, et al: Gastric carcinoids and related endocrine growths. Digestion 35 (Suppl 1):3, 1986

155. Solcia E, Capella C, Vassallo G, Buffa R: Endocrine cells of the gastric mucosa. Int Rev Cytol 42:233, 1975

156. Solcia E, Capella C, Fiocca R, et al: Gastric argyrophil carcinoidosis in patients with Zollinger-Ellison syndrome due to type 1 multiple endocrine neoplasia: a newly recognized association. Am J Surg Pathol 14:503, 1990

157. Friesen SR: The development of endocrinopathies in prospective screening of two families with multiple endocrine adenopathy type I. World J Surg 3:735, 1979

158. Voillemot N, Potet F, Mary JY, Lewin MJM: Gastrin cell distribution in normal human stomachs and in patients with Zollinger-Ellison syndrome. Gastroenterology 75:61, 1978

159. Capella C, Polak JM, Timson CM, Frigerio B, Solcia E: Gastric carcinoids of argyrophil ECL cells. Ultrastruct Pathol 1:411, 1980

160. Dayal Y: Neuroendocrine cells of the gastroin-

testinal tract: introduction and historical perspectives. In Dayal Y (ed): Endocrine Pathology of the Gut and Pancreas. CRC Press, Boca Raton, FL, 1991

161. Challacombe DN, Robertson K: Enterochromaffin cells in the duodenal mucosa of children with celiac disease. Gut 18:373, 1977

162. Sjolund K, Alumets J, Borg N-O, et al: Enteropathy of celiac disease in adults: increased number of enterochromaffin cells in the duodenal mucosa. Gut 23:42, 1982

163. Enerback L, Hallert C, Norrby K: Raised 5-hydroxytryptamine concentration in enterochromaffin cells in adult celiac disease. J Clin Pathol 36:499, 1983

164. Challacombe DN, Dawkins PD, Baker P: Increased tissue concentrations of 5-hydroxytryptamine in the duodenal mucosa of patients with celiac disease. Gut 18:882, 1977

165. Challacombe DN, Brown GA, Black SC, Storrie MH: Increased excretion of 5-hydroxyindolacetic acid in urine of children with untreated celiac disease. Arch Dis Child 47:442, 1972

166. Solcia E, Capella C, Buffa R, et al: Endocrine cells of the gastrointestinal tract and related tumors. p. 163. In Ioachim HL (ed): Pathobiology Annual. Raven Press, New York, 1979.

167. Sherman SP, Chin-Yang L, Carney A: Microproliferation of enterochromaffin cells and the origin of carcinoid tumors of the ileum. Arch Pathol Lab Med 103:639, 1979

168. O'Brian DS, Dayal Y, DeLellis RA, et al: Rectal carcinoids as tumors of the hindgut endocrine cells: a morphological and immunohistochemical analysis. Am J Surg Pathol 6:131, 1982

169. Owen DA, Hwang WS, Thorlakson RH, Walli E: Malignant carcinoid tumor complicating chronic ulcerative colitis. Am J Clin Pathol 76:333, 1981

170. Lindop GBM: Enterochromaffin cell hyperplasia and megacolon: report of a case. Gut 24:575, 1983

171. Dayal Y, O'Briain DS, Wolfe HJ: SRIF and G-cell hyperplasia in duodenal ulcer disease: a morphometric study. Lab Invest 40, No. 2, 1979

172. Arnold R, Hulst MV, Neuhof CH, et al: Antral gastrin-producing G cells and somatostatin-producing D cells in different states of gastric acid secretion. Gut 23:285, 1982

173. Holle GE, Buck E, Pradayrol L, et al: Behavior of somatostatin-immunoreactive cells in the

gastric mucosa before and after selective proximal vagotomy and pyloroplasty in treatment of gastric and duodenal ulcers. Gastroenterology 89:736, 1985

174. Holle GE, Spann W, Eisenmenger W, et al: Diffuse somatostatin-immunoreactive D-cell hyperplasia in the stomach and duodenum. Gastroenterology 91:733, 1986

175. Miller RR, Sumner HW: Argyrophil cell hyperplasia and an atypical carcinoid tumor in chronic ulcerative colitis. Cancer 50:2920, 1982

176. Gledhill A, Enticott ME, Howe S: Variation in the argyrophil cell population of the rectum in ulcerative colitis and adenocarcinoma. J Pathol 149:287, 1986

177. Bishop AE, Pietroletti R, Taat CW, et al: Increased populations of endocrine cells in Crohn's ileitis. Virchows Arch [A] 410, 391, 1987

178. Tehrani MA, Carfrae DC: Carcinoid tumor and Crohn's disease. Br J Clin Pract 29:123, 1975

179. Lampert IA, Thorpe P, Van Noorden S, et al: Selective sparing of enterochromaffin cells in graft versus host diseases affecting the colonic mucosa. Histopathology 9:875, 1985

180. Walker-Smith J: Diseases of the Small Intestine in Childhood. Pitman Medical, London, 1979

181. Williams ED, Sandler M: The classification of carcinoid tumors. Lancet 1:238, 1963

182. Sanders RJ: Carcinoids of the Gastrointestinal Tract. Charles C Thomas, Springfield, IL, 1973

183. Falkmer S, Alumets J, Hakanson R, et al: Occurrence of pancreatic polypeptide, somatostatin, glucagon, insulin, enkephalin, β-endorphin, and substance P cells in rectal carcinoids. p. 351. In Miyoshi A (ed): Gut Peptides, Secretion, Function and Clinical Aspects. Elsevier/North-Holland, Amsterdam, 1977

184. Ritchie AC: Carcinoid tumors. Am J Med Sci 232:311, 1956

185. Black WC, Haffner HE: Diffuse hyperplasia of gastric argyrophil cells and multiple carcinoid tumors: a historical and ultrastructural study. Cancer 21:1080, 1968

186. Goldman H, French S, Burbige E: Kulchitsky cell hyperplasia and multiple metastasizing carcinoids of the stomach. Cancer 47:2620, 1981

187. Morgan JG, Marks C, Hearn D: Carcinoid tumors of the gastrointestinal tract. Ann Surg 180:720, 1974

188. Moertel CG, Sauer WG, Dockerty MB, Bagenstoss AH: Life history of the carcinoid tumor of the small intestine. Cancer 14:901, 1961

189. Zakariai YM, Quan SHQ, Hajdu SI: Carcinoid tumors of the gastrointestinal tract. Cancer 35:588, 1975

190. Kuiper DH, Gracie WA, Pollard HM; Twenty years of gastrointestinal carcinoids. Cancer 25:1424, 1970

191. Brown NK, Smith MP: Neoplastic diathesis of patients with carcinoid; report of a case with four other neoplasms. Cancer: 32:216, 1973

192. Hajdu SI, Winawer SJ, Myers WPL: Carcinoid tumors: a study of 204 cases. Am J Clin Pathol 61:521, 1974

193. Swartzlander FC, Jackman RJ, Dockerty MB: Submucosal rectal nodules: clinicopathologic review. Am J Surg 92:657, 1956

194. Orloff MJ: Carcinoid tumors of the rectum. Cancer 28:175, 1971

195. Weibel LA, Joergenson EJ, Keasbey LE: A clinical study of small bowel tumors. Report of 165 lesions. Am J Gastroenterol 21:466, 1954

196. Spiers RE, Williams ER: Carcinoids of the small bowel. Am J Surg 110:780, 1965

197. McNeal JE: Mechanism of obstruction in carcinoid tumors of the small intestine. Am J Clin Pathol 56:452, 1971

198. Warner TF, O'Reilly G, Lee GA McL: Mesenteric occlusive lesion and ileal carcinoid. Cancer 44:758, 1979

199. Anthony PP, Drury RAB: Elastic vascular sclerosis of mesenteric blood vessels in argentaffin carcinoma. J Clin Pathol 23:110, 1970

200. Dayal Y, O'Brian DS, Wolfe HJ, Reichlin S: Carcinoid tumors: a comparison of their immunocytochemical hormonal profile with morphologic and histochemical characteristics. Lab Invest 42(1):1111, 1980

201. Dayal Y, O'Brian DS, DeLellis RA, Wolfe HJ: Carcinoid tumors in gastrointestinal, and extra intestinal sites: a comparative study of polypeptide hormonal profile. Reg Pept 1:22, 1980

202. Soga J, Tazawa K: Pathologic analysis of carcinoids. Histologic re-evaluation of 62 cases. Cancer 28:990, 1971

203. Murayama H, Imai T, Kikuchi M, Kamio A: Duodenal carcinoid (APUDOMA) with psammoma bodies: a light and electron microscopic study. Cancer 43:1411, 1979

204. Subbuswamy SG, Gibbs NM, Ross CF, Morson BC: Goblet cell carcinoid of the appendix. Cancer 34:338, 1974

205. Klein HZ: Mucinous carcinoid of the vermiform appendix. Cancer 33:770, 1974

206. Jones RA, Dawson IMP: Morphology and staining patterns of endocrine cell tumors in the gut, pancreas and bronchus and their possible significance. Histopathology 1:137, 1977

207. Johnson LA, Weiland L, Geller SA, Dayal Y, et al: Carcinoids: the association of histologic growth pattern and survival in advanced stage disease. Cancer 51:882, 1983

208. Dayal Y, Doos WG, O'Brien MJ, et al: Psammomatous somatostatinomas of the duodenum. Am J Surg Pathol 7:653, 1983

209. Dayal Y, Tallberg KA, Nunnemacher G, et al: Duodenal carcinoids in patients with and without neurofibromatosis: a comparative study. Am J Surg Pathol 10:348, 1986

210. Marcial MA, Pinkus GS, Skarin A, et al: Ampullary somatostatinoma: psammomatous variant of gastrointestinal carcinoid tumor—an immunohistochemical and ultrastructural study. Report of a case and review of the literature. Am J Clin Pathol 80:755, 1983

211. Taccagni GL, Carlucci M, Sironi M, et al: Duodenal somatostatinoma with psammoma bodies: an immunohistochemical and ultrastructural study. Am J Gastroenterol 81: 33, 1986

212. Chen RS, Tang CK, Lee JY, Kurland CL: Duodenal somatostatin-containing tumor with psammoma bodies. Hum Pathol 16:517, 1985

213. Albrecht S, Gardiner GW, Kovacs K, et al: Duodenal somatostatinoma with psammoma bodies. Arch Pathol Lab Med 113:517, 1989

214. Case records of the Massachusetts General Hospital, case 15-1989. N Engl J Med 320: 996, 1989

215. Burke AP, Sobin LH, Shekitka KM, et al: Somatostatin-producing duodenal carcinoids in patients with von Recklinghausen's neurofibromatosis: a predilection for black patients. Cancer 65: 1591, 1990.

216. Abt AB, Carter SL: Goblet cell carcinoid of the appendix. An ultrastructural and histochemical study. Arch Pathol Lab Med 100:301, 1976

217. Chen V, Qizilbash AH: Goblet cell carcinoid tumor of the appendix. Report of five cases and review of the literature. Arch Pathol Lab Med 103:180, 1979

218. Warner TFCs, Seo IS: Goblet cell carcinoid of appendix. Ultrastructural features and histogenic aspects. Cancer 44:1700, 1979

219. Soga J, Tazawa K, Aizawa O, et al: Argentaffin cell adenocarcinoma of the stomach: An atypical carcinoid? Cancer 28:999, 1971

220. Hernandez FJ, Fernandez BB: Mucus-secreting colonic carcinoid tumors: Light and electronmicroscopic study of three cases. Dis Col Rectum 17:387, 1974

221. Warkel RL, Cooper PH, Helwig EB: Adenocarcinoid: a mucin producing carcinoid tumor of the appendix. Cancer 42:2781, 1978

222. Cooper PH, Warkel RL: Ultrastructure of the goblet cell type of adenocarcinoid of the appendix. Cancer 42:2687, 1978

223. Isaacson P: Crypt cell carcinoma of the appendix (so-called adenocarcinoid tumor). Am J Surg Pathol 5:213, 1981

224. Cantor AM, Rigby CC, Beck PR, Mangion D: Neurofibromatosis, pheochromocytoma, and somatostatinoma. Br Med J 285:1618, 1982

225. Giffiths DFR, Jasani B, Newman GR, et al: Glandular duodenal carcinoid—a somatostatin rich tumor with neuroendocrine association, J Clin Pathol 37:163, 1984

226. Kunieda Y, Tamura Y, Sasaki H, et al: Carcinoid of the papilla of Vater—somatostatinoma: a case report. Japn J Cancer Clin 32:831, 1986

227. Goedert M, Otten U, Suda K, et al: Dopamine, norepinephrine and serotonin production by an intestinal carcinoid tumor. Cancer 45:104, 1980

228. Creutzfeldt W, Arnold R, Frerichs H: Insulinomas and gastrinomas. p. 589. In Bloom SR (ed): Gut Hormones. Churchill Livingstone Edinburgh, 1978

229. Kovacs K, Horvath E, Ezrin C, et al: Immunoreactive somatostatin in pancreatic islet-cell carcinoma accompanied by ectopic ACTH syndrome. Lancet 1:1365, 1977

230. Krejs GJ, Orci L, Conlon M, et al: Somatostatinoma syndrome: biochemical, morphologic and clinical features. N Engl J Med 301:285, 1979

231. Galmiche JP, Chayvialle JA, Dubois PM, et al: Calcitonin-producing pancreatic somatostatinoma. Gastroenterology 78:1577, 1980

232. Alumets J, Ekelund G, Hakanson R, et al: Jejunal endocrine tumor composed of somatostatin and gastrin cells and associated with duodenal ulcer disease. Virchows Arch [A] 378:17, 1978

233. Solcia E, Capella C, Buffa R, et al: Pathology of the Zollinger-Ellison syndrome. p. 119. In Fenoglio CM, Wolff M (eds): Progress in Surgical Pathology. Vol. 1. Masson, New York, 1980

234. Bordi C, Ravazzola M, Baetens D, et al: A

study of glucagonomas by light and electronmicroscopy and immunofluorescence. Diabetes 28:925, 1979

235. McDonald RA: A study of 356 carcinoids of the gastrointestinal tract. Am J Med 21:867, 1956

236. Sjoblom SM: Clinical presentation and prognosis of gastrointestinal carcinoid tumors. Scand J Gastroenterol 23:779, 1988

237. Yoshino T, Ohtsuki Y, Shimada Y, et al: Multiple carcinoid tumor combined with mucosal carcinoma of the stomach: a case report. Acta Pathol Jpn 37:1669, 1987

238. Morgan JE, Kaiser CW, Johnson W, et al: Gastric carcinoid (gastrinoma) associated with achlorhydria (pernicious anemia). Cancer May 1983

239. Gueller R, Haddad JK: Gastric carcinoids simulating benign polyps. Two cases diagnosed by endoscopic biopsy. Gastrointest Endosc 21: 153, 1975

240. Dayal Y, Wolfe HJ: Hyperplastic proliferations of gastrointestinal endocrine cells. In Dayal Y (ed): Endocrine Pathology of the Gut and Pancreas. CRC Press, Boca Raton, FL, 1991

241. Soga J, Tazawa K: Pathologic analysis of carcinoids. Histologic re-evaluation of 62 cases. Cancer 28:990, 1971

242. Chejfec G, Gould VE: Malignant gastric neuroendocrinomas. Hum Pathol 8:433, 1977

243. Sweeney EC, McDonnell L: Atypical gastric carcinoids. Histopathology 4:215, 1980

244. Rogers LW, Murphy RC: Gastric carcinoids and gastric carcinoma. Morphologic correlates of survival. Am J Surg Pathol 3:195, 1979

245. Mignon M, Lehy T, Bonnefond A, et al: Development of gastric argyrophil carcinoid tumors in a case of Zollinger-Ellison syndrome with primary hyperparathyroidism during long-term antisecretroy treatment. Cancer 59:1959, 1987

246. Goldfain D, Lebodic MF, Lavergne A, et al: Gastric carcinoid tumors in patients with Zollinger-Ellison syndrome on long term omeprazole. Lancet i:776, 1989

247. Maury CPJ, Tornroth T, Teppo AM: Atrophic gastritis in Sjogren's syndrome: Morphologic, biochemical and immunologic findings. Arthrit Rheum 28:388, 1985

248. Maeda M, Kijima Y, Sakomoto S, Kanayama M: A young female case of myxedema associated with atrophic gastritis (type A) with re-

markable hypergastrinemia. Nippon-Naika-Gakkai Zasshi 73:995, 1984

249. Rooney PJ, Vince M, Dennedy AC, et al: Hypergastrinemia in rheumatoid arthritis. Br Med J 2(869):752, 1973

250. Bruce TA, Azmy M, Earll JM: Gastric carcinoid associated with achlorhydria, hypergastrinemia and Addison's disease. South Med J 81:1595, 1988

251. Leor J, Levartowsky D, Sharon C: Polyglandular autoimmune syndrome, type 2. South Med J 82:374, 1989

252. Spinner MW, Blizzard RM, Gibbs J, et al: Familial distribution of organ specific antibodies in blood of patients with Addison's disease and hypoparathyroidism and their relatives. Clin Exp Immunol 5:461, 1969

253. Adams JF, Glen AIM, Kennedy EH, et al: The histological and secretory changes in the stomach in patients with autoimmunity to gastric parietal cells. Lancet 1:401, 1964

254. Sjoblom SM, Haapianen R, Miettinen M, Jarvinen H: Gastric carcinoid tumors and atrophic gastritis. Acta Chir Scand 153:37, 1987

255. Godwin JD, II: Carcinoid tumors. An analysis of 3837 cases. Cancer 36:560, 1975

256. Stalnikowicz R, Eliakin R, Steiner D, et al: Should gastric carcinoid tumors associated with pernicious anemia be treated aggressively. J Clin Gastroenterol 9:521, 1987

257. Wilander E, Sundstrom CH, Grimelius L: Pernicious anemia in association with argyrophil (Sevier-Munger) gastric carcinoid.t Scand J Hematol 23:415, 1979

258. Goldman H, French S, Burbrige E: Kulchitsky cell hyperplasia and multiple metastasizing carcinoids of the stomach. Cancer 47:2620, 1981

259. Wilander E, Portela-Gomes G, Grimelius L, Westermark P: Argentaffin and argyrophil reactions of human gastrointestinal carcinoids. Gastroenterology 73:733, 1977

260. Wilander E, Grimelius L, Lundquist G, Skoog V: Polypeptide hormones in argentaffin and argyrophil gastroduodenal endocrine tumors. Am J Pathol 96:519, 1979

261. Dayal Y, Wolfe HJ: Regulatory substances in clinically nonfunctioning gastrointestinal carcinoids. p. 497. Falkmer S, Hakanson R, Sundler F (eds): In Evolution and Tumor Pathology of the Neuroendocrine System. Elsevier, Amsterdam, 1984

262. Morgan JE, Kaiser CW, Johnson W, et al:

Gastric carcinoid (gastrinoma) associated with achlorhydria (pernicious anemia). Cancer 51:2332, 1983

263. Black WC III: Enterochromaffin cell types and corresponding carcinoid tumors. Lab Invest 19:473, 1968

264. Creutzfeldt W: The achlorhydria-carcinoid sequence: role of gastrin. Digestion 39:61, 1988

265. Iwafuchi M, Watanabe H, Yanaihara N, Ito S: Immunohistochemical and ultrastructural characteristics of gastric carcinoids. Biomed Res (Suppl 1) 4:307, 1983

266. Solcia E, Capella C, Buffa R, et al: Endocrine cells of the gastrointestinal tract and related tumors. p. 163. In Ioachim HL (ed): Pathobiology Annual. Raven Press, New York, 1979

267. Dische FE: Argentaffin and nonargentaffin carcinoid tumors of the appendix. J Clin Pathol 21:60, 1968

268. Wilander E, Grimelius L, Portela-Gomes G, et al: Substance P and enteroglucagon-like immunoreactivity in argentaffin and argyrophil mid gut carcinoid tumors. Scand J Gastroenterol 14(suppl 53):19, 1979

269. Wilander E, El-Salhy M: Immunocytochemical staining of mid-gut carcinoid tumors with sequence-specific gastrin antisera. Acta Pathol Microbiol Scand (sect A) 89:247, 1981

270. Alumets J, Hakanson R, Ingemansson S, Sundler F: Substance P and 5-HT in granules isolated from an intestinal argentaffin carcinoid. Histochemistry 52:217, 1977

271. Scott JE: Carcinoid tumors of the colon. Br J Surg 60:684, 1973

272. Greenwood SM, Huvos AG, Erlandson RA, Malt SH: Rectal carcinoid and rectal adenocarcinoma: a case report and review of the literature. Dis Colon Rect 17:644, 1974

273. O'Briain DS, Dayal Y, DeLellis RA, et al: Rectal carcinoids as tumors of the hindgut endocrine cells: a morphological and immunohistochemical analysis. Am J Surg Pathol 6:131, 1982

274. Taxy JB, Mendelsohn G, Gupta PK: Carcinoid tumors of the rectum: Silver reactions, fluorescence, and serotonin content of the cytoplasmic granules. Am J Clin Pathol 74:791, 1980

275. Yoshida A, Yano M, Fujinaga Y, et al: Argentaffin carcinoid tumor of the rectum. Cancer 48:2103, 1981

276. Alumets J, Alm P, Falkmer S, et al: Immunohistochemical evidence of peptide hormones in endocrine tumors of the rectum. Cancer 48:2409, 1981

277. Willander E, Portela-Gomes G, Grimelius L, et al: Enteroglucagon and substance P-like immunoreactivity in argentaffin and argyrophil rectal carcinoids. Virchows Arch [B] 25:117, 1977

278. Lembeck F: 5-Hydroxytryptamine in carcinoid tumors. Nature 172:910, 1953

279. Pernow B, Waldenstrom J: Paroxysmal flushing and other symptoms caused by 5-hydroxytryptamine and histamine in patients with malignant tumors. Lancet ii:951, 1954

280. Thorson A: Studies on carcinoid disease. Acta Med Scand Suppl 334:1, 1958

281. Thorson A, Bjork G, Bjorkmann G, Waldenstrom J: Malignant carcinoid of small intestine with metastases to liver, valvular disease of the right side of the heart (pulmonary stenosis and tricuspid regurgitation without septal defects), peripheral vasomotor symptoms, broncho constriction, and an unusual type of cyanosis. Am Heart J 44:795, 1954

282. Grahame-Smith DG: The Carcinoid Syndrome. Heinemann, London, 1972, p. 76

283. Grahame-Smith DG: Natural history and diagnosis of the carcinoid syndrome. p. 575. In Bonfils S (ed): Clinics in Gastroenterology. Vol. 3, No. 3. WB Saunders, London, 1974

284. Azzopardi JG: Systemic effects of neoplasia. p. 98. In Harrison CV (ed): Recent Advances in Pathology. 8th ed. J & A Churchill, London, 1966

285. Sandler M, Snow PJD: An atypical carcinoid tumor secreting 5-hydroxytryptophan. Lancet i:137, 1958

286. Oates JA, Butler TC: Pharmacologic and endocrine aspects of carcinoid syndrome. Adv Pharmacol Chemother 5:109, 1967

287. Sjoerdsma A, Weissbach H, Udenfriend S: Clinical, physiological and biochemical study of patients with malignant carcinoid (argentaffinoma). Am J Med 20:520, 1956

288. Beaton H, Homan W: Gastrointestinal carcinoids and the malignant carcinoid syndrome. SGO 152:268, 1981

289. Peart WS, Porter KA, Robertson JIS, et al: Carcinoid syndrome due to pancreatic-duct neoplasm secreting 5-hydroxytryptophan and 5-hydroxytryptamine. Lancet i:239, 1963

290. Dollinger MR, Ratner LH, Shamoian CA, Blackbourne BD: Carcinoid syndrome associated with pancreatic tumors. Arch Intern Med 120:575, 1967

291. Gordon DL, Lo MC, Schwartz MA: Carcinoid of the pancreas. Am J Med 51:412, 1971

292. Patchefsky AS, Gordon G, Harrer WV, Hoch WS: Carcinoid tumor of the pancreas: ultrastructural observations of a lymph node metastasis and comparison with bronchial carcinoid. Cancer 33:1349, 1974

293. Davis Z, Moertel CG, McIlrath DC: The malignant carcinoid syndrome. Surg Gynecol Obstet 137:637, 1973

294. Chatterjee K, Heather JC: Carcinoid heart disease from primary ovarian carcinoid tumors. Am J Med 45:643, 1968

295. Zollinger RM, Ellison EM: Primary peptic ulceration of the jejunum associated with islet cell tumors of the pancreas. Ann Surg 142:709, 1955

296. Zollinger RM, Coleman DW: The Influences of Pancreatic Tumors on the Stomach. Charles C Thomas, Springfield, IL, 1974, p. 1

297. Dayal Y, O'Briain DS: The pathology of the pancreatic endocrine cells. p. 111. In DeLellis RA (ed): Diagnostic Immunohistochemistry. Masson, New York, 1981

298. Walsh JH, Grossman MI: Gastrin. N Engl J Med 292:1324, 1377, 1975

299. Wolfe MM, Jensen RT: Zollinger-Ellison syndrome: current concepts in diagnosis and management. N Engl J Med 317:1200, 1987

300. Hoffman JW, Fox PS, Wilson SD: Duodenal wall tumors and the Zollinger-Ellison syndrome. Arch Surg 107:334, 1973

301. Antonioli DA, Dayal Y, Dvorak AM, Banks PA: Zollinger-Ellison syndrome secondary to a GRF-containing jejunal gastrinoma: clinical and morphological features. Gastroenterology 92:814, 1987

302. Bhagavan BS, Slavin RE, Goldberg J, Rao RN: Ectopic gastrinoma and Zollinger-Ellison syndrome. Hum Pathol 17:584, 1986

303. Nord KS, Joshi V, Hanna M, et al: Zollinger-Ellison syndrome associated with renal gastrinoma in a child. J Pediatr Gastroenterol Nutr 5:980, 1986

304. Miyata M, Nakao K, Sakamoto T, et al: Removal of mesenteric gastrinoma: A case report. Surgery 99:245, 1986

305. Creutzfeldt W, Arnold R, Creutzfeldt C, Track NS: Pathomorphologic, biochemical and diagnostic aspects of gastrinomas (Zollinger-Ellison syndrome). Hum Pathol 6:47, 1975

306. Royston CMS, Brew DSJ, Garnham JR, et al: The Zollinger-Ellison syndrome due to an infiltrating tumor of the stomach. Gut 13:638, 1972

307. Larsson LI, Ljungberg O, Sundler F, et al: An antropyloric gastrinoma associated with pancreatic nesidioblastosis and proliferation of islets. Virchows Arch [A] 360:305, 1973

308. Bhagavan BS, Hofkin GA, Woel GM, Koss LG: Zollinger-Ellison syndrome: Ultrastructural and histochemical observations in a child with endocrine tumorlets of gastric antrum. Arch Pathol 98:217, 1974

309. Kovacs K, Horvath E, Ezrin C: Pituitary adenomas. p. 341. In Sommers SC, Rosen PP (eds): Pathology Annual 1977, pt 2. Appleton-Century-Crofts, East Norwalk, CT, 1977

310. Larsson LI, Hirsch MA, Holst JJ, et al. Pancreatic somatostatinoma: clinical features and physiologic implications. Lancet 1:666, 1977

311. Ganda OP, Weir GC, Soeldner JS, et al: "Somatostatinoma": a somatostatin-containing tumor of the endocrine pancreas. N Engl J Med 296:963, 1977

312. Pipeleers D, Somers G, Gepts W, et al: Plasma pancreatic hormone levels in a case of somatostatinoma: diagnostic and therapeutic implications. J Clin Endocrinol Metab 49:572, 1979

313. Gerlock AJ, Muhletaler CA, Halter S, Goncharenko V: Pancreatic somatostatinoma: Histologic, clinical, and angiographic features. Am J Radiol 133:939, 1979

314. Kaneko H, Yanaihara N, Ito S, et al: Somatostatinoma of the duodenum. Cancer 44:2273, 1979

315. Dayal Y, Ganda OP: Somatostatin producing tumors. In Dayal Y, (ed): Endocrine Pathology of the Gut and Pancreas. CRC Press, Boca Raton, FL, 1991

316. Alumets J, Ekelund G, Hakanson R, et al: Jejunal endocrine tumor composed of somatostatin and gastrin cells and associated with duodenal ulcer disease. Virchows Arch [A] 378:17, 1978

317. Murayama H, Imai T, Kikuchi M, Kamio A: Duodenal carcinoid (APUDoma) with psammoma bodies: a light and electron microscopic study. Cancer 43:1411, 1979

318. Weichert RF III, Reed R Creech O Jr: Carcinoid-islet cell tumors of the duodenum. Ann Surg 165:660, 1967

319. Vinik AI, Strodel WE, Lloyd RV: Unusual gastroenteropancreatic (GEP) tumors and their hormones. p. 293. In Thompson NW, Vinik AL (eds): Endocrine Surgery Update. Grune & Stratton, Orlando FL, 1983

320. Stamm B, Hedinger Chr. E, Saremaslani P: Duodenal and ampullary carcinoid tumors: a report of 12 cases with pathological characteristics, polypeptide content and relation to the MEN-1 syndrome and von Recklinghausen's

disease (neurofibromatosis). Virchows Arch [A] 408:475, 1986

321. Burke AP, Federspiel BH, Sobin LH, et al: Carcinoids of the duodenum: a histologic and immunohistochemical study of 65 tumors. Am J Surg Pathol 13:828, 1989

322. Ross MD, Dent RI: Foregut APUDomas in Zimbabwe-Rhodesian Africans. Clin Oncol 6: 167, 1980

323. Weder W, Saremaslani P, Maurer P: Calciton-inbildendes duodenal Karzinoid bei Neurofibro-matose von Recklinghausen. Schweiz Med Wochenschr 113:885, 1983

324. Johnson L, Weaver M: von Recklinghausen's disease and gastrointestinal carcinoids. JAMA 245:2496, 1981

325. Hough DR, Chan A, Davidson H: von Reck-linghausen's disease associated with gastroin-testinal carcinoid tumors. Cancer 51:2206, 1983

326. Dawson BV, Kazama R, Paplanus SH: Associa-tion of carcinoid with neurofibromatosis. South Med J 77:511, 1984

327. Gerich JE, Patton GS: Somatostatin, physiol-ogy and clinical applications. Med Clin N Am 62:375, 1978

328. Hibi M, Kato Y, Minura Y, et al: Malignant somatostatinoma of the papilla of Vater with neurofibromatosis. J Jpn Soc Gastroenterol Surg 18:2387, 1985

329. Malone MJ, Silverman ML, Braasch JW, et al: Early somatostatinoma of the papilla of the duct of Santorini. Arch Surg 120:1381, 1985

330. Takegawa S, Hagiwara T, Ishii H, et al: A case of duodenal somatostatinoma and a review of the literature. J Jpn Gastroenterol Soc 82:1780, 1985

331. Kock KF, Sanderman J: A polypoid duodenal somatostatinoma: a case report. Scand J Gas-troenterol 23:100, 1988

332. Axelrod L, Busch MA, Hirsch HJ, Loo SWH: Malignant somatostatinoma: clinical features and metabolic studies. J Clin Endocrinol Metab 52:886, 1981

333. Shirouzu K, Miyamoto Y, Shiramizu T, Mori-matsu M: Somatostatinoma of the pancreas. Acta Pathol Jpn 35:1285, 1985

334. Davis RB, Kennedy BJ: Carcinoid syndrome associated with adrenal hyperplasia. Arch Intern Med 109:192, 1962

335. Hirata Y, Sakamoto N, Yamamoto H, et al: Gastric carcinoid with ectopic production of ACTH and beta-MSH. Cancer 37:377, 1976

336. Marcus FS, Friedman MA, Callen PW, et al: Successful therapy of an ACTH-producing gas-tric carcinoid APUD tumor: report of a case and review of the literature. Cancer 46:1263, 1980

337. Heitz PU, Kloppel G, Polak JM, Staub JJ: Ec-topic hormone production by endocrine tumors: localization of hormones at the cellular level by immunocytochemistry. Cancer 48:2029, 1981

338. Coscia M, Brown RD, Miller M, et al: Ectopic production of antidiuretic hormone, adrenocor-ticotrophic hormone and beta-melanocyte stim-ulating hormone by an oat cell carcinoma of the lung. Am J Med 62:303, 1977

339. Azzopardi JE, Williams FD: Pathology of non-endocrine tumors associated with Cushing's syndrome. Cancer 22:274, 1968

340. DeLellis RA, Wolfe HJ: Multiple endocrine adenomatosis syndromes. p. 1648 In Holland JF, Frei E III (eds): Cancer Medicine. 2nd ed. Lea & Febiger, Philadelphia, 1982

341. Wermer P: Multiple endocrine adenomatosis; multiple hormone-producing tumors, a familial syndrome. p. 671. In Bonfils S (ed): Clinics in Gastroenterology. Vol 3. WB Saunders, Philadelphia, 1974

342. Lee HY, Garber PE: Recklinghausen's disease associated with pheochromocytoma and carci-noid tumor. Ohio St Med J 66:583, 1970

343. Arnesjo B, Idvall I, Ihse I, et al: Concomittant occurrence of neurofibromatosis and carcinoid of the intestine. Scand J Gastroenterol 8:637, 1973

344. Garcia JC, Carney JA, Stickler GB, et al: Zol-linger-Ellison syndrome and neurofibromatosis in a 13-year-old boy. J Pediatr 93:982, 1978

345. Hough DR: Von Recklinghausen's disease as-sociated with gastrointestinal carcinoid tumors. Cancer, May 1983

346. DeLellis RA, Dayal Y, Tischler AS, et al: Mul-tiple endocrine neoplasia (MEN) syndromes: cellular origins and interrelationships. p. 163. In Richter GW, Epstein MA (eds): Review of Experimental Pathology. Vol. 28. Academic Press, San Diego, 1986

347. Wheeler MH, Curley LR, Williams ED: The association of neurofibromatosis, pheochromo-cytoma, and somatostatin-rich duodenal carci-noid tumor. Surgery 100:1163, 1986

348. Griffiths DFR, Williams GT, Williams ED: Duodenal carcinoid tumors, pheochromocy-

toma and neurofibromatosis. Islet cell tumor, pheochromocytoma and the Von-Hipple-Lindau complex: two distinctive neuroendocrine syndromes. Quart J Med 64:769, 1987

349. Simmons TC, Henderson DR, Gletten F, et al: The association of neurofibromatosis, psammomatous ampullary carcinoid tumor and extrahepatic biliary obstruction. J Clin Gastroenterol 9:490, 1987

350. Saurenmann P, Binswanger R, Maurer R, et al: Somatostatin-producing tumor in Recklinghausen's neurofibromatosis. Case report and literature review. Schweiz Med Wochenschr 117:1134, 1987

351. Swinburn BA, Yeong ML, Lane MR, et al: Neurofibromatosis associated with somatostatinoma: a report of two patients. Clin Endocrinol (Oxford) 28:353, 1988

352. Stephens M, Williams GT, Jasani B, Williams ED: Synchronous duodenal neuroendocrine tumors in von Recklinghausen's disease—A case report of co-existing gangliocytic paraganglioma and somatostatin-rich glandular carcinoid. Histopathology 11:1331, 1987

353. Wermer P: Genetic aspects of adenomatosis of endocrine glands. Am J Med 16:363, 1954

354. Gerstein JD, Muir RW: Zollinger-Ellison syndrome: a review. Am Surg 41:230, 1975

355. Isenberg JI, Walsh JH, Grossman MI: Zollinger-Ellison syndrome. Gastroenterology 65:140, 1973

356. Weichert RF, Roth LM, Krementz RL, Drapanas T: Carcinoid-islet cell tumors of the duodenum; report of twenty-one cases. Am J Surg 121:195, 1971

357. Grimelius L, Strand A: Ultrastructural studies of the argyrophil reaction in alpha$_1$ cells in human pancreatic islets. Virchows Arch [A] 364:129, 1974

358. Kubo T, Watanabe H: Neoplastic argentaffin cells in gastric and intestinal adenocarcinomas. Cancer 27:447, 1971

359. Clayton F, Sibley RK, Ordonez NG, Hanssen G: Argyrophilic breast carcinomas; evidence of lactational differentiation. Am J Surg Pathol 6:323, 1982

11

Neoplasms of the Anus

Elson B. Helwig

ANAL CANAL AND ANORECTAL JUNCTION

The histologic patterns of carcinomas involving the anal canal and the anorectal junction are usually diverse. The variations cannot readily be explained on the basis of origin either from the stratified squamous epithelium of the anal canal or from the epithelium of the rectal mucosa.

In 1880 Herrmann and Desfosses[1] wrote in a paper that was later used principally by writers dealing with anal ducts that "the mucosa of the inferior portion of the rectum is not directly continuous with the external tegment. There exists at the level corresponding to the columns of Morgagni a circular zone measuring between 0.6 to 1.2 cm that represents a persistent remnant of the cloaca of the embryo. This cloacal region is covered with a special mucosa that is found limiting the rectum and joining below with skin by a sharp transition." In a separate paper Herrmann[2] wrote in detail about the embryology and histology of the zone and discussed the part played in the proctologic diseases by the junction and the anal ducts that arise from it.

In 1935 Tucker and Hellwig[3] called attention to the inadequate recognition in textbooks that the rectal mucosa does not join directly with the epidermis of the anal canal. They pointed out that a small section of an intermediate zone

of the anal canal might objectively be misinterpreted as urethra with paraurethral ducts, and they stressed the cloacal origin of the region. Tucker in the following year attributed islands of transitional epithelium in anal canals to persistance of embryologic structure of cloacal origin.

In 1956 Grinvalsky and Helwig[4] studied the anorectal junction and anus from 25 consecutive abdominoperineal resections in order to confirm the observations made by Herrmann, by Tucker and Hellwig, and by Tucker and to relate the histologic anal structure to the types of neoplasms occurring in this region. On gross examination (Fig. 11-1) the level of the rectal mucosa is accentuated by the irregular transversely disposed dentate line. The dentate line represents the upper limit of a distinct zone, 0.3 to 1.1 cm wide, also transversely disposed, corresponding to the columns and sinuses of Morgagni, and terminating at the level of the anal valves. The mucosa of this zone is distinguished by the glistening, delicately wrinkled, membranous appearance, which contrasts with the velvety character of the rectal mucosa and the thicker, opaque look of the anal mucosa. In some specimens ridges of opaque anal mucosa, especially on the surface of the columns of Morgagni, interrupt the membranous zone, and the anal mucosa appears to join directly with rectal mucosa. However, in the sinuses of Morgagni the membranous appearance of the zone persists; in these sinuses minute porelike openings of the anal ducts can occasionally be identified.

Histologically the membranous mucosa at the anorectal junction is composed of transitional or stratified columnar epithelium five to seven

The opinions or assertions contained herein are the private views of the author and are not to be construed as official or as reflecting the views of the Department of the Army or the Department of Defense.

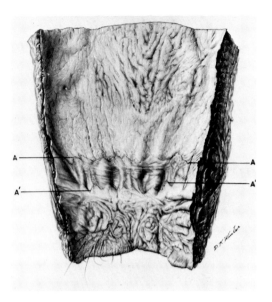

Fig. 11-1. Drawing of a gross specimen showing transversely wrinkled membranous cloacal segment (A–A') interposed between the anal mucosa and rectal mucosa.

cells thick and thrown into broad and crested but delicate folds. The mucosa can be divided into three levels or zones.

The *basal zone* shows a single layer of thin elongated cells with club-shaped nuclei often arranged in a palisaded manner on the connective tissue of the lamina propria. Cells typical of the basal zone are not uniformly present, and cells of the intermediate zone may rest on the lamina propria.

The *intermediate zone* is three to five cells thick and consists of thin elongated or polyhedral cells with fusiform or club shapes. The nuclei may vary in size, but generally the nuclei and cells are oriented perpendicularly to the surface. The cytoplasm is finely granular and may contain minute vacuoles.

The *surface zone* shows a variety of cells. In recesses between folds and on the ascending margins of the folds, a single layer of columnar cells with narrow bases is present. The nuclei are located in the basal position of the cells and aligned to produce a palisaded effect. Fine cytoplasmic processes extend from the surface

cells to between the cells of the intermediate zone. The cytoplasm of the surface columnar cells is progressively more foamy at the free border.

Over the surface of the membranous folds the cells are often flattened or lunate, with their long axis parallel to the surface and forming a cap over two or three columnar cells. The columnar cells, as they gradually ascend, become cuboidal and ultimately lunate with an acidophilic homogeneous cytoplasm. Typical goblet cells are dispersed among the cells of the surface zone and are more numerous among the columnar cells. In scattered foci intramucosal flasklike groups of plump mucinous cells resembling Brunn's nests are present.

Histochemically the columnar cells of the surface mucosa, the goblet cells, and intramucosal clusters of mucous cells stain positive with mucicarmine stain. The surface lunate cells and the more superficial cells of the intermediate zone may stain faintly positive. The periodic acid–Schiff (PAS) preparations with prior diastase digestion shows a more intense positive reaction than is seen in the mucicarmine stain.

The transitional epithelium usually extends from the glandular rectal mucosa to the tips of the anal valves, where it joins the stratified squamous epithelium of the anal mucosa. Sometimes the anal stratified squamous epithelium extends proximally over the anal valves and over the columns of Morgagni. Rarely it involves the sinuses of Morgagni and the superficial segments of the anal ducts arising in this location.

Two types of accessory structures—the anal ducts and aberrant glands—originate in the membranous (transitional) mucosa of the anorectal junction.

The anal ducts are noted in the region of the sinuses of Morgagni. They are long, tubular structures that show little branching but follow a tortuous course through the lamina propria (Fig. 11-2). They usually extend caudad for a short distance in the lamina propria before penetrating the internal anal sphincter muscle. The anal ducts may also extend cephalad under the rectal mucosa for at least several millimeters. The anal ducts penetrate the internal sphincter

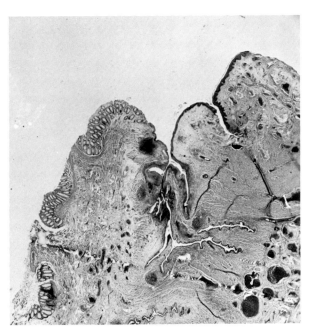

Fig. 11-2. Cloacal zone of the anal canal with branching and deeply penetrating anal duct. (H&E, ×
12.5.)

to various depths and may extend into the adventitial fat.

The anal ducts are lined by transitional or stratified columnar epithelium that is four to six cells thick at the anorectal junction but distally decreases to two or three cells in thickness as it penetrates the internal sphincter muscle. The surface layer cells are sometimes flat but often are mucous cells and distinct goblet cells. Mucicarmine and PAS preparations after diastase are positive. In the most distal regions the lumens of the ducts become less manifest, and in some terminal segments a scalloped configuration of cuboidal epithelium separated by transitional epithelium is found.

Aberrant mucosal glands occur in the recesses between the folds of the membranous anorectal mucosa (Fig. 11-3). The glands rarely branch, and they are composed of an internal layer of cylindrical mucous cells with small basal nuclei surrounded by a layer of 2 to 10 transitional or undifferentiated cells.

The lamina propria is a richly vascularized layer of collagenous fibers oriented parallel to the surface. Among the collagenous fibers and in the columns of Morgagni are smooth muscle cells that sometimes form bundles. A recognizable basement membrane is not noted between the transitional mucosa and the lamina propria.

The cloacogenic segment of the anal canal has characteristics that resemble those seen in regions of the urinary tract. The transitional zone is similar to the mucosa of the urinary bladder neck and prostatic urethra, and the stratified columnar epithelial areas are similar to the mucosa of the membranous urethra. The anal cloacogenic zone is interpreted as a remnant of cloacal entoderm. Gillespie and MacKay[5] by electron microscopy concluded that the cloacogenic transitional epithelium incorporates features of both uroepithelium and squamous epithelium.

CLOACOGENIC CARCINOMA

The histogenetic significance of the anal cloacogenic segment and its related glands and anal ducts is reflected in the varied histologic

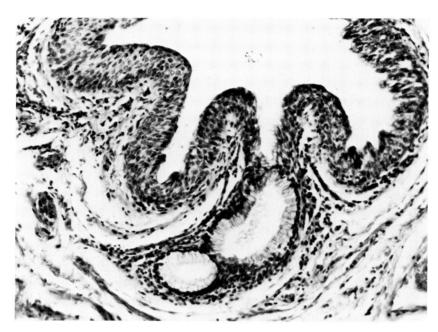

Fig. 11-3. Transitional epithelium of the membranous zone with an aberrant gland lined with cylindrical mucous cells surrounded by undifferentiated cells. (H&E, × 180.)

patterns that occur. The interrelated and complex mingling of the various cell types forming the epithelial components of the cloacogenic zone and accessory structures seems adequate to explain the wide variation in the histologic patterns of tumors involving this region.[4, 6] Another effect of the several histologic pictures identified in the tumors is the corresponding profusion of terms used to designate the neoplasms. These include so-called *basal cell carcinoma, basal-squamous cell epithelioma, basaloid carcinoma, epidermoid carcinoma, cylindroma, anal duct carcinoma, mucoepidermoid carcinoma, adenoacanthoma, atypical carcinoma, cloacogenic carcinoma, and transitional cell carcinoma.*[6] Because carcinomas of the anorectal junction have histologic patterns that relate to the embryologic remnants of the cloaca, the terms *transitional cloacogenic carcinoma* and *cloacogenic carcinoma* seem most appropriate.

Cloacogenic carcinoma is an uncommon but not rare tumor that probably accounts for no more than 3 percent of all anorectal cancers.[7–11] In an unreported study of 231 cases

of cloacogenic carcinoma the average age of the patients was 54 years. The youngest patient at the time of diagnosis was 20 years, and the oldest 90 years. Men were affected slightly more often than women, but the patient population was predominantly male. Others have reported a much greater incidence in women. Ninety percent of the patients were white, 7 percent black, and the remainder of other ethnic groups. The most common signs and symptoms were rectal bleeding (72 percent), rectal pain (50 percent), rectal mass (50 percent), change of bowel habits (36 percent), and weight loss (15 percent). Other signs and symptoms were tenesmus, loss of sphincter control, rectal discharge, burning, a feeling of pressure, and low back pain. Polypoid tumors were infrequent. Sixty-five percent of the carcinomas metastasized. The most common metastatic sites were the regional nodes, including retroperitoneal nodes (59 percent), liver (28 percent), bladder (24 percent), rectal skin and perineum (22 percent), prostate (20 percent), pelvis (19 percent), and pelvic bones (10 percent).

The most common co-existing diseases at the

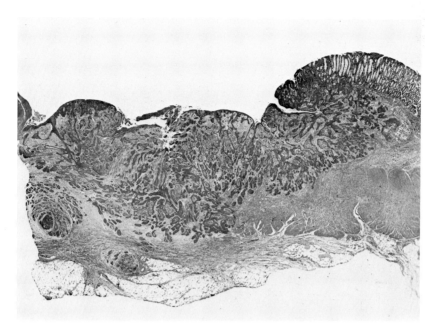

Fig. 11-4. The transitional membranous zone is replaced by a cloacogenic transitional carcinoma invading into the adjacent fibrofatty tissue. (H&E, × 8.)

time of surgery were hemorrhoids (60 percent) and rectal fissure (27 percent).

The size of the tumors ranged from 1 to 13 cm in diameter, with an average of 4.2 cm. Grodsky[7] has emphasized that no typical gross clinical feature aids in differentiating cloacogenic carcinomas arising in the intermediate membranous zone above the anal crypts from mucosal or keratinizing epidermoid malignancy.

The histologic appearance of the cloacogenic tumors may vary because of the complex epithelium from which they arise (Figs. 11-4 and 11-5). The predominant pattern is that of a transitional cell carcinoma similar to that seen in the urinary bladder. The cells vary from distinctly transitional-type elongated cells and nuclei to short cuboidal cells (basaloid) with almost round nuclei.[12] The basaloid cells are considered to represent undifferentiated basal cells probably having origin within the basal layer of anal transitional epithelium and the basaloid tumor a less differentiated form of cloacogenic carcinoma. The tumor cells occur in variable but often large infiltrating masses, and the more

differentiated tumors frequently contain areas of squamoid differentiation with parakeratinization. At the periphery of the epithelial masses the cells are sometimes aligned in palisade fashion but usually not in the distinct manner seen in basal cell carcinoma of the skin. Mitotic figures are present, but marked pleomorphism and multinucleated cells are seldom numerous.

Variations from the strictly transitional pattern take place in which not only islands of squamous cells are noted but in which the whole process is squamoid (Fig. 11-6). The squamous cells mature by parakeratosis. In other tumors irregular islands of transitional cells contain mucous cells stainable with the mucicarmine and PAS techniques. The mucous cells rarely form nests surrounded by the transitional cells.

Of those patients from whom information was obtained, about two-thirds exhibited metastasis at some time during the illness. At the last known follow-up nearly two-thirds of the patients were dead. Approximately 70 percent of the patients were treated by surgical means, 19 percent by radiation therapy, and most of the remaining

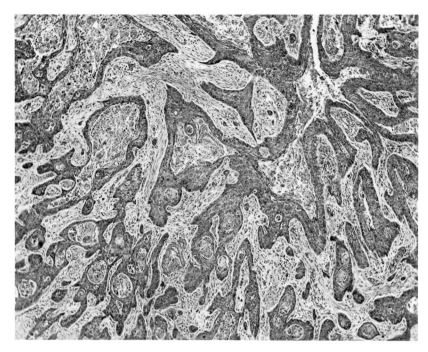

Fig. 11-5. Cloacogenic transitional cell carcinoma with irregular fingerlike projections of atypical transitional epithelium invading the stroma. (H&E, × 50.)

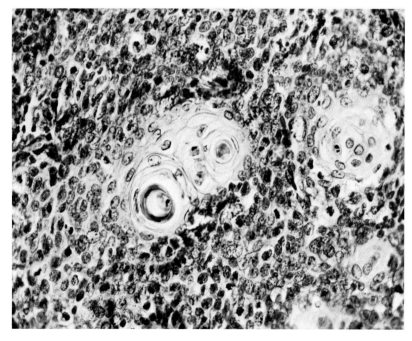

Fig. 11-6. Mass of an atypical transitional tumor cells shows foci of squamoid differentiation. (H&E, × 350.)

by combintaions of surgical therapy, radiation therapy, and chemotherapy. Others have reported poor results with various types and combinations of treatment.[6, 13]

Carbrera et al.[14] noted that in women anal carcinoma may be more than casually associated with cancer of the lower genital tract and that the areas are derived from closely related embryologic anlagen. They recommend careful follow-up of this group of patients.

ANAL DUCT CARCINOMA

Since the genesis of the anal ducts and anal glands is linked to that of the anal cloacogenic membranous zone, similar types of epithelial tumors develop and the necessity of a separate category of carcinoma is questionable.[6] The course of the anal ducts has certain implications in the evaluation of the tumors in this region. The ducts not only extend outward from the cloacogenic membranous zone but also occasionally are directed cephalad or upward beneath the rectal mucosa for a considerable distance. Still more commonly they extend caudad or downward beneath the anal mucosa and even penetrate the surrounding fat. Carcinoma arising in the anal ducts infiltrates not only outward in relation to the anal canal but sometimes also inward, causing a breach filled with tumor in the normal mucosa of either the lower rectum or anal canal.

The histologic patterns of the ductal carcinomas are similar to those arising in the anal cloacogenic zone, including variation of squamous, transitional, and mucinous carcinoma.[15–17] In this manner squamous cell carcinomas may originate externally to the rectum and secondarily appear in the rectal lumen. It is difficult to establish the primary site of the carcinoma in the cloacogenic region when the tumor is large and destructive of the original landmarks. Furthermore, in some small carcinomas the carcinomatous transition is present not only in the anal ducts but also in the anal cloacogenic membranous zone, indicating an inclusive primaary site. Only if the carcinomatous transition is limited

to the ducts is it a strictly ductal carcinoma. In most examples the ductal carcinomas show prolongations of atypical transitional cells arranged in large ductal configurations or solid cords (Fig. 11-7). Central epithelial cells may be parakeratotic and degenerated and appear as if filling a pseudolumen. This histologic picture varies if the epithelial cells exhibit other differentiating features. The tumor tends to infiltrate widely and may induce stenosis of the anal canal.

The anal ducts extending caudad or downward have been recognized as a pathogenic factor in the development of fistula-in-ano and ischiorectal abscess. These fistulous tracts and perianal abscesses are not only relatively common but also are characteristically slowly progressive. The slow insidious clinical course and the lack of obvious gross tumor involving the anal mucosa obscures the presence of any underlying carcinoma.[18–20] Usually the first clue to the presence of a carcinoma happens with the examination of tissue removed in the course of treatment of a fistula or longstanding firm painful masses in the perianus and buttock.

Perianal mucinous carcinomas are uncommon tumors, as indicated by the few reports, with mostly single cases recorded in the literature.[21]

Histologically periductal mucinous carcinomas grow in different patterns. In one pattern the predominant picture is that of collections of mucin infiltrating among and separating the stromal layers. It is more or less easy to discern mucin-secreting cells in association with the mucin. Examination of several fields may be necessary. The mucous cells often show only a minor degree of atypia, making it difficult to judge whether or not they are malignant. This determination rests upon identifying more atypia than would be expected in the cylindrical mucous cells of a benign process such as colitis cystica profunda, in which mucin also infiltrates the stroma.[22] Clumps of atypical mucous cells with hyperchromatic nuclei, especially if situated within the stroma, favor a malignant diagnosis. Other mucinous carcinomas are differentiated with irregular but distinct glandlike patterns lined by pleomorphic cylindrical mucous cells.[17]

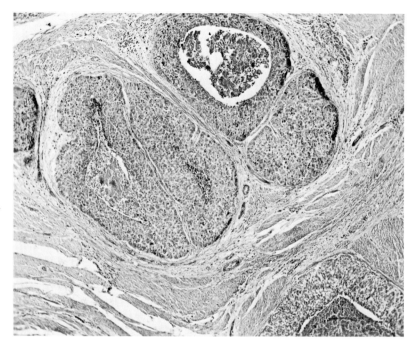

Fig. 11-7. Anal duct cloacogenic transitional cell carcinoma invading the internal sphincter muscle. The tumor cells centrally show degeneration. (H&E, × 50.)

In this type of mucinous adenocarcinoma distinct infiltration of the stroma almost always is present, and the diagnosis of carcinoma is unquestionable.

Another pattern of mucinous carcinoma of the perianal area is the adenocystic type, in which small acinar nests of atypical mucous cells seem to float in a sea of mucus.

Finally, a few perianal mucinous carcinomas contain foci of squamous differentiation and are referred to by some as *muco-epidermoid tumors*.[16]

The clinical behavior of the anal duct carcinomas depends not only on the histologic appearance but also on the anatomic location. The mucinous carcinomas located in the perianal region tend to recur after excision and metastasize to the inguinal lymph nodes.

The question of the origin of carcinoma associated with anal fistula and perianal abscess has not been resolved completely. Most likely it is related to the anal ducts rather than the apocrine glands, which are capable of secreting mucin as demonstrated in anogenital Paget's disease. Histochemical studies also have shown the presence of mucin in the normal apocrine glands of the anogenital region.

SQUAMOUS CELL CARCINOMA

Squamous cell carcinoma (epidermoid carcinoma) of the anal canal arises mostly in the lower segment of the canal at the junction with the perianal skin.[23–25] In this area of junction an overlapping of the endoderm and ectoderm occurs.

Squamous cell carcinoma occurs about twice as frequently as cloacogenic carcinoma.[6] Women are affected three times as often as men, and the peak age for both sexes is in the fifth and sixth decades.

The most frequent clinical sign is rectal bleeding, which commonly appears in association with either flat or verrucous painful tumor masses.

Prior diseases or lesions are alleged factors in the cause of squamous cell carcinoma. These varied conditions include fistula, long-standing irritations, condylomas, syphilis, irradiation change, and infections, such as human papillomavirus (HPV).[26]

Histologically most carcinomas tend to show considerable differentiation toward polygonal squamoid cells with scattered squamous pearls. A few tumors are poorly differentiated and grow in unorganized cell masses with marked cell pleomorphism and many mitotic figures.

According to Singh et al.[6] about one-half of the carcinomas have already invaded the sphincter muscles and one-fourth have metastasized to lymph nodes at the first examination. Recurrence increases with the depth of invasion and commonly occurs in the pelvis and perineum.

The overall survival is slightly less than 50 percent.

CARCINOMA IN SITU

Carcinoma in situ of the anal canal takes place in each of the segments. The incidence in each segment is probably proportional to the incidence of invasive carcinoma.[27, 28]

Histologically the mucosa is usually thickened, and there are cytologic changes similar to those noted in invasive carcinoma (Fig. 11-8). The dysplastic change involves the mucosa in a diffuse manner rather than in the patchy (''salt and pepper'') distribution observed in bowenoid papulosis, from which it must be differentiated. Since keratinization is not a promi-

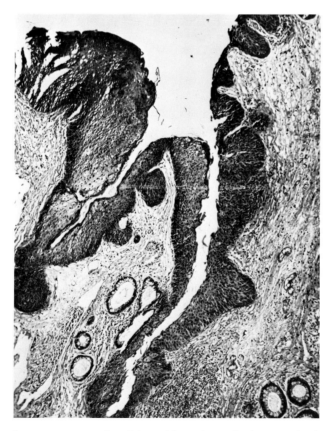

Fig. 11-8. Anal membranous mucosa and anal duct with carcinoma in situ occurring in a male homosexual. (H&E, × 60.)

nent feature of the normal mucosa of the anal canal, it follows that dyskeratosis (individual cell keratinization) is less conspicuous in carcinoma is situ.

Although clinically carcinoma in situ appears as white plaques, the designation of *leukoplakia* pathologically is inappropriate and misleading. Benign entities such as lichen sclerosis et atrophicus also appear as white perianal plaques but histologically are not carcinoma in situ.[29] The characteristic histologic picture of lichen sclerosis et atrophicus is hyperkeratosis and epidermal atrophy without dysplasia, liquefaction of the basal cell layer, and homogenization of the collagen in the upper corium.

VERRUCOUS CARCINOMA

In 1947 Ackerman[30] described a variety of squamous cell carcinoma of the oral cavity with a unique behavior and characteristic gross and microscopic findings. Grossly the tumor had a verrucous appearance and extended over the invaded contiguous surfaces in a manner often associated with infection. Microscopically, at first, keratin piled up on the surface, followed by club-shaped fingers of epithelium pushing rather than infiltrating the deeper tissues. The epithelium was well differentiated, and the basement membrane was intact. With deeper invasion cystic degeneration and formation of inflammatory tissue tracts occurred. Local recurrence was common and invasion of local structures often extensive. Local metastases were rare, with distant metastases not observed.

Apparently similar lesions appear elsewhere in the body, including the skin, but reports of anal lesions are rare even if the few cases of giant condyloma acuminatum are included in this category.[31–33] It is possible that condyloma acuminatum could eventuate as a verrucous carcinoma. Furthermore, it is doubtful that hematoxylin and eosin (H&E)-sections would enable a pathologist to make a distinction between the two.

Kao et al.[33] studied 46 cases of cutaneous verrucous carcinoma but none in the anal area.

They concluded that verrucous carcinoma is low grade but capable of local invasion and rare metastasis. Immunoperoxidase viral studies were negative.

BOWEN'S DISEASE

Bowen's disease is a dermatosis that undergoes malignant change with enough regularity that it is considered a precancerous dermatosis.[34–38] It occurs predominantly in older people. Clinically the lesions appear as variously shaped plaques that may be erythematous, pigmented, crusted, scaly, nodular, verrucous, or fissured. The lesions are single or multiple and may involve the skin of the anogenital region, where, particularly in women, they appear verrucous, polypoid, and pigmented. Excision is the treatment of choice, since recurrence is high with irradiation, curettage, and desiccation and following short periods of treatment with topical 5-fluorouracil 1 to 5 percent.

Graham and Helwig[34] reported that at least 5 percent of patients with Bowen's disease show clinical and microscopic invasive carcinoma from the epidermis or pilary complex into the adjacent corium. Two percent of all patients with Bowen's disease show not only cutaneous invasion but also metastasis to extracutaneous organs. In addition, an average of 6 years after onset of Bowen's disease at least 42 percent of patients develop other cutaneous and mucocutaneous premalignant and malignant lesions, and at least 25 percent develop primary extracutaneous malignant tumors. From the time of diagnosis of Bowen's disease until death 70 percent of the patients will be affected with primary internal and extracutaneous malignant tumors.

Women with anogenital Bowen's disease tend to develop systemic cancer in the pelvic girdle organs, including the vagina, cervix, uterus, ovary, rectum, anus, urethra, and urinary bladder.[34]

The characteristic microscopic features of Bowen's disease include a plaquelike lesion of the epidermis with acanthosis, hyperkeratosis, and/or parakeratosis and usually hypogranulosis. The epithelial cells exhibit a disorientation or withblown appearance throughout, lack normal progression of maturation, and show an atypical epithelial cell proliferation, including multinucleated giant cells, vacuolated cells, mitotic figures, and dyskeratotic cells appearing at all levels of the epidermis.

In addition to involvement of the epidermis, the process in hair-bearing areas shows involvement of the pilary acrotrichium, infundibulum, and sebaceous gland.[34] The atypical cellular proliferation takes place in the outer root sheath and ultimately replaces the cells of the sebaceous gland but does not extend below this level. In contrast the cells of the acrosyringium of the eccrine sweat duct are not involved, although the course of the duct becomes straight rather than spiral. As long as the atypical epithelial proliferation is confined by an intact basement membrane, the Bowen's disease process is regarded as a form of precancerous dermatosis (some prefer to call it *carcinoma in situ*). If the latter term is used it must be recognized that not all forms of cutaneous "carcinoma in situ" have the same biologic behavior.

The upper corium subjacent to the base of the lesion is usually infiltrated with inflammatory cells, mostly lymphocytes and histiocytes.

Bowen's disease is regarded as an invasive carcinoma if the atypical pleomorphic epithelial cells disrupt the basement membrane of either the epidermis or pilary structure and infiltrate the contiguous corium. Caution must be exercised to avoid interpreting pleomorphic cells in a tangential plane of an elongated rete ridge as an area of invasion.

In histochemical studies the vacuolated cells show a negative reaction for mucin with Alcian blue and mucicarmine stains, in contrast to the positive results occurring in anogenital Paget's disease. The vacuolated cells may contain PAS-positive glycogen.

With electron microscopy the lesions of Bowen's disease reveal aggregated tonofilaments and loss of desmosomes.[39] The clumped tonofilaments ultimately occupy a large part of the dyskeratotic cells and enfold organelles, nuclear remnants, and many vacuoles.

Bowen's disease must be differentiated from bowenoid papulosis; this differentiation is described under Bowenoid Papulosis, below.

BOWENOID PAPULOSIS

Bowenoid papulosis is characterized by pigmented papules on or near the anogenitalia, principally in young men and women.[40, 41] Clinicians usually diagnose a benign condition, but the pathologist, on the baisis of cytologic atypia, often interprets the changes as carcinoma in situ or Bowen's disease.[42–45] Although the genital distribution of this condition has been emphasized in the literature, the lesions also occur in the anal and perianal zones.[6]

Bowenoid papulosis occurs in both men and women, and the peak incidence appears during the third decade. The duration of the lesions ranges from a few weeks to several years. The process may be either confined to the perianal area or also involve the genital region. Most lesions are small, measuring only a few millimeters in diameter, and are either single or, more commonly, multiple. Smaller lesions, described as verrucous or pigmented papules, sometimes coalesce to form plaques. Other than pruritus and irritation changes, most patients are free from symptoms. Verruca, nevus, and occasionally condyloma acuminatum are other clinical diagnoses entertained.

Bowenoid papulosis microscopically is characterized by irregular acanthosis, occasional papillomatosis, varying degrees of hyperkeratosis, and frequent parakeratosis.[40] A general orderly maturation of the keratinocytes occurs, but with a scattering of hyperchromatic nuclei, dyskeratotic cells, and mitotic figures at all levels of the epithelium (Figs. 11-9 and 11-10). The "salt and pepper" distribution effect of the dyskeratotic cells and mitotic figures superimposed on a relatively orderly epithelial background is suggestive of bowenoid papulosis. Mitotic figures, occasionally in the same stage, tend to appear within small clusters. The basement membrane at the dermal-epidermal junction is intact and invasive carcinoma is not discernible.

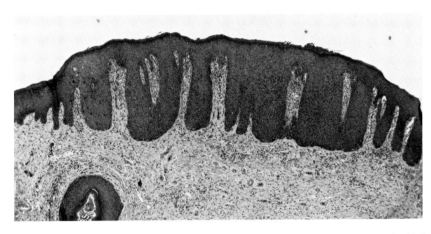

Fig. 11-9. Flat papule of bowenoid papulosis with acanthotic epidermis and elongated, thickened rete ridges. (H&E, × 40.)

In bowenoid papulosis inclusionlike bodies are sometimes noted in the granular and parakeratotic zones and about the follicular ostia.[40, 46] The inclusionlike bodies appear deeply basophilic, rounded, and sometimes with a halo. The squamous cells may appear koilocytotic (koilocytes) with perinuclear cytoplasmic vacuolization and sometimes enlarged and irregular nuclei with hyperchromasia.

Hair follicles present in bowenoid papulosis usually do not show involvement of the acrotrichium and follicular infundibulum, but the intraepidermal sweat duct (acrosyringium) is likely to display full-thickness acrosyringeal involvement. These changes are the reverse of those seen in Bowen's disease, in which full-thickness follicular involvement occurs down to the level of the sebaceous gland and in which the acrosyringium as a rule is spared.

The dermal changes include a mixed infiltrate of mostly lymphocytes and histiocytes, telangiectatic vessels, and incontinence of melanin. Special histochemical stains, including Movat and colloidal iron, may reveal variable amounts of hyaluronic acid in the corium. The PAS stain shows inconsistent epithelial glycogen and an intact basement membrane.

By electron microscopy the dysplastic epithelial cells may show increased intercellular spaces, microvillous protusions of the cytoplasmic membranes, irregular contour of the nuclei, and dispersed irregular chromatin. In 1 of 12 cases examined by Patterson et al.,[40] several small, rounded, electron-dense particles were present within degenerated nuclei and were considered consistent with viral elements. In the same study 1 of 17 cases stained with antibody to HPV using the immunoperoxidase technique detected the presence of HPV antigens. In the whole group of 100 patients, 20 had been treated for viral infection with podophyllum resin from days to years before biopsy.

Sixty patients were treated surgically, including 10 women with vulvectomies. Others were treated with topical 5-fluorouracil and electrodessication. Fifteen patients had one or more recurrences. Follow-up on 48 patients (median of 4 years) disclosed 2 with unrelated causes of death and the remaining patients alive and free of disease. None developed other cutaneous or extracutaneous malignancies. Tissue from these patients was not tested for HPV by DNA probes.

Anal tissue samples of bowenoid papulosis appearing histologically acceptable in H&E-stained sections seldom, in our experience, were positive with the immunoperoxidase method for HPV on the same tissue. In contrast DNA probes on the same histologic bowenoid papulosis tissue as well as on condyloma acuminatum specimens generally detected the HPV types effectively. The DNA probes positive for HPV types

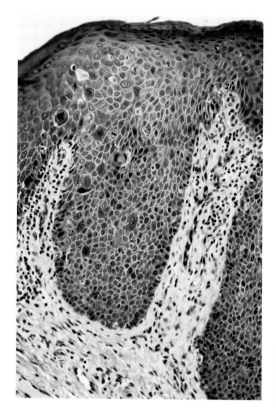

Fig. 11-10. A characteristic microscopic picture of bowenoid papulosis showing atypical dyskeratotic cells and mitoses in a scattered pattern among maturing squamous cells. (H&E, × 160.)

6 and 11 are commonly associated with noninvasive lesions. HPV types 16 and 18 and less well-documented types 31, 35, and 51 associated with potentially malignant lesions.

As Koss[47] pointed out, much is yet to be learned about the cytologic manifestations of HPV infection of the female genital tract and their clinical significance. This situation undoubtedly applies to similar infections and lesions of the anorectal area.

The application and advantages of the in-situ hybridization techniques over that of immunohistochemistry is discussed at length by Grody et al.[48]

CONDYLOMA ACUMINATUM

Condyloma acuminata are papillary, warty, or nodular, usually soft, gray to pink growths with a predilection for warm moist surfaces.[49–51] They commonly appear about the anal and perianal region, perineum, and male and female genitalia as single or multiple growths, sometimes covering a large area.

In condyloma acuminatum the squamous epithelium shows acanthosis, variable degrees of papillomatosis, ordinarily thickening of the stratum corneum, and partial parakeratotic maturation. The rete ridges are irregular, elongated, and often blunt and branching (Figs. 11-11 and 11-12). Typically the epithelial cells show a rather orderly progression of maturation in contrast to the disorganized pattern common to squamous carinoma. However, the often present scattered dysplastic cells and mitotic figures alone, without general epithelial disorganization, do not indicate carcinoma in situ. The contiguous supporting stroma of the condyloma is well defined, suggesting a compressed pushing margin. It may contain an infiltrate of inflammatory cells, usually of chronic variety.

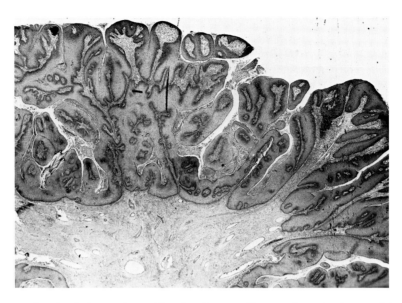

Fig. 11-11. Broadened and elongated rete ridges forming a papillary configuration in a condyloma acuminatum. Demarcation of the condyloma and adjacent stroma is sharp. (H&E, × 9.)

Considerable diagnostic importance is placed on the presence of clear vacuolated squamous epithelial cells (koilocytes), usually located in the superficial epithelial zone, as a signal of a viral cause.[47] However, not all condylomas show appreciable koilocytosis. Using the technique of DNA probes as described in bowenoid papulosis, the examples of condyloma acuminata, especially in areas of koilocytosis, show positive staining for HPV, including types 6 and 11 (usually a benign association) and types 16, 18, 30, 35, and 51 (of malignant potential). Curiously, the histologic examination of the surface epithelium in the vicinity of a typical condyloma acuminatum may disclose foci similar to those seen in bowenoid papulosis.

The distinction between condyloma acuminatum and carcinoma in situ may be difficult. Tangential cuts of a branching condyloma may mimic infiltrating squamous cell carcinoma but lack the diffuse pleomorphism and dysplasia of carcinoma. Completely disorganized, irregular masses of epithelium with dysplastic and mitotic cells favor a diagnosis of carcinoma. Treatment with podophyllin resin as a cause of mitoses and dyskeratosis is seldom verified.[49]

Although examples of malignant transformation of condyloma acuminatum are reported,[51] controversy of the degree of malignancy and whether it is cytologic or biologic is not always clear.

HPV has been indentified in vulvar condylomas by the peroxidase-antiperoxidase test. From a practical standpoint viral antigens are not detected in all histologically apparent viral "warts," making results of routinely processed surgical tissue unreliable. Alternative tests such as DNA probes are type specific and more reliable.[26, 48] Multiple types of HPV may be present to confuse the situation in regard to potential aggressive growth.

GIANT CONDYLOMA ACUMINATUM (BUSCHKE-LOEWENSTEIN TUMOR)

In 1925 Buschke and Loewenstein[52] described condylomata acuminata of the penis that simulated cancer. Since that time similar tumors have been described with a predilection for the prepuce.[53] Giant condylomata acuminata are

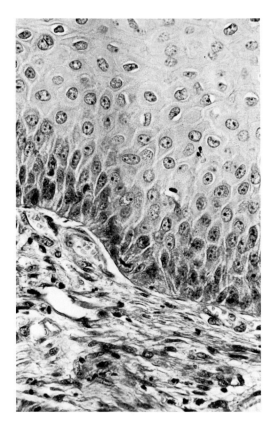

Fig. 11-12. The base of the condyloma acuminatum is sharply defined. Minimal dysplasia is present near the base. (H&E, × 300.)

large warty growths that ulcerate, become infected, penetrate, and burrow into deeper tissues to form ureterocutaneous fistulas. Massive cauliflowerlike ulcerative, friable, bleeding growths may develop along the penile shaft. Paradoxically histopathologic changes of malignancy and invasion of blood and lymphatic vessels are absent.

In 1967 Knoblich and Failing[54] described a rectal tumor located 8 cm above the anus with perirectal involvement and the histologic characteristics of a Buschke-Loewenstein tumor. Since that time four patients both male and female, with lesions of the Buschke-Loewenstein type have been recorded.[55–57] Histologically tumors of this type show acanthotic squamous epithelium thrown up into folds, scallops, and papillae

that are supported by a core of vascularized connective tissue stroma. The cells in the basal layer assume a more squamoid appearance, but the junction of the epithelium and stroma always appears distinct, as if a basement membrane were present. Maturation of the squamous cells tends to occur in an orderly manner, with parakeratosis and varying degrees of hyperkeratosis and koilocytosis of the malpighian cells. In general the squamous epithelial cells do not show appreciable pleomorphism.

According to Knoblich and Failing[54] only a few minor histologic differences exist between condyloma acuminatum and the giant condyloma acuminatum. These are mainly an exaggeration of the features seen in condyloma acuminatum, such as the accentuation of acanthosis and papillomatosis, and the thickened, elongated rete ridges. It is claimed that mitotic activity is more prominent and that individual cell keratinization and keratin pearls may be seen in the giant form. We have noted these changes in both types of lesions. Perhaps the clinical picture or gross appearance is the best clue as to the type of lesions, and the histologic examination confirms the basic nature of the process. Sturm et al.[57] reported a squamous cell carcinoma arising in a giant condyloma acuminatum of the anus of a 49-year-old man.

MALIGNANT MELANOMA

Primary anorectal melanoma may puzzle both clinicians and pathologists.[59–61] The anorectum accounts for 1 to 3 percent of all melanomas and is the third most common site for melanoma, preceded only by skin and eye. It is one-eighth as common as squamous cell carcinoma in the anal region.

The anatomy of the anorectal region is clouded by the difficulty in establishing clearcut landmarks. The lower end of the anal canal is lined by squamous mucous membrane that merges with the perianal skin. Interposed between the squamous mucous membrane and the glandular mucosa of the distal rectum is a distinct circular zone 3 to 11 mm wide lined by transitional or cloacogenic epithelium. Walls[62] defined the upper limits of the anal canal as the *anorectal ring*—the insertion of the levatores ani muscles—thus including 4 to 16 mm of rectal-type mucosa in the anal canal. The intersphincteric distance may be as much as 40 mm; unless the relationship to the levatores ani is known, no tumor that is closer than 4 cm to the anal orifice can be unquestionably accepted as within the rectum.

Under these guidelines only a few examples qualify as rectal melanoma. According to Walls[62] melanin is present in the pecten but decreases proximally and is absent a short distance below the anal valves. Fenger and Lyon[63] occasionally found melanin-containing cells in the transitional zone of the normal anal mucosa, and I rarely have noted melanocytes as high as the distal rectal mucosa.

In a study of 17 cases of anorectal melanomas, only 1 was clearly within the rectum, 1 was marginal, 1 indeterminate, and 14 regarded as anal.[58, 64]

Although some reports have shown a preponderant incidence in men, probably no sex difference exists. The age incidence roughly corresponds to that of rectal cancer.

Patients with anorectal melanoma have symptoms and signs that are confused with those of hemorrhoids, including bleeding, pain, and a mass.

Many patients develop a polypoid tumor that has been used as a sign in differentiation from carcinoma. Pigment may be absent or obscured by hemorrhage.

The cell types comprising the tumors can be broadly divided into polygonal and spindle, but mixed types and small cell types occur. Occasionally large giant cells are present. The pattern of growth ranges from monotonous sheets of cells simulating lymphoma to nesting cells, usually elongated, and occasionally arranged in radial palisades (Figs. 11-13 and 11-14). Less commonly the cells mimic a carcinoid tumor, with which it would be easy to confuse.

A divergence of opinion exists in the literature

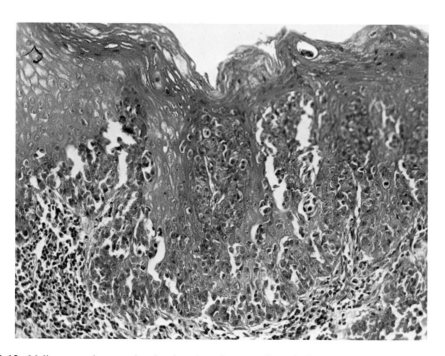

Fig. 11-13. Malignant melanoma showing junction change and atypical melanocytes within the squamous mucosa. (H&E, × 165.)

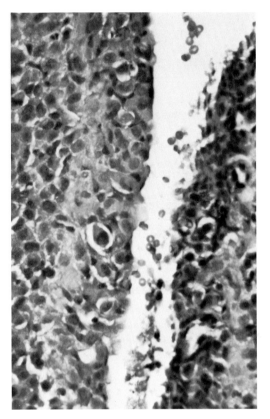

Fig. 11-14. Melanoma cells involve an anal duct. (H&E, × 400.)

as to the occurrence of junction change in the anal mucosa. Most reports include a percentage of tumors in which junction change cannot be identified, but this probably happens because the anal mucosa is ulcerated. Melanoma cells located in the stroma and separated from the squamous mucosa probably represents seeding. Similarly a primary melanoma in the squamous mucosa seeds to the glandular mucosa and submucosa. Primary melanoma may involve the transitional zone as well as the contiguous anal ducts. In support of the origin of primary melanoma in this zone is the occurrence of mucosal melanocytes.

In primary melanoma the distribution of the melanoma cells shows a pattern of either nodular melanoma or superficial spreading melanoma and occasionally of a lentiginous melanoma.

Regardless of pattern, anorectal melanoma is a deadly tumor.[65] Wanebo et al.[61] reported 23 deaths among 26 patients with tumor measuring 2 mm or more in thickness; 1 patient with a tumor measuring 2 mm in thickness is alive with metastases and 3 patients with tumors measuring 1.7 mm or less are alive 13 or more years after diagnosis.

Investigators have commented on both the comparative rarity of melanin pigment and the frequent occurrence in the melanomas.[63] Melanin can be demonstrated by the Warthin-Starry stain pH 3.2 and premelanin by anti S-100 and HMB 45 antigens using immunohistochemical identification.

At the present time excision is the treatment of choice, but survival is very limited regardless of the methods used for those lesions measuring greater than 1.7 mm in depth. As with melanomas of the skin the frequency of local infiltration and extent of metastases is often unpredictable.

PERIANAL PAGET'S DISEASE

Perianal Paget's disease is so unusual that it is seldom diagnosed correctly prior to biopsy.[66, 67] Most patients complain of combinations of ulceration, crusting, scaling, and, more rarely, bleeding. Some perianal lesions also involve the perineum and the genitalia (Fig. 11-15). The disease affects older age groups and usually is present for many years prior to diagnosis.

Microscopically the main changes in perianal Paget's disease in H&E-stained sections are hyperkeratosis, parakeratosis, acanthosis, and pale vacuolated epithelial cells within the epidermis.[66] The vacuolated cells contain vesicular nuclei either centrally located or compressed to the cell periphery by clear or pale basophilic cytoplasm (mucin) (Fig. 11-16).

The Paget's cells appear more numerous at the tips or margins of the rete ridges, with a tendency to flatten as the surrounding essentially normal squamous cells mature. Paget's cells occur in the outer root sheath of the pilary complex and in the sweat ducts. Invariably serial

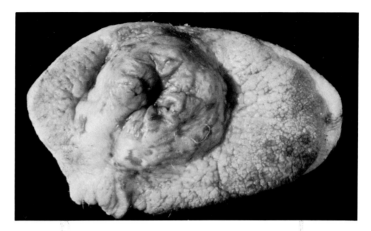

Fig. 11-15. Perianal Paget's disease showing an elevated papillary picture. Microscopically an underlying infiltrating adnexal carcinoma involving apocrine glands is present.

sections will reveal intraepidermal glandular and ductlike structures of the Paget's cells. Sometimes the rete ridges are greatly extended, mimicking changes of basal cell or squamous cell carcinoma.

A mixed inflammatory infiltrate usually is concentrated immediately beneath the epidermis. In occasional lesions there is a "dropping off" of melanin pigment into the upper corium, where it is found both free and within melano-

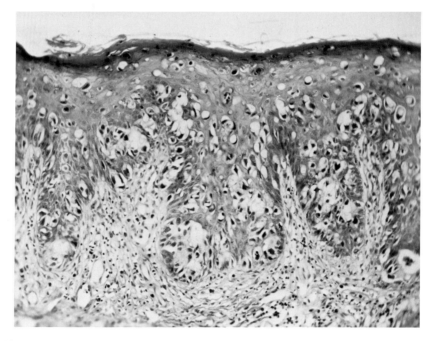

Fig. 11-16. Anogenital Paget's disease showing vacuolated cells in single and suggestive acinar arrangements within the epidermis. By special stains the clear cells contain mucin. (H&E, × 125.)

phages. This picture must be differentiated from that of melanoma.

When the Paget's cells involve the sweat glands but are confined by an intact basement membrane, the process is regarded as an insitu change. Only those examples in which infiltration of the Paget's cells into the contiguous corium occurs is the picture interpreted as adnexal carcinoma. Apocrine glands are usually the glands involved, but in some instances the eccrine glands participate.

Paget's cells confined by the basement membrane of the epidermis, sweat glands, and pilary complex are considered as a form of carcinoma in situ. An infiltrating carcinoma occurs when the basement membrane is voided by infiltrating Paget's cells into the adjacent stroma.

Histochemical stains help to identify perianal Paget's disease.[66] With the colloidal iron (AMP) and Alcian blue stains the Paget's cells stain blue and the positive mucin is resistant to hyaluronidase digestion indicating that it is not hyaluronic acid. Malignant melanoma cells may show a feeble but similar response. In Bowen's disease and erythroplasia of Queyrat the stains for mucin are negative. The positive Alcian blue stain in Paget's cells is digested with sialidase, indicating the presence of sialic acid (sialomucin). The PAS stain in Bowen's disease and erythroplasia of Queyrat may be positive but digests with diastase, indicating glycogen. Some melanoma cells contain PAS-positive resistant material. Confusion in diagnosis may occur with stains for melanin (Warthin-Starry pH 3.2) because intraepidermal Paget's cells may contain secondary melanin granules. With immunohistochemical stain, anal-perianal Paget's cells show a strong positive reaction of carcinoembryonic antigen (CEA).

In perianal Paget's disease there is a greater chance of finding an associated subjacent glandular adnexal carcinoma, breast carcinoma, or regional internal cancer with or without metastasis than with Paget's disease located on the genital area, pubis, and thighs.[66, 68, 69] In Paget's disease confined within the basement membranes of the epidermis or adnexa the prognosis is highly favorable, but when infiltration of Pag-

et's disease from the epidermis or subjacent adnexal structures or a regional internal carcinoma is present the prognosis is grave. Of 14 patients with perianal Paget's disease, 12 developed either underlying adnexal carcinoma, carcinoma of rectum, or carcinoma of the breast, and 9 died. The cause of the high incidence of associated carcinoma in this region is not apparent. The histogenesis of extramammary Paget's disease remains controversial. The two principal concepts are (1) epidermotropic migration of Paget's cells into the epidermis from an underlying carcinoma and (2) origin of the Paget's cells in the epidermis independently or concomitantly with an underlying carcinoma. Our data support the concept that the neoplasia may involve the epidermis alone, both the epidermis and the underlying adnexa, or both epidermis and adjacent internal organs. There is probably a multicentric effect rather than migration of carcinoma cells into the epidermis. Ultrastructural studies are at variance and have not clarified the issue.[69–71]

Surgical excision of the lesion is the treatment of choice, since the process tends to recur or fail to respond to radiation therapy, curettement, or chemotherapy.

KERATOACANTHOMA

Keratoacanthoma is a benign epithelial tumor of the skin first described by Hutchinson[73] in 1888 as a "crater form ulcer." Characteristically it enlarges rapidly over a period of a few weeks to form a cup-shaped nodule covered marginally by skin and centrally by a crater filled with keratin. At full development it measures up to 2 cm in diameter. After a static period it usually regresses. Although the common site of involvement is the skin of the head and hands, the perianal skin is sometimes involved.[74]

It is, of course, extremely important to distinguish a keratoacanthoma from a squamous cell carcinoma histologicaly.[75] In the histologic examination of a keratoacanthoma it is essential that the microscopic sections include full cross-

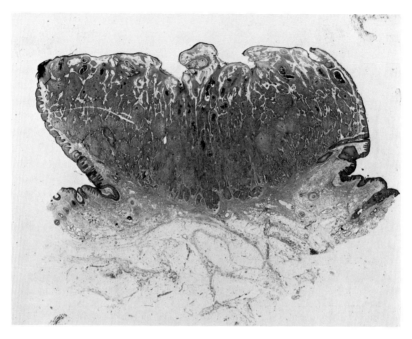

Fig. 11-17. Keratoacanthoma showing a hemispherical cup-shaped configuration with central squamous proliferation and keratinization. (H&E, × 7.)

sections and the base of the lesion. A small biopsy of the process may be misleading and misinterpreted as a squamous cell carcinoma. On the basis of examination of the complete lesion, the correct diagnosis should be made.

In the usual histologic picture the epidermis, which may be acanthotic but not dysplastic, covers the margins of the cup-shaped lesion and then centrally turns inward, where it is continuous with a mass of intercommunicating foci of squamous cells (Figs. 11-17 and 11-18). The masses of squamous cells generally show a tendency to mature with the formation of a central nidus of keratin. The intercommunication of the masses of squamous cells is of considerable importance in recognition of lesion, since a squamous cell carcinoma tends to show separate individual nests of pleomorphic cells. In keratoacanthoma pleomorphism in the main mass of squamous cells is absent, and the presence of rare dysplastic cells near the margins should not eliminate the diagnosis of keratoacanthoma

if the overall configuration is characteristic. The presence of foreign body giant cells in relation to the deeper keratin masses and the transmigration of leukocytic cells through the epithelial masses in the absence of radiation or other traumatic insults favors a diagnosis of keratoacanthoma. The base of all keratoacanthomas irregularly protrudes into the contiguous stroma; this feature is of no value in distinguishing the lesion from squamous cell carcinoma. In most de novo cutaneous squamous cell carcinomas the involved epidermis of the lesion shows dysplasia.

Exceptional keratoacanthomas persist for many months, which always raises the question as to whether or not the lesions are really keratoacanthomas even though they are histologically acceptable as such. Keratoacanthomas may recur, but recurrence does not mean the lesions are malignant.[76] A few keratoacanthomas invade the perineural space, but in our experience the invasion does not adversely affect the biologic behavior and the prognosis.[77]

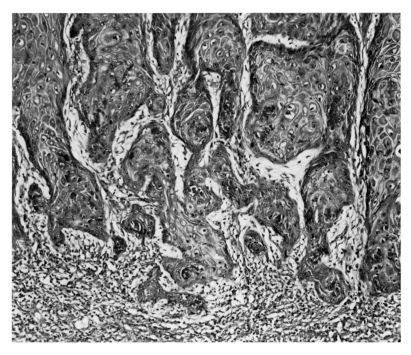

Fig. 11-18. Keratoacanthoma with interconnecting masses of maturing squamous cells extending into the adjacent stroma. (H&E, × 100.)

HIDRADENOMA PAPILLIFERUM

Hidradenoma papilliferum, an uncommon tumor, occurs in the anogenital area almost exclusively in white women.[78, 79] The average age of patients with perianal tumors (45 years) is greater than that of patients with vulvar lesions (39 years).

Most patients have noticed the presence of the tumor for less than 1 year and complain of a lump. Other complaints include bleeding, itching, swelling at menstrual period, pain, erosion, and ulceration.

The tumor seldom measures greater than 1 cm. It appears clinically as a circumscribed, firm, freely movable, slightly elevated nodule. It is usually called a "cyst" and in the perianal area a hemorrhoid, polyp, or fibroma. Only rarely do the tumors form an everted red mass.

Microscopically the tumors are usually spherical and circumscribed, but a few are located within a cystic space.[78] The tumors exhibit both glandular and papillary patterns. The glandular areas frequently manifest a double layer of epithelial cells resting on a well-defined thin basement membrane (Fig. 11-19). The papillary structures are usually slender, with a scanty connective tissue core supporting a single or double layer of cells.

Two general types of epithelium are present. Most frequently the epithelial cells are tall and columnar, with nipplelike cytoplasmic projections, and they rest on a layer of smaller cuboidal cells. The second type of epithelium is composed of large cuboidal cells with brightly eosinophilic cytoplasm that contains a few coarse eosinophilic granules at the cell apex. These cells resemble apocrine metaplasia. Cellular and nuclear pleomorphism are sometimes present in the papillary foci.

Histochemically PAS-reactive diastase resistant granules are often present in the layer of

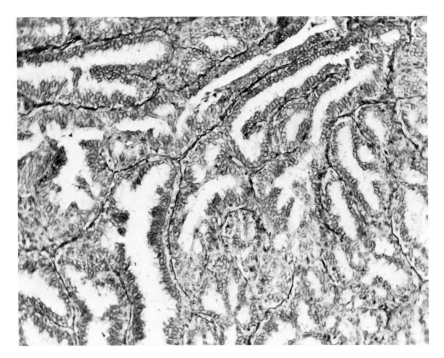

Fig. 11-19. Hidradenoma showing cylindrical cells sometimes resting on a flat layer of cells and a delicate stroma arranged in a complex papillary pattern. Some cells resemble apocrine cells. (H&E, × 180.)

eosinophil cells. In a frozen section an Oil red O stain exhibits sudanophilic material within the apical portion of the large eosinophil cells.

Various tissues, including sweat gland, Wolfian duct remnants, and accessory mammary gland, have been suggested as the tissue of origin. Most microscopic and histochemical changes favor origin from sweat gland.

In a study of 44 patients with follow-up information all lesions behaved in a benign manner.[78]

The one lesion that most closely resembles hidradenoma papilliferum is the intraductal papilloma of the breast, but the latter is often multiple and the former single.

Syringocystadenoma papilliferum is usually a verrucous lesion more common on the head and often associated with nevus sebaceus. The papillary processes are broad, and the stroma is densely infiltrated with plasma cells, in contrast to the delicate complex papillae without plasma cells seen in hidradenoma papilliferum.

GRANULAR CELL TUMOR

The granular cell tumor (granular cell myoblastoma) described by Abrikossoff[80] in 1926 uncommonly occurs in the gastrointestinal tract. In a study of 75 granular cell tumors involving the gastrointestinal tract 16 occurred in the perianal area near the anal verge.[81] Most tumors presented as a painless lump and in some instances were mistaken for an abscess or hemorrhoid.

Granular cell tumors are characterized by plump polygonal or sometimes fusiform cells containing eosinophilic granules (Figs. 11-20 and 11-21). The granules exhibit well-described histochemical reactions. The most characteristic occurs with the PAS stain, in which the cytoplasmic granules stain red even after prior digestion with diastase. With Masson's trichrome stain the granules stain red and the tumors are clearly demonstrated. With the Movat penta-

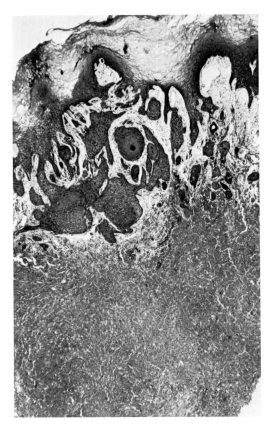

Fig. 11-20. Granular cell tumor made up of mostly polygonal cells with an eosinophilic granular cytoplasm. The covering epidermis shows pseudoepitheliomatous hyperplasia mimicking squamous cell carcinoma. (H&E, × 51.)

chrome stain the granules appear brown, and with the Alcian blue preparation the granules stain at pH 2.5 but are negative at pH 0.5. Other stains for mucin as well as silver stains are negative. A positive immunohistochemical reaction occurs in the cytoplasm of the granular cells when subjected to anti-S-100 antigen.[82]

The electron microscopic appearance is controversial. The tumor cells usually show distinct basement membranes and are packed with granules that are most likely lysosomes. Occasional tumors contain myelic figures. These changes suggest that the cells resemble Schwann cells, but other authors do not recognize such changes and doubt the validity of the concept.

Among the different origins proposed, the Schwann cell theory has gained the most support on the basis of the probable lysosomal nature of the granules and the reaction of the cells with anti-S-100 antigen, which resembles that occurring in normal Schwann cells.

Prominent pseudoepitheliomatous hyperplasia is a commonly associated change of the covering epidermis, and in many instances it extends into the granular cell tumor.[81, 83] None of the pseudoepitheliomatous hyperplasias or the granular cell tumors has shown a malignant transition.

BENIGN LYMPHOID POLYP AND MALIGNANT LYMPHOMA

Benign lymphoid polyps are more common in the rectal mucosa but also are encountered in the upper anal canal.[84] Clinically the polyps show various shapes, and except for occasional ulcers and erosions they are covered with gray mucosa.

Histologically the anal polyps are covered with squamous or a mixture of squamous and glandular mucosa. For a satisfactory examination the complete polyp in an ideal fixed state must be examined. The lymphoid tissue is not encapsulated and is usually divided into lobules by thin septa. Lymphoid follicles of varying distinctness and size surrounded by mature lymphocytes form the characteristic picture. Phagocytic cells and occasional plasma cells may be present. Mitotic figures are confined mostly to the follicular center. Simple excision effects a cure.

In contrast malignant lymphoma of the anus is extremely rare and is practically always associated with a systemic lymphoma. The lymphoid infiltrate is characterized by a diffuse pattern without lymphoid follicles, and phagocytic histiocytes are essentially absent. The lymphoid infiltrate obliterates the normal architecture, and the margins are infiltrating rather than expanding. A lobular pattern with dividing septa is absent.

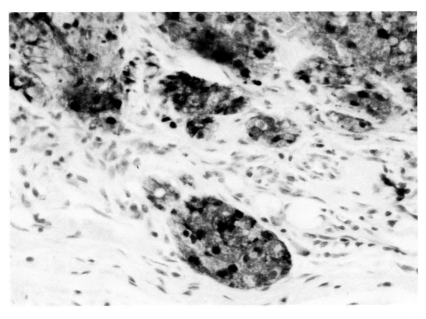

Fig. 11-21. With the immunoperioxidase technique and anti-S-100 the granular cells stain brown. (×400.)

HEMORRHOIDS AND CONCOMITANT TUMORS

Patients with hemorrhoids experience intense discomfort and a tendency to recurrent bleeding. The pathologic changes are usually but not invariably bland. Hemorrhoids should be examined microscopically.

The most perplexing change met with on histologic examination is the sudden discovery of the cytologic appearance of marked epithelial dysplasia or carcinoma in situ of the mucosa and sometimes invasive carcinoma. Associated epithelial hyperplasia and dysplasia, particularly of the transitional type, together with tangential sections of the hemorrhoidal tissue, cause difficulty in deciding about invasion. If a basement membrane appears intact and regular, it probably is not invasion.

Another rare and usually unexpected concomitant lesion in a hemorrhoid is a nevus. Most are compound nevi and as a rule are only lightly pigmented. The determination of benignity follows the same microscopic criteria as used for cutaneous nevi.

Granuloma pyogenicum occurs as an elevated hemorrhagic nodule. It is composed of lobules of small, well-formed blood vessels similar to those seen in granulation tissue. The stroma is infiltrated with inflammatory cells.

Kaposi's sarcoma of the anorectal area is characterized histologically by the typical vascular slit pattern, usually congested, and frequently accompanied by partially obscuring inflammation. It may occur as a concomitant change in human immunodeficiency virus infections.[85, 86]

INFLAMMATORY CLOACOGENIC POLYP

Lobert and Appelman[87] and Saul[88] described the clinical and pathologic features of eight examples of an inflammatory polyp arising from the transitional zone of the anal cancal. Histologically the surface epithelium may be mostly squamous, but the core of the polyp has a tubulovillous pattern with displaced groups of crypts into the submucosa and extension of inflammatory fibromuscular stroma into the lamina propria. Simple resection appears to be the treatment of choice.

BASAL CELL CARCINOMA

Basal cell carcinoma of the perianal skin clinically appears similar to basal cell carcinoma developing elsewhere, including the superficial spreading type. Histologically an occasional anal Paget's lesion with greatly prolonged rete ridges mimics basal cell carcinoma. The cells of Paget's lesions are immunohistochemically CEA positive. Similarly nevus-melanoma cells are S100 and HMB45 positive.

MISCELLANEOUS TUMORS

Leiomyomas and leiomyosarcomas arising from the internal sphincter muscle rarely develop. Even more rare is the occurrence of sarcoma botryoides (embryonal rhabdomyosarcoma) of the anus.[89]

Other mesenchymal tumors and tumorlike conditions include fibroma, neurofibroma, hemangioma, endometrioma, and tailgut cyst.[90]

Lastly, metastatic carcinomas, particularly from the lower genitourinary structures, may involve the anus.

ACKNOWLEDGMENT

I wish to sincerely thank Ann Gordon for her editorial and secretarial assistance.

REFERENCES

1. Herrmann G, Desfosses L: Sur la muqueuse de la region cloacle du rectum. C R Acad Sci 90:1301, 1880
2. Herrmann G: Sur la structure et developpement de la muqueuse anale. J Anat Physiol 16:434, 1880
3. Tucker C, Hellwig CA: Anal ducts: comparative and developmental histology. Arch Surg 31:521, 1935
4. Grinvalsky H, Helwig EB: Carcinoma of the anorectal junction: histologic considerations. Cancer 9:480, 1956
5. Gillespie JJ, MacKay B: Histogenesis of cloacogenic carcinoma. Hum Pathol 9:579, 1978
6. Singh R, Nime F, Mittelman A: Malignant epithelial tumors of the anal canal. Cancer 48:411, 1981
7. Grodsky L: Cloacogenic cancer of the anorectal junction. Report of seven cases. Dis Colon Rectum 6:37, 1963
8. Cullen PK Jr, Pontius EE, Sanders J: Cloacogenic anorectal carcinoma. Dis Colon Rectum 9:1, 1966
9. Klotz RG, Pamukcoglu T, Souilliard DH: Transitional cloacogenic carcinoma of the anal canal. Cancer 20:1727, 1967
10. Kheir S, Hickey RC, Martin RG, et al: Cloacogenic carcinoma of the anal canal. Arch Surg 104:407, 1972
11. Levin SE, Cooperman H, Freilich M, et al: Transitional cloacogenic carcinoma of the anus. Dis Colon Rectum 20:17, 1977
12. Pang LSC, Morson BC: Basaloid carcinoma of the anal canal. J Clin Pathol 20:28, 1967
13. Svenson EW, Montague ED: Results of treatment in transitional cloacogenic carcinoma. Cancer 46:828, 1980
14. Cabrera A, Jsukada Y, Pickren JW, et al: Development of lower genital carcinomas in patients with anal carcinoma. Cancer 19:470, 1966
15. Close AS, Schwab RL: A history of the anal ducts and anal duct carcinoma. Cancer 8:979, 1955
16. Morson BC, Volkstadt H: Mucoepidermoid tumours of the anal canal. J Clin Pathol 16:200, 1963
17. Winkelman J, Grosfeld J, Bigelow B: Colloid carcinoma of anal-gland origin. Am J Clin Pathol 42:395, 1964
18. Mosary SH, Tayebi SA: Carcinoma arising in a perianal sinus tract: report of a case. Dis Colon Rectum 18:416, 1975
19. Fogler R, Lanter B, Stern G, Weiner E: Mucoepidermoid carcinoma in an ''anal fistula'' with associated adenocarcinoma in a villous adenoma of the descending colon. Dis Colon Rectum 20:428, 1977
20. Kline RJ, Spencer RJ, Harrision EG Jr: Carcinoma associated with fistula-in-ano. Arch Surg 89:989, 1964
21. Prioleau PG, Allen MS Jr, Roberts T: Perianal mucinous adenocarcinoma Cancer 39:1295, 1977

22. Wayte DM, Helwig EB: Colitis cystica profunda. Am J Clin Pathol 48:159, 1967

23. Clark J, Petrelli N, Herrera L, Mittelman A: Epidermoid carcinoma of the anal canal. Cancer 57:400, 1986

24. Kuehn PG, Eishenberg H, Reed JF: Epidermal carcinoma of the perianal skin and anal canal. Cancer 22:932, 1968

25. Boman BM, Moertel CG, O'Connell MJ, et al: Carcinoma of the anal canal. A clinical and pathologic study of 188 cases. Cancer, 54:114, 1984

26. Gal AA, Saul SH, Stoles MH: In situ hybridization analysis of human papillomavirus in anal squamous cell carcinoma. Mod Pathol 2:439, 1989

27. Moreno FR: Carcinoma in situ of the anal canal. Dis Colon Rectum 9:218, 1964

28. Vickers PM, Jackman RJ, McDonald JR: Anal carcinoma in situ. South Surg 8:503, 1939

29. Hart WR, Norris HJ, Helwig EB: Relation of lichen scherosis et atrophicus of the vulva to development of carcinoma. Obstet Gynecol 45:369, 1975

30. Ackerman LV: Verrucous carcinoma of the oral cavity. Surgery 23:670, 1948

31. Gingrass PJ, Bubrick MP, Hitchcock CR, et al: Anorectal verrucose squamous carcinoma: report of two cases. Dis Colon Rectum 21:120, 1978

32. Drut R, Ontiveros R, Cabral DH: Perianal verrucose carcinoma spreading to the rectum. Dis Colon Rectum 18:516, 1975

33. Kao GF, Graham JH, Helwig EB: Carcinoma cuniculatum (verrucous carcinoma of the skin). A clinicopathologic study of 46 cases with ultrastructural observations. Cancer 49:2395, 1982

34. Graham JH, Helwig EB: Bowen's disease and its relationship to systemic cancer. Arch Dermatol 80:133, 1959

35. Graham JH, Helwig EB: Premalignant cutaneous and mucocutaneous diseases. p. 581. In Graham JH, Johnson WC, Helwig EB (eds): Dermal Pathology. Harper & Row, Hagerstown, MD, 1972

36. Gilmour IEW, Ross CF: A case of anal intraepidermal carcinoma of Bowen's type. Gastroenterology, 26:108, 1954

37. Grodsky L: Bowen's disease of the anal region. Am J Surg 88:710, 1954

38. Scoma JA, Levy EI: Bowen's disease of the anus. Dis Colon Rectum 18:137, 1975

39. Sato A, Seiji M: Electron microscopic observations of malignant dyskeratosis in leukoplakia and Bowen's disease. Acta Derm Venereol (Stockh) 73:101, 1973

40. Patterson JW, Graham JH, Kao, GF, Helwig EB: Bowenoid papulosis. A clinicopathologic study with ultrastructural observations. Cancer 57:823, 1986

41. Wade TR, Kopf AW, Ackerman AB: Bowenoid papulosis of the penis. Cancer 42:1890, 1978

42. Oriel JD, Whimster IW: Carcinoma in isut associated with virus-containing anal warts. Br J Dermatol 84:71, 1971

43. Berger BW, Hori Y: Multicentric Bowen's disease of the genitalia. Arch Dermatol 114:1698, 1978

44. Lloyd LM: Multicentric pigmented Bowen's disease of the groin. Arch Dermatol 101:48, 1970

45. Lupulescu A, Mehregan AH, Rahbari H, et al: Venereal warts vs Bowen's disease. A histologic and ultrastructural study of five cases. JAMA 237:2520, 1977

46. Zelickson AS, Prawer SE: Bowenoid papulosis of the penis. Demonstration of intranuclear viral-like particles. Am J Dermatopathol 2:305, 1980

47. Koss LG: Cytologic and histologic manifestations of human papillomavirus infection of female genital tract and their clinical significance. Cancer 60:1942, 1987

48. Grody WW, Gatti RA, Naeim F: Diagnostic molecular pathology. Mod Pathol 2:553, 1989

49. Fitzgerald DW, Hamet HF: The variable significance of condyloma acuminata. Am J Surg 179:328, 1974

50. Jenson AB, Sommer BA, Payling-Wright C, et al: Human papilloma virus. Lab Invest 47:491, 1982

51. Kovi J, Tillman RC, Lee SM: Malignant transformation of condyloma acuminatum. A light microscopic and ultrastructural study. Am J Clin Pathol 61:702, 1974

52. Buschke A, Lowenstein L: Uber carcinomahnliche Condylomata Acuminata des Penis. Kein Wschr 4:1726, 1925

53. Dawson DF, Duckworth JK, Beinhardt H, et al: Giant condyloma and verrucous carcinoma of the genital area. Arch Pathol 79:225, 1965

54. Knoblich R, Failing JF Jr: Giant condyloma acuminatum (Buschke-Lowenstein tumor) of the rectum. Am J Clin Pathol 48:389, 1967

55. Judge JR: Giant condyloma acuminatum involving rectum and anus. Arch Pathol 88:46, 1969

56. Alexander RM, Kaminsky DB: Giant condyloma acuminatum (Buschke-Lowenstin tumor) of the

anus: case report and review of the literature. Dis Colon Rectum 22:561, 1979

57. Sturm JT, Christenson CE, Uecker JH, Perry JF Jr: Squamous cell carcinoma of the anus arising in a giant condyloma acuminatum: report of a case. Dis Colon Rectum 18:147, 1975

58. Mason JK, Helwig EB: Ano-rectal melanoma. Cancer 19:39, 1966

59. Morson BC, Volkstadt H: Malignant melanoma of the anal canal. Clin Pathol 16:126, 1963

60. Alexander RM, Cone LA: Malignant melanoma of the rectal ampula: report of a case and review of the literature. Dis Colon Rectum 20:53, 1977

61. Wanebo, HJ, Woodruff JM, Gist AF, Quan SH: Anorectal melanoma. Cancer 47:189, 1981

62. Walls EW: Observations of the microscopic anatomy of the human anal canal Br J Surg 45:504, 1958

63. Fenger C, Lyon H: Endocrine cells and melanin-containing cells in the anal canal epithelium. Histochem J 14:631, 1982

64. Werdin C, Limas C, Knodell RG: Primary melanoma of the rectum. Evidence for origin from rectal mucosal melanocytes. Cancer 61:1364, 1988

65. Cooper PH, Mills Se, Allen MS: Malignant melanoma of the anus: report of 12 patients and analysis of 225 additional cases. Dis Colon Rectum 25:693, 1982

66. Helwig EB, Graham JH: Anogenital (extramammary) Paget's disease. A clinicopathological study. Cancer 16:387, 1963

67. Grodsky L: Extramammary Paget's disease of the perianal region. Dis Colon Rectum 3:502, 1960

68. Rabson AS, Van Scott EJ, Smith R: Carcinoma of the anorectal junction with "extramammary Paget's disease." Arch Pathol 65:432, 1958

69. Arminski TC, Pollard RJ: Paget's disease of the anus secondary to a malignant papillary adenoma of the rectum. Dis Colon Rectum 16:46, 1973

70. Ordonex NG, Await H, MacKay B: Mammary and extramammary Paget's disease. An immunocytochemical and ultrastructural study. Cancer, 59:1173, 1987

71. Medenica M, Sahihi T: Ultrastructural study of a case of extramammary Paget's disease of the vulva. Arch Dermatol 105:236, 1972

72. Ferenczy Z, Richard RM: Ultrastructure of perianal Paget's disease. Cancer 29:1141, 1972

73. Hutchinson JA: Smaller Atlas of Illustrations of Clinical Surgery, Vol. 2. Blakeston, Philadelphia, 1888, Plate 921

74. Elliott GB, Fisher BK: Perianal keratoacanthoma. Arch Dermatol 95:81, 1967

75. de Moragan JM, Montgomery H, McDonald JR: Keratoacanthoma versus squamous-cell carcinoma. Arch Dermatol 77:390, 1958

76. Silberberg I, Kopf AW, Baer R: Recurent keratoacanthoma of the lip. Arch Dermatol 86:44, 1962

77. Lapins, NA, Helwig EB: Perineural invasion of keratoacanthoma. Arch Dermatol 116:791, 1980

78. Meeker JR, Neubecker RD, Helwig EB: Hidradenoma papilliferum. Am J Clin Pathol 37:182, 1962

79. Cooper WL, McDonald JR: Adenoma of apocrine sweat glands (hidradenoma of the anal canal). Arch Pathol 38:155, 1944

80. Abrikossoff AI: Uber myome ausgehend von der quergestneiften willkurlichen Muskulatur. Virchows Arch [A] 260:214, 1926

81. Johnston J, Helwig EB: Granular cell tumors of the gastrointestinal tract and perianal region. A study of 74 cases. Dig Dis Sci 26:807, 1981

82. Armin A, Connelly EM, Rowden G: An immunoperoxidase investigation of $100 protein in granular cell myoblastomas: evidence for Schwann cell derivation. Am J Clin Pathol 79:37, 1983

83. Rickert RR, Larkey IG, Kantor EB: Granular-cell tumors (myoblastomas) of the anal region. Dis Colon Rectum 21:413, 1978

84. Helwig EB, Hansen J: Lymphoid polyps (benign lymphoma) and malignant lymphoma of the rectum and anus. Surg Gynecol Obstet 92:233, 1951

85. Cox FH, Helwig EB: Kaposi's sarcoma. Cancer 12:289, 1959

86. Santucci M, Pimpinelli N, Moretti S, Giannotti B: Classic and immunodeficiency-associated Kaposi's sarcoma. Arch Pathol Lab Med 112:1214, 1988

87. Lobert PF, Appelman HD: Inflammatory cloacogenic polyp. A unique inflammatory lesion of the anal transitional zone. Am J Surg Pathol 5:761, 1981

88. Saul SH: Inflammatory cloacogenic polyp. Hum Pathol 18:1120, 1987

89. Sharp WC, Helwig EB: Sarcoma botryoides (embryonal rhabdomyosarcoma) of the anus. J Dis Child 97:845, 1959

90. Hjermstad BM, Helwig EB: Tailgut cysts. Report of 53 cases. Am J Clin Pathol 89:139, 1988

Index

Page numbers followed by f denote figures; those followed by t denote tables.

AAD. *See* Antibiotic-associated diarrhea (AAD)
Aberrant mucosal glands, in anorectal mucosa, 369, 370f
Acquired immunodeficiency syndrome (AIDS)
  Candida infection in, 172
  CMV colonic ulcers in patients with, 25, 26f
  Crohn's disease remission in, case study, 76
  Crytosporidium infection in, 36
  exploding crypt cells and, 161
  herpes simplex virus colitis in patients with, 23–24
  histoplasmosis in gastrointestinal tract, 34
  macrophage distinction, Whipple's disease and, 165
  microsporidia causing diarrhea in, 170
ACTH. *See* Adrenocorticotropic hormone (ACTH)
Acute self-limited colitis (ASLC)
  due to *Campylobacter* infection, 29f
  due to *Shigella* infection, 28f
  versus IBD, 27t, 27
    immunoglobulin-containing cells in differential diagnosis of, 69–72, 70f
ADCC. *See* Antibody-dependent cell-mediated cytotoxicity (ADCC)

Addison's disease, gastric carcinoids associated with, 335
Adenocarcinoid tumor appendiceal, 296. *See also* Goblet cell carcinoid tumors
  biologic behavior of, 300
  clinical characteristics, 299–300
  histogenesis of, 296, 299
  microscopic features of, 292, 293f–294f
  periappendiceal lymphatic permeation and, 296, 298f
  tumor nests, 295f–296f, 297f
  of the colon and rectum, 236–237
  metastasizing versus non-metastasizing, 301
Adenocarcinoma
  colorectal
    histologic grades of, 229, 231, 230f–232f
    and small cell carcinoma differentiation, 236, 236t
  invasive, of the appendix, 284, 285f–286f, 287
  of large bowel, 230f
  linitis plastica-type, 230f
Adenoma(s)
  association with adenosquamous carcinoma of colon and rectum, 234–235
  Brunner's gland type, 209
  of the colon
    associated with polyposis

  syndromes, 219
  and malignancy relationship, 220–221, 220f–221f
  and dysplasia in IBD compared, 87–88
  familial adenomatous, colorectal cancer and, 250, 251
  mixed or intermediate form. *See* Tubulovillous adenomas
  multiple, polyposis syndromes and, 214–215
  nodular lymphoid hyperplasia mimicking, 219, 219f
  noncystic localized, in the appendix, 267, 267f–268f
  papillary. *See* Tubulovillous adenomas
  pseudoinvasion of, in early colorectal cancer, 248, 249f, 250
  tubular. *See* Adenomatous polyp
  tubulovillous. *See* Tubulovillous adenomas
  in ulcerative colitis, management of, 115
  villoglandular. *See* Tubulovillous adenomas
  villous. *See* Villous adenoma
Adenomatoid hyperplasia, as stage in ECL cell hyperplasia-neoplasia sequence, 319, 321f
Adenomatous epithelium, appendiceal, 269, 270f, 271, 271f–273f

Adenomatous polyp
  appendiceal, 267, 267f–268f
  of the colon
    behavior of, 196–197
    carcinoma occurring in, fre-
      quency of, 200t
    gross pathology, 192–193,
      193f
    incidence by age and sex,
      196
    location of, 195–196
    microscopic pathology, 193,
      194f–195f, 195, 196f
    pathogenesis of, 195–196
  of small intestine, 209–210
Adenosquamous carcinoma, of
    colon and rectum,
    234–235
Adrenocorticotropic hormone
    (ACTH)
  Cushing's syndrome and, 350
  as secretory product of
    endocrine cells, 306,
    307t
AGCH. *See* Antropyloric G cell
    hyperplasia (AGCH)
AIDS. *See* Acquired immunode-
    ficiency syndrome
    (AIDS)
AJCC. *See* American Joint
    Commission of Cancer
    (AJCC)
Alkaline phosphatase-immuno-
    globulin complexes, in
    IBD, 65
Allelic deletions, colorectal can-
    cer and, 251
Allergic proctitis, 52–53
  Ige-containing cells in, 70–71,
    71f
Amebiasis, colitis and, 34–35
American Joint Commission of
    Cancer (AJCC), univer-
    sal staging system for
    colorectal cancer pro-
    posed by, 238, 238t–239t
Amoebic colitis, 34–35, 35f
Ampicillin, colitis induced by,
    42
Amyloidosis, associated with
    diagnostic normal villi,
    181

Anal canal
  carcinoma of
    carcinoma in situ, 375–376,
      376f
    cloacogenic segment. *See*
      Cloacogenic carcinoma
    squamous cell, 374–375
  cloacal segment
    and accessory structures,
      368–369, 369f
    gross pathology of, 367, 368f
    historical review of studies on,
      367
    mucosal zones, 368
Anal ducts, 368–369, 369f
  carcinoma of, 373–374, 374f
Anogenital Paget's disease, 383,
    384f
Anogenital region
  Bowenoid papulosis of,
    377–379, 378f–379f
  Bowen's disease and, 376–377
  condyloma acuminatum of,
    379–380, 380f–381f
  hidradenoma papilliferum of,
    387–388, 388f
Anorectal junction
  accessory structures, 368–369,
    369
  historical review of studies on,
    367
  mucosal levels of, 368
Anorectal melanoma, primary,
    381–383, 382f–383f
Anthraquinone purgatives,
    catharctic colon syn-
    drome and, 41
Antibiotic-associated diarrhea
    (AAD), *Clostridium dif-
    ficile* associated with, 30
Antibiotic therapy
  diagnostic variably abnormal
    villi and, 175
  effect on UC and CCD, 16
  for Whipple's disease, 165
Antibody-dependent cell-medi-
    ated cytotoxicity
    (ADCC), in IBD, 68–69
  schematic representation of,
    68f
Antibody production, local, in
    IBD, 69–72, 70f, 71f

Anti-inflammatory drugs
  effect in UC and CCD, 15
  nonsteroidal. *See* Nonster-
    oidal anti-inflammatory
    drugs (NSAIDs)
Antimetabolites, associated with
    diagnostic variably
    abnormal villi, 175
Antioncogenes, colorectal can-
    cer and, 250–251
α_1–antitrypsin, classic inflam-
    matory reactions and, 62
Antropyloric G cell hyperplasia
    (AGCH)
  clinical conditions associated
    with, 317t
  primary, 315–316
    differential diagnosis of,
      316f
  secondary to clinical condi-
    tions, 316–318
    pernicious anemia, 317f
    Zollinger-Ellison syndrome,
      318f
Anus. *See also under Anal*
  giant condyloma acuminatum
    in, 381
  histopathology of, in non-
    caseating epithelioid cell
    granuloma, 8, 9f
  malignant lymphoma of, 389
  metastatic carcinoma involv-
    ing, 391
  sarcoma botryoides of, 391
Aphthoid ulcers, in colonic
    Crohn's disease, 4f, 5,
    13
Apoptosis, in GVHD, 150f, 161
Appendix
  carcinoid tumor of, 341f
  epithelial proliferations in. *See
    also individually named
    neoplasms*
    adenomas
      circumferential, of villous
        or undulating patterns,
        267–269, 270f, 271,
        271f–273f
      colonic-type noncystic
        localized, 267,
        267f–268f
      cystadenoma and mucocele

relationship, 271, 274–279, 274f–278f

goblet cell carcinoid tumor, 291–301, 293f–294f, 295f–300f

hyperplastic polyps or mucosa, 264, 265f–266f, 267

literature status on, 263–264

noncarcinoid, 263, 264t

pseudomyxoma peritonei secondary to, 288, 289f–290f, 291

questions relating to, 263

invasive carcinoma of, 279, 281, 283f–286f, 287–288

actuarial survival curves in, 287f

involvement in ulcerative colitis, 4

vermiform, involvement in CCD and UC, 8

APUD characteristics

carcinoid syndrome and, 344

of endocrine cells in the gut, 310

Argentaffinomas, 327

histogenesis of, 332–334

in the midgut, 340

Argyrophil cells

in atrophic gastritis

linear hyperplasia of, 320f

micronodular hyperplasia of, 320f

simple hyperplasia of, 319f

and carcinoid tumor classification, 327

in midgut carcinoid, 340f

Armed adenocarcinoid tumor nomenclature, 292, 301

metastases and survival studies, 300

Arthus reaction, classic inflammatory reactions and, 61–62, 62f

ASLC. *See* Acute self–limited colitis (ASLC)

Astler-Coller staging system, for colorectal carcinoma, 237–238, 238t

five-year survival percentages

compared, 239–240, 240t

Atrophic gastritis

ECL cell hyperplasia in, 319, 319f–321f

gastric carcinoids associated with, 334, 335t

Autocytotoxic phenomena, in IBD

cellular, 68–69

humoral, 67–68

Autoimmune disorders, gastric carcinoids associated with, 335

Autoimmune thyroiditis, gastric carcinoids associated with, 335

Azothioprine, effect on UC and CCD, 15–16

Azulfidine therapy, effect on UC and CCD, 16

"Backwash ileitis"

mimicking Crohn's ileitis, 184

in ulcerative colitis, 4, 12

Bacterial infections, in differential diagnosis of IBD, 26–28

Campylobacter fetus ss. jejuni, 28, 29f, 30

Clostridium difficile, 30–32, 31f

Escherichia coli 0157:H7, 30

Yersinia spp., 32, 33f

Basal cell carcinoma, of perianal skin, 391

B cells, suppressed production in IBD, 73–74

Behçet's disease, colitis associated with, 49

Biopsy

in CCD and UC. *See under* Endoscopic biopsy

of duodenal bulb, 182–183, 183f

endoscopic. *See* Endoscopic biopsy

ileal, 183–185, 184f

proximal jejunal, normal, 181, 181t

of small bowel. *See* Small bowel biopsy

Bisacodyl, colitis induced by, 41, 42f

Blood flow, in ischemic bowel disease, experimental models, 121–122, 122f, 126

Blood groups, tumor associated antigens related to, 255t

Blood vessel invasion, in colorectal cancer evaluation, 241

Bone marrow transplantation, colitis following, 45

Bowel. *See also* Large bowel; Small bowel

obstruction and perforation, in colorectal cancer evaluation, 242

wall of

histopathological findings in UC and CCD differential diagnosis, 7–8, 9f

thickening in CCD, 5

Bowenoid papulosis, of anogenital region, 377–379, 378f–379f

Bowen's disease, of anogenital region, 376–377

Brunner gland artifact, in small bowel biopsy, 140, 142f

Brunner's gland "adenoma," of small intestine, 209

and malignancy relationship, 220

Buschke-Lowenstein tumor, 380–381

Bypass, small intestinal, colitis following, 45, 47, 47f

Calcium, ischemic bowel disease and, 130–131

Campylobacter spp., stain selection for, 10

Campylobacter fetus ss. jejuni, enteric infection with, 28, 29f, 30

Campylobacter jejuni, and IBD association, 61

Candida spp., in AIDS patients, 172

Capillaria philippinensis, 170

Capillariasis, associated with diagnostic variably abnormal villi, 170
Carcinoembryonic antigen (CEA)
in differential diagnosis of undifferentiated colorectal tumors, 236, 236t
Paget's cells and, 385
and tumor classification, 231
Carcinoid syndrome, 344–345
atypical versus classic, 345
Carcinoid tumors
biologically functioning, general characteristics of, 344
classification of, 327
clinical conditions associated with
carcinoid syndrome, 344–345
Cushing's syndrome, 350
gastrinoma syndrome, 345–346, 347f, 348
somatostatinoma syndrome, 348–350, 349
other conditions, 350–351
diagnosis of, 351–352
in ECL cell hyperplasia-neoplasia sequence, 321, 323f
of the foregut, 334. *See also* Gastric carcinoids
immunoreactivity frequency, 343f
gastric, 334–338. *See also* Gastric carcinoids
general characteristics, 325–326
goblet cell. *See* Goblet cell carcinoid tumors
of the hindgut, 341–343, 342f
immunoreactivity frequency, 343f
histogenesis of, 332–334
histologic features of
glandular pattern, 329, 330f
insular pattern, 327, 328f, 329
mixed pattern, 331, 331f
psammomatous pattern, 331–332, 333f

trabecular pattern, 329, 329f
undifferentiated pattern, 329, 330f, 331
immunoreactivity frequency comparisons, 343
of the midgut, 338–341, 340f–341f
immunoreactivity frequency, 343f
psammomatous, 331–332, 333f
of the rectosigmoid, 207, 208f
secretory products, 326–327
Carcinoma
of anal ducts, 373–374, 374f
basal cell, of perianal skin, 391
Bowen's disease as, 376–377
cloacogenic. *See* Cloacogenic carcinoma
of colon and rectum. *See* Colorectal cancer
dyspalsia in IBD as aid to predicting, 86
invasive
absence of dysplasia with, 89–90
of the appendix, 279, 281, 283f–286f, 287–288
metastatic, involving anus, 391
small intestinal polyp potential for, 219–221
squamous cell, of anal canal, 374–375
verrucous, of oral cavity, 376
Carcinoma in situ
in anal canal, 375–376, 376f
malignant changes in intestinal adenoma as, 220
Carcinosarcoma, of the colon, 236
Cartilaginous exostoses, colon adenomas associated with, 219
Castor oil, catharctic colon syndrome and, 41
Cathartic colon syndrome, 41
C3b INA (C3b inactivator), complement system and, 65
CCD. *See* Colonic Crohn's disease (CCD)
CEA. *See* Carcinoembryonic antigen (CEA)

Celiac sprue, 146f, 147–148, 149f–150f
abnormal biopsy findings in, 146f
EC cell hyperplasias in, 323, 324f
in infectious gastroenteritis, 146f, 151–152
versus infectious gastroenteritis, 151, 151f
Cell-mediated immunity, in IBD, 72–74
Cellular immunity, in IBD, 68–69
Chemotherapeutic agents
colitis induced by, 42, 43f
diagnostic variably abnormal villi and, 173
necrotizing enterocolitis in cancer patients, 52
Chlamydia psittaci, gastrointestinal disease caused by, IBD differential diagnosis and, 25
Chlamydia trachomatis, gastrointestinal disease caused by, IBD differential diagnosis and, 25
Choriocarcinoma, in colonic tumor and hepatic metastases, 236
Chromogranins, in neuroendocrine cell identification, 312–314
Chromosomes, alterations in colorectal tumors, 221–222
Chronic granulomatous disease, of childhood
colitis associated with, 48
flat small bowel biopsy and, 155, 156f
Chronic renal failure, gastric carcinoids associated with, 335
Cimetidine, gastric carcinoids associated with, 335
C1 INH (C1 esterase inhibitor), complement system and, 65
Circumferential villous adenoma, appendiceal, 264, 266f, 267–271, 270f

growth patterns, 268
Circumferential villous cystade-
    noma, 271, 271f
Clinical staging system, for rec-
    tal carcinoma, 228
Clinoril, associated with diag-
    nostic variably abnormal
    villi, 175
Cloacogenic carcinoma
    in anal duct, 373, 374f
    incidence of, 370–371
    nomenclature for, 370
    transitional, 371, 371f–372f,
        373
        and squamoid differentia-
            tion, 371, 372f
    tumor size in, 371
Cloacogenic polyp, inflamma-
    tory, 390–391
Clostridium difficile
    enteric infection with, 30–32
    pseudomembranous colitis due
        to, 31f, 31
Clostridium difficile toxin-
    induced inflamma-tory
    disease,
antibiotic and azulfidine therapy
    linked, 16
c-myc oncogenes, colorectal
    cancer and, 250–251
Coagulative necrosis
    in severe ischemic colitis, 124,
        125f
    stress ulceration and, 130
"Cobblestone" mucosa, in co-
    lonic Crohn's disease, 5
Coccidiosis, associated with
    diagnostic variably
    abnormal villi, 169–170,
    170f, 171f
Colchicine, associated with for
    considering, 113
Colitis
    amoebic, 34–35, 35f
    collagenous. *See* Collagenous
        colitis
    in differential diagnosis of IBD
        acute self–limited type, 27t,
            27
        collagenous type, 49–51, 50f
        eosinophilic type and aller-
            gic proctitis, 52–53

motor disorders associated
    with
    diverticulitis, 37–38, 38f
    solitary rectal ulcer syn-
        drome, 39f, 39–40
    necrotizing enterocolitis, 52
    nonspecific (idiopathic)
        ulcer, 51–52
    secondary to vascular
        hypoperfusion, 40–41
    systemic disease asso-ciated
        Behçet's disease, 49
        chronic granulomatous
            disease of childhood, 48
        hemolytic-uremic syn-
            drome, 49
        immunodeficiency syn-
            dromes, 48–49
    therapeutic intervention
        induced drug therapies,
            41–42, 43f
        enemas and laxatives, 41,
            42f
        following bone marrow
            transplantation, 45
        intestinal bypass/fecal
            stream diversion, 45,
            47f, 47
        radiation therapy, 43–45,
            44f, 46f
    fulminant. *See* Fulminant coli-
        tis
    of indeterminate type, 15
    ischemic. *See* Ischemic colitis
    pseudomembranous type, due
        to *Clostridium difficile*,
        31
    ulcerative. *See* Ulcerative coli-
        tis (UC)
    uremic, ischemic etiology for,
        130–131, 131f
Collagenous colitis, 49–51, 50f
    lymphocytic colitis and, 51
    microscopic colitis and, 51
Collagenous sprue, 152–153
Colloid carcinomas, versus
    mucinous, 231,
    232f–233f, 234
Colon
    adenomas of, and polyposis
        syndrome association,
        219

cancer of
    and adenoma relationship,
        220–221, 220f–221f
    and rectum involvement. *See*
        Colorectal cancer
    classification of disorders of,
        24t
    effect of chronic radiation on,
        45, 46f
    endoscopic biopsies, in inac-
        tive UC, 12f, 12
    nonspecific (idiopathic) ulcers
        of, 51–52
    obstruction of, colitis compli-
        cating, 40–41
    shortening of
        as laxative effect, 41
        in UC and CCD, 5
Colonic Crohn's disease (CCD)
    diagnosis of, 1–2
    and diverticulitis, 37–38, 38f
    effects of therapy on, 15–16
    in endoscopic biopsy speci-
        mens, 8, 10–15. *See also*
        Endoscopic biopsy
    and fulminant UC
        mimicking features, 17–18,
            18t
        misclassification of CCD, 17
    granulomatous inflammation
        in, 7, 8f
    in resection specimens, 2–8.
        See also Resection speci-
        mens
    and ulcerative colitis
        differential diagnosis of, 1
        versus colitis of indetermi-
            nate type, 15
        future directions for, 19–20
        in inactive stage, 16
        using endoscopic biopsy
            specimens, 11, 15t
        using resection specimens,
            4t
        histopathology compared,
            7f, 8f
            in endoscopic biopsies, 11t
            in resection specimens, 6t
Colon polyps. *See also under*
    individually named
    polyps
    adenomatous, 192–197

Colon polyps *(Continued)*
  carcinoid, 207, 208f
  hyperplastic, 190–192
  inflammatory, 206, 206f–207f
  juvenile, 200–203
  leiomyoma of the muscularis
    mucosa, 207, 208f
  lipoma, 207–208
  lymphoid, 206–207
  Peutz–Jeghers, 203–205
  tubulovillous adenomas,
    199–200
  villous adenoma, 197–199
Colorectal cancer
  cytometric DNA analysis in,
    252, 254–256
  distribution of
    by age, 226–227
    by sex, 226
    by site, 225–226
  early stage, 242, 243f–244f,
    246–250, 249f
  epidemiology, 225
  incidence of, 225
  molecular genetics of, 250–252
  prognosis factors
    bowel obstruction and perfo-
      ration, 242
    histopathologic characteris-
      tics, 228–229
    lymphatic infiltration, 242
    tumor classification,
      229–240. *See also*
      Colorectal tumors, clas-
      sification of; Staging
      systems
    tumor resection, 227–228
    vascular invasion, 240–242
  risk in IBD, 1
  tumor associated antigens,
    252, 253f–254f
    blood group-related, 255t
Colorectal tumors
  classification of
    adenocarcinoma, 229, 231,
      230f–232f
    goblet cell carcinoid,
      236–237
    mucinous or colloid, 231,
      232f–233f, 234
    small cell undifferentiated,
      235–236, 235f

squamous and adenosqua-
      mous, 234–235
  genetic alteration in, 221–222
  staging of. *See* Staging systems
  tumor associated antigens,
    252, 253f–254f
Common variable hypogamma-
    globulinemia (CVH),
    153–154, 154f
  nodular lymphoid hyperplasia
    association with, 219
Complement system, inhibitors
    of, in IBD, 65
Condyloma acuminatum
  of anogenital region, 379–380,
    380f–381f
  giant, 380–381
  of the penis, 380
Contrast media, colitis induced
    by, 41
Cowden's syndrome, 218
  and malignancy relationship,
    220
Crohn's disease
  associated with diagnostic nor-
    mal villi, 178, 180, 180f
  endocrine cell hyperplasias in,
    325
  Ige-containing cells in, 70–71,
    71f
  response to cyclosporine thera-
    py, 76t
Cronkhite-Canada syndrome,
    218
  associated with diagnostic
    variably abnormal villi,
    176, 177f
  and malignancy relationship,
    220
Crypt abscesses
  anti-inflammatory drugs effect
    on, 15
  in colonic Crohn's disease,
    6–7
Crypt architecture
  in celiac sprue, 148
  destroyed in UC, 5, 7f, 13f, 13
  distorted in fulminant UC, 18,
    18f
  distorted in IBD, 63, 64f
  maintained in CCD, 5, 7f
Crypt cell(s)

carcinoma of. *See* Goblet cell
    carcinoid tumor
  exploding, in GVHD, 150f,
    161
Cryptosporidiosis, 36f
Cryptosporidium spp.
  colitis and, 35–36
  intestinal mucosal abnormali-
    ties produced by, 169,
    170f
Crypt(s)
  dysplasia involving one part
    of, 105–106
  serrated, as problem in dyspla-
    sia diagnosis, 103–105,
    107f
Cushing's syndrome, 350
CVH. *See* Common variable
    hypogammaglobuline-
    mia (CVH)
Cyclosporine therapy, response
    in Crohn's disease, 76t
Cystadenocarcinoma
  appendiceal, 281, 284f
  as neoplastic mucocele, 275
Cystadenoma, 273f
  circumferential villous, 271,
    271f
  mucinous. *See* Mucinous cyst-
    adenoma
  and mucocele relationship,
    271–279
  rupture of, pseudomyxoma
    peritonei and, 291
  undulating, 271, 272f
Cyst(s)
  lymphangiectatic, of small
    intestine, 211, 212f
  sebaceous, colon adenomas
    associated with, 219
  tailgut, 391
Cytomegalovirus (CMV)
  associated with diagnostic
    variably abnormal villi,
    172
  exploding crypt cells and, 161
  gastrointestinal disease caused
    by, IBD differential
    diagnosis and, 25, 26f
Cytometric DNA analysis, in
    colorectal cancer, 252,
    254–256

D cells, of the antrophylonic mucosa, 306
hyperplasias of, 324
Dermatitis herpetiformis, celiac sprue and, 146f, 151–152
Devon family syndrome, 219
Diabetes mellitus, gastric carcinoids associated with, 335
Diarrhea
antibiotic-associated, 30
Giardia lamblia causing, 167
infectious, tuberculosis versus Crohn's disease, 33
microsporidia causing, 170
Dinitrochlorobenzene (DNCB)
cell-mediated hypersen-sitivity model and, in IBD, 76
cutaneous anergy to, in IBD, 73
Discrete ulcers
in colonic Crohn's disease, 4f, 5, 13
in fulminant colitis, 19
Dispersed endocrine system (DES), endocrine cell population of gut as, 305
Diverticulitis, 37
combined with Crohn's disease, 37–38, 38f
DNA analysis, cytometric, in colorectal cancer, 252, 254–256
DNCB. *See* Dinitrochlor benzene (DNCB)
Drug injury, associated with diagnostic variably abnormal villi, 173–175
Dukes' staging system, for rectal carcinoma, 237t, 237
five-year survival percentages compared, 239–240, 240t
Dulcolax. *See* Bisacodyl
Duodenal bulb
with Brunner gland artifact, 142f
endoscopic biopsy of, 182
normal histology, 182–183, 183f
Duodenum
psammomatous carcinoid of, 333f

ulcer disease of, gastric carcinoids associated with, 335
Dysplasia, in IBD
absence with invasive carcinoma, 89–90
and adenomas compared, 87–88
biopsy for
dysplasia in one part only, 106
factors in examining, 116, 117–118
endoscopy preparation, effects of, 117
fixatives effect on interpretation, 117
orientation, 116–117
implications, 111
indefinate for dysplasia
original classification modification, 97, 97t, 98f, 99, 99f, 100f
patient management in, 112
negative for dysplasia, 90
active colitis in resolving phase, 90–93, 93f, 94f
changes associated with active regeneration, 93–96, 95f, 96f
patient management in, 111
positive for dysplasia. *See* Dysplastic biopsies
reproducibility of results, 111
classification of mucosal change in, 90, 90t
indefinate, 97–99
negative, 90–96
positive, 99–103. *See also* Dysplastic biopsies
concept of, 87
cumulative incidence of, 85–86, 86f
defined, 90
diagnosis of
difficult situations in, 103
acute inflammation effect, 108, 110f, 111

biopsy partially involved, 106
crypt partially involved, 105–106
follicular inflammation, 105, 108f
inflammatory polyps and, 106–107, 109f, 110f
serrated crypts, 103–105, 107f
negative resection specimens following, 115–116
evolution of, 88–89
and application to patient management, 89
high-risk groups for, 86–87
lesions and masses, 89
prevalence of, 85
Dysplastic biopsies
diagnosis of, 99–100
high-grade dysplasia, 103, 105f, 106f
low-grade dysplasia, 100–103, 101f, 102f
management of, 112–113
confirming results, 113
in high-grade dysplasia, 114
in low-grade dysplasia, 114
options for, 113–114
surgical, 114–115
problems involving focality of dysplasia and sampling, 113
Dysplastic lesions, as stage in ECL cell hyperplasia-neoplasia sequence, 321, 322f

ECAC. *See* Epithelial cell-associated component (ECAC)
Ectasia, as non-neoplastic mucocele, 275
Edema
mucosal, anti-inflammatory drugs causing, 15
in severe ischemic colitis, 126, 126f
EMA. *See* Epithelial membrane antigen (EMA)

Embedding procedure, for endoscopic biopsy specimens,
10
Endocrine cells
characteristics of, 305–308,
306f
ultrastructural, 306–308,
307t
closed-type, 305
gastrointestinal carcinoids
arising from. *See*
Carcinoid tumors
goblet cell carcinoid tumor
and, 294
gut hormone identification and
nomenclature and, 308,
309f
histogenesis of, 310
hyperplasias of, 314–315
antral G cell. *See also*
Antropyloric G cell
hyperplasia (AGCH)
primary, 315–316, 316t
secondary, 316–318, 317t,
317f–318f
D cells, 325
enterochromaffin cells,
323–324, 324f
enterochromaffin-like cells,
318–319, 319f–324f,
321–323
other cell types, 325
misnaming of, 305
open-type, 305
peptidergic innervation of the
gut and, 308, 310
Endometrioma, anal, 391
Endoscopic biopsy
in CCD and UC
anatomic distribution of
findings, 12f, 12
histopathology
characteristics of inflammation, 11t, 12–13
distribution of nonspecific
active inflammation,
13–15
limitations and advantages,
11, 11t
of duodenal bulb, 182
normal histology, 182–183,
183f

Enemas
colitis induced by, 41
steroid, effect on UC and
CCD, 16
Entamoeba histolytica, colitis
and, 34–35
Enteric pathogens, identified in
population-based stud-
ies, 28, 29t
Enterochromaffin (EC) cells,
305. *See also* Endocrine
cells
hyperplasias of, 323–324, 324f
in Lausanne classification, 308
Enterochromaffin-like (ECL)
cells. *See also* Endocrine
cells
hyperplasias of, 318–323
clinical significance,
322–323
hyperplasia-neoplasia
sequence, 319, 321,
319f–322f
in Lausanne classification, 308
Enterocolitis, necrotizing. *See*
Necrotizing enterocolitis
Enzyme-immunoglobulin complexes, disease associa-
tion and, 65
Eosinophilic colitis, 52–53
Eosinophilic gastroenteritis,
associated with diagnos-
tic variably abnormal
villi, 165–166, 166f
Epithelial cell-associated component (ECAC), humoral
immunity against in
IBD, 67
Epithelial membrane antigen
(EMA), in differential
diagnosis of undif-feren-
tiated colorectal tumors,
236, 236t
Epithelium
adenomatous, appendiceal,
269, 270f, 271,
271f–273f
in small bowel biopsy
abnormal findings, 144
normal findings, 139f, 141
Escherichia coli
0157:H7 strain

enteric infection with, 30
ischemic bowel disease and,
130
and IBD association, 61
Excision, local, colorectal carcinoma and, 228
Exostoses, cartilaginous, colon
adenomas associated
with, 219
Exploding crypt cells, in GVHD,
150f, 161

Fabry's disease, vacuolated ganglion cells in, 180
FAL. *See* Fractional allelic loss
(FAL)
Familial adenomatous adenomas
(FAP), colorectal cancer
and, 250, 251
Familial enteropathy, 158
Familial polyposis coli,
211–212
behavior of, 214
gross pathology, 212, 213f
incidence by age and sex,
213–214
location and multiplicity of,
212
microscopic pathology, 212
pathogenesis of, 212
FAP. *See* Familial adenomatous
adenomas (FAP) *fap*
locus, colorectal tumors
and
and genetic alterations,
221–222
mapping of, 251
Fibroma, anal, 391
Fibronectin, classic inflammatory reactions and, 62
Fissuring ulcer, in fulminant colitis, 17, 17f
with necrotic tissue, 17f, 19
Fixatives
effect on interpretation of
biopsy, 117
selecting for endoscopic biopsy specimens, 10
Flat small bowel biopsy
diagnostic and nonspecific,
147t
diseases associated with

adult immunodeficiency syndromes, 153–155, 154f

celiac sprue, 146f, 147–148, 149f–150f, 151–152

childhood kwashiorkor, 156–158

chronic granulomatous disease, 155, 156f

collagenous sprue, 152–153, 153f

familial enteropathy, 158

other protein injury, 152

refractory sprue and ulcerative jejunoileitis, 152

tropical sprue syndrome, 155–156, 157f

Fleets Phospho-Soda. *See* Hypertonic phosphate enemas

FMLP. *See* Formyl-methionyl-leucyl-phenylalanine (FMLP)

Folic acid therapy, diagnostic variably abnormal villi and, 173

Follicular inflammation, as problem in dysplasia diagnosis, 105, 108f

"Follicular proctitis," in ulcerative colitis, 5, 7f, 13

Foregut, carcinoids of, 334. *See also* Gastric carcinoids immunoreactivity in, 343f, 343

Formalin-induced fluorescence, in neuroendocrine cell identification, 311

Formyl-methionyl-leucyl-phenylalanine (FMLP), classic inflammatory reactions and, 63

Fractional allelic loss (FAL), colorectal cancer and, 251–252

Fulminant colitis, 16–19 in colonic Crohn's disease, 29

Fulminant ulcerative colitis, 16f–17f, 17 versus colonic Crohn's disease mimicking features, 17–18, 18t misclassification of, 17 fissuring ulcer in, 17, 17f

Fungal infections diagnostic variably abnormal villi and, 172 in differential diagnosis of IBD, 34 *Paracoccidioides brasiliensis*, 33–34

Gangliocytic paragangliomas, 211

Ganglion cells, vacuolated, 180

Ganglioneuromas, in Cowden's syndrome, 218

Gardner's syndrome, 214

Gastric carcinoids classification of, 334–335, 335t diagnosis of, 334 diseases associated with increased risk for, 334–335, 335t in hyper- and normogastrinemic patients, 335, 336t immunocytochemical profiles in, 337–338, 337t, 338f incidence of, 334 silver staining in, 335–337, 336t ultrastructural appearances of, 338, 339f

Gastrin ECL cell hyperplasia and, 318 as secretory product of endocrine cells, 306, 307t

Gastrinomas differential diagnosis of, 346 histogenesis of, 332–334 ultrastructural characteristics of, 348

Gastrinoma syndrome, 345–346, 347f, 348

Gastritis, atrophic, ECL cell hyperplasia in, 319, 319f–321f

Gastroenteritis eosinophilic, associated with diagnostic variably abnormal villi, 165–166, 166f infectious. *See* Infectious gastroenteritis

viral, in differential diagnosis of IBD, 23–26

Gastrografin, colitis induced by, 41

Gastrointestinal tract anatomic distribution of endocrine cell types in, 309f carcinoids of. *See* Carcinoid tumors

Gastrointestinal Tumor Study Group (GITSG), colorectal cancer staging and, 238

G cells, of antral mucosa, 306 differentiation of, pre- and postnatal, 310 hyperplasias. *See* Antropyloric G cell hyperplasia (AGCH)

Giant condyloma acuminatum, 380–381

Giardia lamblia, immunodeficiency malabsorptive states and, 153

Giardiasis, diagnostic variably abnormal villi and, 167–169, 169f

GITSG. *See* Gastrointestinal Tumor Study Group (GITSG)

Glandular pattern carcinoid tumors, histologic features of, 329, 330f

Gluten-sensitive enteropathy. *See* Sprue

Glycoproteins, mucosal, as aid in UC and CCD pathologic distinction, 19t, 19

Goblet cell carcinoid tumors, 301, 332. *See also* Adenocarcinoid tumor appendiceal actuarial survival curves in, 287–288, 287f biologic behavior of, 300 clinical characteristics of, 299–300 gross pathology of, 292 histogenesis of, 296, 299 metastases from, 300, 300f microscopic features, 292, 293f

Goblet cell carcinoid tumors
  (Continued)
  nomenclature for, 291–292
  Paneth cells and, 292, 294f,
    294
  therapeutic options, 300–301
  tumor cell nests, 294,
    295f–296f, 296,
    297f–299f
  of the colon and rectum,
    236–237
  histologic features of, 332
Gold salt therapy, enterocolitis
    as complication of, 42
Goodpasture's disease, classic
    inflammatory reactions
    and, 62
Graft-versus-host disease
    (GVHD)
  associated with nonspecific
    variably abnormal villi,
    150f, 160–162
  colitis in, 45
Granular cell tumor, 388–389,
    389f, 390f
  pseudoepitheliomatous hyper-
    plasia and, 389
Granuloma(s)
  in colonic Crohn's disease, 6,
    13
    noncaseating epitheloid cell.
      See Non-caseating epith-
      eloid cell granuloma
  pyogenicum, hemorrhoids and,
    390
Granulomatous disease, chronic,
    of childhood, colitis
    associated with, 48
Granulomatous inflammation
  Campylobacter infection caus-
    ing, 30
  in colonic Crohn's disease, 7,
    8f, 7, 8f, 13
GVHD. *See* Graft-versus-host
    disease (GVHD)

Hamartoma(s)
  of the colon, congenital
    anomalies and, 219
  multiple, 218
Hamartomatous polyps, 190
Hand lens, use in small bowel

biopsy examination,
    144–145
Helicobacter spp. *See*
    Campylobacter spp.
Hemangioma, anal, 391
Hemolytic-uremic syndrome,
    colitis associated with,
    49
Hemorrhagic necrosis, of small
    intestine, 129–130, 129f,
    130f
Hemorrhoids, 390
Hemosiderin, in severe ischemic
    colitis, 124
Henoch-Schönlein purpura,
    associated with diagnos-
    tic variably abnormal
    villi, 175
Herpes simplex virus
  associated with diagnostic
    variably abnormal villi,
    172
  gastrointestinal disease caused
    by, IBD differential
    diagnosis and, 23–25
5-HIAA. *See* 5-hydroxyin-
    doleacetic acid (5-
    HIAA)
Hidradenoma papilliferum, of
    anogenital area,
    387–388, 388f
High-grade dysplasia
  biopsy management in, 114
  diagnosis of, 103, 105f, 106f
  management of, 114
Hindgut, carcinoids of, 341
  electron microscopic studies
    of, 341–342, 342f
  immunocytochemical studies
    of, 341–342, 342f
  immunoreactivity in, 343f, 343
  trabecular pattern, 329f
Histoplasma capsulatum, gas-
    trointestinal involvement
    by, 34
Histoplasmosis
  versus IBD, 34
  macrophage distinction,
    Whipple's disease and,
    165
HPV. *See* Human papillo-
    mavirus (HPV)

5-HT. *See* Serotonin (5-HT)
Human leukocyte antigen
    (HLA), IBD and Crohn's
    disease association with,
    77
Human papillomavirus (HPV),
    Bowenoid papulosis and,
    378–379
Humoral immunity, in IBD,
    67–68
Hyalinosis, associated with diag-
    nostic variably abnor-
    mal villi, 175–176
Hydrogen peroxide, colitis
    induced by, 41
Hydroxychloroquine, effect on
    immune complex-medi-
    ated colitis, 64
5-hydroxyindoleacetic acid (5-
    HIAA)
  carcinoid syndrome and,
    344–345
  and EC cell hyperplasias asso-
    ciation, 323–324
5-hydroxytryptamine. *See*
    Serotonin (5-HT)
Hypergastrinemic states
  ECL cell hyperplasia in, 318
  oxyntic mucosa and, 321,
    324f
  gastric carcinoids in, 335, 336t
Hyperplasia
  endocrine cell. *See under*
    Endocrine cells; *individ-
    ually named cells*
  pseudoepitheliomatous, granu-
    lar cell tumor and, 389
Hyperplastic mucosa, in the
    appendix, 264, 265f
Hyperplastic polyp
  of the colon, 189, 190
    behavior of, 192
    gross pathology, 190, 191f
    incidence by age and sex,
      192
    location and multiplicity of,
      192
    and malignancy relationship,
      220
    microscopic pathology, 190,
      191f, 192
    pathogenesis of, 192

morphology and frequency of, 189, 190

Hypertonic phosphate enemas, colitis induced by, 41, 42f. *See also* Enemas

Hyperviscosity syndrome, necrotizing enterocolitis and, 129

Hypovolemic shock, in ischemic bowel disease, 121–122, 122f

IBD. *See* Idiopathic inflammatory bowel disease (IBD)

Idiopathic inflammatory bowel disease (IBD)
  autocytotoxic phenomena
    cellular, 68–69
    humoral, 67–68
  cell-mediated immunity in, 72–74
  definition of, 1–2
  differential diagnosis of, 23
    classification of disorders of the colon in, 24t
    colitis
      acute self–limited type, 27t, 27, 69–72, 70f
      miscellaneous types, 49–53
      systemic disease associated, 48–49
      therapeutic intervention induced, 41–47
    inflammation
      infectious agents causing, 23–37
      motor disorders associated, 37–40
      secondary to vascular hypoperfusion, 40–41
  etiologic agents of, 61
  experimental models for, 61–64
  forms of, 1
    colitis of indeterminate type, 15
    Crohn's disease. *See* Colonic Crohn's disease (CCD)
    ulcerative colitis. *See* Ulcerative colitis (UC)
  genetic linkage in, 76–77

hypersensitivity model, cell-mediated, 76
immune complexes in, role of, 64
inflammatory mediators in, 65–66
  classic reactions, 62–63
local antibody production in, 69–72
local lymphocyte function in the gut, 74–76
phagocyte function in 66–67

Ileum
  biopsy of, 183–185, 184f
  endoscopic biopsy, in CCD, 12, 13f
  glandular carcinoid of, 330f
  inflammatory-type 64–65

Immunodeficiency syndromes
  acquired. *See* Acquired immunodeficiency syndrome (AIDS)
  colitis associated with acquired, 49. *See also* Acquired immunodeficiency syndrome (AIDS)
  hereditary, 48–49
  late-onset (common variable hypogammaglobulinemia), 153–154, 154f
  selective IgA deficiency, 154–155

Immunoglobulins
  heavy chain (Gm) allotypes, and Crohn's disease association, 77
  selective IgA deficiency, 154–155
  used to distinguish ASLC from IBD, 69–72

Immunoproliferative small intestinal disease (IPSID), associated with diagnostic variably abnormal villi, 166–167

Immunoreactivity, frequency in carcinoid tumors of the gut, 343f

Infectious agents, as aid in UC and CCD pathologic distinction, 19t, 19–20

Infectious diarrhea, tuberculosis versus Crohn's disease, 33

Infectious gastroenteritis associated with nonspecific variably abnormal villi, 158–159
  celiac sprue versus, 151, 151f

Infectious proctitis, agents isolated in, 33

Inflammation. *See also* Colitis
  acute, as problem in dysplasia diagnosis, 108, 110f, 111
  follicular, dysplasia diagnosis and, 105, 108f
  histopathologic characteristics of, 12–13
  infectious agent caused, in differential diagnosis of IBD
    bacterial, 26–33
    fungal, 33–34
    parasitic, 34–37
    viral, 23–26
  nonspecific active
    in colonic Crohn's disease, 14f, 14–15
    in ulcerative colitis, 13–14

Inflammatory bowel disease. *See* Idiopathic inflammatory bowel disease (IBD)

Inflammatory cell populations, as aid in UC and CCD pathologic distinction, 19

Inflammatory mediators
  as aid in UC and CCD pathologic distinction, 19
  in IBD, 65–66, 66f

Inflammatory polyps
  cloacogenic, 390–391
  of the colon, 206, 206f–207f
  dysplasia in, 106–107, 109f–110f
  fibroid, of small intestine, 209, 210f, 211f
  and malignancy relationship, 220
  of stomach and ileum, polyposis syndrome association with, 219
  in UC, 5–6

Insular pattern carcinoid tumors, histologic features of, 327, 328f, 329
Interleukin 1 (IL-1), production in normal and IBD mucosa, 74–75
Interleukin 2 (IL-2)
  alteration in gut mucosa, 75
  lamina propria cells cytotoxic activity and, 75–76, 75t
Intestinal bypass, colitis following, 45, 47, 47f
Intestines. *See* Bowel; Large bowel; Small bowel
Intramucosal carcinoma, malignant changes in intestinal adenoma as, 221
Intrarectal steroid therapy, effect on UC and CCD, 16
IPSID. *See* Immunoproliferative small intestinal disease (IPSID)
Ischemia, associated with diagnostic variably abnormal villi, 175, 176f–167f
Ischemic bowel disease
  blood flow experimental models, 121–122, 122f
  etiology of, 121
  gastrointestinal tract responses and, 131–132
    impact on diagnostic practices, 132–133
  outcome in, 121
  pathogenesis of, 121
  pathologic response in, 121
  spectrum of, 122–123, 122t
    ischemic colitis, 123–127
    necrotizing enterocolitis of premature infants, 127–129
    other pathologic lesions, 129–131
Ischemic colitis
  clinical forms of, 123, 123f
  experimental studies, 126
  gross pathology, 123–124, 124f
  histologic examination, 124, 125f
  pathogenesis of, 123–124, 123f

biochemical studies in, 126–127
  severe forms, findings in, 124, 125f, 126
Isoretinoin, colitis induced by, 41–42
Isospora belli
  colitis and, 35–36
  intestinal mucosal abnormalities produced by, 169, 171f
Isospora natalensis, colitis and, 35–36

Jass classification of rectal carcinoma, 239, 239t
  corrected five-year survival, 239, 239t
  updated, 239, 240t
Jejunoileitis, ulcerative, 152
Juvenile polyp, of the colon, 200
  behavior of, 203
  gross pathology of, 200, 202f
  incidence by age and sex, 203
  location and multiplicity of, 203
  and malignancy relationship, 220
  microscopic pathology of, 200, 202, 202f
  pathogenesis of, 202–203
Juvenile polyposis syndrome
  clinical course and classification of, 215
  gross pathology, 215, 216f
  incidence by age and sex, 216–217
  microscopic pathology, 215
  pathogenesis of, 217

Kala azar, associated with diagnostic variably abnormal villi, 170–172
Kaposi's sarcoma, of anorectal area, 390
Keratoacanthoma, 385–386, 386f–387f
Kultschitzky cells, 305. *See also* Endocrine cells
Kwashiorkor, in childhood, 156, 158

Lactic dehydrogenase-immunoglobulin complexes, in IBD, 65
Lamina propria
  cellular cytotoxic activities following Il-2 activation, 75–76, 75t
  chronic inflammation of, in UC, 5, 13
  proliferating endocrine cells in, 322f
  in small bowel biopsy
    abnormal findings, 144
    normal findings, 141
Large bowel
  adenocarcinoma of, 230f
  carcinoma incidence in, 225. *See also* Colorectal cancer
  classification of mucosal changes in, 90t
  linitis plastica-type adenocarcinoma of, 230f
  normal mucosa in, 91f
  scirrhous infiltration of, colorectal cancer and, 229
Late-onset immunodeficiency. *See* Common variable hypogammaglobulinemia (CVH)
Lausanne classification, of endocrine cells, 308
Laxatives
  colitis induced by, 41, 42f
  effect on colon length, 41
  implicated in cathartic colon syndrome, 41
LCA. *See* Leukocyte common antigen (LCA)
Leiomyomas
  anal canal and, 391
  of the muscularis mucosa, 207, 208f
    and malignancy relationship, 220
Leiomyosarcomas, anal canal and, 391
Leishmania spp., 171
Leishmaniasis, associated with diagnostic variably abnormal villi, 170–172

Leukocyte common antigen (LCA), in differential diagnosis of undifferentiated colorectal tumors, 236, 236t
Leukotrienes
classic inflammatory reactions and, 62–63
B₄, 63
Linear hyperplasia, as stage in ECL cell hyperplasia-neoplasia sequence, 319, 320f
Linitis plastica, colorectal cancer and, 229, 230f
Lipid storage disease, associated with diagnostic normal villi, 180–181
Lipoma, of the colon, 207, 208f
and malignancy relationship, 220
Lipomatosis, of small intestine, and malignancy relationship, 220
a-β-lipoproteinemia, associated with diagnostic normal villi, 176, 178, 179f
Local antibody production, in IBD, 69–72, 70f, 71f
Local excision, colorectal carcinoma and, 228
Low-grade dysplasia
biopsy management in, 114
diagnosis of, 100–103, 101f, 102f
management of, 114
Lumen
appendiceal, dilation of, 279
endocrine cell communication with, 305–306, 306
Lymphangiectasia, associated with diagnostic variably abnormal villi, 173, 175f
Lymphangiectatic cyst, of small intestine, 211, 212f
and malignancy relationship, 220
Lymphatic vessel invasion
in colorectal cancer evaluation, 241–242
malignant polyp with, outcome in, 247, 247t

Lymphocytic colitis, 51
Lymphocytic infiltration, in colorectal cancer evaluation, 242
Lymphogranuloma venereum (LGV), *Chlamydia trachomatis* induced, in differential diagnosis of IBD, 25–26
Lymphoid cells, local function in the gut, 74–75
Lymphoid nodules, proliferation of, in UC, 5, 7f
Lymphoid polyposis. *See* Nodular lymphoid hyperplasia
Lymphoid polyps, of the colon, 206–207
Lymphoma
malignant, of the anus, 389
primary intestinal, associated with diagnostic associated with diagnostic variably abnormal villi, 173–175

Macroglobulinemia
associated with diagnostic variably abnormal villi, 172–173, 174f
macrophage distinction, Whipple's disease and, 165
Macrophages, in Whipple's disease, 165
Major histocompatibility complex (MHC), and genetic linkage in disease, 76–77
Malabsorptive states
duodenal bulb biopsy in, 182–183, 183f
flat small bowel biopsy associated
celiac sprue, 146f, 147–148, 149f–150f, 151–152
childhood kwashiorkor, 156–158
chronic granulomatous disease, 155, 156f
collagenous sprue, 152–153, 153f
familial enteropathy, 158

other protein injury, 152
refractory sprue and ulcerative jejunoileitis, 152
tropical sprue syndrome, 155–156, 157f
ileal biopsy in, 183–185
normal villi associated, diagnostic
a-β-lipoproteinemia, 176, 178, 179f
amyloidosis, 181
Crohn's disease, 178, 180f
lipid storage diseases, 180
melanosis, 181
proximal jejunal biopsy in, 181, 181t
small bowel biopsy in. *See also* Small bowel biopsy
abnormal findings, 141–147
severe. *See* Flat small bowel biopsy
normal findings, 138–141
processing methods, 137–138
variably abnormal villi associated
diagnostic
drug and irradiation therapy, 173–175
eosinophilic gastroenteritis, 165–166, 166f
fungal diseases, 172
ischemia, 175–176, 176f–177f
lymphangiectasia, 173, 175f
macroglobulinemia, 172–173, 174f
parasitic diseases, 167–172, 169f–171f
polyposis syndromes, 176, 177f
primary intestinal lymphoma, 166–167
viral diseases, 172
Whipple's disease, 162, 163f–164f, 165
nonspecific
graft-versus-host disease, 150f, 160–162
infectious gastroenteritis, 151f, 158–159

Malabsorptive states
(*Continued*)
stasis syndromes, 159,
160f
Zollinger-Ellison syn-
drome, 159–160, 161f
Malignant lymphoma, anal, 389
Malignant melanoma, anorectal,
381–383, 382f–383f
Malignant polyp, in early colorectal cancer, 242–243
extent of, 243
morphology of, 243,
244f–245f
outcome of
in grade III carcinoma,
246–247, 247t
with lymphatic vessel invasion, 247, 247t
polypectomy, adequacy indicators, 248
postpolypectomy bowel resection, 248
and surgical resection findings, 243, 246, 246t
therapeutic options, 221
Mastocytosis, associated with
diagnostic normal villi,
181
Mediators, of inflammation, in
IBD, 65–66, 66f
Mediterranean lymphoma, associated with diagnostic
variably abnormal villi,
166–167
Melanoma, primary anorectal,
381–383, 382f–383f
Melanosis, associated with diagnostic normal villi, 181
MEN. *See* Multiple endocrine
neoplasia (MEN) syn-
drome
MEr-29, diagnostic variably
abnormal villi and, 174
Metaplastic polyp or mucosa.
See Hyperplastic polyp;
Hyperplastic mucosa
Metastatic carcinoma
involving anus, 391
peritoneal, pseudomyxoma
secondary to, 300,
300f

Methyldopa, colitis induced by,
41–42
MHC. *See* Major histocompatibility complex (MHC)
Microcirculation, in severe
ischemic colitis, 124,
125f
Microglandular carcinoma. *See*
Goblet cell carcinoid
tumor
Micronodular hyperplasia, as
stage in ECL cell hyper-
plasia-neoplasia
sequence, 319, 320f
Microscopic colitis, 51
Microsporidia, causing diarrhea,
170
Microsporidiosis, associated
with diagnostic variably
abnormal villi, 170
Microvillous inclusion disease,
158
Midgut, carcinoids of, 338–339
immunocytochemical studies
of, 339–340
immunoreactivity in, 343f, 343
insular pattern, 328f
ultrastructural characteristics
of, 340–341, 341f
Mixed pattern carcinoid tumors,
histologic features of,
331, 331f
Molecular genetics, of colorectal
cancer, 250–252
Morgagni
columns of, muscle cells and,
368, 369
sinuses of, anal ducts and, 368
Motor disorders, colitis associated with
diverticulitis, 37–38, 38f
solitary rectal ulcer syndrome,
39f, 39–40
Mucin, in resolving phase of
active UC, 91–92
Mucinous carcinoid tumor. *See*
Goblet cell carcinoid
tumor
Mucinous carcinomas
appendiceal, 281
versus colloid, 231,
232f–233f, 234

grading of, 234
Mucinous cystadenoma
mucus herniation and, 279,
283f
as neoplastic mucocele, 275,
276f–278f, 278
Mucocele, 271
and cystadenoma relationship,
271–279
described, 271, 274f
multiloculated, 271, 275f
neoplastic and non-neoplastic
forms of, 274–275
Muco-epidermoid tumors, 374
Mucopenic depression, amoebic
colitis and, 34–35, 35f
Mucosa
anorectal junction, zones of,
368
characteristic features in CCD,
5
edema of, anti-inflammatory
drugs causing, 15
hyperplastic, in the appendix,
264, 265f
in large bowel
changes classified, 90t
normal, 91f, 92f
morphometry of, as aid in UC
and CCD pathologic dis-
tinction, 19t, 19
oxyntic, ECL cell hyperplasias
and, 321, 324f
rectal and colonic, effect of
chronic radiation on, 45,
46f
regenerated, in quiescent UC,
90, 91f. *See also*
Regeneration, of mucosa
Mucus glycoproteins, as aid in
UC and CCD pathologic
distinction, 19t, 19
Multiple adenomas, polyposis
syndromes and, 214–215
Multiple endocrine neoplasia
(MEN) syndrome, 316
ECL cell carcinoids and,
321–322
type III, 351
type 1 (Wermer's syndrome),
350
Multiple hamartoma, 218

Muscularis mucosa
leiomyoma of, 207, 208f
and malignancy relationship,
220
normal findings in small
bowel biopsy, 141
Mycocele, rupture of, pseudomyxoma peritonei
and, 288

National Surgical Adjuvant
Breast and Bowel
Projects (NSABP), col-
orectal cancer staging
and, 238–239
Natural killer lymphocytes,
activity in IBD, 73
Necrosis
coagulative. *See* Coagulative
necrosis
hemorrhagic, of small intestine, 129–130, 129f,
130f
Necrotizing enterocolitis
in cancer patients, 52
in normal birthweight infants,
129
in premature infants, 127
autopsy findings, 127, 127f,
128f
diagnostic practices, 132
experimental models,
127–129
gross pathology, 127, 128f
Neomycin, diagnostic variably
abnormal villi and, 175
Neoplastic polyps, 189
Neuroendocrine cells
histochemical staining
methods
formalin-induced fluores-
cence, 311
silver-staining techniques,
311–312
immunocytochemical markers,
312–313
chromogranins, 313–314
neuron-specific enolase, 313
synaptophysin, 314
staining techniques to identify,
310–311
Neurofibroma, anal, 391

Neurogenic polyps
and malignancy relationship,
220
of small intestine, 210–211
Neuron-specific enolase (NSE)
in differential diagnosis of
undifferentiated colorec-
tal tumors, 236, 236t
in neuroendocrine cell identification, 311–312, 313
Neuropeptides, as aid in UC and
CCD pathologic distinc-
tion, 19t, 19
Nevus, hemorrhoids and, 390
Niemann-Pick disease, vacuolated ganglion cells in, 180
Nodular lymphoid hyperplasia,
218–219
associated with immunodeficiency malabsorptive
states, 154
etiologic categories, 219
and malignancy relationship,
220
mimicking adenomas, 219,
219f
Nonargentaffin carcinoid
tumors, 327
Noncaseating epitheloid cell
granuloma, in colonic
Crohn's disease, 6, 7f,
13
anal histopathology, 8, 9f
Nonspecific active inflammation, histopathologic distribution in UC and
CCD, (NSAIDs)
associated with diagnostic
variably abnormal villi,
175
colitis induced by, 41–42
Norwalk-like viruses
associated with diagnostic
variably abnormal villi,
172
gastroenteritis and, 23
NSABP. *See* National Surgical
Adjuvant Breast and
Bowel Projects
(NSABP)
NSE. *See* Neuron-specific enolase (NSE)

Nutritional blood flow, in
ischemic bowel disease,
experimental models,
121–122, 122f, 126

Obstruction, colonic, colitis
complicating, 40–41
Oldfield's syndrome, 219
Omeprazole, gastric carcinoids
associated with, 335
Oncogenes, colorectal cancer
and, 250–251
Oral cavity, verrucous carcinoma of, 376
Oxyntic mucosa, ECL cell
hyperplasias and, 319,
319f–321f, 321, 324f

PAGCH. *See* Primary antral G
cell hyperplasia
(PAGCH)
Paget's disease
anogenital, 383, 384f
perianal, 383–385, 384f
Pancreas, somatostatinomas of,
348–349
Paneth cells, goblet cell carcinoid tumor and, 292,
294f, 294
Papillary adenoma. *See* Tubulovillous adenomas
Papilliferum
hidradenoma, 387–388, 388f
syringocystadenoma, 388
Paracoccidioides brasiliensis,
gastrointestinal in-volve-
ment by, 33–34
Paracoccidioidomycosis, versus
IBD, 33–34
Paragangliomas, gangliocytic,
211
Paraneuron concept, gut endocrine cells and, 310
Paraphenylenediamine (PPD),
impaired skin test
responses to, in IBD, 73
Parasitic infestations
associated with diagnostic
variably abnormal villi,
167–172, 169f–171f
in differential diagnosis of
IBD, 34–37

Parasitic infestations *(Continued)*
amebiasis, 34–35, 35f
anisakidae, 37
crytosporidium, 35–36, 36f
schistosoma, 36–37
Penicillin, colitis induced by, 42
Peptidergic innervation, in the gut
Perianal Paget's disease,
383–385, 384f
histogenesis of, 385
Perianal skin, basal cell carcinoma of, 391
Pernicious anemia
antropyloric G cell hyperplasia
(AGCH) in, 317–318,
317f
ECL cell hyperplasia in, 319
gastric carcinoids associated
with, 334, 335t
Peutz-Jeghers polyp, of the
colon, 203
behavior of, 205
gross pathology of, 203, 204f
incidence by age and sex, 205
location and multiplicity of,
205
and malignancy relationship,
220
microscopic pathology of, 203,
204f–205f
pathogenesis of, 204–205
Peutz-Jeghers syndrome
behavior of, 217–218
conditions present in, 217
gross and microscopic pathology, 217
incidence by age and sex, 217
location of, 217
and malignancy relationship,
220
pathogenesis of, 217
Phagocytes, function in IBD,
66–67
Phenolphthalein, cathartic
colon syndrome and, 41
PMC. *See* Pseudomembranous
colitis (PMC)
Polycythemia vera, necrotizing
enterocolitis and, 129
Polyglandular autoimmune syndrome, gastric carcinoids
associated with, 335

Polymorphonuclear (PMN)
leukocytes, within lami-
na propria
abnormal findings, 144
normal findings, 141
Polyp-carcinoma sequence,
219–221
Polypectomy
for malignant polyp, 221
adequacy indicators, 248
specimen handling, 220f–221f,
221
Polyposis syndromes, 211
associated with diagnostic
variably abnormal villi,
176, 177f
Cowden's syndrome, 218
Cronkhite-Canada syndrome,
218
familial polyposis coli,
211–214, 213f
Gardner's syndrome, 214
juvenile polyposis syndrome,
215–217, 216f
multiple adenomas, 214–215
nodular lymphoid hyperplasia,
218–219
Peutz-Jeghers syndrome,
217–218
Turcot's syndrome, 214
other, 219
Polyp(s)
anorectal, benign lymphoid,
389
of the colon. *See* Colon
polyps
defined, 189
inflammatory
cloacogenic, 390–391
in UC, 5–6
intestinal. *See also* Small
intestinal polyps
and carcinoma relationship,
220–221, 220f–221f
classification and frequency
of, 189–190, 190t
malignant. *See* Malignant
polyp
in polyposis syndromes. *See*
Polyposis syn-
dromes;*individually
named syndromes*

Potassium-induced stenotic
ulcer, in ischemic bowel
disease, 130, 131f
Premature infants, necrotizing
enterocolitis of,
127–129, 127f, 128f
Primary antral G cell hyperplasia (PAGCH), 315–316
differential diagnosis of,
315–316
Primary intestinal lymphoma,
associated with diagnos-
tic variablyabnormal
villi, 166–167, 168f
Proctitis
allergic. *See* Allergic proctitis
"follicular," in ulcerative colitis, 5, 7f, 13
following fecal stream diversion, 45, 47, 47f
infectious, agents isolated in,
33
radiation inducing acute
episode, 44f
Proctocolectomy
for dysplasia in IBD, 114–115
and patient management in
dysplasia, 89
Prostaglandins
role in inflammatory reaction
mediation, 65
E$_2$, inhibition of, 65–66, 66f
Protein injury, in malabsorptive
states, 152
Proximal jejunal biopsy, normal
findings, diseases associated with, 181, 181t
Psammomatous carcinoids,
331–332, 333f
of the duodenum, 333f
Pseudoepitheliomatous hyperplasia, granular cell
tumor and, 389
Pseudoinvasion, adenoma showing, in early colorectal
cancer, 248, 249f, 250
Pseudolipomatosis, hydrogen
peroxide causing, 41
Pseudolymphoma, 167
Pseudomembrane, produced in
solitary rectal ulcer syndrome, 39

Pseudomembranous colitis (PMC), due to *Clostridium difficile*, 31, 130
Pseudomyxoma peritonei, 268, 279, 288
 behavior of, 291
 epithelium types encountered in, 288, 289f–290f
 incidence by age and sex, 291
 mycocele and cystadenoma rupture and, 288, 291
 secondary to metastatic adeno-carcinoid tumors, 300, 300f
 survival rates in, 291
Pseudo-Zollinger-Ellison syn-drome. *See* Primary antral G cell hyperplasia (PAGCH)

Radiation, therapeutic
 associated with diagnostic variably abnormal villi, 173–175
 colitis induced by, 43–45, 44f, 46f
"Railroad track" ulcers, in colonic Crohn's disease, 5
Raji cell technique, immune complexes in IBD and, 64
"Rake ulcers," in colonic Crohn's disease, 5
Ranitidine, gastric carcinoids associated with, 335
ras-gene mutations, colorectal tumors and, and genetic alterations, 221–222
 model, 251
ras oncogenes, colorectal cancer and, 250
Reactive oxygen metabolites (ROMs), ischemic colitis and, 127
Rectum
 carcinoid tumor of, 207, 208f, 342f
 mixed pattern, 331f
 undifferentiated pattern, 330f

carcinoma of
 and colon involvement. *See* Colorectal cancer
 incidence, 225
 staging systems for. *See under* Staging systems
 treatment alternatives, 227–228
 effect of chronic radiation on, 45, 46f
 endoscopic biopsy, in inactive UC, 13, 13f
 prolapse of, in solitary rectal ulcer syndrome, 39
Refractory sprue, 148, 152
Regeneration, of mucosa, in biopsy negative for dys-plasia
 changes associated with, 93–96
 differential diagnosis, 94–96, 95f, 96f
 in resolving UC, 92, 94f
Resection specimens
 colorectal carcinoma and, 227. *See also* Surgical resec-tion
 ulcerative colitis and colonic Crohn's disease in
 gross pathology, 3t, 3–5, 4f
 histopathology, 5–8, 6t, 7f–8f
 laboratory procedures, 2
 pathologic features distin-guishing between, 9t
Retention cyst, as non-neoplastic mucocele, 275
Retention polyp. *See* Juvenile polyp
Rheumatoid arthritis, gastric car-cinoids associated with, 335
ROMs. *See* Reactive oxygen metabolites (ROMs), ischemic colitis abnor-mal villi, 172
 gastroenteritis and, 23
Ruvalcaba-Myhre-Smith syn-drome, 219

Salicylazosulfapyridine, effect on UC and CCD, 15

Salmonella colitis, microgranu-lomas in, 32–33
Sampling problems, in dysplasia biopsy, 113
Sarcoma botryoides, anal, 391
Schistosomiasis, associated with diagnostic variably abnormal villi, 170
Schizogony, 169–170
Scirrhous infiltration, of the bowel, colorectal cancer and, 229
Sebaceous cysts, colon adeno-mas associated with, 219
Secondary antropyloric G cell hyperplasia, 316–318, 317f, 318f
Secretory granules
 of endocrine cells, 306
 ultrastructural characteristics of, 307t
Selective IgA deficiency, 154–155
Senna, cathartic colon syn-drome and, 41
Serial sectioning, in small bowel biopsy, 138, 139f
Serotonin (5-HT)
 carcinoid syndrome and, 344–345
 and EC cell hyperplasias asso-ciation, 323–324
Serpiginous ulcers, in fulminant colitis, 19
Serrated crypts, as problem in dysplasia diagnosis, 103–105, 107f
Signet ring cell mucinous carci-noma
 appendiceal, 287
 of the colon, 233f, 234
Silver staining techniques
 of gastrointestinal carcinoids, 336, 336t
 in neuroendocrine cell identifi-cation, 311–312
Simple hyperplasia, as stage in ECL cell hyperplasia-neoplasia sequence, 319, 319f
Simple mucocele, as non-neo-plastic mucocele, 275

Sjögren's syndrome, gastric carcinoids associated with, 335
"Skip lesions," in colonic Crohn's disease, 4
Small bowel
  hemorrhagic necrosis of, 129–130, 129f, 130f
  polyps. See Small intestinal polyps
Small bowel biopsy
  epithelium
    abnormal findings, 144
    normal findings in, 139f, 141
  lamina propria, normal findings in, 141, 143f
  muscularis mucosa, normal findings in, 141
  processing methods, 137–138
  specimen misinterpretation, sources of, 137
  villous architecture in
    abnormal findings, 141–142
    classification and interpretation of, 145, 147, 147f
    mild lesion, 142, 144, 144f
    moderate lesion, 144, 145f
    severe lesion, 144, 146f
    normal findings, 138–141, 139f, 140f, 142f–143f
  villous architecture in, severe lesion. See also Flat small bowel biopsy
Small cell undifferentiated carcinoma, of colon and rectum, 235–236, 235f
  differential diagnosis of, 236, 236t
Small intestinal polyps, 208–209
  adenomatous, 209–210
  Brunner's gland "adenoma," 209
  inflammatory fibroid, 209, 210f, 211f
  lymphangiectatic cyst, 211, 212f
  neurogenic, 210–211
Small intestinal polyps
  polyposis syndromes. See Polyposis syndromes; individually named syndromes

potential for malignancy, 219–221
  villous adenoma, 210
Soap, colitis induced by, 41
Solitary rectal ulcer syndrome, 39f, 39–40
Somatostatinomas
  histogenesis of, 332–334
  immunocytochemical studies of, 349
  pancreatic, associated with somatostatinoma syndrome, 348–349
  ultrastructural characteristics of, 349–350, 349f
Somatostatinoma syndrome, 348–350, 349f
Sprue
  celiac. See Celiac sprue
  collagenous, 152–153
  refractory (unclassified), 148, 152
  tropical, 155–156, 157f
Squamous cell carcinoma
  of anal canal, 374–375
  of colon and rectum, diagnostic criteria for, 234–235
  and keratoacanthoma, distinguishing between, 386–387
Staging systems
  for colorectal cancer
    Astler-Coller, 237–238, 238t
    five-year survival percentages compared, 239–240, 240t
    universal system using TNM criteria, 238–239, 238t–239t
  for rectal carcinoma
    clinical, 228
    Dukes' system, 237t, 237
    Jass classification, 239, 239t
    corrected five-year survival, 239, 239t
    updated, 239, 240t
Stasis syndromes, associated with nonspecific variably abnormal villi, 159, 160f
Stenotic ulcer, potassium-induced, in ischemic bowel disease, 130, 131f

Steroid enemas, effect on UC and CCD, 16
Steroid therapy, intrarectal, effect on UC and CCD, 16
Stomach, inflammatory-type polyps of, 219
Stress ulceration, in ischemic bowel disease, 130–131, 131f, 132f
Strongyloides stercoralis, 170
Strongyloidiasis, associated with diagnostic variably abnormal villi, 170
Sulfasalazine, prostaglandin synthesis inhibition by, 65–66
Sulfasalazine-azulfidine, effect on UC and CCD, 15
Sulindac, associated with diagnostic variably abnormal villi, 175
Suppressor T cells, in IBD, 73–74
Surgical resection, in colorectal cancer, 227–228
  malignant polyp and, 243, 246, 246t
  new method for, 228
  postpolypectomy, 248
Sweat glands, Paget's cells involvement of, 385
Synaptophysin, in neuroendocrine cell identification, 314
Syringocystadenoma papilliferum, 388

TAA. See Tumor associated antigens (TAA)
Tailgut cyst, 391
Tangential sectioning, in small bowel biopsy, 140, 140f
Tangier disease, 180–181
T cells, responses in IBD patients, 72–74
Terminal complement components (C5b-9), classic inflammatory reactions and, staining for, 63f
T helper cells, in IBD, 74–76

Therapeutic intervention, colitis induced by
  drug therapies, 41–42, 43
  enemas and laxatives, 41, 42f
  following bone marrow transplantation, 45
  following small intestinal bypass and fecal stream diversion, 45, 47, 47f
  radiation therapy, 43–45, 44f, 46f
T lymphocytes
  activity in IBD, 72–74
  local function in the gut, 74–76, 75f
TNM criteria, in colorectal cancer staging system, 238t
  five-year survival percentages compared, 239–240, 240t
"Toxic megacolon." *See* Fulminant colitis
Trabecular pattern carcinoid tumors, histologic features of, 329, 329f
Transitional cloacogenic carcinoma, 371, 371f–372f, 373
Transitional membranous zone with aberrant mucosal gland, 369, 370f
  cloacogenic transitional carcinoma invading, 371f, 371, 372f
Transplantation, of bone marrow, colitis following, 45
Triparanol, associated with diagnostic variably abnormal villi, 174
Tropical sprue syndrome, 155–156, 157f
  moderate villous abnormality in, 145f
Trypanosomatidae, kala azar and, 171
Tuberculosis, infectious diarrhea and, 33
Tubular adenoma. *See* Adenomatous polyp
Tubulovillous adenomas, of the colon, 199–200
  behavior of, 201f

carcinoma occurring in, frequency of, 199, 200t
  pedunculated, 201f
  sessile, 201f
Tumor associated antigens (TAA)
  blood group-related, 255t
  colorectal cancer and, 252, 253f–254f
Tumor(s)
  of colon and rectum, classification of
    adenocarcinoma, 229, 231, 230f–232f
    mucinous versus colloid, 231, 232f–233f, 234
  colorectal, genetic alteration in, 221–222
  concomitant in a hemorrhoid, 390
  of gastrointestinal tract, biologically functioning, general characteristics of, 344. *See also* Carcinoid tumors
  granular cell, in gastrointestinal tract, 388–389, 389f, 390f
  surgical resection in colorectal carcinoma, 227–228
Turcot's syndrome, 214

UC. *See* Ulcerative colitis (UC)
Ulcerative colitis (UC)
  adenoma management in, 115
  and colonic Crohn's disease
    differential diagnosis of, 1
      versus colitis of indeterminate type, 15
      future directions for, 19–20
      in inactive stage, 16
      using endoscopic biopsy specimens, 11, 15t
      using resection specimens, 4t
    histopathology compared, 7f, 8f
      in endoscopic biopsies, 11t
      in resection specimens, 6t
  diagnosis noncolitic patients compared, 88

effects of therapy on, 15–16
  in endoscopic biopsy specimens, 8, 10–15. *See also* Endoscopic biopsy
  "follicular proctitis" in, 5, 7f, 13
  fulminant form. *See* Fulminant ulcerative colitis
  IgE-containing cells in, 70–71, 71f
  quiescent, 90, 91f
  in resection specimens, 2–8. *See also* Resection specimens
  resolving phase in, 90–93, 93f, 94f
  surveillance in, 87
Ulcerative jejunoileitis, 152
Ulcer(s)
  of CMV colitis, 25, 26f
  in colonic Crohn's disease, 4f, 5
    histopatholic features of, 6–7
  in fulminant colitis
    fissuring type, 17, 17f
    with necrotic tissue, 17f, 19
    with transmural inflammation, 17, 18f
  in ischemic bowel disease
    potassium-induced stenotic, 130, 131f
    stress ulceration, 130–131, 131f, 132f
  nonspecific (idiopathic), of the colon, 51–52
  serpiginous, in fulminant colitis, 19
Undifferentiated pattern carcinoid tumors, histologic features of, 329, 330f, 331
Undulating cystadenoma, 271, 272f
Union Internationale Contra le Cancer (UICC), universal staging system for colorectal cancer proposed by, 238, 238t–239t
Uremic colitis, ischemic etiology for, 130–131, 131f

Vascular invasion, in colorectal cancer evaluation, 240–242

Vasoactive intestinal peptides (VIP), as aid in UC and CCD pathologic distinction, 19t, 19

Verapamil, for stress ulcer reduction, 131

Vermiform appendix, involvement in CCD and UC, 8

Vero cells, cytotoxin active against, 30

Verotoxin, production of, 30

Verrucous carcinoma, of oral cavity, 376

Villoglandular adenoma. *See* Tubulovillous adenomas

Villous adenoma
circumferential appendiceal, 264, 266f, 267–271, 270f
of the colon
behavior of, 199
carcinoma occurring in, frequency of, 200t
gross pathology, 197, 197f
incidence by age and sex, 198
location and multiplicity of, 198
microscopic pathology, 197–198, 198f, 199f
pathogenesis of, 198
of small intestine, 210

Villous architecture
abnormal findings, 141–142
classification and interpretation of, 145, 147, 147f
diseases associated with
variably abnormal villi—diagnostic, 162t, 162–176
variably abnormal villi—nonspecific, 158t, 158–162
mild lesion, 142, 144, 144f
moderate lesion, 144, 145f
severe lesion, 144, 146f. *See also* Flat small bowel biopsy
in giardial infestation, 168–169
normal findings, 138–141, 139f, 140f, 142f–143f
diseases associated with, variably normal villi—diagnostic, 176, 178t, 178–181

Villous cystadenoma, appendiceal, 273f
evolution of, 278, 280f–282f
herniation of mucosa in, 279, 282f. *See also* Pseudomyxoma peritonei

VIP. *See* Vasoactive intestinal peptides (VIP), as aid in UC and CCD pathologic distinction

Viral diseases, associated with diagnostic variably abnormal villi, 172

Viral gastroenteritis, in differential diagnosis of IBD, 23–26

Viral infections, in differential diagnosis of IBD, 23
chlamydiae and, 25–26
cytomegalovirus, 25, 26f
herpes simplex, 23–25

Vitamin B_{12}, associated with diagnostic variably abnormal villi, 173

von Recklinghausen's disease gastrointestinal carcinoids associated with, 350–351
and malignancy relationship, 220

Wermer's syndrome, gastrointestinal carcinoids associated with, 350

Whipple bacilli, 162, 165

Whipple's disease, associated with diagnostic variably abnormal villi, 162, 163–164f, 165

Yersinia enterocolitica, enteric infection with, 32
colonic involvement, 33f

Yersinia pseudotuberculosis, enteric infection with, 32

Zanca's syndrome, 219

Zollinger-Ellison syndrome
antropyloric G cell hyperplasia (AGCH) in, 318f
associated with nonspecific variably abnormal villi, 159–160, 161f
diagnostic criteria, 346
ECL cell carcinoids and, 321–322
ECL cell hyperplasia in, 319
gastric carcinoids associated with, 335
gastrinoma syndrome associated with, 345–346, 347f, 348